Contents

Preface/Acknowledgments

Nutrition therapy is the implementation of evidence-based nutrition recommendations and interventions. As new discoveries in the science of nutrition and diabetes are reported, nutrition therapy, if needed, changes. In 1971, the American Diabetes Association (ADA) published its first report on diabetes nutrition recommendations (ADA 1971). These recommendations have been updated in five position statements (ADA 1979, 1987, 1994, 2002, 2008), technical reviews (Franz 1994, 2002), and a systematic review (Wheeler 2012). A summary of the position statements is also incorporated into the annual ADA Standards of Care. The 1994 recommendations perhaps drew the most attention by the public when they reported that total, not the type of, carbohydrate affected blood glucose levels and sugary foods could be substituted for starchy foods. Additionally, before the 1994 recommendations, all position statements attempted to identify an "ideal" nutrition prescription with ideal percentages of carbohydrate, protein, and fat that would apply to everyone with diabetes. Although the need for individualization was stressed in all prior position papers, nutrition prescriptions, which were commonly given by physicians, for specific calorie levels and/or percentages of macronutrients, really did not allow for much, if any, individualization. The 1994 position statement also recommended that individualized nutrition prescriptions be based on metabolic profiles, treatment goals, and, perhaps most importantly, changes the person with diabetes is willing and able to make.

The Academy of Nutrition and Dietetics (Acad Nutr Diet, formerly the American Dietetic Association) published its first set of nutrition practice guidelines for type 2 and type 1 diabetes in 1995 and 1998, respectively (Monk 1995; Kulkarni 1998). Both sets of guidelines were field-tested in randomized clinical trials and shown to be effective (Franz 1995; Kulkarni 1998). Updates were published in 2001 and in the Acad Nutr Diet Evidence Analysis Library (American Dietetic Association 2001; Acad Nutr Diet 2008a). The guidelines for nutrition therapy for gestational diabetes were also published and field-tested (Reader 2006) and updated (Acad Nutr Diet 2008b). Nutrition practice guidelines for type 1 and type 2 diabetes in adults also have been updated and published (Franz 2010). Medical nutrition therapy has repeatedly been shown to be effective and essential in the prevention of diabetes and in the management of diabetes and its complications. However, just as there is no one medication or insulin therapy that applies to all people with diabetes, there is no one nutrition therapy intervention that applies to all people with diabetes. A goal of this guide is to assist health care providers in the selection of appropriate individualized nutrition therapy interventions.

The 1999 *American Diabetes Association Guide to Medical Nutrition Therapy for Diabetes* served as the basis for this guide. Authors were asked to update the available 1999 chapters by reviewing the evidence published after 1998. If evidence analysis was available in the current reviews by the Acad Nutr Diet and ADA (www.adaevidence; Franz 2010; Acad Nutr Diet 2008), they were asked to briefly summarize this evidence. Chapter authors also conducted a literature search for evidence published after these summaries. Chapters include tables of the new evidence, conclusions from the evidence, and recommendations for integrating diabetes nutrition therapy into the management of diabetes and its complications or for the prevention of diabetes. This guide is intended to serve as a resource for all health care professionals interested in the evidence supporting nutrition therapy interventions, not just for macro- and micronutrients, but for all the related areas of diabetes management in which nutrition therapy is essential.

It has been an honor and a pleasure to edit this text. We are truly indebted to the talented chapter authors for the thoroughness and thoughtfulness given to writing their chapters. They truly represent the many excellent clinicians and researchers interested in the field of diabetes nutrition. We also thank the reviewers, especially Stephanie Dunbar, Director of Nutrition and Clinical Affairs for the ADA, who directed the review. Special thanks go to Victor Van Beuren, our editor, who kept us on target and committed to the proposed timeline. And, of course, thanks go to the American Diabetes Association for its ongoing recognition of the integral role of nutrition therapy in the treatment of diabetes and its dedication to providing professionals with the latest available evidence.

Marion J. Franz, MS, RD, CDE
Alison B. Evert, MS, RD, CDE

BIBLIOGRAPHY

Academy of Nutrition and Dietetics: Evidence Analysis Library. Available at http://www.adaevidencelibrary.com. Accessed January 2012

Academy of Nutrition and Dietetics: Diabetes Type 1 and 2 for Adults Evidence-Based Nutrition Practice Guidelines, 2008a. Available at http://www.adaevidencelibrary.com/topic.cfm?=3251. Accessed January 2012

Academy of Nutrition and Dietetics: Gestational Diabetes Mellitus (GDM) Evidence-Based Nutrition Practice Guidelines, 2008b. Available at http://adaevidencelibrary.com/topic.cfm?=3731. Accessed January 2012

American Diabetes Association: Evidence-based nutrition principles and recommendations for the treatment and prevention of diabetes and related complications. *Diabetes Care* 25:202–212, 2002

American Diabetes Association: Nutrition recommendations and interventions for diabetes: a position statement of the American Diabetes Association. *Diabetes Care* 31 (Suppl. 1):S61–S78, 2008

American Diabetes Association: Nutrition recommendations and principles for individuals with diabetes mellitus: 1986 (Position Statement). *Diabetes Care* 10:126–132, 1987

American Diabetes Association: Nutrition recommendations and principles for people with diabetes mellitus (Position Statement). *Diabetes Care* 17:519–522, 1994

American Diabetes Association: Principles of nutrition and dietary recommendations for individuals with diabetes mellitus: 1979 (Special Report). *Diabetes* 28:1027–1030, 1979

American Diabetes Association: Principles of nutrition and dietary recommendations for patients with diabetes mellitus: 1971 (Special Report). *Diabetes* 9:633–634, 1971

American Dietetic Association: *Nutrition Practice Guidelines for Type 1 and Type 2 Diabetes* [CD-ROM]. Chicago, American Dietetic Association, 2001

Franz MJ, Bantle JP, Beebe CA, Brunzell JD, Chiasson J-L, Garg A, Holzmeister LA, Hoogwerf B, Mayer-Davis E, Mooradian AD, Purnell JQ, Wheeler M: Evidence-based nutrition principles and recommendations for the treatment and prevention of diabetes and related complications (Technical Review). *Diabetes Care* 25:148–198, 2002

Franz MJ, Horton ES, Bantle JP, Beebe CA, Brunzell JD, Coulston AM, Henry RR, Hoogwerf BJ, Stacpoole PW: Nutrition principles for the management of diabetes and related complications (Technical Review). *Diabetes Care* 17:490–518, 1994

Franz MJ, Monk A, Barry B, McLain K, Weaver T, Cooper N, Upham P, Bergenstal R, Mazze RS: Effectiveness of medical nutrition therapy provided by dietitians in the management of non-insulin-dependent diabetes mellitus: a randomized, controlled clinical trial. *J Am Diet Assoc* 95:1009–1017, 1995

Franz MJ, Powers MA, Leontos C, Holzmeister LA, Kulkarni K, Monk A, Wedel N, Gradwell E: The evidence for medical nutrition therapy for type 1 and type 2 diabetes in adults. *J Am Diet Assoc* 110:1852–1889, 2010

Kulkarni K, Castle G, Gregory R, Holmes A, Leontos C, Powers M, Snetselarr L, Splett P, Wylie-Rosett J: Nutrition practice guidelines for type 1 diabetes mellitus positively affect dietitian practices and patient outcomes. *J Am Diet Assoc* 98:62–70, 1998

Monk A, Barry B, McClain K, Weaver T, Cooper N, Franz MJ: Practice guidelines for medical nutrition therapy by dietitians for persons with non-insulin-dependent diabetes. *J Am Diet Assoc* 95:999–1008, 1995

Reader D, Splett P, Gunderson EP, for the Diabetes Care and Education Dietetic Practice Group: Impact of gestational diabetes nutrition practice guidelines implemented by registered dietitians on pregnancy outcomes. *J Am Diet Assoc* 106:1426–1433, 2006

Wheeler ML, Dunbar SA, Jaacks LM, Karmally W, Mayer-Davis EJ, Wylie-Rosett J, Yancy WS Jr: Macronutrients, food groups, and dietary patterns in the management of diabetes mellitus: a systematic review of the literature, 2010. *Diabetes Care* 35:434–445, 2012

Foreword

JOHN P. BANTLE, MD

Optimal treatment of diabetes mellitus requires nutrition therapy, an exercise program, and, for most patients, medication(s). When patients fail to achieve diabetes treatment goals, it is usually because one or more of these fundamental treatment modalities has not been effectively implemented. For many patients, the most challenging part of the treatment program (and thus the part of the program that often is not done well) is nutrition therapy. Patients often have difficulty understanding nutrition therapy. Moreover, many have difficulty putting their plan into action.

There are at least five reasons why understanding and adhering to nutrition therapy is difficult. First, nutrition recommendations have changed over time, with new recommendations sometimes contradicting previous recommendations. The contradictions have usually resulted from recommendations made in the absence of scientific evidence. The recommendations must then be modified or even abandoned when evidence becomes available. This creates confusion and erodes confidence in the recommendations. Second, many physicians do not themselves understand the principles of nutrition therapy and do not emphasize the importance of strategies to achieve food and nutrition goals. Thus, patients often do not recognize the importance of nutrition therapy. A third reason that nutrition therapy is difficult is that adhering to any eating pattern is challenging if that eating pattern differs from the usual eating pattern followed by family, friends, and cultural group. Even the most motivated of patients is likely to develop a sense of deprivation if asked to avoid foods that others are eating and enjoying. Any recommendation to depart from usual eating habits should be made only if there is compelling scientific evidence of potential benefit. Fourth, in our society, food has many purposes in addition to meeting biological needs. Food is often the focus of social activities and is frequently used as a reward, as a means of expressing affection, and as a way to help cope with stress. We are constantly exposed to appealing advertisements for food that exploit these factors. Even the most motivated of patients can be expected to occasionally succumb to these influences. Fifth, and very importantly, it is now clear that energy intake, energy expenditure, and body weight are regulated in the central nervous system. Thus, when we ask overweight or obese patients with diabetes to reduce energy intake and lose weight, we are asking them to override a powerful biological control system. Most of us have great difficulty making this change.

Although nutrition therapy is difficult and there are barriers to overcome, we should still do everything we can to implement it effectively. Healthy eating patterns are a key element in establishing good control of glycemia and lipemia and thereby preventing the complications of diabetes and its companion atherosclerosis. Without a strong nutrition component, most treatment plans will fall short. However, we must keep in mind that only a limited number of dietary strategies have documented efficacy. Marion Franz and Alison Evert and their chapter authors have done an outstanding job of describing these strategies in the *American Diabetes Association Guide to Nutrition Therapy for Diabetes*. They also carefully point out gaps in our knowledge, allowing us to avoid making unsubstantiated recommendations. I believe this volume belongs in the bookshelf of every health care provider who deals with patients who have diabetes mellitus.

John P. Bantle is Professor of Medicine and Director, Division of Endocrinology and Diabetes, University of Minnesota, Minneapolis, MN.

Chapter 1
Effectiveness of Medical Nutrition Therapy in Diabetes

Joyce Green Pastors, MS, RD, CDE, and Marion J. Franz, MS, RD, CDE

Highlights

Background on Diabetes Nutrition Therapy

Evidence for the Clinical Effectiveness of MNT in Diabetes

Summary

Highlights
Effectiveness of Medical
Nutrition Therapy in Diabetes

■ Medical nutrition therapy (MNT) for the treatment of diabetes is effective, with the greatest impact at the initial onset of diabetes. Randomized control and observational studies have shown that within the first 6 months of diagnosis, A1C can be reduced up to ~3% point reductions (range 0.23–2.6%), depending on the type and duration of diabetes. However, MNT is effective throughout the diabetes disease process, with an average reduction of A1C levels of 1–2% point reductions.

■ Because type 2 diabetes is a progressive disease, an evaluation of nutrition interventions should be completed at 3 months, and if no clinical improvement has occurred, a change in treatment plan should be recommended, including the addition of oral glucose-lowering medication(s) and/or insulin.

■ MNT is a process that includes a nutrition assessment, nutrition diagnosis, nutrition interventions (education, counseling, and goal-setting), and nutrition monitoring and evaluation.

■ MNT provided by a registered dietitian is effective in promoting positive clinical outcomes, especially with multiple follow-up encounters involving nutrition education and counseling.

■ There are many types of nutrition interventions that are effective, including decreased calorie and fat intake, carbohydrate counting, use of insulin-to-carbohydrate ratios, healthy food choices, individualized meal planning, and behavioral strategies.

■ Other clinical outcomes such as improved lipid profiles, weight loss, decreased blood pressure, decreased need for medication, and decreased risk of onset and progression of comorbidities can be achieved with MNT.

Effectiveness of Medical Nutrition Therapy in Diabetes

Since the discovery of "sweet urine," people with diabetes have been given advice on what to eat and drink, often based more on theories or beliefs than on facts. Food and nutrition advice has ranged from "starvation diets" to high- or low-carbohydrate or low-fat diets to nutritional supplements that will provide a cure.

Over the years, various diabetes organizations have published nutrition recommendations on the basis of available research and clinical observations. In recent years, the goal in the development of diabetes nutrition therapy recommendations has been to have the recommendations be based on evidence rather than theories. For example, it was longstanding advice that people with diabetes should not eat sugar or foods containing sugars. This information was based on the assumption that because sugars were small molecules, they would be absorbed rapidly, causing blood glucose levels to increase at a greater rate than starches (which are larger molecules). When research first revealed that total amounts of carbohydrate were more important than the source (Bantle 1983), the public, and many health professionals, were surprised. However, almost all diabetes nutrition recommendations now acknowledge that sugary foods can be substituted for starchy foods.

The primary goals of diabetes medical nutrition therapy (MNT) are to support the achievement and maintenance of as normal blood glucose levels as safely possible, a lipid profile that reduces the risk for cardiovascular disease, blood pressure in an ideal range, and improved or continued quality of life. Important questions then become, what is the evidence that diabetes MNT can achieve these goals and what types of MNT interventions are effective? It is important that clinicians, regardless of their field of practice, know expected outcomes from their interventions, when to evaluate such outcomes, and what interventions contribute to successful outcomes.

BACKGROUND ON DIABETES NUTRITION THERAPY

Attempts have been made to identify the efficacy and method of delivery of diabetes nutrition therapy. For example, a Cochrane review reported on a total of 18 randomized controlled trials of nutrition approaches for individuals with type 2 diabetes and, not surprisingly, could not identify one type of nutrition advice that was most effective (Nield 2007). They did report that nutrition therapy advice plus exercise was associated with a statistically significant mean decrease in A1C of 0.9% (CI 0.4–1.3) at 6 months and of 1.0% (CI 0.4–1.5) at 12 months.

A systematic review of healthy eating by the American Association of Diabetes Educators also did not reveal a clear pattern of food and nutrition interventions leading to outcomes of weight, fat intake, saturated fat, and carbohydrate. However, this review did conclude that there is a tendency for successful healthy eating interventions to include an exercise dimension and group work (Povey 2007).

Therefore, it seems clear that a single approach to diabetes MNT does not exist, just as there is no one medication or insulin regimen that applies to all people with diabetes. Instead of asking about specific eating patterns or food/nutrient interventions, this review examines the effectiveness of diabetes MNT provided by nutrition professionals (registered dietitians [RDs] or dietitians in many countries and nutritionists in some countries) and what interventions contribute to successful outcomes.

MNT for diabetes incorporates a process that, when implemented correctly, includes the following steps: *1*) assessment and reassessment (for follow-up nutrition care); *2*) nutrition diagnosis to identify the specific nutrition-related problems; *3*) nutrition interventions that include education, counseling, and goal-setting; and *4*) nutrition monitoring and evaluation, which involves monitoring progress and measuring outcome indicators (Lacey 2003). The fourth step requires that expected outcomes of nutrition interventions be known.

EVIDENCE FOR THE CLINICAL EFFECTIVENESS OF MNT IN DIABETES

The evidence for diabetes MNT comes from randomized controlled trials and observational and outcome studies showing that nutrition interventions improve metabolic outcomes, such as blood glucose and A1C, in individuals with diabetes. Randomized controlled trials are considered the gold standard for evidence. However, when assessing the impact of an intervention in clinical practice, these trials have limitations. First and foremost, subjects are selected (and rejected) usually on their perceived ability to complete the study. In clinical practice, patients are generally offered care regardless of their interest and ability to make lifestyle changes. Outcome or observational studies usually provide outcome data from all patients entered into patient care and thus are often a more realistic report on expected outcomes from clinical care. However, these studies are frequently criticized for their lack of rigorous study design. In general, useful data can be collected from both types of study designs.

Metabolic outcomes are improved in nutrition intervention studies, both when provided as independent MNT or when nutrition therapy is provided as part of overall diabetes self-management education (DSME) (Table 1.1). Studies in Table 1.1 were identified from the literature search published in the Academy of Nutrition and Dietetics (formerly the American Dietetic Association) Evidence Analysis Library (Acad Nutr Diet 2008a) and previously published articles (Franz 2008; Pastors 2002; Pastors 2003). MNT studies report the outcomes of nutrition interventions provided by an RD (or nutritionist). DSME is provided by a multidisciplinary team, which in these studies included a minimum of an RD providing nutrition therapy and a registered nurse. Studies include randomized clinical trials and longitudinal, retrospective, cohort, time series, descriptive, and observational

Table 1.1 Summary of Evidence for Effectiveness of MNT in Diabetes

	Population/ Type of Study	Number of Interventions (study length)	Nutrition Therapy Intervention	A1C and Other Outcomes from MNT Interventions
MNT studies				
UKPDS 1990 and 2000	n = 3,044 adults with type 2 diabetes/RCT	3 at 1–month intervals (3 months)	↓ Energy, 50% carbohydrate, 20% protein, 30% fat	A1C: ↓ 1.9%* Weight: ↓ 4.5 kg (P < 0.001) TC: ↓ 7.8 mg/dL LDL cholesterol: ↓ 7.8 mg/dL TG: ↓ 28.4 mg/dL (all P < 0.001)
Laitinen 1993	n = 86 adults with type 2 diabetes/RCT	6 at 2-month intervals (15 months)	Nutrition education focusing on fat, carbohydrates, fiber, sweeteners, behavior modification	A1C: ↓ 0.6% (P < 0.053) Weight: ↓ 5.1 kg (P < 0.05)
Delahanty 1993	n = 623 with type 1 diabetes/observational study	Quarterly visits during DCCT (9 years; average 4.1 years)	Intensive MNT; exchange lists; carbohydrate counting	A1C: ↓ 0.9% (P < 0.001)
Franz 1995	n = 179 adults with type 2 diabetes/RCT	3 within first 6 weeks (6 months)	Individualized MNT	A1C: ↓ 0.9% (4-year duration of diabetes) (P < 0.001) A1C: ↓ 1.9% (newly diagnosed) (P < 0.001) Weight: ↓ 1.4 kg (P > 0.001) TC: ↓ 7.8 mg/dL (P < 0.05) TG: ↓ 15.0 mg/dL (P < 0.05)
Miller 2002	n = 90 adults with type 2 diabetes/RCT	10 weekly sessions (1 year)	Nutrition education, emphasis on food labeling	A1C: ↓ 0.5% (P < 0.001)
Maislos 2002	n = 492 adults with type 2 diabetes/time series study	2 (up to 2 years)	Nutrition education, energy balance	A1C: ↓ 0.9% (P < 0.0001)

Table 1.1 Summary of Evidence for Effectiveness of MNT in Diabetes (*continued*)

	Population/ Type of Study	Number of Interventions (study length)	Nutrition Therapy Intervention	A1C and Other Outcomes from MNT Interventions
Ash 2003	*n* = 51 adults with type 2 diabetes/RCT	12 weekly for 3 months; follow-up at 18 months	Individualized MNT; decreased energy intake	A1C: ↓ 1.2% (12 weeks) (*P* < 0.001) A1C: ↑ 0.4% (18 months) (NS)
Goldhaber-Fiebert 2003	*n* = 75 adults with type 2 diabetes/RCT	11 weekly 90-min nutrition classes (3 months)	Portion control and healthy food choices	A1C: ↓ 1.8% Weight: ↓ 1.0 kg (both *P* = 0.028)
Ziemer 2003	*n* = 648 adults with type 2 diabetes/RCT	4 initial at 1, 2, and 4 weeks (6 months)	Healthy food choices and exchange lists	A1C: ↓ 1.9% (*P* < 0.0001) TG: ↓ 35.5 mg/dL (*P* < 0.001) HDL cholesterol: ↑ 2.3 mg/dL (*P* < 0.005)
Wilson 2003	*n* = 7,490 adults with type 2 diabetes (Indian Health Service)/retrospective cohort study	2 or more (~132 days)	Individualized MNT by RD	A1C: ↓ 0.23 % (*P* < 0.0001)
Lemon 2004	*n* = 244 adults with type 2 diabetes/time series study	1–6; avg 2 times and 111 min (6 months)	Individualized MNT; carbohydrate counting and simplified meal plans	A1C: ↓ 1.7% Weight: ↓ 3 kg TC: ↓ 27.5 mg/dL SBP: ↓ 5.4 mmHg (all *P* < 0.001) Lifestyle index and exercise ↑ (*P* < 0.0001)
Gaetke 2006	*n* = 175 adults with type 2 diabetes/retrospective cohort study	1 (3 months)	Individualized counseling session	A1C: ↓ 2.6% (*P* < 0.01)

	Population/ Type of Study	Number of Interventions (study length)	Nutrition Therapy Intervention	A1C and Other Outcomes from MNT Interventions
Barnard 2006	n = 99 adults with type 2 diabetes/RCT	1-h individual; 1-h weekly group meetings (22 weeks)	Low-fat vegan diet or ADA diet (15–20% protein, 60–70% carbohydrate and monounsaturated fat)	A1C: ↓ 0.96 in vegan diet ($P < 0.0001$) and 0.56 in ADA diet ($P < 0.001$) Weight: ↓ 6.5 kg in vegan diet and 3.1 kg in ADA diet (both $P < 0.0001$) SBP: ↓ ~3.7 in both ($P < 0.05$) TC: ↓ ~25 mg/dL in both ($P < 0.0001$) LDL cholesterol: ↓ ~16 mg dL in both ($P < 0.001$) TG: ↓ ~27 mg/dL in both ($P < 0.05$)
Coppell 2010	n = 93 adults with type 2 diabetes/RCT	7; 2 within 1 month, 5 at 1-month intervals (6 months)	↓ Energy for 5% weight loss; 45–50% carbohydrate, 10–20% protein, <30% fat (<10% saturated), 40 g fiber/day	A1C: ↓ 0.5% ($P = 0.007$) Weight: ↓ 2.1 kg ($P = 0.032$)
Andrews 2011	n = 246 adults with newly diagnosed type 2 diabetes/RCT	Usual care (initial dietitian session, follow-up every 6 months) vs. intensive diet intervention (dietitian session every 3 months, monthly nurse support) vs. latter with physical activity program (6 months)	↓ Energy for 5–10% weight loss; individualized U.K. dietary guidelines; goal-oriented motivational interviews	A1C: ↓ 0.3% in both intervention groups ($P < 0.001$) Insulin resistance ↓ ($P < 0.0001$) Weight: ↓ 4.8 kg ($P < 0.0001$) Waist circumference: ↓ 4 cm ($P < 0.0001$) Reduced need for drug treatment

Table 1.1 Summary of Evidence for Effectiveness of MNT in Diabetes (*continued*)

	Population/ Type of Study	Number of Interventions (study length)	Nutrition Therapy Intervention	A1C and Other Outcomes from MNT Interventions
MNT/DSME Studies				
DAFNE Study Group 2002	*n* = 169 individuals with type 1 diabetes/RCT	5-day course (follow-up at 6 months)	Advanced carbohydrate counting; insulin-to-carbohydrate ratios	A1C: ↓ 1.0% (*P* < 0.0001) ↑ Dietary freedom (*P* < 0.0001) and overall quality of life (*P* < 0.01)
Graber 2002	*n* = 350 patients with diabetes/ observational study	Weekly for 3 months (3 months)	Individualized MNT	A1C: ↓ 1.7% (*P* < 0.0001)
Rickheim 2002	*n* = 170 individuals with newly diagnosed type 2 diabetes/RCT	4 initial, 3 weeks, 3 months, 6 months (6 months)	Carbohydrate counting, portion control	A1C: ↓ 2.0% (*P* < 0.01)
Banister 2004	*n* = 70 adults with type 2 diabetes/longitudinal study	4-h class; 1–2 individual RD consults; monthly groups (1 year)	Basic nutrition; individualized meal plans	A1C: ↓ 1.5% (*P* < 0.001)
Bray 2005	*n* = 160 adults with type 2 diabetes (convenience sample)/time series study	4 sessions in 6 months (1 year)	9 nutrition education sessions + nurse case management	A1C: ↓ 1.1% (*P* < 0.0001)
Chima 2005	*n* = 430 adults with type 2 diabetes/ descriptive study	3 2-h group classes + 2–3 individual MNT sessions (90 days to 3 years)	Individual MNT sessions; heart-healthy foods	A1C: ↓ 1.6% (*P* < 0.001)
Sämann 2005	*n* = 1,592 type 1 diabetes/ time series	5-day classes (follow-up at 3 years)	Carbohydrate counting; insulin-to-carbohydrate ratios	A1C: ↓ 0.7% (*P* < 0.001) Severe hypoglycemia: ↓ 0.2 events/ patient-year (*P* < 0.0001)

	Population/ Type of Study	Number of Interventions (study length)	Nutrition Therapy Intervention	A1C and Other Outcomes from MNT Interventions
Lowe 2008	n = 82 individuals with type 1 and 55 with type 2 diabetes/time series	Intensive self-management course (follow-up at 12 months)	Carbohydrate counting; insulin-to-carbohydrate ratios	A1C: ↓ 0.6% ↑ Empowerment and quality of life
Huang 2010	n = 154 adults with type 2 diabetes/RCT	Individualized sessions with RD every 3 months	Nutrition education; ↓ energy intake; portion control	A1C: ↓ 0.7% (in subjects with baseline A1C > 7%, n = 60) (P = 0.007)

*All A1C percentages indicate point reductions.

ADA, American Diabetes Association; MNT, MNT provided by RDs, dietitians, or nutritionists; MNT/DSME, MNT provided by RDs, dietitians, or nutritionists in diabetes self-management programs. RCT, randomized controlled trial; SBP, systolic blood pressure; TC, total cholesterol; TG, triglycerides. Adapted from Franz 2008.

studies. Because A1C is consistently reported across all studies, these values are included in Table 1.1. Other outcomes, as available, are also reported in Table 1.1.

In the past decade, at least two other randomized controlled trials have been conducted involving lifestyle intervention, with both MNT and physical activity as the primary components (Look AHEAD 2007; Wolf 2004). These studies are not included in the summary of evidence in Table 1.1 because they were combined interventions and did not focus primarily on MNT as the intervention. Also, the goals for each of these studies focused on weight loss (Wolf 2004) and cardiovascular risk reduction (Look AHEAD 2007, 2010) as primary outcomes. In addition, other nutrition intervention studies have been published in the literature but are not reported in the summary of evidence because of high dropout rates or incomplete data.

Providing hospitalized patients with nutritionist visits and education can also be highly cost-effective for the health care system. In an evaluation of different types of educational visits for patients with diabetes (n = 18,404) at eight Philadelphia Health Care Centers, a total of 31,657 hospitalizations were recorded for 7,839 patients in the cohort. For patients who had at least one type of educational visit, the hospitalization rate was 34% lower than for patients who had no educational visit. Patients who had at least one visit with a nutritionist had hospitalization rates 45% lower than the rate of patients who had no educational visit. The average annual hospital charges for patients who received any educational visit were 39% less than the per-year average for patients who had no such visits (Robbins 2008).

Randomized controlled trials and other outcome studies of MNT document mean decreases in A1C of ~1–2% (up to ~3% in newly diagnosed patients), depending on the type and duration of diabetes and at what time point outcomes are reported. The evidence suggests that MNT is most beneficial at initial diagnosis, but is effective at any time during the disease process, and that ongoing evaluation and intervention are essential. Outcomes resulting from nutrition interventions are generally known in 6 weeks to 3 months, and evaluation should be performed at these times. At 3 months, if no clinical improvement has been seen in metabolic outcomes (glucose, lipids, blood pressure), usually a change in medication(s) is needed. Type 2 diabetes is a progressive disease, and as β-cell function decreases, glucose-lowering medication(s), including insulin, must be combined with MNT to achieve target goals.

Examples of Type 2 Diabetes Studies

The U.K. Prospective Diabetes Study (UKPDS) was a randomized controlled trial that involved 3,044 newly diagnosed patients with type 2 diabetes at 15 centers. All treatment and control subjects received nutrition counseling, usually from a dietitian on study entry until 3 months, at which time they were randomized into intensive or conventional therapy. During the initial period when nutrition counseling was the primary intervention, the mean A1C decreased by 1.9% (from ~9 to ~7%), and there were average weight losses of 4.5 kg (UKPDS 7 1990; UKPDS 2000). UKPDS researchers concluded that, for improved glycemia, a reduction in energy intake was at least as important, if not more important, than the actual weight lost. At 2 years, the conventional group, whose primary therapy was diet, maintained an A1C of ~7%, and even at study end, the A1C was still slightly less than at diagnosis. However, because of the progressive deterioration of diabetes control, the majority of patients needed multiple therapies to attain glycemic target levels in the longer term.

Also in the U.K. and in newly diagnosed individuals with type 2 diabetes (n = 593), the Early ACTID (Early Activity in Diabetes) trial compared usual care (initial dietitian consultation and follow-up every 6 months; control group) to an intensive nutrition intervention (dietitian consultation every 3 months with monthly nurse support) or to the latter plus a pedometer-based activity program (Andrews 2011). Baseline A1C levels were 6.7, 6.6, and 6.7%, respectively. At 6 months, A1C had not improved in the usual care group but had improved in the two intensive nutrition intervention groups (–0.3%). These differences persisted to 12 months despite the use of fewer diabetes drugs. Improvements were also seen in body weight and insulin resistance between the intervention and control groups. Of interest, adding the physical activity program created no additional benefit.

In individuals with an average duration of diabetes of 4 years, intensive nutrition therapy provided by RDs resulted in a decrease in A1C of 0.9% (8.3 to 7.4%) and in subjects with a duration of diabetes <1 year of 1.9% (8.8 to 6.9%) (Franz 1995). By 6 weeks to 3 months, it was known if nutrition intervention had achieved target goals; if it had not, the RD notified the referral source that changes in medication were needed. A1C values were maintained to 6 months.

Of interest is a randomized controlled trial of individuals with an average duration of diabetes of 9 years who had A1C levels >7% despite optimized drug therapy (Coppell 2010). The intervention group received intensive nutrition therapy resulting in a difference in A1C between the intervention and control groups at 6 months (–0.5%). This difference was highly significant, as were changes in anthropometric measurements, documenting the effectiveness of nutrition therapy even in diabetes of long duration. Furthermore, the reduction in A1C is comparable with that seen in clinical trials when a new drug, often a third, is added to conventional agents.

In another smaller randomized control trial, obese subjects receiving intensive nutrition interventions experienced a decrease in A1C of 0.6% every 2 months for up to 15 months (Laitinen 1993). Also reported was a decrease in A1C of 0.5% in patients ≥65 years of age after 10 weekly sessions with an RD emphasizing goal-setting and using learning and social cognitive theory (Miller 2002). In a study of patients with type 2 diabetes in rural Costa Rica, a decrease in A1C value of 1.8% at 3 months was reported after nutrition and exercise interventions (Goldhaber-Fiebert 2003). Also, in a study of urban African Americans, decreases in A1C at 6 months of 1.9% were shown from interventions using healthy food choices and exchange-based meal plans (Ziemer 2003). In a randomized controlled trial conducted in Taiwan, decreases of 0.7% in A1C were reported in subjects after quarterly sessions with an RD for 1 year compared to a routine care control group (Huang 2010).

A study that monitored outcomes illustrates the effectiveness of nutrition interventions in clinical practice (Lemon 2004). Data were collected from 221 patients with type 2 diabetes who were referred for nutrition education/counseling to 59 RDs working in 31 outpatient settings in the state of Wisconsin. To minimize selection bias, the RD recruited the first two patients meeting inclusion criteria each day, up to six per week. Data were collected at baseline, 3 months, and 6 months. RDs spent an average of 111 ± 55 min with each subject, they met with subjects an average of 2.1 ± 1.0 times, and 33 intervention topics were reported. Clinical outcomes (A1C, lipids, blood pressure, weight) improved significantly between baseline and 3 or 6 months, while stabilizing between 3 and 6 months. A1C decreased by 1.4% over 3 months and by 1.7% at 6 months (54% of subjects were newly diagnosed).

Examples of Type 1 Diabetes Studies

The Dose Adjusted for Normal Eating (DAFNE) trial was another study conducted in Great Britain to evaluate whether a 5-day course teaching how to adjust mealtime insulin based on planned carbohydrate intake can improve both glycemia and quality of life in individuals with type 1 diabetes (DAFNE Study Group 2002). In this study, individuals using routinely prescribed insulin therapy, in which the insulin regimen is determined first and eating must then be consistent and matched to the time actions of insulin, were either immediately provided the skills needed to determine mealtime bolus insulin doses based on desired carbohydrate intake on a meal-to-meal basis or they attended the training 6 months later. In the group receiving the DAFNE training, A1C levels were significantly improved by 1%, with no significant increase in severe hypoglycemia, along with positive effects on quality of life, satisfaction with treatment, and psychological well-being. These results occurred despite an increase in the number of insulin injections (but not in total amount of insulin) and an increase in blood glucose monitoring compared with the control subjects who received the training later.

A follow-up of original trial participants at a mean of 44 months documented a mean improvement in A1C from baseline of 0.4%, remaining significant but less than the 12-month levels. Improvements in quality of life seen at 12 months were well maintained over ~4 years (Speight 2010). Of interest is another follow-up report examining changes in food and eating practices in DAFNE trial participants after changing to flexible, intensive insulin therapy. Concern had originally been expressed that individuals with type 1 diabetes, if given the freedom to adjust insulin doses based on carbohydrate intake, would overeat or make unhealthy food choices. These concerns were unfounded, since individuals using flexible, intensive insulin therapy did not engage in more excessive or unhealthy eating. Instead, many of the participants reported making few eating changes and, in some cases, actually reported being more rigid in their eating habits (Lawton 2011).

A group in Germany reported a 1.5% lower A1C level 1 year after a 5-day intensive training course (after which the DAFNE trial was modeled) teaching participants how to match insulin doses to their food choices while keeping their blood glucose level close to normal. The course was taught by specially trained dietitians and nurse educators (Pieber 1995). Improvements were maintained to 3 years without increasing the risk of hypoglycemia (Sämann 2005). A similar program in Australia teaching carbohydrate counting and insulin dose adjustment to patients with type 1 or type 2 diabetes and taught by dietitians and doctors also prompted good results. Participants reported A1C levels fell from 8.7% initially to 8.1% at 12 months (Lowe 2008).

The role of nutrition behaviors in achieving glycemic control in 623 intensively treated patients in the Diabetes Control and Complications Trial (DCCT) was examined. The four nutrition behaviors associated with a clinically significant reduction in A1C (0.9%) were as follows: adhering to the prescribed meal and snack plan, adjusting insulin dose in response to meal size, promptly treating hyperglycemia, and avoiding overtreatment of hypoglycemia (Delahanty 1993).

Nutrition Therapy Clinical Effectiveness Studies

Nutrition therapy for diabetes is clinically effective. Randomized controlled trials and observational outcome studies have documented decreases in A1C of ~1–2% (range –0.5% to –2.6%), depending on the type and duration of diabetes. These outcomes are similar to those from oral glucose-lowering medications.

Although attempts are often made to identify one approach to diabetes MNT, a single approach does not exist. Research shows that there are many types of nutrition interventions that are effective. Interventions include reduced energy/fat intake, carbohydrate counting, simplified meal plans, healthy food choices, individualized meal-planning strategies, exchange choices, use of insulin-to-carbohydrate ratios, physical activity, and behavioral strategies. In reviewing consistent themes for nutrition intervention, it appears that, for individuals with type 2 diabetes, reducing the energy content of usual food intake is central to successful outcomes. For individuals with type 1 diabetes, adjusting insulin doses for planned carbohydrate intake is of primary importance.

Central to these interventions are multiple encounters to provide education and counseling initially and on a continued basis. The number and duration of MNT encounters may need to be greater if the patient has language, ethnic, or cultural concerns; if changes in medications (such as addition of glucose-lowering medications or insulin therapy in type 2 diabetes or changes in insulin regimens in type 1 or type 2 diabetes) are made; or for weight management. Nutrition education and counseling must be sensitive to the personal needs and cultural preferences of the individual and his or her ability and willingness to make changes.

At ~6 weeks after the initial nutrition encounter, it should be determined whether the individual is making progress toward personal goals. If there is no evidence of progress, the individual and nutrition professional need to reassess and consider possible revisions to the nutrition care plan. At 3 months, changes in medical therapy (medications added or adjusted) need to be made if blood glucose concentrations or A1C percentages have not shown a downward trend; the patient has lost weight with no improvement in glucose; the patient is doing well with lifestyle changes and further interventions are unlikely to improve medical outcomes; or if the patient has done all that he or she can or is willing to do.

How often nutrition education and counseling needs to be implemented is unknown at this time. Evaluating the effectiveness of diabetes MNT is performed at 3, 6, or 12 months and usually includes the initial series of encounters. The number of initial and follow-up sessions varies in all the studies. It can be speculated that just as it is important for individuals with diabetes to be seen on a regular basis for medical care, it is also important for individuals to receive continuing education, counseling, and support for lifestyle changes. The Academy of Nutrition and Dietetics nutrition practice guidelines for type 1 and type 2 diabetes recommends at least one follow-up encounter annually to reinforce lifestyle changes and to evaluate and monitor outcomes that affect the need for changes in MNT (or medication) (Acad Nutr Diet 2008a). For example, children and adolescents often require MNT changes because of growth or other lifestyle factors. Patients with type 2 diabetes often require the addition of or changes in medication. The RD can also assist physicians and other health care providers by helping patients understand and accept the reasons for management changes.

Other important clinical outcomes that need to be evaluated, in addition to A1C levels, are lipids and blood pressure. In studies done primarily in individuals without diabetes, cardioprotective nutrition therapy implemented by RDs resulted in a reduction of serum total cholesterol by 7 to 21%, LDL cholesterol by 17 to 22%, and triglycerides 11 to 31% (Acad Nutr Diet 2011). Pharmacological therapy changes should be considered if goals are not achieved between 3 and 6 months after initiating MNT.

Nutrition therapy is also effective in reducing blood pressure in both normotensive and hypertensive adults. Substantial reductions in blood pressure that are clinically relevant are reported from implementation of multiple lifestyle interventions (Appel 2006). Nutrition therapy recommendations (weight loss, sodium reduction, increased physical activity, and following the DASH diet [Dietary Approaches to Stop Hypertension] [rich in fruits, vegetables, and low-fat dairy products but low in saturated and total fat]) in hypertensive individuals not on medication reduced systolic blood pressure by 14.2 mmHg and diastolic blood pressure by 7.4 mmHg and in nonhypertensive individuals reduced systolic blood pressure by 9.2 mmHg and diastolic blood pressure by 5.8 mmHg (Appel 2003). However, generally, studies implementing MNT for hypertension implemented by RDs report an average reduction in blood pressure of ~5 mmHg in both systolic and diastolic blood pressure (Acad Nutr Diet 2008b).

SUMMARY

- For individuals with type 2 diabetes, attention to food intake and patterns of eating are important for the management of diabetes, even if on medications, including insulin.
- For individuals with type 1 diabetes, matching insulin doses to planned carbohydrate intake is important for the management of diabetes.
- Nutrition education and counseling is best provided in a series of encounters—usually one initial encounter with two or three follow-up encounters, which can be implemented individually or in groups. The dietitian (or nutritionist) should determine if and when additional encounters are needed.
- Ongoing nutrition education and counseling is needed yearly, or more often as required or requested, or when changes in medication are made.
- A variety of nutrition interventions can be implemented depending on which are best suited to the needs of the individual patient. For patients with type 2 diabetes, the focus should be on reducing or maintaining a reduced energy intake. For patients with type 1 diabetes, a primary focus for educating patients is on how to adjust insulin doses on the basis of planned carbohydrate intake.
- Blood glucose monitoring and A1C results can be used to evaluate the effectiveness of MNT; lipids and blood pressure outcomes also require monitoring and evaluation.
- To successfully integrate MNT into overall diabetes management, an interdisciplinary team approach is essential.

BIBLIOGRAPHY

Academy of Nutrition and Dietetics: Disorders of lipid metabolism evidence-based nutrition practice guideline, 2011. Available from http://adaevidencelibrary.com/topic.cfm?cat=4528. Accessed 5 June 2011

Academy of Nutrition and Dietetics: Effectiveness of MNT for hypertension, 2008b. Available from http://www.adaevidencelibrary.com/conclusion.cfm?conclusion_statement_id=251204. Accessed 5 June 2011

Academy of Nutrition and Dietetics: Type 1 and type 2 diabetes evidence-based nutrition practice guidelines for adults, 2008a. Available from http://adaevidencelibrary.com/topic.cfm?cat=3253. Accessed 5 June 2011

Andrews RC, Cooper AR, Montgomery AA, Norcross AJ, Peters TJ, Sharp DJ, Jackson N, Fitzsimons K, Bright J, Coulman K, England CY, Gorton J, McLenaghan A, Paxton E, Polet A, Thompson C, Dayan CM: Diet or diet plus physical activity versus usual care in patients with newly diagnosed type 2 diabetes: the Early ACTID randomized controlled trial. *Lancet* 378:129–139, 2011

Appel LJ, Brands MW, Daniels SR, Karanja N, Elmer PJ, Sacks FM: Dietary approaches to prevent and treat hypertension: a scientific statement from the American Heart Association. *Hypertension* 47:296–308, 2006

Appel LJ, Champagne CM, Harsha DW, Cooper LS, Obarzanek E, Elmer PJ, Stevens JV, Vollmer WM, Lin PH, Svetkey LP, Stedman SW, Young DR, for the Writing Groups of the PREMIER Collaborative Research Group: Effects of comprehensive lifestyle modification on blood pressure control: main results of the PREMIER clinical trial. *JAMA* 289:2083–2093, 2003

Ash S, Reeves MM, Yeo S, Morrison G, Carey D, Capra S: Effect of intensive dietetic interventions on weight and glycaemic control in overweight men with type II diabetes: a randomized trial. *Int J Obes* 27:797–802, 2003

Banister NA, Jastrow ST, Hodges V, Loop R, Gilham MG: Diabetes self-management training program in a community clinic improves patient outcomes at modest cost. *J Am Diet Assoc* 104:807–810, 2004

Bantle JP, Laine DC, Castle GW, Thomas JW, Hoogwerf BJ, Goetz FC: Postprandial glucose and insulin responses to meals containing different carbohydrates in normal and diabetic subjects. *N Engl J Med* 309:7–12, 1983

Barnard ND, Cohen J, Jenkins DJA, Turner-McGrievy G, Gloede L, Jaster B, Seidl K, Green AA, Talpers S: A low-fat vegan diet improves glycemic control and cardiovascular risk factors in a randomized clinical trial in individuals with type 2 diabetes. *Diabetes Care* 29:1777–1783, 2006

Bray P, Thompson D, Wynn JD, Cummings DM, Whetstone L: Confronting disparities in diabetes care: the clinical effectiveness of redesigning care management for minority patients in rural primary care practices. *J Rural Health* 21:317–321, 2005

Chima CS, Farmer-Dziak N, Caradwell P, Snow S: Use of technology to track program outcomes in diabetes self-management programs. *J Am Diet Assoc* 105:1933–1938, 2005

Coppell KJ, Kataoka M, Williams SM, Chisholm AW, Vorgers SM, Mann JI: Nutritional intervention in patients with type 2 diabetes who are hyperglycaemic despite optimized drug treatment: Lifestyle Over and Above Drugs in Diabetes (LOADD) study: randomized controlled trial. *BMJ* 341:c3337, 2010

DAFNE Study Group: Training in flexible, intensive insulin management to enable dietary freedom in people with type 1 diabetes: Dose Adjusted for Normal Eating (DAFNE) randomized controlled trial. *BMJ* 325:746–752, 2002

Delahanty LM, Halford BN: The role of diet behaviors in achieving improved glycemic control in intensively treated patients in the Diabetes Control and Complications Trial. *Diabetes Care* 16:1453–1458, 1993

Franz MJ, Boucher JL, Pastors JG, Powers MA: Evidence-based nutrition practice guidelines for diabetes and scope and standards of practice. *J Am Diet Assoc* 108:S52–S58, 2008

Franz MJ, Monk A, Barry B, McClain K, Weaver T, Cooper N, Upham P, Bergenstal R, Mazze RS: Effectiveness of medical nutrition therapy provided by dietitians in the management of non-insulin-dependent diabetes mellitus: a randomized controlled trial. *J Am Diet Assoc* 95:1009–1017, 1995

Gaetke LM, Stuart MA, Truszczynska H: A single nutrition counseling session with a registered dietitian improves short-term outcomes for rural Kentucky patients with chronic disease. *J Am Diet Assoc* 106:109–112, 2006

Goldhaber-Fiebert JD, Goldhaber-Fiebert SM, Tristan ML, Nathan DM: Randomized controlled community-based nutrition and exercise intervention improves glycemia and cardiovascular risk factors in type 2 diabetic patients in rural Costa Rica. *Diabetes Care* 26:24–29, 2003

Graber AI, Elasy TA, Quinn D, Wolff K, Brown A: Improving glycemic control in adults with diabetes mellitus: shared responsibility in primary care practices. *South Med J* 95:684–690, 2002

Huang MC, Hsu CC, Wang HS, Shin SJ: Prospective randomized controlled trial to evaluate effectiveness of registered dietitian-led diabetes management on glycemic and diet control in a primary care setting in Taiwan. *Diabetes Care* 33:233–239, 2010

Lacey K, Pritchett E: Nutrition care process model: ADA adopts road map to quality care and outcomes management. *J Am Diet Assoc* 103:1061–1072, 2003

Laitinen JH, Ahola IE, Sarkkinen ES, Winberg RL, Harmaakorpi-Livonen PA, Uusitupa MI: Impact of intensified dietary therapy on energy and nutrient intakes and fatty acid composition of serum lipids in patients with recently diagnosed non-insulin-dependent diabetes mellitus. *J Am Diet Assoc* 93:276–283, 1993

Lawton J, Rankin D, Cooke DD, Clark M, Elliot J, Heller S, for the UK NIHR DAFNE Study Group: Dose adjustment for normal eating: a qualitative longitudinal exploration of the food and eating practices of type 1 diabetes patients converted to flexible intensive insulin therapy in the UK. *Diabetes Res Clin Pract* 91:87–93, 2011

Lemon CC, Lacey K, Lohse B, Hubacher DO, Klawitter B, Palta M: Outcomes monitoring of health, behavior, and quality of life after nutrition intervention in adults with type 2 diabetes. *J Am Diet Assoc* 104:1805–1815, 2004

Look AHEAD Research Group: Long-term effects of a lifestyle intervention on weight and cardiovascular risk factors in individuals with type 2 diabetes mellitus: four-year results of the Look AHEAD trial. *Arch Intern Med* 170:1566–1575, 2010

Look AHEAD Research Group: Reduction in weight and cardiovascular disease risk factors in individuals with type 2 diabetes: one year results of the Look AHEAD trial. *Diabetes Care* 30:1374–1382, 2007

Lowe J, Linjawi S, Mensch M, James K, Attia J: Flexible eating and flexible insulin dosing in patients with diabetes: results of an intensive self-management course. *Diabetes Res Clin Pract* 80:439–443, 2008

Maislos M, Weisman D, Sherf M: Western Negev Mobile Diabetes Care Program: a model for interdisciplinary diabetes care in a semi-rural setting. *Acta Diabetol* 39:49–53, 2002

Miller CK, Edwards L, Kissling G, Sanville L: Nutrition education improves metabolic outcomes among older adults with diabetes mellitus: results from a randomized controlled trial. *Prev Med* 34:252–259, 2002

Nield L, Moore H, Hooper L, Cruickshank K, Vyas A, Whittaker V, Summerbell CD: Dietary advice for treatment of type 2 diabetes mellitus in adults. *Cochrane Database Syst Rev* CD004097, 2007

Pastors JG, Franz MJ, Warshaw H, Daly A, Arnold MS: How effective is medical nutrition therapy in diabetes care? *J Am Diet Assoc* 103:827–831, 2003

Pastors JG, Warshaw H, Daly A, Franz M, Kulkarni K: The evidence for the effectiveness of medical nutrition therapy in diabetes management. *Diabetes Care* 25:608–613, 2002

Phillips LS: A simple meal plan emphasizing healthy food choices is as effective as an exchange-based meal plan for urban African Americans with type 2 diabetes. *Diabetes Care* 26:1719–1724, 2003

Pieber TR, Brunner GA, Schnedl WJ, Schattenberg S, Kaufmann P, Krejs GJ: Evaluation of a structured outpatient group education program for intensive insulin therapy. *Diabetes Care* 18:625–630, 1995

Povey RC, Clark-Carter D: Diabetes and healthy eating: a systematic review of the literature. *Diabetes Educ* 33:931–959, 2007

Rickheim PL, Weaver TW, Flader JL, Kendall DM: Assessment of group versus individual diabetes education. *Diabetes Care* 25:269–274, 2002

Robbins JM, Thatcher GE, Webb DA, Valdmanis VG: Nutritionist visits, diabetes classes, and hospitalization rates and charges: The Urban Diabetes Study. *Diabetes Care* 31:655–660, 2008

Sämann A, Mühlhauser I, Bender R, Kloos C, Müller UA: Glycemic control and severe hypoglycaemia following training in flexible, intensive insulin therapy to enable dietary freedom in people with type 1 diabetes: a prospective implementation study. *Diabetologia* 48:1965–1970, 2005

Speight J, Amiel SA, Bradley C, Heller S, Oliver L, Roberts S, Rogers H, Taylor C, Thompson G: Long-term biomedical and psychosocial outcomes following DAFNE (Dose Adjustment for Normal Eating) structured education to promote intensive insulin therapy in adults with sub-optimally controlled type 1 diabetes. *Diabetes Res Clin Pract* 89:22–29, 2010

U.K. Prospective Diabetes Study (UKPDS) 7: Response of fasting plasma glucose to diet therapy in newly presenting type II diabetic patients. *Metabolism* 39:905–912, 1990

U.K. Prospective Diabetes Study Group, prepared by Manley SE, Stratton IM, Cull CA, Frighi V, Eeley A, Matthews DR, Holman RR, Turner RC, Neil HAW: Effects of three months' diet after diagnosis of type 2 diabetes on plasma lipids and lipoproteins (UKPDS 45). *Diabet Med* 17:518–523, 2000

Wilson C, Brown T, Acton K, Gilliland A: Effects of clinical nutrition education and educator discipline on glycemic control outcomes in the Indian Health Service. *Diabetes Care* 26:2500–2504, 2003

Wolf AM, Conaway MR, Crowther JQ, Hazen KY, Nadler JL, Oneida B, Bovbjerg VE: Translating lifestyle intervention to practice in obese patients with type 2 diabetes: Improving Control with Activity and Nutrition (ICAN) study. *Diabetes Care* 27:1570–1576, 2004

Ziemer DC, Berkowitz KJ, Panayioto RM, El-Kebbi IM, Musey VC, Anderson LA, Wanko NX, Fowke ML, Brazier CW, Dunbar VG, Slocum W, Bacha GM, Gallina DL, Cook CB, Phillips LS: A simple meal plan emphasizing healthy food choices is as effective as an exchange-based meal plan for urban African Americans with type 2 diabetes. *Diabetes Care* 26:1719–1724, 2003

Joyce Green Pastors, MS, RD, CDE, is an Assistant Professor of Education, Internal Medicine, Virginia Center for Diabetes Professional Education, University of Virginia Health System, Charlottesville, VA. Marion J. Franz, MS, RD, CDE, is a Nutrition/ Health Consultant at Nutrition Concepts by Franz, Inc., Minneapolis, MN.

Chapter 2

Macronutrients and Nutrition Therapy for Diabetes

Marion J. Franz, MS, RD, CDE

Highlights

Macronutrient Distribution in the Nutrition Prescription

Carbohydrates and Diabetes Nutrition Therapy

Protein and Diabetes Nutrition Therapy

Dietary Fat and Diabetes Nutrition Therapy

Summary of Recommendations for Macronutrients

Highlights
Macronutrients and Nutrition
Therapy for Diabetes

■ No ideal distribution of macronutrients—carbohydrate, protein, or fat—for a diabetes nutrition prescription has been identified. Instead, as for all Americans, a healthy eating pattern is recommended. For guidelines on healthy eating patterns, the Dietary Reference Intakes or the *Dietary Guidelines for Americans, 2010*, are helpful resources.

■ Available evidence does not show an adverse effect on insulin sensitivity from carbohydrate intake; a higher carbohydrate intake may instead improve insulin resistance.

■ Three 1-year studies in individuals with type 2 diabetes comparing higher-carbohydrate diets to lower-carbohydrate, low-fat, or high–monounsaturated fat diets found no differences in A1C, LDL cholesterol, or triglyceride levels; blood pressure; or weight at study end. Therefore, total energy intake and a healthy eating pattern should take precedence over the distribution of macronutrients.

■ Sucrose-containing foods can be substituted for other carbohydrates in the food/meal plan. However, as for the general public, excessive intake of sugars should be avoided in a healthy eating pattern. Whenever possible, nutrient-dense foods containing whole grains and fiber should be selected.

■ In people with type 2 diabetes, ingestion of protein does not increase postprandial glucose or lipid responses but does cause an acute insulin response. This response does not result in a long-term effect on insulin levels.

■ Although it is commonly stated that fats slow absorption and delay peak glycemic responses, evidence as to the magnitude of this effect is difficult to find.

■ Chronic intakes of higher total and saturated fats are associated with an increase in insulin resistance, and consumption of saturated and *trans* fatty acids is associated with an adverse effect on lipid/lipoprotein profile and increased risk of cardiovascular disease. It is recommended that saturated fats be replaced with unsaturated fats and intake of *trans* fat be minimized. Ingestion of omega-3 fatty acids from fish is recommended.

Macronutrients and Nutrition Therapy for Diabetes

Nutrition therapy implemented appropriately contributes to important and essential outcomes in the management of diabetes. However, just as there is no one medical therapy appropriate for all individuals with type 1 or type 2 diabetes, there is no one prescription for nutrition therapy appropriate for all people with diabetes. It is clear, as outlined in Chapter 1, that a variety of nutrition interventions lead to positive outcomes. What is essential is that health care professionals select nutrition therapy interventions that will lead to positive outcomes in the patients they are counseling. Agreement from diabetes patients as to their willingness and ability to implement nutrition interventions is equally essential.

Primary goals of nutrition therapy for diabetes are to improve glycemic, lipid, and blood pressure control, thus contributing to reduced risk for potential long-term complications of diabetes and heart disease, and to improve the quality of life for individuals with diabetes. How best to achieve these goals has been, and remains, controversial. Because all fields of medicine have moved toward evidence-based recommendations, so has the field of nutrition therapy and diabetes. In 2008, the Academy of Nutrition and Dietetics (Acad Nutr Diet; formerly the American Dietetic Association) published evidence-based nutrition practice guidelines (EBNPG) for adults with type 1 and type 2 diabetes in the Acad Nutr Diet Evidence Analysis Library (Acad Nutr Diet 2008). Subsequently, a review of the research leading to the EBNPG, a summary of the research published after the completion of the Evidence Analysis Library (through 1 September 2009), and evidence-based diabetes nutrition recommendations were published (Franz 2010). In 2008, the American Diabetes Association (ADA) also published a position statement titled "Nutrition Recommendations and Interventions for Diabetes" (ADA 2008). These recommendations are integrated into their annual standards of medical care in diabetes and updated as new evidence becomes available (ADA 2012).

This chapter reviews and summarizes previously published macronutrient (carbohydrate, protein, and fat) evidence, incorporates research published after 1 September 2009, and summarizes key recommendations related to the role of macronutrients in nutrition therapy for diabetes. A literature search was conducted using PubMed MEDLINE, and additional articles were identified from reference lists. Search criteria included the following: carbohydrate, protein, fat, research in human subjects with diabetes, English language articles, and publication after completion of the literature search for the Acad Nutr Diet EBNPG review. The initial search produced 58 articles, of which 42 were excluded because titles or abstracts did not meet inclusion criteria. Sixteen articles were retrieved for more detailed evaluation. Six of these articles are included and four were added from the review of reference lists, making a total of 10 studies (8 clinical trials and 2 observational studies) that met inclusion criteria. These studies are summarized in Table 2.1. Evidence published before September 2009 is included in the tables in "The Evidence for Medical Nutrition Therapy for Type 1 and Type 2 Diabetes in Adults" (Franz 2010) and in the Acad Nutr Diet Evidence Analysis Library (http://www.adaevidencelibrary.com). Evidence from the *Report of the Dietary Guidelines Advisory Committee (DGAC) on the Dietary Guidelines for Americans, 2010,* is also referenced and is publicly available at http://www.cnpp.usda.gov/ dgas2010-dgacreport.htm and at http://www.nutritionevidencelibrary.gov.

MACRONUTRIENT DISTRIBUTION IN THE NUTRITION PRESCRIPTION

The ADA 2008 nutrition position statement concluded that it is unlikely that there is an optimal mix of macronutrients for the diabetic diet (ADA 2008). For guidance on macronutrient distribution, the Institute of Medicine's dietary reference intakes (DRIs) for a healthy eating pattern for adults may be helpful (Institute of Medicine 2002). The DRI acceptable macronutrient distribution ranges for carbohydrate, fat, and protein are 45–65, 20–35, and 10–35% of total energy, respectively. The position statement also notes that regardless of the macronutrient distribution, total energy intake must be appropriate for weight management. The mix of macronutrients is adjusted to meet metabolic goals and individual preferences of the person with diabetes (ADA 2012).

A 2012 ADA systematic review of the literature regarding macronutrients, food groups, and eating patterns in the management of diabetes concluded that several different macronutrient distributions may lead to improvement in glycemic and/or cardiovascular disease (CVD) risk factors and that many different approaches to medical nutrition therapy and eating patterns effectively improve glycemic control and reduce cardiovascular risk among individuals with diabetes (Wheeler 2012).

The Acad Nutr Diet EBNPG reviewed a total of 18 studies using differing percentages of carbohydrate, fat, or protein and also concluded that research does not support an ideal percentage of energy from macronutrients in the food/meal plan for people with diabetes. It is recommended that registered dietitians encourage consumption of macronutrients on the basis of DRIs (Acad Nutr Diet 2008; Franz 2010).

The *Dietary Guidelines for Americans, 2010* can be used to identify a healthy eating pattern that is not a rigid prescription, but rather includes options that can accommodate cultural, ethnic, traditional, and personal preferences as well as food costs and availability. Although healthy eating patterns that meet nutrient needs over time at an appropriate calorie level can be diverse, some key elements exist: an abundance of vegetables and fruits, an emphasis on whole grains, moderate amounts and a variety of protein foods, limited amounts of foods high in added sugars, and more oils than solid fats. Research is available on beneficial health outcomes from examples of healthy eating patterns, such as the Dietary Approaches to Stop Hypertension (DASH), a Mediterranean-style eating pattern, and a vegetarian eating pattern (U.S. Department of Agriculture and U.S. Department of Health and Human Services 2010).

Table 2.1 Studies on Macronutrients (Carbohydrate, Protein, and Fat) Published After September 2009

	Population/ Duration of Study	Intervention (type of study)	Major Findings	Comments
Carbohydrate				
Strychar 2009	$n = 30$ adults with type 1 diabetes/6 months	Eucaloric diets, higher in CHO (54–57%)/lower in fat (27–30%) vs. higher in MUFAs (20%)/lower in CHO (43–46%) (RCT)	6 months: nonsignificant differences in insulin doses, A1C, total, LDL, and HDL cholesterol, TG, BP; lower CHO group: ↑ weight (2.4 kg) and ↓ plasminogen activator inhibitor 1 (both $P < 0.05$)	
Esposito 2009	$n = 215$ overweight newly diagnosed patients with type 2 diabetes and not treated with drug therapy/4 years	Mediterranean-style diet, energy-restricted (1,500 kcal/day for women, 1,800 kcal/day for men), low-CHO (<50% total kcal) vs. low-fat diet (<30% total kcal) (RCT)	After 4 years, 44% of Mediterranean-style and 70% of the low-fat groups required drug therapy ($P < 0.001$); Mediterranean group: A1C, HDL cholesterol, and TG improved more vs. low-fat group (all $P < 0.05$)	Actual intake: Mediterranean-style, ~1,900 kcal, ~44% CHO, ~39% fat; low-fat diet, ~1,900 kcal, ~52% CHO, ~30% fat
De Natale 2009	$n = 18$ adults with type 2 diabetes on diet or diet plus metformin/4 weeks	Plant-based high-CHO (52%)/high-fiber (28 g/1,000 kcal) diet versus a lower plant-based CHO (45%)/high-MUFA (23%) diet (RCT)	High-CHO/high-fiber diet ↓ total, LDL, and HDL cholesterol, postprandial TG, glucose, and insulin vs. high-MUFA diet (all $P < 0.05$)	Authors concluded that a diet based on legumes, vegetables, fruits, and whole cereals has multiple beneficial effects on CVD risk factors
He 2010	$n = 7,822$ women with type 2 diabetes in the Nurses' Health Study/up to 26-year follow-up	Association with whole grains and components (cereal fiber, bran, and germ) in relation to all-cause and CVD-specific mortality (cohort study)	853 all-cause deaths and 295 CVD deaths; after adjustment for age, the highest vs. the lowest fifth of intakes were associated with 16–31% lower all-cause mortality; bran had the strongest association (P for trend = 0.01)	
Powers 2010	$n = 14$ with type 2 diabetes on metformin only/2 test meals	4-h glycemic response to moderate-CHO (45 g) vs. high-CHO (90 g) lunch measured by CGM (crossover study)	90 g CHO-fixed lunch: higher peak glucose (210 vs. 190 mg/dL), longer time to return to preprandial glucose (201 vs. 163 min)	Consuming twice as much CHO did not double any of the responses

	Population/ Duration of Study	Intervention (type of study)	Major Findings	Comments
Protein				
Papak-onstanti-nou 2010a	$n = 23$ subjects, newly diagnosed, untreated, with type 2 diabetes and 26 without type 2 diabetes/ 2 meals	30% protein, 51% CHO, 19% fat, vs. 15% protein, 51% CHO, 34% fat, meals, equal in kcal and fiber (crossover study)	Nonsignificant meal effect on postprandial glucose and insulin responses within groups	
Papak-onstanti-nou 2010b	$n = 17$ adults with newly diagnosed, untreated, type 2 diabetes/4 weeks	30% protein, 50% CHO, 20% fat, vs. 15% protein, 50% CHO, 35% fat, meals, both diets ↓700 kcal/day (crossover study)	Nonsignificant difference in ↓ weight loss, fasting blood glucose, postprandial glucose and insulin, total and LDL cholesterol; high protein diet ↓ TG ($P = 0.04$) and BP ($P < 0.001$)	
Gannon 2010	$n = 8$ men with untreated type 2 diabetes/10 weeks	Weight-maintaining, non-ketogenic diet, 30% CHO, 30% protein, 40% fat (LoBAG$_{30}$), outcomes, food provided (time series)	Fasting plasma glucose ↓ 28%, 24-h total glucose area ↓ 35%, mean GHb ↓ 25% (10.0 to 8.7 at 5 weeks to 7.5%); no change in weight, insulin, lipids, BP, or kidney function	No control group, only eight subjects
Fats/Cholesterol				
Stirban 2010	$n = 34$ subjects with type 2 diabetes/6 weeks	2 g omega-3 fatty acids vs. olive oil (placebo) supplements (RCT)	Omega-3 fatty acids vs. placebo prevented deterioration of postprandial macrovascular function and improved postprandial microvascular function	
Pearce 2011	$n = 65$ adults with type 2 diabetes or impaired glucose tolerance/12 weeks	HPHchol vs. HPLchol (40% CHO, 30% protein, 30% fat; 590 mg cholesterol or 213 mg cholesterol [eggs vs. lean meat]); hypoenergetic (RCT)	Both diets: ↓ weight 6 kg ($P < 0.001$), total cholesterol ($P < 0.001$), non-HDL cholesterol ($P < 0.001$), apolipoprotein B ($P < 0.01$), A1C ($P < 0.001$), fasting plasma glucose ($P < 0.01$), fasting insulin ($P < 0.01$), BP ($P < 0.001$); HDL cholesterol ↑ on HPHchol and ↓ on HPLchol ($P < 0.05$)	

BP, blood pressure; CHO, carbohydrate; CGM, continuous glucose monitoring; HPHchol, high-protein, high-cholesterol diet; HPLchol, high-protein, low-cholesterol diet; LoBAG$_{30}$, low biologically available glucose diets, 30 indicates % CHO; MUFA, monounsaturated fatty acid; RCT, randomized controlled trial; TG, triglyceride.

CARBOHYDRATES AND DIABETES NUTRITION THERAPY

Carbohydrates consist of sugars, starches, and fibers. These are the preferred names for carbohydrate categories rather than simple or complex carbohydrates, since they are based on chemical composition (DGAC 2010). Along with the acceptable macronutrient distribution ranges, the DRIs set a recommended dietary allowance (RDA) for carbohydrates of at least 130 g/day for adults and children (Institute of Medicine 2002). This RDA is based on the estimated average requirement for carbohydrate ingestion that will provide the brain with adequate glucose without additional glucose from protein or triglycerides stored in the fat cells (100 g/day) and a coefficient of variation of 15% based on the variation in brain glucose utilization. The RDA is equal to the estimated average requirement plus twice the coefficient of variation to cover the needs of 97–98% of individuals. Therefore, the RDA for carbohydrate is at least 130% of the estimated average requirement, or at least 130 g/day of carbohydrate. The ADA notes the following: "Although brain fuel needs can be met on lower-carbohydrate diets, long-term metabolic effects of very-low-carbohydrate diets are unclear, and such diets eliminate many foods that are important sources of energy, fiber, vitamins, and minerals and that are important in dietary palatability" (ADA 2012).

Definitions of carbohydrate intake have not been well defined. A high-carbohydrate intake is often defined as a carbohydrate intake ≥55% of total energy. A low-carbohydrate intake may be defined as <25% of total energy or <130 g/day. A very-low-carbohydrate ketogenic diet is defined as <20 g/day. However, differing definitions for carbohydrate intake are used. For example, a meta-analysis used 9–45% of total energy as carbohydrate as a definition of low-carbohydrate intake (Kirk 2008). As a result of this definition, there was an overlap of carbohydrate intake in the low- and high-carbohydrate groups (carbohydrate in the high-carbohydrate group ranged from 40 to 70%). Of interest is a Mediterranean-style eating pattern in subjects with type 2 diabetes that was considered to be low carbohydrate, with <50% of daily calories from carbohydrate (actual intake ~44%) (Esposito 2009), whereas for most individuals with type 2 diabetes, this intake of carbohydrate would be considered a moderate-carbohydrate intake.

It is important to note that most individuals with diabetes do not eat a low- or high-carbohydrate diet but rather report a moderate intake; studies reported an intake of ~46% in individuals with type 1 diabetes (Delahanty 2009) and ~44% in individuals with type 2 diabetes (Vitolins 2009). Furthermore, it appears difficult for people with type 2 diabetes to eat a high-carbohydrate diet. In the U.K. Prospective Diabetes Study, despite receiving individual education from dietitians on the recommended carbohydrate intake of 50–55%, patients reported a carbohydrate intake of 43% energy intake, which was similar to the general public (Eeley 1996).

Carbohydrate and Insulin Resistance

If consuming a high-carbohydrate intake contributed to insulin resistance, carbohydrate intake should be reduced, especially in people at risk for or with type 2 diabetes. Although evidence is limited, available evidence does not report an adverse effect on insulin sensitivity from carbohydrate intake; instead, carbohydrate may improve insulin sensitivity. A review compared short-term intervention studies with higher (>50% of total energy) versus lower carbohydrate intake in subjects with and without diabetes (McClenaghan 2005). Of 11 studies in subjects without diabetes, 7 reported an increase in insulin sensitivity from the higher-carbohydrate diet and 5 reported no differences. Of eight studies in subjects with diabetes, five reported improvement in insulin sensitivity from the higher-carbohydrate diet and three reported no difference. The author concluded that higher-carbohydrate diets do not adversely affect insulin sensitivity and may offer some benefits. Longer-term clinical trials and epidemiological studies in people without diabetes have also reported no adverse effects on insulin sensitivity from higher-carbohydrate diets (Ard 2004; Bessesen 2001; Howard 2006).

However, examining the effect of carbohydrate on insulin action is difficult because any change in one component of the diet is accompanied by changes in other components of the diet. Therefore, as carbohydrate intake is increased, fat is generally decreased, and vice versa. Chronic consumption of foods high in fat, especially saturated fats, as will be reviewed later, is reported to increase insulin resistance. Therefore, it is unknown if the benefit on insulin sensitivity is due to the higher carbohydrate intake or the lower fat intake.

Carbohydrates and Glycemia

The balance between digestible carbohydrate and available insulin is a major determinant of postprandial glucose levels. However, other intrinsic and extrinsic variables also influence the effect of carbohydrate on glucose levels. Continuous glucose monitoring systems can be used to better understand the postprandial effects of carbohydrate. For example, in people with type 2 diabetes, a lunch meal containing double the carbohydrate content did not double the glycemic response (Powers 2010). Under debate is what amount of carbohydrate intake best facilitates glycemic control in people with diabetes.

Type 1 Diabetes

In people receiving intensive treatment in the Diabetes Control and Complications Trial, a lower carbohydrate (37%) intake and higher total (45%) and saturated (17%) fat intakes were associated with worse glycemic control at year 5 compared to a higher carbohydrate (56%) intake (A1C values of 7.5 versus 7.0%, respectively), independent of exercise and BMI (Delahanty 2009). The authors suggest that the carbohydrate content is less critical than the total and saturated fat content, to which it is usually inversely related. They note that high-fat meals have been shown to interfere with indexes of insulin signaling, which results in a transient increase in insulin resistance (Savage 2007), and that a lower-fat diet reduces basal free fatty acid concentrations and improves peripheral insulin sensitivity in type 1 diabetes (Rosenfalck 2006).

To determine the effects on CVD risk factors in people with type 1 diabetes, a eucaloric diet higher in carbohydrate and lower in fat was compared to a diet lower in carbohydrate and higher in monounsaturated fatty acids (MUFAs). After 6 months, there were no significant differences between groups other than decreased plasminogen activator inhibitor 1 and weight gain in the lower-carbohydrate/MUFA group. This result suggests that if individuals choose to lower carbohydrate intake, these calories should be replaced with unsaturated fats rather than saturated fats and special attention should be paid to total energy intake (Strychar 2009).

Type 2 Diabetes

A cross-sectional study of American Indians with type 2 diabetes in the Strong Health Study assessed dietary intake in 1,284 participants. Lower intake of carbohydrate (<35–40% of energy) and higher intakes of total (>25–30% of energy) and saturated fats (>13% of energy) were associated with poorer glycemic control. A lower fiber intake and a higher protein intake were marginally associated with poor glycemic control (Xu 2007).

Clinical trials in individuals with diabetes have compared lower carbohydrate intakes and higher total fat and saturated fat intakes to higher carbohydrate intakes and lower total fat and saturated fat intakes. A meta-analysis of 19 short-term studies (10 days to 6 weeks) with 306 individuals with type 2 diabetes compared lower-carbohydrate, higher-fat diets (40%/40%) to higher-carbohydrate, lower-fat diets (58%/24%) and found no significant differences between diets in the reduction in A1C and total and LDL cholesterol. The higher-carbohydrate diets did increase triglyceride levels and decrease HDL cholesterol. However, the higher-carbohydrate diet did not elevate triglycerides when energy restriction was prescribed. Therefore, total energy intake is a factor when determining the effect of carbohydrate on triglyceride levels. Studies in which glucose-lowering medications were changed and that included an increase in fiber and whole grains were excluded from the meta-analysis because such diets are high in fiber, which in itself has beneficial effects on glycemia and lipemia, regardless of the carbohydrate-to-fat ratio (Kodama 2009). In general, total and LDL cholesterol change more favorably in individuals assigned to low-fat/higher-carbohydrate diets, whereas, HDL cholesterol and triglyceride values change more favorably in individuals randomized to low-carbohydrate diets (Nordmann 2006).

Since publication of the meta-analysis, three 1-year studies in people with type 2 diabetes comparing higher-carbohydrate diets to lower-carbohydrate, low-fat, or high-MUFA diets have been published and reported no differences in A1C, weight loss, LDL cholesterol, triglycerides, or blood pressure (Brehm 2009; Davis 2009; Wolever 2008). Vegetarian and vegan diets are high in carbohydrate. A vegetarian diet (52% energy from carbohydrate) was compared to a diet high in MUFAs, with reported beneficial effects from the vegetarian diet on lipids (total cholesterol, LDL cholesterol, postprandial triglycerides), glucose, and insulin levels (De Natale 2009). A 22-week low-fat vegan diet (75% carbohydrate) compared to a control diet (60–75% carbohydrate and MUFAs) showed greater improvements in A1C levels (~1% point reduction), body weight, and lipids (total and LDL cholesterol, triglycerides) from the vegan diet in secondary analysis. The intent-to-treat analyses, however, showed no significant differences between groups (Barnard 2006).

In summary, in observational studies in people with type 1 and type 2 diabetes, higher-carbohydrate diets compared to diets higher in total fat and saturated fat are associated with lower A1C levels. However, in clinical trials, both high- and low-carbohydrate diets lead to similar improvements in A1C and body weight. It appears likely that the total energy intake of the eating pattern outweighs the distribution of carbohydrates. High-carbohydrate diets, which are generally low in fat, tend to have beneficial effects on total and LDL cholesterol, whereas low-carbohydrate diets tend to have beneficial effects on triglycerides and HDL cholesterol. Because of beneficial and/or similarities in outcomes, it would seem prudent to recommend an eating pattern with moderate amounts of carbohydrate (which is how many people with diabetes already eat) and that includes fruits, vegetables, whole grains, and low-fat dairy foods—all carbohydrate sources—in appropriate amounts and portion sizes.

Types of Carbohydrate

Sucrose. After reviewing 15 studies in which sucrose was substituted for isocaloric amounts of starch, the Acad Nutr Diet EBNPG concluded the following: "If persons with diabetes choose to eat foods containing sucrose, the sucrose-containing foods can be substituted for other carbohydrate foods. Sucrose intakes of 10% to 35% of total energy do not have a negative effect on glycemic or lipid level responses when substituted for isocaloric amounts of starch" (Acad Nutr Diet 2008; Franz 2010). The ADA also concluded, "sucrose-containing foods can be substituted for other carbohydrates in the meal plan, or, if added to the food/meal plan, covered with insulin or other glucose-lowering medications" (ADA 2008). However, as with the general public, care should be taken to avoid excess energy intake, and excessive intake of sugars should be avoided in a healthier eating pattern. The DGAC recommends a maximal intake level of ≤25% of total energy from added sugars, based on research showing that people with intakes of added sugars at or above this level are more likely to have poorer intakes of important essential nutrients (DGAC 2010). For a daily energy intake of ~2,000 kcal, this would be about 10 teaspoons of added sugars; however, average intake for all individuals in the U.S. is ~22 teaspoons per day. (One 12-ounce can of cola contains ~8 teaspoons of added sugar, for ~130 kcal.) In general, it is recommended that most women should eat or drink no more than 100 kcal/day from added sugars and most men no more than 150 kcal/day (Johnson 2011).

There is a natural liking of sweet tastes and, in that regard, people with diabetes are similar to people without diabetes. Unfortunately, people with diabetes are often made to feel guilty if they choose foods that contain added sugars. Knowing the total carbohydrate content, including sugars, of foods can assist people with diabetes to make appropriate food choices that they will enjoy while maintaining glycemic control.

High-fructose corn syrup. High-fructose corn syrup is composed of either 42 or 55% fructose and is similar in composition to table sugar (sucrose). Therefore, the recommendations discussed above related to sucrose also apply to high-fructose corn syrup. High-fructose corn syrup does not differ uniquely from sucrose and other nutritive sweeteners in metabolic effects (glucose, insulin, and triglycerides), subjective effects (hunger, satiety, and energy intake at subsequent meals), and adverse effects such as weight gain (Acad Nutr Diet 2012). It is the sweetener commonly used by the beverage industry.

Fiber and whole grains. Foods containing fiber and whole grains are also recommended. After reviewing 15 studies reporting on the effect of fiber intake on glycemic and lipid outcomes in individuals with diabetes, the Acad Nutr Diet EBNPG concluded the following: "While diets containing 44 to 50 g fiber daily are reported to improve glycemia in persons with diabetes, more usual intakes (up to 24 g/day) have not shown beneficial effects on glycemia. Recommendations for fiber intake for people with diabetes are similar to the recommendations for the general public (DRI: 14 g/1,000 kcal)" (Acad Nutr Diet 2008; Franz 2010). However, the guidelines do recommend including foods containing 25–30 g fiber per day, with special emphasis on soluble fiber sources (7–13 g) because of their beneficial effect on lipids.

The ADA also recommends that people with diabetes choose a variety of fiber-containing foods such as legumes, fiber-rich cereals (≥5 g fiber/serving), fruits, vegetables, and whole-grain products because they provide vitamins, minerals, and other substances important for good health. The first priority is to achieve fiber-intake goals set for the general population of 14 g/1,000 kcal (ADA 2008). Interestingly, the DGAC notes that it is difficult to meet dietary fiber recommendations with a low carbohydrate intake (DGAC 2010).

However, consumption of whole-grain foods is likely to be of equal importance in reducing CVD risk as fiber. Whole-grain foods contain fiber, vitamins, minerals, phenolic compounds, phytoestrogens, and other unmeasured constituents, which have been shown to lower serum lipids and blood pressure, improve glucose and insulin metabolism and endothelial function, and alleviate oxidative stress and inflammation in the general population (He 2010). In a prospective study of 7,822 women with type 2 diabetes, intakes of whole grain, cereal fiber, and bran were inversely associated with all-cause and CVD mortality during a 26-year follow-up (He 2010). Bran intake had the strongest association, and germ intake, which was also evaluated, was not associated with all-cause or CVD mortality.

Glycemic index/glycemic load. The glycemic index (GI) measures the relative area under the glucose curve of 50 g digestible carbohydrate compared with 50 g of a standard food, either glucose or bread. The GI index does not measure how rapidly blood glucose levels increase after eating different types of carbohydrate-containing foods, which implies that a high-GI food peaks quickly and a low-GI food peaks later. In a review of studies comparing different types of low- and high-GI foods and glucose, in people without diabetes, glucose peaks occurred consistently at ~30 minutes, regardless of whether the food was categorized as low-, medium-, or high-GI, with a modest difference in glucose peak values between high- and low-GI foods (Brand-Miller 2009). In contrast to what is often stated, low-GI foods did not produce a slower rise in blood glucose, nor did they produce an extended, sustained glucose response.

The estimated glycemic load of foods, meals, and eating patterns is calculated by multiplying the GI by the amount of carbohydrate in each food and then totaling the values for all foods in a meal or eating pattern. The glycemic load is used most often in research studies, especially in epidemiological studies, but because of the calculations needed, it is not likely a practical approach for individuals to use for planning meals or prandial insulin doses.

After reviewing 15 studies reporting on the relationship between the GI values of foods/diets and metabolic outcomes, the Acad Nutr Diet EBNPG concluded the following: "Studies comparing high- versus low-GI diets report mixed effects on A1C levels. These studies are complicated by differing definitions of high-GI or low-GI diets or quartiles, as well as possible confounding dietary factors" (Acad Nutr Diet 2008; Franz 2010). The guidelines note that definitions of low- versus high-GI diets range from 38 to 77% for low-GI diets and from 63 to 98% for high-GI diets. Other problems include the variability of GI responses from carbohydrate-containing foods within and among individuals. As with carbohydrate, most individuals with diabetes appear to consume a moderate-GI diet, and it is unknown whether reducing the usual GI by a few units will result in improved glycemic control. Of the 15 studies reviewed, 12 are of short duration (<3 months) with a limited number of subjects. Only three studies were of 1-year duration. After 1 year, one study reported no difference in actual GI between the low-GI and control groups, and two studies reported no differences in A1C between the low-GI and control groups.

The ADA also noted the conflicting evidence of randomized clinical trials of low- versus high-GI diets and also expressed concern about the variability in responses to specific carbohydrate-containing foods. ADA also noted that most individuals already consume a moderate-GI diet; however, for individuals consuming a high-GI diet, consuming a low-GI diet may result in a modest benefit in postprandial hyperglycemia (ADA 2008).

Nonnutritive sweeteners and sugar alcohols. Five nonnutritive sweeteners are approved by the U.S. Food and Drug Administration (FDA) as food additives: aspartame, saccharine, acesulfame K, neotame, and sucralose; one other—stevia—is approved as Generally Recognized As Safe (GRAS). The FDA also sets a sweetener Acceptable Daily Intake (ADI), which is the level a person can safely consume on average every day over a lifetime without risk. The ADI is typically 1/100th of the amount of the nonnutritive sweeteners shown to be safe in animal studies. The ADA notes that before being allowed on the market, all nonnutritive sweeteners undergo rigorous scrutiny and are shown to be safe when consumed by the public, including people with diabetes and women during pregnancy (ADA 2008). The Acad Nutr Diet EBNPG note that although nonnutritive sweeteners independently do not effect changes in glycemic responses, some of the products sweetened with nonnutritive sweeteners contain energy and carbohydrate from other foods, and these foods need to be taken into consideration (Acad Nutr Diet 2008; Franz 2010).

Reduced-calorie sweeteners approved by the FDA include sugar alcohols (polyols) such as erythritol, isomalt, lactitol, maltitol, mannitol, sorbitol, xylitol, tagatose, and hydrogenated starch hydrolysates. They produce lower postprandial glucose responses than sucrose or glucose and contain on average about 2 calories/g. There is no evidence that the amount of sugar alcohols likely to be consumed will reduce glycemia, energy intake, or weight. Although safe to use, they may cause diarrhea, especially in children (ADA 2008).

Carbohydrate Summary

Carbohydrates eaten and available insulin are the primary determinants of postprandial glucose levels. Foods containing carbohydrate—fruits, vegetables, whole grains, legumes, and low-fat dairy foods—are important components of a healthy eating pattern. For people with diabetes, these foods should be included in appropriate amounts and portion sizes in their food/meal plan. In addition, nutrient-dense foods are recommended. Nutrient-dense foods are foods and beverages that have not been "diluted" with the addition of added solid fats and added sugars. Monitoring carbohydrates, whether by carbohydrate counting, choices, or experience-based estimation, remains a key strategy in achieving glycemic control (ADA 2012). Although some individuals may note improvements in postprandial glucose responses with the use of the GI/glycemic load, the concept of the GI/glycemic load adds an additional level of complexity to nutrition therapy recommendations and is perhaps best used for fine-tuning postprandial responses after first focusing on total carbohydrate.

The Acad Nutr Diet EBNPG recommend the following: "In persons receiving either medical nutrition therapy alone, glucose-lowering medications, or fixed insulin doses, meal and snack carbohydrate should be consistently distributed throughout the day on a day-to-day basis." Nutrition therapy for people with type 2 diabetes is discussed in Chapter 6. The Acad Nutr Diet EBNPG also recommend the following: "In persons with type 1 (or type 2) diabetes who adjust their mealtime insulin doses or who are on insulin pump therapy, insulin doses should be adjusted to match carbohydrate intake (insulin-to-carbohydrate ratios). This can be accomplished by comprehensive nutrition education and counseling on interpretation of blood glucose patterns, nutrition-related medication adjustment, and collaboration with the health care team" (Acad Nutr Diet 2008; Franz 2010). Nutrition therapy for people using insulin therapy is discussed in Chapters 5, 7, and 21.

PROTEIN AND DIABETES NUTRITION THERAPY

In people with type 1 or type 2 diabetes with normal renal function, both the Acad Nutr Diet EBNPG and the ADA currently have not found adequate evidence to support recommending a change in the usual protein intake of 15–20% of total daily energy intake (Acad Nutr Diet 2008; ADA 2008). Exceptions for change in protein intake are in individuals who consume excessive amounts of protein foods high in saturated fatty acids, in people who have a protein intake less than the RDA of 0.8 g good-quality protein/kg body weight/day (on average ~10% of energy intake), or in patients with diabetic nephropathy.

In people with type 2 diabetes, ingestion of protein results in acute insulin and glucagon responses with minimal, if any, postprandial glucose or lipid responses (Acad Nutr Diet 2008; Papakonstantinou 2010a). Studies lasting 5–12 weeks comparing high-protein diets to lower-protein diets showed no differences in longer-term insulin response despite the acute insulin response.

Studies in people with type 1 diabetes and protein intake are limited. In a study in which a standard lunch (450 kcal) was compared with a protein-added (+200 kcal) lunch, the early glucose response was similar, but the late glucose response (2–5 h) was slightly increased and required 3–4 units of additional insulin. However, the total insulin requirement over the 5 h was not increased (Peters 1993). Large amounts of protein appear to have the potential to modestly increase postprandial glucose levels and may require additional small amounts of prandial insulin. If protein is lowered, insulin doses may also have to be decreased. Perhaps the best assumption is that prandial bolus insulin doses cover the meal carbohydrate needs for insulin and the protein needs for insulin are covered by basal insulin doses. Generally, an individual's protein intake is fairly consistent, and the need for extra insulin only becomes an issue when excessive protein is included in meals. Evidence does not support recommendations that suggest protein slows absorption of carbohydrate, contributes to a sustained elevation of glucose levels, or is helpful in the treatment of hypoglycemia (Franz 2002). Because protein does not increase circulating blood glucose levels and, in people with type 2 diabetes, increases insulin levels, it should not be used to treat acute hypoglycemia or to prevent overnight hypoglycemia (e.g., by adding protein to bedtime snacks) (ADA 2008).

Recent research has focused on higher-protein diets and lower-carbohydrate diets for beneficial effects on glycemia and CVD risk factors. In a small crossover study, a high-protein, low-fat (30% protein, 50% carbohydrate, 20% fat) diet was compared to a low-protein, high-fat (15% protein, 50% carbohydrate, 35% fat) diet, each for 4 weeks. Both diets had beneficial effects on weight loss, fasting glucose, and total and LDL cholesterol, with no differences in postprandial glucose and insulin responses. However, the high-protein, low-fat diet improved both triglyceride levels and blood pressure (Papakonstantinou 2010b). In two small 5-week and 10-week studies of men with untreated diabetes, weight-maintaining diets containing 30% protein, 30% carbohydrate, and 40% fat decreased glycated hemoglobin (% GHb) by 13% at 5 weeks and 25% at 10 weeks with no changes in insulin, glucagon, and blood pressure and without the addition of glucose-lowering medications (Gannon 2010).

Studies thus far on high-protein diets for people with type 2 diabetes have been of short duration and with small numbers of subjects with diabetes. Although beneficial outcomes have been reported, studies on higher protein intakes are usually conducted in research centers or food is provided to subjects, and the ability of individuals to increase protein intake long term is unknown (Brinkworth 2004).

DIETARY FAT AND DIABETES NUTRITION THERAPY

Dietary fats are said to slow glucose absorption and delay the peak glycemic response after consuming carbohydrate foods. However, evidence to support this statement is difficult to find. In an early study in subjects with type 2 diabetes, 5, 15, 30, or 50 g fat (butter) were added to 50 g carbohydrate (potato), resulting in a mean glucose area response that was similar after ingestion of the potato with or without the differing amounts of butter (Gentilcore 2006). In another study, 50 g potato alone or with 100 g butter or 80 g olive oil were compared, and the addition of both fats had no effect on glucose or insulin postprandial responses (Thomsen 2003). In subjects with type 1 diabetes, the addition of 200 kcal (22 g fat) to a standard meal also did not affect the glucose response or insulin requirements (Peters 1993). Therefore, in acute studies, with a limited number of subjects, the addition of fat to meals appears to have minimal effects on postprandial glucose.

Epidemiological data and controlled clinical trials have reported that long-term higher levels of total fat intake results in greater whole-body insulin resistance. However, obesity may complicate the relationship (Lovejoy 2002). The data further support an adverse effect of saturated fatty acids on insulin sensitivity. The DGAC reviewed the evidence for the effect of saturated fatty acid intake on type 2 diabetes or increased risk of CVD and concluded that intake of saturated fatty acids increases total and LDL cholesterol, increases risk of CVD, and increases markers of insulin resistance and risk of type 2 diabetes. The committee concluded from 12 studies published since 2000 and reviewed in the nutrition evidence library that a 5% energy decrease in saturated fatty acids, replaced by MUFAs or polyunsaturated fatty acids, decreases risk of CVD and type 2 diabetes in healthy adults and improves insulin responsiveness in insulin-resistant individuals and individuals with type 2 diabetes (DGAC 2010).

The risk of CVD associated with *trans* fatty acids is due to their positive association with LDL cholesterol and the reverse association with HDL cholesterol, the effect on inflammatory processes, and their interference with fat metabolism. The majority of *trans* fatty acids come from hydrogenation of unsaturated fats industrially, but ~1–2% (<2% of total energy intake) is found naturally in the gastrointestinal tracts of ruminant animals, ending up in meats and dairy products. The DGAC concluded that avoiding industrial *trans* fats is important, but small amounts of ruminant *trans* fats in the diet is acceptable (DGAC 2010).

The DGAC also reviewed the evidence for the effect of dietary cholesterol. From a review of 16 studies published since 1991, the committee concluded that consumption of one egg per day is not associated with risk of CVD or stroke in healthy adults, although consumption of more than seven eggs per week has been associated with increased risk. They note, however, that in three methodologically strong prospective cohort studies, in individuals with type 2 diabetes, egg consumption (one egg/day) does have negative effects on serum lipids and lipoproteins and does increase risk of CVD. Therefore, it is recommended that dietary cholesterol be limited to <200 mg/day for people with type 2 diabetes (DGAC 2010). Conflicting evidence comes from a study in 65 adults with type 2 diabetes or impaired glucose tolerance comparing a hypoenergetic high-protein, high-cholesterol diet (two eggs/day) to a high-protein, low-cholesterol diet (100 g lean animal protein). At 12 weeks, weight loss was similar and LDL cholesterol was unchanged. All the subjects experienced a reduction in total cholesterol, A1C, and blood pressure (Pearce 2011).

Consumption of n-3 fatty acids (omega-3 fatty acids) from fish or from supplements has been shown to reduce adverse CVD outcomes in persons with and without diabetes. A Cochrane Systematic Review and a second systematic review and meta-analysis concluded that omega-3 supplementation in persons with type 2 diabetes lowers triglyceride levels, but may raise LDL cholesterol and have no effect on glycemic control or fasting insulin (Hartweg 2008; Hartweg 2009) (see Chapter 13).

Endothelial dysfunction precedes the onset of atherosclerosis and the occurrence of CVD risk. The correction of fasting endothelial dysfunction with n-3 fatty acids is reported, but in people with type 2 diabetes, postprandial vascular dysfunction is also of concern. Supplementation with 2 g n-3 fatty acids or olive oil in people with type 2 diabetes revealed that n-3 fatty acids also improved post-

prandial vascular function (Stirban 2010). The DGAC concluded that two servings of fatty seafood per week (4-oz servings) providing an average of 250 mg/day
of n-3 fatty acids decreases risk of CVD (DGAC 2010). The ADA also recommends two or more servings of fatty fish per week (with the exception of com-
mercially fried fish filets) (ADA 2008).

The Acad Nutr Diet EBNPG reviewed a total of 43 studies related to the
prevention and treatment of CVD in people with diabetes. It is recommended
that cardioprotective nutrition interventions be implemented in the initial series
of nutrition therapy encounters, since both glycemic control and cardioprotective
nutrition interventions improve the lipid profile, reduce CVD risk, and improve
CVD outcomes (Acad Nutr Diet 2008; Franz 2010). Nutrition interventions
include reduction in saturated and *trans* fatty acids and dietary cholesterol and
interventions to improve blood pressure. Chapter 13 reviews nutrition therapy for
lipid disorders.

SUMMARY OF RECOMMENDATIONS FOR MACRONUTRIENTS

Since no ideal percentages of macronutrients—carbohydrate, protein, and
fat—appear to exist, it would seem prudent to base the nutrition prescription for
individuals with diabetes on an appropriate energy intake and a healthy eating
pattern. Individuals with both type 1 and type 2 diabetes report eating a moderate
carbohydrate eating pattern (~45–50% of total kcal), which would appear to be of
less importance than total energy intake. However, nutrition interventions must
always be based on changes that the individual with diabetes is willing and able to
make. Even small changes in food/nutrient intake can result in beneficial outcomes.

Although total carbohydrate intake appears to determine glycemic responses
more than the type of carbohydrate (i.e., starch vs. sugar or high- vs. low-GI foods)
and because of similarities and conflicting metabolic outcomes from differing
amounts of macronutrients, attention to a healthy eating pattern appears more
appropriate. A healthy eating pattern includes the following: a caloric intake that
attains and maintains a healthy weight for adults and appropriate weight gain in
children and adolescents; foods from all food groups in nutrient-dense forms and in
recommended amounts; replacement of solid fats with oils when possible; reduced
intake of added sugars, refined grains (replaced with whole grains), and sodium; and
if consumed, moderate alcohol intake (DGAC 2010). Intake of vegetables and fruits,
whole grains, fat-free or low-fat milk and milk products, and seafood should be
increased and foods containing saturated fat and *trans* fatty acid decreased.

For all people with diabetes, monitoring total carbohydrate intake remains a
key strategy for achieving glycemic control. Individuals on nutrition therapy
alone, glucose-lowering medications, or fixed insulin doses appear to do better
when carbohydrate intake is kept consistent on a day-to-day basis. Medical therapy then needs to be adjusted appropriately to cover the carbohydrate. Individuals
self-adjusting their insulin doses can use insulin-to-carbohydrate ratios and correction factors (Chapter 5) to meet their glucose goals.

There is no conclusive evidence that changing usual protein intake in people
with diabetes would be beneficial. The effect of protein on glycemia depends on
the state of insulinization and the degree of glycemic control. In people with well-

controlled diabetes, consistent amounts of protein will have minimal acute effects on glucose or insulin.

The ADA recommends limiting saturated fat intake to <7% of total energy intake, minimizing intake of *trans* fat, and limiting dietary cholesterol to <200 mg/day (ADA 2008). They note that reducing saturated fatty acids may also reduce HDL cholesterol, but importantly, the ratio of LDL cholesterol to HDL cholesterol is not adversely affected. Major sources of saturated fatty acids in the American diet include regular cheese, pizza, grain-based desserts, dairy-based desserts, chicken and chicken mixed dishes, and sausage, franks, bacon, and ribs (DGAC 2010). Saturated fatty acids can be replaced with foods containing monounsaturated and polyunsaturated fatty acids. Solid fats can be replaced with vegetable oils such as canola, olive, safflower, soybean, corn, or cottonseed oils. Synthetic *trans* fatty acids are found in partially hydrogenated oils used in some margarines, snack foods, and prepared desserts and should be avoided. Natural *trans* fatty acids are present in meat, milk, and milk products, and eliminating them is not recommended.

In summary, *1*) focus nutrition interventions on nutrition therapy strategies shown to improve metabolic outcomes—glycemia, lipids, blood pressure—and quality of life, prioritizing goals for each individual with diabetes; *2*) negotiate with individuals on lifestyle changes they are willing and able to make; and, perhaps the best advice, *3*) instruct patients on appropriate portion sizes of foods shown to have health benefits.

BIBLIOGRAPHY

Academy of Nutrition and Dietetics: Nutritive and nonnutritive sweeteners evidence analysis project, 2011. Available from http://www.adadevidencelibrary.com/topic.cfm?cat=4. Accessed 12 May 2011

Academy of Nutrition and Dietetics: Type 1 and type 2 diabetes evidence-based nutrition practice guidelines for adults, 2008. Available from http://www.adaevidencelibrary.com/topic.cfm?=3252. Accessed 12 May 2011

American Diabetes Association: Nutrition recommendations and interventions for diabetes (Position Statement). *Diabetes Care* 31 (Suppl. 1):S61–S78, 2008

American Diabetes Association: Standards of medical care in diabetes: 2012. *Diabetes Care* 35 (Suppl. 1):S11–S63, 2012

Ard JD, Grambow SC, Liu D, Slentz CA, Kraus WE, Svetkey LP; PREMIER Study: The effect of the PREMIER interventions on insulin sensitivity. *Diabetes Care* 27:340–347, 2004

Barnard ND, Cohen J, Jenkins DJA, Turner-McGrievy G, Gloede L, Jaster B, Seidl K, Green AA, Talpers S: A low-fat vegan diet improves glycemic control and cardiovascular risk factors in a randomized trial in individuals with type 2 diabetes. *Diabetes Care* 29:1777–1783, 2006

Bessesen DH: The role of carbohydrate in insulin resistance. *J Nutr* 131:2782S–2786S, 2001

Brand-Miller JC, Stockmann K, Atkinson F, Petocz P, Denyer G: Glycemic index, postprandial glycemia, and the shape of the curve in healthy subjects: analysis of a database of more than 1000 foods. *Am J Clin Nutr* 89:97–105, 2009

Brehm BJ, Lattin BL, Summer SS, Boback JA, Gilchrist GM, Jandacaek RJ, D'Alessio DA: One-year comparison of a high-monounsaturated fat diet with a high-carbohydrate diet in type 2 diabetes. *Diabetes Care* 32:215–220, 2009

Brinkworth GD, Noakes M, Keogh JB, Luscombe ND, Wittert GA, Clifton PM: Long-term effects of a high-protein, low-carbohydrate diet on weight control and cardiovascular risk markers in obese hyperinsulinemic subjects. *Int J Obes Relat Metab Disord* 28:661–670, 2004

Davis NJ, Tomuta N, Schechter C, Isasi CR, Segal-Isaacson CJ, Stein D, Zonszein J, Wylie-Rosett J: Comparative study of the effects of a 1-year dietary intervention of a low-carbohydrate diet versus a low-fat diet on weight and glycemic control in type 2 diabetes. *Diabetes Care* 32:1147–1152, 2009

De Natale C, Annuzzi G, Bozzetto L, Mazzarella R, Costabile G, Ciano O, Riccardi G, Rivellese AA: Effects of a plant-based high-carbohydrate/high-fiber diet versus high-monounsaturated fat/low-carbohydrate diet on postprandial lipids in type 2 diabetic patients. *Diabetes Care* 32:2168–2173, 2009

Delahanty LM, Nathan DM, Lachin JM, Hu FB, Cleary PA, Ziegler GA, Wylie-Rosett J, Wexler DJ, for the Diabetes Control and Complications Trial/Epidemiology of Diabetes: Association of diet with glycated hemoglobin during intensive treatment of type 1 diabetes in the Diabetes Control and Complications Trial. *Am J Clin Nutr* 89:518–524, 2009

Dietary Guidelines Advisory Committee (DGAC) Report on the Dietary Guidelines for Americans, 2010. Available at: http://www.cnpp.usda.gov/dgas2010-dgacreport.htm. Accessed 12 May 2011

Eeley EA, Stratton IM, Hadden DR, Turner RC, Holman RR: UKPDS 18: Estimated dietary intake in type 2 diabetic patients randomly allocated to diet, sulphonylurea or insulin therapy. UK Prospective Diabetes Study Group. *Diabet Med* 13:656–662, 1996

Esposito K, Maiorino MI, Ciotola M, Di Palo C, Scognamiglio P, Gicchino M, Petrizzo M, Saccomanno F, Beneduce F, Ceriello A, Giugliano D: Effects of a Mediterranean-style diet on the need for antihyperglycemic drug therapy in patients with newly diagnosed type 2 diabetes: a randomized trial. *Ann Intern Med* 151:306–314, 2009

Franz MJ: Protein and diabetes: much advice, little research. *Curr Diab Rep* 2:457–464, 2002

Franz MJ, Powers MA, Leontos C, Holzmeister LA, Kulkarni K, Monk A, Wedel N, Gradwell E: The evidence for medical nutrition therapy for type 1 and type 2 diabetes in adults. *J Am Diet Assoc* 110:1852–1889, 2010

Gannon MC, Hoover H, Nuttall FQ: Further decrease in glycated hemoglobin following ingestion of a LoBAG$_{30}$ diet for 10 weeks compared to 5 weeks in people with untreated type 2 diabetes. *Nutr Metab* 7:64, 2010

Gentilcore D, Chaikomin R, Jones KL: Effects of fat on gastric emptying of and the glycemic, insulin, and incretin responses to a carbohydrate meal in type 2 diabetes. *Am J Clin Nutr* 91:2062–2067, 2006

Hartweg J, Perera R, Montori V, Dinneen S, Neil HA, Farmer A: Omega-3 polyunsaturated fatty acids (PUFA) for type 2 diabetes mellitus. *Cochrane Database Syst Rev* CD003205, 2008

Hartweg J, Farmer AJ, Holman RR, Neil A: Potential impact of omega-3 treatment on cardiovascular disease in type 2 diabetes. *Curr Opin Lipidol* 20:30–38, 2009

He M, van Dam RM, Rimm E, Hu FB, Qi L: Whole-grain, cereal fiber, bran, and germ intake and the risks of all-cause and cardiovascular disease-specific mortality among women with type 2 diabetes mellitus. *Circulation* 121:2162–2168, 2010

Howard BV, Van Horn L, Hsia J, Manson JE, Stefanickk ML, Wassertheil-Smoller S: Low-fat dietary pattern and risk of cardiovascular disease: the Women's Health Initiative Randomized Controlled Dietary Modification Trial. *JAMA* 295:655–666, 2006

Institute of Medicine, Food and Nutrition Board: *Dietary Reference Intakes: Energy, Carbohydrates, Fiber, Fat, Fatty Acids, Cholesterol, Protein, and Amino Acids.* Washington, DC, National Academies Press, 2002

Johnson RI, Appel LJ, Brands M, Howard BV, Lefevre M, Lustig RH, Sacks F, Steffen LM, Wylie-Rosett J: Dietary sugars intake and cardiovascular health: a scientific statement from the American Heart Association. *Circulation* 120:1011–1020, 2011

Kirk JK, Graves DE, Craven TE, Lipkin EW, Austin M, Margolis KL: Restricted-carbohydrate diets in patients with type 2 diabetes: a meta-analysis. *J Am Diet Assoc* 108:91–100, 2008

Kodama S, Saito K, Tanaka S, Maki M, Yachi Y, Sato M, Sugawara A, Totsuka K, Shimano H, Ohashi Y, Yamada N, Sone H: Influence of fat and carbohydrate proportions on the metabolic profile in patients with type 2 diabetes: a meta-analysis. *Diabetes Care* 32:959–965, 2009

Lovejoy JC. The influence of dietary fat on insulin resistance. *Curr Diab Rep* 2:435–440, 2002

McClenaghan NH: Determining the relationship between dietary carbohydrate and insulin resistance. *Nutr Res Rev* 18:222–240, 2005

Nordmann AJ, Nordmann A, Briel M, Keller U, Yancy WS, Brehm BJ, Bucher HC: Effects of low-carbohydrate vs low-fat diets on weight loss and cardiovascular risk factors. *Arch Intern Med* 166:285–293, 2006

Papakonstantinou E, Triantafillidou D, Panagiotakos DB, Iraklianou S, Berdanier CD, Zampelas A: A high protein low fat meal does not influence glucose and insulin responses in obese individuals with or without type 2 diabetes. *J Hum Nutr Diet* 23:183–189, 2010a

Papakonstantinou E, Triantafilidou D, Panagioitakos DB, Koutsovasilis A, Saliaris M, Manolis A, Melidonis A, Zampelas A: A high-protein low-fat diet is more effective in improving blood pressure and triglycerides in calorie-restricted obese individuals with newly diagnosed type 2 diabetes. *Eur J Clin Nutr* 64:595–602, 2010b

Pearce KL, Clifton PM, Noakes M: Egg consumption as part of an energy-restricted high-protein diet improves blood lipid and blood glucose profiles in individuals with type 2 diabetes. *Br J Nutr* 105:584–592, 2011

Peters AL, Davidson MB: Protein and fat effects on glucose responses and insulin requirements in subjects with insulin-dependent diabetes mellitus. *Am J Clin Nutr* 58:555–560, 1993

Powers MA, Cuddihy RM, Wesley D, Morgan B: Continuous glucose monitoring reveals different glycemic responses of moderate- vs high-carbohydrate lunch meals in people with type 2 diabetes. *J Am Diet Assoc* 110:1912–1915, 2010

Rosenfalck AM, Almdal T, Biggers L, Madsbad S, Histed J: A low-fat diet improves peripheral insulin sensitivity in patients with type 1 diabetes. *Diabet Med* 23:384–392, 2006

Savage DB, Petersen KF, Shulman GI: Disordered lipid metabolism and the pathogenesis of insulin resistance. *Physiol Rev* 87:507–520, 2007

Stirban A, Nandrean S, Götting C, Tamler R, Pop A, Negrean M, Gawlowski T, Stratmann B, Tschoepe D: Effects of n-3 fatty acids on macro- and microvascular function in subjects with type 2 diabetes mellitus. *Am J Clin Nutr* 91:808–813, 2010

Strychar IS, Cohn JS, Renier G, Rivard M, Aris-Jilwan N, Beauregard H, Meltzer S, Belanger A, Dumas R, Ishac A, Radwan F, Yale J-F: Effects of a diet higher in carbohydrate/lower in fat versus lower in carbohydrate/higher in monounsaturated fat on postmeal triglyceride concentrations and other cardiovascular risk factors in type 1 diabetes. *Diabetes Care* 32:1597–1599, 2009

Thomsen C, Storm H, Holst JJ, Hermansen K: Differential effects of saturated and monounsaturated fats on postprandial lipemia and glucagon-like peptide 1 responses in patients with type 2 diabetes. *Am J Clin Nutr* 77:605–611, 2003

U.S. Department of Agriculture and U.S. Department of Health and Human Services: *Dietary Guidelines for Americans, 2010.* 7th ed. Washington, DC, U.S. Government Printing Office, 2010 (www.dietaryguidelines.gov)

Vitolins MZ, Anderson AM, Delahanty L, Raynor H, Miller GD, Mobley C, Reeves R, Yamamoto M, Champagne C, Wing RR, Mayer-Davis W, the Look AHEAD Research Group: Action for Health in Diabetes (Look AHEAD) Trial: baseline evaluation of selected nutrients and food group intake. *J Am Diet Assoc* 109:1367–1375, 2009

Wheeler ML, Dunbar SA, Jaacks LM, Karmally W, Mayer-Davis EJ, Wylie-Rosett J, Yancy WS: Macronutrients, food groups and eating patterns in the management of diabetes: a systematic review of the literature, 2010. *Diabetes Care* 35:434–445, 2012

Wolever TSM, Gibbs AL, Mehlin C, Chiasson J-L, Connelly PW, Jesse RG, Leiter LA, Maheux P, Rabasa-Lhoret R, Rodger NW, Ryan EA: The Canadian Trial of Carbohydrates in Diabetes (CCD), a 1-y controlled trial of low-glycemic index dietary carbohydrate in type 2 diabetes: no effect on glycated hemoglobin but reduction in C-reactive protein. *Am J Clin Nutr* 87:114–125, 2008

Xu J, Eilat-Adar S, Loria CM, Howard BV, Fabsitz RR, Begum M, Zephier EM, Lee ET: Macronutrient intake and glycemic control in population-based sample of American Indians with diabetes: The Strong Heart Study. *Am J Clin Nutr* 86:480–487, 2007

Marion J. Franz, MS, RD, CDE, is a Nutrition/Health Consultant at Nutrition Concepts by Franz, Inc., Minneapolis, MN.

Chapter 3
Micronutrients and Diabetes

Joshua J. Neumiller, PharmD, CDE, CGP, FASCP

Highlights

Requirements for Micronutrients: Dietary Reference Intakes

Requirements for Micronutrients in Diabetes

Micronutrient Effects on Glucose and Insulin Homeostasis

Definition and Regulation of Supplements

Summary

Highlights
Micronutrients and Diabetes

■ Dietary reference intakes (DRIs) are reference values that are quantitative estimates of nutrient intakes to be used for planning and assessing diets for healthy people. DRIs consist of four reference intakes: Recommended Dietary Allowance (RDA), Estimated Average Requirement (EAR), Adequate Intake (AI), and Tolerable Upper Intake Level (UL).

■ Many micronutrients are involved in carbohydrate and/or glucose metabolism as well as with insulin release and sensitivity. This information, however, is frequently extrapolated beyond what is supported by research findings, and clinical data for most micronutrients for the treatment of diabetes are inconclusive.

■ Supplements are defined as any product that is intended to supplement the diet. Dietary supplements contain one or more of the following: vitamin, mineral, herb or other botanical, or amino acid. Unlike drugs, supplements do not need to undergo efficacy or safety testing before being marketed.

■ Currently, there is insufficient evidence to support the routine use of supplements for the treatment of diabetes. There are, however, select groups of individuals who may benefit, such as people with poor glycemic control and/or people with a documented deficiency of a given micronutrient or vitamin. Compelling data from well-designed, long-term studies are needed before supplement products can be recommended for widespread use in people with diabetes.

Micronutrients and Diabetes

Micronutrients are vitamins and minerals that are required in small quantities for specific physiological functions. Micronutrients often function as coenzymes or cofactors essential for metabolic processes (glycolysis, lipid metabolism, amino acid metabolism, etc.) and are thus essential to sustaining life (Shils 2005). Vitamins and minerals have been studied in the prevention and treatment of both type 1 and type 2 diabetes, as well as for the treatment of diabetes complications (Mooradian 1994). "Natural" medicines, including micronutrients, are widely used by people with diabetes. Some surveys indicate that as many as 60% of people with diabetes use some form of alternative medicine (Yeh 2002). Accordingly, it is not uncommon for consumers with diabetes to ask a variety of questions about the utility of micronutrients and supplements in the management of their diabetes.

The objective of this chapter is to assist health care professionals in answering some of the questions posed by people with diabetes concerning micronutrients. This chapter, which focuses on micronutrients for the treatment of diabetes, begins with a summary of dietary intake requirements for micronutrients for people with diabetes from the book *American Diabetes Association Guide to Medical Nutrition Therapy of Diabetes* (Franz 1999). The chapter then reviews and updates currently available data for select micronutrients and antioxidants on carbohydrate/glucose metabolism and/or insulin activity and reviews the U.S. Food and Drug Administration (FDA) regulation processes for supplement products.

REQUIREMENTS FOR MICRONUTRIENTS: DIETARY REFERENCE INTAKES

Before addressing the role of vitamins and minerals in diabetes, it is helpful to review requirements for micronutrients and how they are determined. Vitamins and minerals are substances required in very small amounts to promote essential biochemical reactions in cells. Together, vitamins and minerals are called micronutrients. At low nutrient levels (deficiency), dependent biological functions are impaired. In contrast, high intakes can result in toxicity and decreased absorption of other micronutrients because of competitive inhibition.

Micronutrients are specific in their functions, and most cannot be made by the body or be replaced by chemically similar elements. They must come from food or supplements. Small amounts of micronutrients are needed for optimal performance, yet lack of a micronutrient for a prolonged period can result in disease seemingly disproportionate to the amount missing. For example, although only small amounts of vitamins are needed, lack of vitamin C results in scurvy, lack of adequate thiamin in beriberi, and lack of adequate niacin in pellagra.

Several factors make determining exact individual requirements for micronutrients difficult. First, metabolism and use of micronutrients are homeostatically regulated, making requirements and the effect of supplementation dependent on an individual's nutritional status. For example, if intake of a particular micronutrient is low, absorption may be increased, and when intake is adequate, excess nutrient may be excreted in the feces and in small amounts in the urine.

Assessment of micronutrient status is difficult. It is assumed that levels of micronutrients in body fluids (plasma) reflect tissue and intracellular status and, therefore, that decreased serum levels indicate suboptimal status. However, plasma levels generally do not reflect intracellular status. Correlations between plasma levels and tissue status, especially in marginal deficiencies, are not always apparent.

Furthermore, metabolism and use of nutrients in general is highly integrated with other nutrients, hormones, and physiological factors. With excessive (or deficient) intakes of a particular micronutrient, the balance of this highly orchestrated

---

Table 3.1 Terms for Nutrient Requirements

■ Adequate Intake (AI): An AI is provided instead of an RDA when sufficient scientific evidence is not available to calculate an EAR. The AI is a recommended daily intake level based on observed or experimentally determined approximations of nutrient intake by a group of healthy people that are assumed to be adequate (Yates 1998). The primary use of the AI is as a goal for the nutrient intake of individuals.

■ Daily Value (DV): This term is used for nutrient levels on food and supplement labels. DVs are derived from RDAs (or AIs) to represent both sexes and most age-groups.

■ Dietary Reference Intakes (DRIs): This is an umbrella term for a set of four reference values: EAR, RDA, AI, and UL.

■ Estimated Average Requirement (EAR): The process for setting the RDA depends on being able to set the EAR. The EAR is the amount of nutrient that is estimated to meet the nutrient requirements of half the healthy individuals in a life stage and gender group (Yates 1998). When selecting the EAR, reduction of disease risk is considered, along with many other health parameters. No RDA is proposed if it is determined that an EAR cannot be set. The EAR is used to assess adequacy of intakes of population groups.

■ Recommended Dietary Allowance (RDA): The RDA is the average daily dietary intake level of a nutrient that is sufficient to meet the nutrient requirement of nearly all (97–98%) healthy individuals in a particular life stage (life stage considers age and, when applicable, pregnancy or lactation) and gender group (Yates 1998). The RDA includes a generous safety factor related to a bell-shaped curve. The majority of the population actually requires only approximately two-thirds of the RDA. This is in contrast to energy requirements, which are based on average needs.

■ Tolerable Upper Intake Level (UL): The UL is the highest level of nutrient intake that is likely to pose no risks or adverse health effects to almost all individuals in the general population. As intake increases above the UL, the risk of adverse effects increases. The UL is not intended to be a recommended level of intake. There is no established benefit for healthy individuals if they consume nutrient intakes above the RDA or AI (Yates 1998). The UL applies to chronic daily use. It is useful because of the increased interest in availability of fortified foods and the increased use of dietary supplements.

Adapted from Yates 1998.

scheme is disrupted, which leads to a cascade of effects. For example, calcium use is affected by a high protein intake, phosphorus and vitamin D intakes, and parathyroid hormone. Changes in any of these factors may affect dietary calcium requirements.

Requirements for micronutrients have been historically based on the 10th edition of *Recommended Dietary Allowances* (RDAs) (Food and Nutrition Board 1989). However, the RDAs, published since 1941 by the Food and Nutrition Board of the Institute of Medicine, National Academy of Sciences, are being replaced by a new approach called Dietary Reference Intakes (DRIs) (Yates 1998). The DRIs are developed by the Food and Nutrition Board in partnership with Health Canada and Canadian scientists. DRIs are reference values that are quantitative estimates of nutrient intakes to be used for planning and assessing diets for healthy people. The standards are for apparently healthy people and are not meant to be applied to those with acute or chronic disease or for the replacement of nutrient levels in previously deficient individuals. For individuals with specific needs, adjustments in the values may need to be made. They consist of four reference intakes: RDA, Adequate Intake (AI), Tolerable Upper Intake Level (UL), and Estimated Average Requirement (EAR).

The four primary uses of the DRIs are for assessing intakes of individuals, assessing intakes of population groups, planning diets for individuals, and planning diets for groups. RDAs and AIs both may be used as goals for individual intakes, whereas EARs may be used to examine the possibility of inadequacy and ULs the possibility of overconsumption for individuals. EARs are also used as guides to limit individual intake and to set goals for the mean intake of groups or of a specific population, as well as for the assessment of inadequate intakes within a group. Table 3.1 summarizes the definitions for the various reference values.

REQUIREMENTS FOR MICRONUTRIENTS IN DIABETES

The literature on the micronutrient status of people with diabetes contains conflicting reports depending on the population studied and because of the uncertainties in methodologies (Mooradian 1994; Mooradian 1987). Adequately controlled studies that establish the role of trace elements in the pathogenesis of carbohydrate intolerance are not available. Although animal studies have suggested that deficiencies in many of the trace elements—including zinc, chromium, magnesium, copper, manganese, and vitamin B_6—may lead to glucose intolerance, evidence for their role in the pathogenesis of glucose intolerance in humans is not definitive.

Many of the studies are done in animals in the laboratory, where diets can be manipulated easily in comparison to the diet of free-living subjects. The result of animal studies should not be extrapolated to humans without studies being performed in humans to validate the findings.

One of the problems with human studies in individuals with diabetes is that trace-metal and water-soluble vitamin urinary losses are increased during uncontrolled hyperglycemia with glycosuria; therefore, the effect of the response to micronutrients may depend on the degree of glucose tolerance. Furthermore, in some studies, the initial glucose tolerance varies from normal to glucose intolerant to diabetes. Results from all of these subjects may be combined, which would minimize the effects of a micronutrient. Furthermore, often, the effect of micronutrients on insulin secretion is biphasic. Low concentrations of the vitamin may stimulate insulin secretion, and high concentrations may have an inhibitory effect.

In human studies, the amount of the micronutrient being studied in the diet eaten is often unknown. For example, studies have reported beneficial effects of chromium on glucose and/or lipid metabolism in subjects eating varied diets with unknown chromium contents. To further confuse the role of micronutrients and diabetes, serum or tissue content of certain elements—copper, manganese, iron, and selenium—can be higher in people with diabetes than in control subjects without diabetes. On the other hand, serum ascorbic acid (vitamin C), B vitamins, and vitamin D may be lower in individuals with diabetes, whereas vitamins A and E have been reported to be normal or increased.

Regardless of the research problems, many micronutrients are intimately involved in carbohydrate and/or glucose metabolism as well as in insulin release and sensitivity. Unfortunately, this information is frequently extrapolated beyond what the research supports. The American Diabetes Association (ADA) recommends that individualized meal planning include optimization of food choices to meet RDA and DRI intakes for all micronutrients (ADA 2012).

MICRONUTRIENT EFFECTS ON GLUCOSE AND INSULIN HOMEOSTASIS

The 1999 chapter of *American Diabetes Association Guide to Medical Nutrition Therapy for Diabetes* concluded that data available did not justify routine supplementation of vitamins and minerals for people with diabetes. However, it was concluded that there are select groups of people who may benefit, such as patients in poor glycemic control and patients deficient in water-soluble micronutrients. An update on chromium, magnesium, vitamin D, and antioxidant supplementation in the treatment of diabetes is provided below. Table 3.2 summarizes research related to carbohydrate and/or glucose metabolism and the known effects related to the treatment of diabetes for additional selected micronutrients.

Chromium

The biologically active complex of elemental chromium is the glucose tolerance factor, which is a complex composed of chromium bound to two molecules of nicotinic acid and single molecules of the amino acids glutamic acid, glycine, and cysteine. Food sources of chromium include canned foods, meats, fish, brown sugar, coffee, tea, some spices, whole-wheat bread, rye bread, and brewer's yeast. The glucose tolerance factor has a role in glucose homeostasis, with chromium deficiency in animals being associated with an increase in blood glucose, cholesterol, and triglycerides. Mechanistically, the glucose tolerance factor acts as a cofactor for insulin and may facilitate insulin–membrane receptor interaction. However, the glucose tolerance factor lowers plasma glucose only in the presence of insulin (fed state) and not in 24-h fasting animals (Truman 1977). Chromium supplements are available in several forms, with the most common forms being chromium picolinate, chromium nicotinate, chromium polynicotinate, and chromium chloride. The picolinate and nicotinate salts demonstrate better absorption

Table 3.2 Effects of Select Vitamins and Minerals on Carbohydrate and/or Glucose Metabolism or Insulin and the Effects of Supplementation on Diabetes

Nutrient (Reference)	Effect on Carbohydrate/ Glucose Metabolism or Insulin	Effect of Supplementation
Zinc (Zn): (Thurman 1997; Arquilla 1978; Kinlaw 1983; Niewoehner 1986; Hallbook 1972; Blostein-Fujii 1997; Walter 1991; Martin Mateo 1978; Lau 1984)	Insulin stored as inactive Zn crystals in β-cells	Zn deficiency may occur in people with uncontrolled diabetes because of increased Zn loss in the urine. Supplementation has not been shown to be beneficial, except for small studies in older adults, suggesting a benefit in healing skin ulcerations.
Copper (Cu): (Walter 1991; Martin Mateo 1978; Lau 1984; Failla 1983)	Cu plasma levels are elevated in patients with retinopathy, hypertension, or macrovascular disease. Levels are normal in people without complications.	Supplementation is not recommended because of elevated plasma levels seen in patients with complications.
Manganese (Mn): (Walter 1991; Everson 1968; Bond 1983)	No evidence of altered Mn states in patients with diabetes	Supplementation has not shown a glucose-lowering effect.
Vanadium: (Goldfine 1995; Cohen 1995; Halberstam 1996; Boden 1996)	Appears to affect insulin signaling and may lead to upregulation of the insulin receptor and subsequent intracellular signaling pathways	Increased insulin sensitivity, increased glycogen synthesis, and suppressed hepatic glucose output in some, but not all, studies in patients with type 2 diabetes
Niacin (nicotinic acid): (Garg 1990; Molnar 1964)	Niacin lowers total and very-low-density lipoprotein cholesterol, and glucose and elevates HDL cholesterol.	Niacin can lead to deterioration of glycemic control in patients with diabetes.
Nicotinamide: (Elliott 1996; Polo 1998; Pozzilli 1997; Visalli 1999; Pozzilli 1995; Pozzilli 1996; European Nicotinamide Diabetes Intervention Trial Group 2004)	In animal studies, nicotinamide prevented autoimmune diabetes, suggesting it may preserve residual β-cell function in newly diagnosed type 1 diabetes patients.	In relatives with confirmed islet cell antibody levels in 18 countries, nicotinamide vs. placebo for 5 years did not prevent the onset of type 1 diabetes.
Thiamin: (Rabbani 2009; Saito 1987)	Daily requirements depend on amount of carbohydrate consumed.	Preliminary clinical research suggests that high-dose thiamine (100 mg three times daily) decreases urinary albumin excretion in type 2 diabetes patients.

Table 3.2 Effects of Select Vitamins and Minerals on Carbohydrate and/or Glucose Metabolism or Insulin and the Effects of Supplementation on Diabetes *(continued)*

Nutrient (Reference)	Effect on Carbohydrate/ Glucose Metabolism or Insulin	Effect of Supplementation
Pyridoxine, Vitamin B$_6$: (Rao 1980; Solomon 1989; Kaplan 1981; Head 2006)	Deficiency in animals and humans has been associated with glucose intolerance and impaired secretion of insulin and glucagon. Poor glucose control may decrease levels of vitamin B$_6$.	Supplementation has no demonstrated benefits on glucose metabolism. Pyridoxine has been used to treat diabetic neuropathy, but evidence is conflicting. Mega-doses are associated with toxic effects, including neuropathy.

Adapted from Franz 1999.

and retention of chromium compared to inorganic salt forms such as chromium chloride (Lanca 2002; Kaats 1996).

As with many micronutrients, evidence is conflicting regarding the role of chromium in the treatment of diabetes. Chromium levels can be below normal in people with diabetes (Davies 1997; Morris 1985), and epidemiological studies have linked lower levels of chromium measured within toenails with an increased risk of diabetes and cardiovascular disease (Rajpathak 2004). In regard to the treatment of type 2 diabetes, several clinical studies have shown that supplementation with oral chromium picolinate improves insulin sensitivity, decreases fasting plasma glucose, and improves A1C (Anderson 1997; Lee 1994; Martin 2006; Rabinovitz 2004). Additional benefits include reductions in total cholesterol and triglyceride levels (Anderson 1997; Lee 1994) and weight reduction in type 2 diabetes patients being treated with a sulfonylurea (Martin 2006). Glycemic benefits have likewise been described with chromium supplementation in people with type 1 diabetes and corticosteroid-induced hyperglycemia (Fox 1998; Ravina 1999).

Despite the promising findings described above, other studies have not demonstrated benefits with chromium supplementation (Abraham 1992; Althius 2002; Kleefstra 2006; Uusitupa 1983; Wise 1978). Even in studies that have shown benefit, the extrapolation of study findings to all people with diabetes is questionable. It has been speculated that chromium supplementation may be primarily beneficial in individuals with poor nutritional status or low chromium levels as opposed to all people with diabetes. For example, one of the largest studies performed that demonstrated clinical benefit was performed in China, where poor nutritional status is more likely, potentially accounting for the clinical benefit observed (Anderson 1997; Kleefstra 2006). Of note, a systematic review on the effect of chromium supplementation on glucose metabolism and lipids concluded that larger effects were more commonly observed in poor-quality studies and that evidence is limited by poor study quality, and heterogeneity in methodology and results (Balk 2007). Table 3.3 provides a summary of select clinical chromium supplementation studies (including results of English language randomized controlled trials [RCTs] including ≥10 human subjects with diabetes in each study arm).

Confounding the interpretation of chromium supplementation studies is the lack of an accurate and reliable measurement of chromium status, thus making chromium deficiency and characterization of study populations based on chromium status difficult to demonstrate (Guerrero-Romero 2005). Whereas chromium supplementation is generally considered safe, it must also be considered that high doses of chromium have been associated with chromosomal damage, psychiatric disturbances, rhabdomyolysis, and renal and hepatic toxicity in some cases (Guerrero-Romero 2005). On the basis of currently available evidence and considerations of potential toxicity with long-term use, current opinion states that chromium supplements can be considered for short-term use in patients suspected of having a chromium deficiency, based on dietary history (Cefalu 2004). Because of inconclusive clinical evidence, however, the use of routine chromium supplementation in people with diabetes is controversial (Cefalu 2004). After reviewing the evidence, the ADA concluded that benefit from chromium supplementation in individuals with diabetes or obesity has not been clearly demonstrated and therefore cannot be recommended (ADA 2008).

Magnesium

Magnesium is a divalent cation that is intimately involved in numerous important biological reactions that take place within the body. Magnesium is a cofactor for over 300 metabolic reactions in the body, including protein synthesis, adenylate cyclase synthesis, cellular energy production and storage, preservation of cellular electrolyte composition, cell growth and reproduction, DNA and RNA synthesis, and stabilization of mitochondrial membranes (Volpe 2008). Magnesium is unevenly distributed in the body, with ~50–60% residing in the skeleton, nearly 50% present in muscle and soft tissues, and only ~1% present in the extracellular compartment, such as serum or interstitial body fluids. Serum magnesium measures only 0.3% of total body magnesium and does not provide a sensitive index of magnesium deficiency.

Low levels of magnesium have been associated with a variety of illnesses, including hypertension, cardiac arrhythmias, congestive heart failure, retinopathy, and insulin resistance (McNair 1978; Paolisso 1990; Resnick 1989; Shattock 1987; Whelton 1989; Yajnik 1984). Of note, magnesium has been shown to play a significant role in glucose and insulin metabolism (Barbagallo 2003; Paolisso 1997). Likewise, decreased magnesium intake has been correlated to an increased risk of type 2 diabetes and metabolic syndrome (Dong 2011; Guerrero-Romero 2002; He 2006; Murakami 2005). Poorly controlled diabetes has been shown to lead to enhanced osmotic diuresis and increased urinary loss of magnesium (de Leeuw 2004), and severe hyperglycemia can decrease tubular reabsorption of magnesium, resulting in lower magnesium levels due to increased excretion (Barbagallo 2003). Additional research indicates that physiological stressors (such as type 2 diabetes) may act to deplete magnesium within the body, which, in turn, may impair normal metabolism and exacerbate the disease state (Bohl 2002).

Research to date indicates that low magnesium blood levels may play a role in insulin resistance (He 2006; Song 2004). Insulin is known to be involved in the

Table 3.3 Select Clinical Evidence Available for Chromium Supplementation as a Treatment for Diabetes

	Population/ Duration of Study	Intervention (type of study)	Major Findings	Comments
Abraham 1992	n = 76 adults with established athero-sclerotic disease (25 with type 2 diabetes and 51 with cardio-vascular disease only)/7–16 months	Placebo vs. Cr chloride, 250 mg/day (RCT)	No effects on fasting blood glucose between groups; TG ($P < 0.02$) and VLDL ($P < 0.05$) ↓ and HDL ($P < 0.005$) ↑ in Cr group	
Lee 1994	n = 28 adults with type 2 diabetes treated with diet, oral therapies, and/or insu-lin/2 months	Placebo vs. Cr pico-linate 200 mg/day (randomized crossover study)	No effects on fasting plasma glucose, A1C, LDL, or HDL; TG levels ↓ with Cr ($P < 0.05$)	
Anderson 1997	n = 180 adults with type 2 diabetes treated with diet, oral therapies, and/or insu-lin/4 months	Placebo vs. Cr pico-linate 200 or 1,000 mg/day (RCT)	↓ in fasting blood glu-cose ($P < 0.05$) in the 1,000 mg/day group; A1C ↓ ($P < 0.05$) at 4 months in both Cr groups; 2-h oral glu-cose tolerance test ↓ ($P < 0.05$) in 1,000 mg/day Cr group	Baseline Cr status and dietary Cr intake unknown
Kleefstra 2006	n = 46 adults with type 2 diabetes treated with insulin/6 months	Placebo vs. Cr pico-linate 500 or 1,000 mg/day (RCT)	No effects on A1C between groups	Weak rela-tionship between an increasing serum Cr concentration and improve-ment of the lipid profile observed
Martin 2006	n = 37 adults with type 2 diabetes; sub-jects started on glipi-zide plus placebo for 3 months and then randomized to pla-cebo or Cr/6 months	Placebo plus glipi-zide vs. Cr picolinate 1,000 mg/day (RCT)	Insulin sensitivity improved with Cr treat-ment ($P < 0.05$)	Authors con-cluded that Cr treatment attenuated sulfonylurea-associated (i.e., glipizide) weight gain and visceral fat accumula-tion

Cr, chromium; RCT, randomized controlled trial; TG, triglyceride; VLDL, very-low-density lipoprotein.

shift of magnesium intracellularly. Likewise, intracellular magnesium is likely involved in the regulation of insulin activity on oxidative glucose metabolism. This result is evidenced by the finding that low intracellular magnesium leads to disorders in tyrosine kinase activity at the insulin receptor level, resulting in decreased insulin sensitivity and insulin-mediated glucose uptake (Barbagallo 2003).

So what role does magnesium supplementation have in the treatment of diabetes? Hypomagnesemia occurs in an estimated 25–38% of people with type 2 diabetes and is more common in individuals with poorly controlled diabetes (de Lordes Lima 1998). Evidence from clinical studies evaluating magnesium supplementation in people with type 2 diabetes or insulin resistance has been conflicting. Some clinical studies suggest that magnesium supplementation is effective in decreasing fasting blood glucose levels and improving measures of insulin sensitivity (Rodriguez-Moran 2003; Yokota 2004; Paolisso 1992; Guerrero-Romero 2004). In contrast, other studies have reported no effect of magnesium supplementation on insulin or glucose levels (de Lordes Lima 1998; de Valk 1998; Eibl 1995; Gullestad 1994; Paolisso 1994). The discrepancies in data could be due to a variety of factors, including differences in magnesium salts or doses used, differences in magnesium status in study participants at baseline, or differences in study methodologies used. Please see a summary of select clinical studies (including results of English language RCTs including ≥10 human subjects with diabetes in each study arm) in Table 3.4.

Vitamin D

Epidemiological research indicates that people with low vitamin D levels have a significantly higher risk of type 2 diabetes than individuals with higher levels (Martins 2007; Pittas 2007). Animal studies have shown that vitamin D deficiency inhibits pancreatic insulin secretion (Nyomba 1986), and the pancreatic β-cell expresses vitamin D receptors (Bland 2004). In turn, vitamin D has been posited as a potential therapeutic agent in both the prevention and treatment of type 1 and type 2 diabetes (Mathieu 2005).

Vitamin D deficiency has been associated with higher risks for metabolic syndrome and type 2 diabetes (Chiu 2004; Scragg 2008; Scragg 2004), and current evidence indicates that vitamin D treatment improves glucose tolerance and insulin resistance (Parekh 2010; von Hurst 2010). Of note, the National Health and Nutrition Examination Survey showed an inverse relationship between serum 25-hydroxyvitamin D and the incidence of type 2 diabetes and insulin resistance (Ford 2005; Scragg 2004).

Ultimately, current evidence does not definitively show that daily vitamin D supplementation is effective in the treatment or prevention of type 1 or type 2 diabetes (Mitri 2011; Pittas 2007; Takiishi 2010). A review of vitamin D and type 2 diabetes included eight observational cohort studies and 11 RCTs. In three small underpowered trials ($n = 32$–62) in individuals with type 2 diabetes, there was no effect of vitamin D supplementation on glycemic outcomes (Mitri 2011). Although preclinical data and observational studies are suggestive of a benefit of vitamin D supplementation in people with diabetes, large prospective, randomized, placebo-controlled trials that measure blood 25-hydroxyvitamin D concentration and clinically relevant glycemic outcomes are needed. Indeed, a great deal of research

Table 3.4 Select Clinical Evidence Available for Magnesium Supplementation as a Treatment for Diabetes

	Population/ Duration of Study	Intervention (type of study)	Major Findings	Comments
Gullestad 1994	*n* = 56 adults with type 2 diabetes treated with diet, oral agents, and/or insulin/16 weeks	Placebo vs. Mg lactate-citrate 15 mmol/day (RCT)	No effects on glucose or insulin levels between groups	
Eibl 1995	*n* = 40 adults with type 2 diabetes treated with diet and oral agents/12 weeks	Placebo vs. Mg citrate 384 g/day (RCT)	No effects on glucose or insulin levels between groups	
de Lordes Lima 1998	*n* = 128 adults with type 2 diabetes treated with diet and/or oral agents/4 weeks	Placebo vs. Mg oxide 41.4 mmol/day (RCT)	No effects on glucose levels between groups	Authors concluded that longer-term studies with Mg at higher-than-usual doses needed to establish routine administration in type 2 diabetes
de Valk 1998	*n* = 50 adults with type 2 diabetes treated with oral agents and insulin use/12 weeks	Placebo vs. Mg aspartate 15 mmol/day (RCT)	No effects on glucose or insulin levels between groups; lipid levels also unchanged with Mg treatment	
Rodriguez-Morán 2003	*n* = 63 adults with type 2 diabetes treated with diet, exercise, and oral agents/16 weeks	Placebo vs. Mg chloride 2.5 g/day (RCT)	Mg treatment resulted in ↓ HOMA-IR index (P = 0.005), fasting plasma glucose (P = 0.01), and A1C (P = 0.04) vs. placebo	

HOMA-IR, homeostasis model of assessment–insulin resistance; Mg, magnesium; RCT, randomized controlled trial.

is currently underway concerning the role of vitamin D in the treatment and prevention of diabetes; however, at the time of this publication, results from large, prospective, randomized trials were not available. The use of vitamin D in deficient individuals is well founded, particularly in regard to bone health. The Institute of Medicine (IOM) concluded in its 2010 report (IOM 2010) that the evidence for a benefit of vitamin D in bone health is compelling, but that for other conditions such as cancer and cardiovascular disease, the evidence is inconclusive and insufficient to drive specific nutritional requirements for vitamin D intake. Table 3.5 provides a summary of DRI recommendations for vitamin D supplementation per the 2010 IOM recommendations (IOM 2010). For a more detailed discussion of vitamin D supplementation for the treatment and prevention of diabetes, please refer to the reviews by Takiishi and Mitri and colleagues (Mitri 2011; Takiishi 2010).

Antioxidants

The 1999 chapter concluded that while there is no justification for the routine supplementation of vitamins and minerals for people with diabetes, antioxidant supplements, such as vitamin E, may be proven to play a role in preventing oxidative damage to tissues and may be recommended for use in the future. Oxidative stress has been implicated in contributing to the pathogenesis of a variety of conditions including coronary artery disease, cancer, and the onset and progression of diabetes and its complications (Sheikh-Ali 2011). Oxidative stress results from free radical production. Free radicals are toxic compounds generated in the process of normal metabolism that contain one or more unpaired electrons. Unpaired electrons have a strong affinity for electrons from other molecules. Because of their reactive nature, free radicals can initiate a chain of oxidative events leading to toxic cellular damage. Antioxidants are compounds that are able to neutralize free radicals. In people with diabetes, depletion of cellular antioxidant defense systems occurs, and the disease is associated with an increase in the production of free radicals. Glucose has been shown to promote oxidative stress in endothelial cell cultures, where elevated ambient dextrose concentrations increased superoxide production (Horani 2004), with elevated plasma glucose levels correlating with superoxide production and increased oxidation of LDLs (Ceriello 2003). For a detailed discussion of the role of oxidative stress in diabetes, refer to the review by Sheikh-Ali and colleagues (Sheikh-Ali 2011).

While a variety of antioxidants are used by people with diabetes, some of the most common products used include vitamin E, vitamin C, and β-carotene. Table 3.6 summarizes research related to carbohydrate and/or glucose metabolism and/or inflammation and the known effects related to the treatment of diabetes for selected antioxidants. Interestingly, while there exists a great deal of empiric evidence that supplementation with antioxidant vitamins is beneficial in people with

---

Table 3.5 Current DRIs for Vitamin D

Infants	0–6 months: 7–12 months:	AI: 400 IU (10 mg/day) AI: 400 IU (10 mg/day)
Children	1–3 years: 4–8 years:	600 IU (15 mg/day) 600 IU (15 mg/day)
Older Children and Adults	9–70 years: Adults >70 years:	600 IU (15 mg/day) 800 IU (20 mg/day)
Pregnancy and lactation		600 IU (15 mg/day)

Adapted from Institute of Medicine Food and Nutrition Board 2010.

diabetes, intervention trials with antioxidants in this population have thus far failed to demonstrate clinical benefit. The Physician's Health Study II, for example, showed that 400 IU vitamin E every other day and 500 mg vitamin C daily conveyed no benefit in regard to decreasing the incidence of major cardiovascular events, with vitamin E actually being associated with an increased risk of hemorrhagic stroke (Stampfer 1993). In another trial, vitamin E dosed at 600 mg every other day did not protect a cohort of healthy women from myocardial infarction, stroke, or cancer (Yochum 2000). Interestingly, a meta-analysis of 68 randomized trials concluded that treatment with vitamin A, vitamin E, and β-carotene may actually place people at an increased risk of mortality (Qiao 1999).

Another popular antioxidant supplement used by people with diabetes is α-lipoic acid. Doses of 600–1,800 mg of oral and 500–1,000 mg of intravenous α-lipoic acid have been shown to improve insulin resistance and glucose effectiveness after 4 weeks and 1–10 days of administration, respectively (Jacob 1996; Jacob 1999; Konrad 1999). Endogenous α-lipoic acid acts as a coenzyme involved in carbohydrate metabolism (Beitner 2003). Perhaps most notably, α-lipoic acid at doses ranging from 600 to 1,200 mg/day appears to improve the symptoms of peripheral neuropathy such as numbness, burning, and pain in the extremities (Ziegler 1999; Reljanovic 1999; Ziegler 1995; Ruhnau 1999; Ametov 2003; Ziegler 2004). Experimental models suggest that α-lipoic acid increases neuronal glucose uptake and blood flow, improves neuronal conduction velocity, and increases the amount of reduced glutathione available within neurons (Kishi 1999; Nagamatsu 1995).

Overall, the contrast between strong experimental evidence of the increased oxidative load in diabetes and its contribution to the pathogenesis of the disease and the lack of clinical benefit shown in clinical trials to date is curious. This "antioxidant paradox," as coined by Sheikh-Ali and colleagues (Sheikh-Ali 2011), is certainly unexpected and cannot be presently explained. Routine supplementation with antioxidants, such as vitamins E and C and carotene, is not advised by the ADA because of lack of evidence of efficacy and concern related to long-term safety (ADA 2012).

DEFINITION AND REGULATION OF SUPPLEMENTS

The FDA defines a dietary supplement as any product (other than tobacco) that is intended to supplement the diet. Dietary supplements contain one or more of the following: vitamin, mineral, herb or other botanical, amino acid, or other dietary substance (which could include phytochemicals, concentrates, metabolites, extracts, or combinations of any of the above) (Dietary Supplement Health and Education Act [DSHEA] 1994). Medical foods are exempt from this definition and are defined as foods used under medical supervision and intended for the specific dietary management of a disease or condition for which distinctive nutritional requirements, based on recognized scientific principles, are established by medical evaluation. Examples are enteral and parental products (DSHEA 1994).

Dietary supplements, although often sold as foods, are used more like drugs. However, unlike drugs, they do not have to be proven effective before being marketed. A drug is formally defined as a substance used as (or in the preparation of) a medication, and the FDA has clear premarket jurisdiction over these substances.

Table 3.6 Effects of Select Antioxidants on Carbohydrate and/or Glucose Metabolism or Insulin and the Effects of Supplementation on Diabetes

Antioxidant (Reference)	Effect on Carbohydrate/ Glucose Metabolism, Insulin, and/or Inflammation	Effect of Supplementation
α-Lipoic acid: (Konrad 1999; Jacob 1996; Jacob 1999; Beitner 2003; Ziegler 1999; Reljanovic 1999; Ziegler 1995; Ruhnau 1999; Ametov 2003; Ziegler 2004; Ziegler 2011)	Coenzyme involved in carbohydrate metabolism; may also suppress vascular inflammation	4-Year treatment with α-lipoic acid (600 mg) vs. placebo showed no significant difference between treatment groups but resulted in improvements of neuropathic sensory symptoms.
β-Carotene: (Montonen 2004; Omenn 1998; Erlinger 2001; Kris-Etherton 2004)	Suggested that β-carotene possesses antioxidant activity that prevents lipid peroxidation, with serum levels inversely related to C-reactive protein levels and white blood cell count	American Heart Association (AHA): the evidence does not justify use of antioxidants for reducing the risk of cardiovascular disease; increased intake does not decrease the risk of developing type 2 diabetes.
Vitamin C: (Montonen 2004; Simon 2000; Kris-Etherton 2004)	Vitamin C is involved in a variety of metabolic processes including oxidation-reduction reactions and carbohydrate metabolism and is used as an antioxidant and for maintaining immune function.	AHA: the evidence does not justify use of antioxidants for reducing the risk of cardiovascular disease; increased intake does not decrease the risk of developing type 2 diabetes.
Vitamin E: (Jiang 2001; Lonn 2002; Kris-Etherton 2004)	Major function is believed to be due to prevention of free radical formation, with therapeutic uses primarily attributed to antioxidant effects.	Supplementation not shown to be cardioprotective or beneficial in treatment of cardiovascular disease in patients with diabetes; dose greater than RDA may be harmful.

Supplements are designed to cure deficiencies, but do not further improve normal status unless proven to be useful as therapeutic agents. If they are to be used as therapeutic agents, their efficacy should be proven by the same standards required for drugs.

Although the FDA is responsible for ensuring that supplements are safe for human consumption, the FDA cannot intervene until damage or harm is documented. Under the Nutrition Labeling and Education Act of 1990, it was proposed that supplements should be required to meet the same requirements as conventional foods to qualify for a health claim and that they should follow the same labeling requirements. However, a Dietary Supplement Act, Title II of Prescription Drug User Free Act of 1992, prohibited the FDA from taking action against supplements for unauthorized health claims until December 1993 (FDA 1993a; FDA 1993b). Finally, in October 1994, Congress passed the Dietary Supplement Health and Education Act (DSHEA 1994), a compromise between the supplement industry and the original intent of the Nutrition Labeling and Education Act of 1990.

There are several key provisions of DSHEA. This act allows supplements to bypass the premarket FDA regulations for drugs or food additives. Supplement manufacturers or companies that sell supplements do not have to prove their products are effective or safe before they go to market. Instead, the burden of proof for an unsafe supplement is placed on the FDA. The FDA can intervene only after an illness or injury occurs. After complaints are received, the FDA is required to prove that the supplement causes harm when taken "as directed" on the label before a product can be restricted. Herbal remedies also may be sold without any knowledge of their mechanism of action (Angell 1998).

Supplements must have the same type of nutritional labeling found on foods, and they cannot carry claims that mention a specific disease unless the claims are backed by scientific evidence. Labels on vitamins, minerals, herbs, amino acids, and other supplements are allowed to make claims about maintaining a healthy body. To protect consumers, the law requires that supplement packages let shoppers know that these types of claims "have not been evaluated by the Food and Drug Administration" and are "not intended to diagnose, cure, or prevent any disease." The law also prohibits point-of-sale information, such as an article or book chapter supporting a dietary supplement claim, without prior FDA review.

Finally, the standards used to prepare and package supplements are left up to the company. Therefore, the product's purity or the amount of the active ingredients in a supplement cannot be certain, even from one package to the next of the same product. DSHEA included the recommendation that good manufacturing practices be used in the development of supplements; however, this protocol is not enforced by the FDA. Good manufacturing practices include a host of activities that are important for manufacturing a product that is free of defects and can include the following: quality assurance surrounding the use of raw materials, strict recordkeeping guidelines, high standards for cleanliness and safety, employment of qualified personnel, in-house testing and production and process controls, and guidelines regarding storage and distribution of products. Patients would be well advised to seek supplements manufactured by reputable companies that follow good manufacturing practices. People should be counseled to purchase products that have been independently evaluated and contain the United States Pharmacopeial Convention (USP), ConsumerLab (CL), or Natural Products Association seal of approval.

SUMMARY

Until reliable studies document the therapeutic benefit of pharmacological dosages of vitamins and minerals, the prudent approach is to supplement with micronutrients only when a specific deficiency status is documented (Chehade 2009). Patients should be educated about the toxicity of mega-doses of micronutrients and be counseled regarding acquiring daily vitamin and mineral requirements by means of a balanced, healthful eating pattern.

People with poorly controlled diabetes are susceptible to several micronutrient deficiencies (Franz 2002). The first step in identifying a deficiency is an evaluation of the nutritional state, including the individual's food and eating habits, food preferences, and overall health status. Healthy adults can receive all the necessary nutrients from foods, but certain high-risk groups, such as growing and developing children and youths, women during pregnancy and lactation, individuals eating <1,200 kcal/day, elderly individuals (especially people with low socioeconomic status), patients in intensive care units or long-term nursing facilities, and total vegetarians, may benefit from an appropriate vitamin-mineral supplement.

On the basis of current evidence, there is presently no justification for routine supplementation of vitamins and minerals for people with diabetes (Chehade 2009). However, there are select groups of people who may benefit, such as patients with diabetes in poor glycemic control, who are more likely to have deficiencies in magnesium, zinc, vitamin D, and water-soluble vitamins. While vitamin and mineral supplements should not be substituted for a healthful eating pattern, there is likely no harm in taking a multivitamin supplement with dose levels no higher than 100% of the RDA. Doses above that do not convey extra protection, but they do increase the risk of toxic side effects. Furthermore, it is likely that the response to supplements is determined by nutritional state, so people with micronutrient deficiencies will likely respond favorably.

Micronutrients are intimately involved in the metabolism of carbohydrates and other nutrients and with the body's use of glucose and insulin. However, without well-designed clinical trials to prove efficacy, the benefit of pharmacological doses of supplements is unknown, and findings from small clinical and animal studies is frequently extrapolated to clinical practice. Presently, there is no evidence of benefit from vitamin or mineral supplementation in people with diabetes without underlying evidence of a deficiency.

BIBLIOGRAPHY

Abraham AS, Brooks BA, Eylath U: The effects of chromium supplementation on serum glucose and lipids in patients with and without non-insulin dependent diabetes. *Metabolism* 41:768–771, 1992

Althius MD, Jordon NE, Ludington EA, Wittes JT: Glucose and insulin responses to dietary chromium supplements: a meta-analysis. *Am J Clin Nutr* 76:148–155, 2002

American Diabetes Association: Nutrition recommendations and interventions for diabetes (Position Statement). *Diabetes Care* 31 (Suppl. 1):S61–S78, 2008

American Diabetes Association: Standards of medical care in diabetes: 2012. *Diabetes Care* 35 (Suppl. 1):S11–S63, 2012

Ametov AS, Barinov A, Dyck PJ, Hermann R, Kozlova N, Litchy WJ, Low PA, Nehrdich D, Novosadova M, O'Brien PC, Reljanovic M, Samiqullin R, Schuette K, Strokov I, Tritschler HJ, Wessel K, Yakhno N, Ziegler D; SYDNEY Trial Study Group: The sensory symptoms of diabetic polyneuropathy are improved with alpha-lipoic acid: the SYDNEY trial. *Diabetes Care* 26:770–776, 2003

Anderson RA, Cheng N, Bryden NA, Polansky MM, Cheng N, Chi J, Feng J: Elevated intakes of supplemental chromium improve glucose and insulin variables in individuals with type 2 diabetes. *Diabetes* 46:1786–1791, 1997

Angell M, Kassirer JP: Alternative medicine-the risks of untested and unregulated remedies. *N Engl J Med* 339:839–841, 1998

Arquilla ER, Packer S, Tarmas W, Miyamoto S: The effect of zinc on insulin metabolism. *Endocrinology* 103:1440–1449, 1978

Balk EM, Tatsioni A, Lichtensetin AH, Lau J, Pittas AG: Effect of chromium supplementation on glucose metabolism and lipids. *Diabetes Care* 30:2154–2163, 2007

Barbagallo M, Dominguez LJ, Galioto A, Ferlisi A, Cani C, Malfa L, Pineo A, Busardo A, Paolisso G: Role of magnesium in insulin action, diabetes and cardio-metabolic syndrome X. *Mol Aspects Med* 24:39–52, 2003

Beitner H: Randomized, placebo controlled, double-blind study on the clinical efficacy of a cream containing 5% alpha-lipoic acid related to photoaging of facial skin. *Br J Dermatol* 149:841–849, 2003

Bland R, Markovic D, Hills CE, Hughes SV: Expression of 25-hydroxyvitamin D3-1 alpha-hydroxylase in pancreatic islets. *J Steroid Biochem Mol Biol* 121:89–90, 2004

Blostein-Fujii A, DiSilvestro RA, Frid D, Katz C, Malarkey W: Short-term zinc supplementation in women with non-insulin dependent diabetes mellitus: effects on plasma 5'-nucleotidase activities, insulin-like growth factor I concentrations, and lipoprotein oxidation rates in vitro. *Am J Clin Nutr* 66:639–642, 1997

Boden G, Chen X, Ruiz J, van Rossum GD, Turco S: Effects of vanadyl sulfate on carbohydrate and lipid metabolism in patients with non-insulin dependent diabetes mellitus. *Metabolism* 45:1130–1135, 1996

Bohl CH, Volpe SL: Magnesium and exercise. *Crit Rev Food Sci Nutr* 42:533–563, 2002

Bond JS, Failla ML, Unger DF: Elevated manganese concentration and arginase activity in livers of streptozotocin-induced diabetic rats. *J Biol Chem* 258:8004–8009, 1983

Cefalu WT, Hu FB: Role of chromium in human health and in diabetes. *Diabetes Care* 27:2741–2751, 2004

Ceriello A: The possible role of postprandial hyperglycaemia in the pathogenesis of diabetic complications. *Diabetologia* 46 (Suppl. 1):M9–M16, 2003

Chehade JM, Sheikh-Ali M, Mooradian AD: The role of micronutrients in managing diabetes. *Diabetes Spectrum* 22:214–218, 2009

Chiu KC, Chu A, Go VL, Saad MF: Hypovitaminosis D is associated with insulin resistance and beta cell dysfunction. *Am J Clin Nutr* 79:820–825, 2004

Cohen N, Halberstam M, Schilmovich P, Chang CJ, Shamoon H, Rosetti L: Oral vanadyl sulfate improves hepatic and peripheral insulin sensitivity in patients with non-insulin dependent diabetes mellitus. *J Clin Invest* 95:2501–2509, 1995

Davies S, Howard JM, Hunnisett A, Howard M: Age-related decreases in chromium levels in 51,665 hair, sweat, and serum samples from 40,872 patients: implications for the prevention of cardiovascular disease and type II diabetes mellitus. *Metabolism* 46:469–473, 1997

de Leeuw I, Engelen W, De Block C, Van Gaal L: Long term magnesium supplementation influences favourably the natural evolution of neuropathy in Mg-depleted type 1 diabetic patients (T1DM). *Magnes Res* 17:109–114, 2004

de Lordes Lima M, Cruz T, Pousada JC, Rodrigues LE, Barbosa K, Cangucu V: The effect of magnesium supplementation in increasing doses on the control of type 2 diabetes. *Diabetes Care* 21:682–686, 1998

de Valk HW, Verkaaik R, Van Rijn HJ, Geerdink RA, Struyvenberg A: Oral magnesium supplementation in insulin-requiring type 2 diabetic patients. *Diabet Med* 15:503–507, 1998

Dietary Supplement Health and Education Act of 1994 (DSHEA). Public Law 103-417

Dong J-Y, Xun P, He K, Qin L-Q: Magnesium intake and risk of type 2 diabetes: meta-analysis of prospective cohort studies. *Diabetes Care* 34:2116–2122, 2011

Eibl NL, Kopp HP, Nowak HR, Schnack CJ, Hopmeier PG, Schernthaner G: Hypomagnesemia in type II diabetes: effect of a 3-month replacement therapy. *Diabetes Care* 18:188–192, 1995

Elliott RB, Pilcher CC, Fergusson DM, Stewart AW: A population based strategy to prevent insulin-dependent diabetes using nicotinamide. *J Pediatr Endocrinol Metab* 9:501–509, 1996

Erlinger TP, Guallar E, Miller ER, Stolzenberg-Solomon R, Appel LJ: Relationship between systemic markers of inflammation and serum beta-carotene levels. *Arch Intern Med* 161:1903–1908, 2001

European Nicotinamide Diabetes Intervention Trial Group: European Nicotinamide Diabetes Intervention Trial (ENDIT): a randomized controlled trial of intervention before the onset of diabetes. *Lancet* 363:925–931, 2004

Everson GJ, Shrader RE: Abnormal glucose tolerance in manganese deficient guinea pigs. *J Nutr* 94:89–94, 1968

Failla ML, Kiser RA: Hepatic and renal metabolism of copper and zinc in the diabetic rat. *Am J Physiol* 244:E115–E121, 1983

Food and Drug Administration: Food labeling: mandatory status of nutrition labeling and nutrient content, revision, format for nutrition label. *Federal Register* 58:2151, 1993a

Food and Drug Administration: Regulation of dietary supplements. *Federal Register* 58:33692, 1993b

Food and Nutrition Board, Institute of Medicine, National Academy of Sciences: *Recommended Dietary Allowances.* 10th ed. Washington, DC, National Academies Press, 1989

Ford ES, Ajani UA, McGuire LC, Liu S: Concentrations of serum vitamin D and the metabolic syndrome among U.S. adults. *Diabetes Care* 28:1228–1230, 2005

Fox GN, Sabovic Z: Chromium picolinate supplementation for diabetes mellitus. *J Fam Pract* 46:83–86, 1998

Franz MJ: 2002 Diabetes nutrition recommendations: grading the evidence. *Diabetes Educ* 28:756–766, 2002

Franz MJ: Micronutrients and diabetes. In *American Diabetes Association Guide to Medical Nutrition Therapy for Diabetes.* Franz MJ, Bantle JP, Eds. Alexandria, VA, American Diabetes Association, 1999, p. 165–191

Garg A, Grundy SM: Nicotinic acid as therapy for dyslipidemia in noninsulin-dependent diabetes. *JAMA* 264:723–726, 1990

Goldfine A, Simonson D, Folli F, Patti ME, Kahn R: Metabolic effects of sodium metavanadate in humans with insulin-dependent and non-insulin dependent diabetes mellitus in vivo and in vitro studies. *J Clin Endocrinol Metab* 80:3311–3320, 1995

Guerrero-Romero F, Rodriquez-Moran M: Complementary therapies for diabetes: the case for chromium, magnesium, and antioxidants. *Arch Med Res* 36:250–257, 2005

Guerrero-Romero F, Rodriguez-Moran M: Low serum magnesium levels and metabolic syndrome. *Acta Diabetol* 39:209–213, 2002

Guerrero-Romero F, Tamez-Perez HE, Gonzalez-Gonzalez G, Salinas-Martinez AM, Montes-Villarreal J, Trevino-Ortiz JH, Rodriguez-Moran M: Oral magnesium supplementation improves insulin sensitivity in non-diabetic subjects with insulin resistance: a double-blind placebo-controlled randomized trial. *Diabetes Metab* 30:253–258, 2004

Gullestad L, Jacobsen T, Dolva LO: Effect of magnesium treatment on glycemic control and metabolic parameters in NIDDM patients. *Diabetes Care* 17:460–461, 1994

Halberstam M, Cohen N, Shlimovich P, Rossetti L, Shamoon H: Oral vanadyl sulfate improves insulin sensitivity in NIDDM but not obese nondiabetic subjects. *Diabetes* 45:659–666, 1996

Hallbook T, Lanner E: Serum-zinc and healing of venous leg ulcers. *Lancet* 2:780–782, 1972

He K, Liu K, Daviglus ML, Morris SJ, Loria CM, Van Horn L, Jacobs DR, Savage PJ: Magnesium intake and incidence of metabolic syndrome among young adults. *Circulation* 113:1675–1682, 2006

Head KA: Peripheral neuropathy: pathogenic mechanisms and alternative therapies. *Altern Med Rev* 11:294–329, 2006

Horani MH, Haas MJ, Mooradian AD: Rapid adaptive down regulation of oxidative burst induced by high dextrose in human umbilical vein endothelial cells. *Diabetes Res Clin Pract* 66:7–12, 2004

Institute of Medicine Food and Nutrition Board: *Dietary Reference Intakes for Calcium, Phosphorous, Magnesium, Vitamin D, and Fluoride.* Washington, DC, National Academies Press, 2010

Jacob S, Henriksen EJ, Tritschler HJ, Augustin HJ, Dietze GJ: Improvement of insulin-stimulated glucose-disposal in type 2 diabetes after repeated parenteral administration of thioctic acid. *Exp Clin Endocrinol Diabetes* 104:284–288, 1996

Jacob S, Ruus P, Hermann R, Tritschler HJ, Maerker E, Renn W, Augustin HJ, Dietze GJ, Rett K: Oral administration of RAC-alpha-lipoic acid modulates insulin sensitivity in patients with type-2 diabetes mellitus: a placebo-controlled pilot trial. *Free Radic Biol Med* 27:309–314, 1999

Jiang Q, Christen S, Shigenaga MK, Ames BN: Gamma-tocopherol, the major form of vitamin E in the US diet, deserves more attention. *Am J Clin Nutr* 74:714–722, 2001

Kaats GR, Blum K, Fisher JA, Adelman JA: Effects of chromium picolinate supplementation on body composition: a randomized, double-masked, placebo-controlled study. *Cur Ther Res* 57:747–756, 1996

Kaplan WE, Abourizk NN: Diabetic peripheral neuropathies affecting the lower extremity. *J Am Podiatry Assoc* 71:356–362, 1981

Kinlaw WB, Levine AS, Morley HE, Silvis SE, McClain CJ: Abnormal zinc metabolism in type II diabetes mellitus. *Am J Med* 75:273–277, 1983

Kishi Y, Schmelzer JD, Yao JK, Zollman PJ, Nickander KK, Tritschler HJ, Low PA: Alpha-lipoic acid: effect on glucose uptake, sorbitol pathway, and energy metabolism in experimental diabetic neuropathy. *Diabetes* 48:2045–2051, 1999

Kleefstra N, Houweling ST, Jansman FG, Groenier KH, Gans RO, Meyboom-de Jong B, Bakker SJ, Bilo HJ: Chromium treatment has no effect in patients with poorly controlled, insulin-treated type 2 diabetes in an obese Western population: a randomized, double-blind, placebo-controlled trial. *Diabetes Care* 29:521–525, 2006

Konrad T, Vicini P, Kusterer K, Hoflich A, Assadkhani A, Bohles HJ, Sewell A, Tritschler HJ, Cobelli C, Usadel KH: Alpha-lipoic acid treatment decreases serum lactate and pyruvate concentrations and improves glucose effectiveness in lean and obese patients with type 2 diabetes. *Diabetes Care* 22:280–287, 1999

Kris-Etherton PM, Lichtenstein AH, Howard BV, Steinberg D, Witztum JL: AHA Science Advisory: Antioxidant vitamin supplements and cardiovascular disease. *Circulation* 110:637–641, 2004

Lanca S, Alves A, Vieira AL, Barata J, de Freitas J, de Carvalho A: Chromium-induced toxic hepatitis. 13:518–520, 2002

Lau AL, Failla ML: Urinary excretion of zinc, copper and iron in the streptozoto-cin-diabetic rat. *J Nutr* 114:224–233, 1984

Lee NA, Reasner CA: Beneficial effect of chromium supplementation on serum triglyceride levels in NIDDM. *Diabetes Care* 17:1449–1452, 1994

Lonn E, Yusuf S, Hoogwerf B, Pogue J, Yi Q, Zinman B, Bosch J, Dagenais G, Mann JFE, Gerstein H, on behalf of the Health Outcomes Prevention (HOPE) Investigators: Effects of vitamin E on cardiovascular and microvascular outcomes in high-risk patients with diabetes. *Diabetes Care* 25:1919–1927, 2002

Martin J, Wang ZQ, Zhang XH, Wachtel D, Volaufova J, Matthews DE, Cefalu WT: Chromium picolinate supplementation attenuates body weight gain and increases insulin sensitivity in subjects with type 2 diabetes. *Diabetes Care* 29:1826–1832, 2006

Martin Mateo MC, Bustamante J, Gonzalez Cantalapiedra MA: Serum zinc, copper and insulin in diabetes mellitus. *Biomedicine* 29:56–58, 1978

Martins D, Wolf M, Pan D, Zadshir A, Tareen N, Thadhani R, Felsenfeld A, Levine B, Mehrotra R, Norris K: Prevalence of cardiovascular risk factors and the serum levels of 25-hydroxyvitamin D in the United States: data from the Third National Health and Nutrition Examination Survey. *Arch Intern Med* 167:1159–1165, 2007

Mathieu C, Gysemans C, Giulietti A, Bouillon R: Vitamin D and diabetes. *Diabetologia* 48:1247–1257, 2005

McNair P, Christiansen C, Madsbad S, Lauritzen E, Faber O, Binder C, Transbol I: Hypomagnesemia, a risk factor in diabetic retinopathy. *Diabetes* 27:1075–1077, 1978

Mitri J, Muraru MD, Pittas AG: Vitamin D and type 2 diabetes: a systematic review. *Eur J Clin Nutr* 65:1005–1015, 2011

Molnar GD, Berge KG, Rosevear JW, McGuckin WF, Achor RP: The effect of nicotinic acid in diabetes mellitus. *Metabolism* 13:181–189, 1964

Montonen J, Knekt P, Jarvinen R, Reunanen A: Dietary antioxidant intake and risk of type 2 diabetes. *Diabetes Care* 27:362–366, 2004

Mooradian AD, Faila M, Hoogwerf B, Isaac R, Maryniuk M, Wylie-Rosett J: Selected vitamins and minerals in diabetes mellitus (Technical Review). *Diabetes Care* 17:464–479, 1994

Mooradian AD, Morley JE: Micronutrient status in diabetes mellitus. *Am J Clin Nutr* 45:877–895, 1987

Morris BW, Kemp GJ, Hardisty CA: Plasma chromium and chromium excretion in diabetes. *Clin Chem* 31:334–335, 1985

Murakami K, Okubo H, Sasaki S: Effect of dietary factors on incidence of type 2 diabetes: a systematic review of cohort studies. *J Nutr Sci Vitaminol* 51:292–310, 2005

Nagamatsu M, Nickander KK, Schmelzer JD, Rava A, Wittrock DA, Tritschler H, Low PA: Lipoic acid improves nerve blood flow, reduces oxidative stress, and improves distal nerve conduction in experimental diabetic neuropathy. *Diabetes Care* 18:1160–1167, 1995

Niewoehner CB, Allen JI, Boosalis M, Levine AS, Morley JE: The role of zinc supplementation in type II diabetes mellitus. *Am J Med* 81:63–68, 1986

Nyomba BL, Auwerx J, Bormans V, Peeters TL, Pelemans W, Reynaert J, Bouillon R, Vantrappen G, De Moor P: Pancreatic secretion in man with subclinical vitamin D deficiency. *Diabetologia* 29:34–38, 1986

Omenn GS: Chemoprevention of lung cancer: the rise and demise of beta-carotene. *Annu Rev Public Health* 19:73–99, 1998

Paolisso G, Barbagallo M: Hypertension, diabetes mellitus, and insulin resistance: the role of intracellular magnesium. *Am J Hypertens* 10:346–355, 1997

Paolisso G, Scheen A, Cozzolino D, Di Maro G, Varricchio M, D'Onofrio F, Lefebvre PJ: Changes in glucose turnover parameters and improvement of glucose oxidation after 4-week magnesium administration in elderly noninsulin-dependent (type II) diabetic patients. *J Clin Endocrinol Metab* 78:1510–1514, 1994

Paolisso G, Scheen A, D'Onofrio E, Lefebvre P: Magnesium and glucose homeostasis. *Diabetologia* 33:511–514, 1990

Paolisso G, Sgambato S, Gambardella A, Pizza G, Tesauro P, Varricchio M, D'Onofrio F: Daily magnesium supplements improve glucose handling in elderly subjects. *Am J Clin Nutr* 55:1161–1167, 1992

Parekh D, Sarathi V, Shivane VK, Bandgar TR, Menon PS, Shah NS: Pilot study to evaluate the effect of short-term improvement in vitamin D status on glucose tolerance in patients with type 2 diabetes. *Endocr Pract* 16:600–608, 2010

Pittas AG, Lau J, Hu FB, Dawson-Hughes B: The role of vitamin D and calcium in type 2 diabetes: a systematic review and meta-analysis. *J Clin Endocrinol Metab* 92:2017–2029, 2007

Polo V, Saibene A, Pontiroli AE: Nicotinamide improves insulin secretion and metabolic control in lean type 2 diabetic patients with secondary failure to sulphonylureas. *Acta Diabetol* 35:61–64, 1998

Pozzilli P, Browne PD, Kolb H: Meta-analysis of nicotinamide treatment in patients with recent-onset IDDM: the Nicotinamide Trialists. *Diabetes Care* 19:1357–1363, 1996

Pozzilli P, Visalli N, Cavallo MG, Signore A, Baroni MG, Buzzetti R, Fioriti E, Mesturino C, Fiori R, Romiti A, Giovannini C, Lucentini L, Matteoli MC, Crino A, Teodonio C, Paci F, Amoretti R, Pisano L, Suraci C, Multari G, Suppa M, Sulli N, De Mattia G, Faldetta MR: Vitamin E and nicotinamide have similar effects in maintaining residual beta cell function in recent onset insulin-dependent diabetes. *Eur J Endocrinol* 137:234–239, 1997

Pozzilli P, Visalli N, Signore A, Baroni MG, Buzzetti R, Cavallo MG, Boccuni ML, Fava D, Gragnoli C, Andreani D: Double blind trial of nicotinamide in recent-onset IDDM (the IMDIAB III study). *Diabetologia* 38:848–852, 1995

Qiao LY, Goldberg JL, Russell JC, Sun XJ: Identification of enhanced serine kinase activity in insulin resistance. *J Biol Chem* 274:10625–10632, 1999

Rabbani N, Alam SS, Riaz S, Larkin JR, Akhtar MW, Shafi T, Thornalley PJ: High-dose thiamine therapy for patients with type 2 diabetes and microalbuminuria: a randomized, double-blind placebo-controlled pilot study. *Diabetologia* 52:201–212, 2009

Rabinovitz H, Friedensohn A, Leibovitz A, Gabay G, Rocas C, Habot B: Effect of chromium supplementation on blood glucose and lipid levels in type 2 diabetes mellitus elderly patients. *Int J Vitam Nutr Res* 74:178–182, 2004

Rajpathak S, Rimm EB, Li T, Morris JS, Stampfer MJ, Willett WC, Hu FB: Lower toenail chromium in men with diabetes and cardiovascular disease compared with healthy men. *Diabetes Care* 27:2211–2216, 2004

Rao RH, Vigg BL, Jaya Rao KS: Failure of pyridoxine to improve glucose tolerance in diabetics. *J Clin Endocrinol Metab* 50:198–200, 1980

Ravina A, Slezak L, Mirsky N, Bryden NA, Anderson RA: Reversal of corticosteroid-induced diabetes mellitus with supplemental chromium. *Diabet Med* 16:164–167, 1999

Reljanovic M, Reichel G, Rett K, Lobisch M, Shuette K, Moller W, Tritschler HJ, Mehnert H: Treatment of diabetic polyneuropathy with the antioxidant thioctic acid (alpha-lipoic acid): a two year multicenter randomized double-blind placebo-controlled trial (ALADIN II): Alpha Lipoic Acid in Diabetic Neuropathy. *Free Radic Res* 31:171–179, 1999

Resnick LM: Hypertension and abnormal glucose homeostasis: possible role of divalent ion metabolism. *Am J Med* 87 (Suppl. 6A):17–22, 1989

Rodriguez-Moran M, Guerrero-Romero F: Oral magnesium supplementation improves insulin sensitivity and metabolic control in type 2 diabetic subjects: a randomized double-blind controlled trial. *Diabetes Care* 26:1147–1152, 2003

Ruhnau KJ, Meissner HP, Finn JR, Reljanovic M, Lobisch M, Schutte K, Nehrdich D, Tritschler HJ, Mehnert H, Ziegler D: Effects of 3-week oral treatment with the antioxidant thioctic acid (alpha-lipoic acid) in symptomatic diabetic polyneuropathy. *Diabet Med* 16:1040–1043, 1999

Saito N, Kimura M, Kuchiba A, Itokawa Y: Blood thiamine levels in outpatients with diabetes mellitus. *J Nutr Sci Vitaminol* 33:421–430, 1987

Scragg R: Vitamin D and type 2 diabetes: are we ready for a prevention trial? *Diabetes* 57:2565–2566, 2008

Scragg R, Sowers M, Bell C: Serum 25-hydroxyvitamin D, diabetes, and ethnicity in the Third National Health and Nutrition Examination Survey. *Diabetes Care* 27:2813–2818, 2004

Shattock MJ, Hearse DJ, Fry CH: The ionic basis of the anti-ischemic and anti-arrhythmic properties of magnesium in the heart. *J Am Coll Nutr* 6:27–33, 1987

Sheikh-Ali M, Chehade JM, Mooradian AD: The antioxidant paradox in diabetes mellitus. *Am J Ther* 18:266–278, 2011

Shils ME, Olson JA, Shike M, Ross AC, Caballero B, Cousins RJ (Eds.): *Modern Nutrition in Health and Disease*. 10th ed. Philadelphia, PA, Lippincott, 2005

Simon JA, Hudes ES: Serum ascorbic acid and gallbladder disease prevalence among US adults. *Arch Intern Med* 160:931–936, 2000

Solomon LR, Cohen K: Erythrocyte O_2 transport and metabolism and effects of vitamin B_6 therapy in type II diabetes mellitus. *Diabetes* 38:881–886, 1989

Song Y, Manson JE, Buring JE, Liu S: Dietary magnesium intake in relation to plasma insulin levels and risk of type 2 diabetes in women. *Diabetes Care* 27:59–65, 2004

Stampfer MJ, Hennekens CH, Manson JE, Colditz GA, Rosner B, Willett WC: Vitamin E consumption and the risk of coronary disease in women. *N Engl J Med* 328:1444–1449, 1993

Takiishi T, Gysemans C, Bouillon R, Mathieu C: Vitamin D and diabetes. *Endocrinol Metab Clin North Am* 39:419–446, 2010

Thurman J, Mooradian AD: Vitamin supplementation therapy in the elderly. *Drugs Aging* 11:433–449, 1997

Truman RW, Doisy RJ: Metabolic effects of the glucose tolerance factor (GTF) in normal and genetically diabetic mice. *Diabetes* 26:820–826, 1977

Uusitupa MI, Kumpulainen JT, Voutilainen E, Hersio K, Sarlund H, Pyorala KP, Koivistoinen PE, Lehto JT: Effect of inorganic chromium supplementation on glucose tolerance, insulin response, and serum lipids in noninsulin-dependent diabetics. *Am J Clin Nutr* 38:404–410, 1983

Visalli N, Cavallo MG, Signore A, Baroni MG, Buzzetti R, Fioriti E, Mesturino C, Fiori R, Lucentini L, Matteoli MC, Crino A, Corbi S, Spera S, Teodonio C, Paci F, Amoretti R, Pisano L, Suraci C, Multari G, Sulli N, Cervoni M, De Mattia G, Faldetta MR, Boscherini B, Pozzilli P: A multi-centre randomized trial of two different doses of nicotinamide in patients with recent-onset type 1 diabetes (the IMDIAB VI). *Diabetes Metab Res Rev* 15:181–185, 1999

Volpe SL: Magnesium, the metabolic syndrome, insulin resistance, and type 2 diabetes mellitus. *Crit Rev Food Sci Nutr* 48:293–300, 2008

Von Hurst PR, Sonehouse W, Coad J: Vitamin D supplementation reduces insulin resistance in South Asian women living in New Zealand who are insulin resistant and vitamin D deficient: a randomized, placebo-controlled trial. *Br J Nutr* 103:549–555, 2010

Walter RM, Uriu-Hare JY, Olin KL, Oster MH, Anawalt BD, Critchfield JW, Keen CL: Copper, zinc, manganese, and magnesium status and complications of diabetes mellitus. *Diabetes Care* 14:1050–1056, 1991

Whelton PK, Klag MJ: Magnesium and blood pressure: review of the epidemiologic and clinical trial experience. *Am J Cardiol* 63:26G–30G, 1989

Wise A: Chromium supplementation and diabetes. *JAMA* 240:2045–2046, 1978

Yajnik CS, Smith RF, Hockaday TDR, Ward NI: Fasting plasma magnesium concentrations and glucose disposal in diabetes. *Br Med J* 288:1032–1034, 1984

Yates AA, Schlicker SA, Suitor CW: Dietary reference intakes: the new basis for recommendations for calcium and related nutrients, B vitamins, and choline. *J Am Diet Assoc* 98:699–706, 1998

Yeh GY, Eisenberg DM, Davis RB, Phillips RS: Use of complementary and alternative medicine among persons with diabetes mellitus: results of a national survey. *Am J Public Health* 92:1648–1652, 2002

Yochum LA, Folsom AR, Kushi LH: Intake of antioxidant vitamins and risk of death from stroke in postmenopausal women. *Am J Clin Nutr* 72:476–483, 2000

Yokota K, Kato M, Lister F, Li H, Hayakawa T, Kikuta T, Kageyama S, Tajima N: Clinical efficacy of magnesium supplementation in patients with type 2 diabetes. *J Am Coll Nutr* 23:506S–509S, 2004

Ziegler D, Hanefeld M, Ruhnau K, Hasche H, Lobisch M, Schutte K, Kerum G, Malessa R: Treatment of symptomatic diabetic polyneuropathy with the antioxidant alpha-lipoic acid: a 7-month, multicenter, randomized, controlled trial (ALADIN III Study). *Diabetes Care* 22:1296–1301, 1999

Ziegler D, Hanefeld M, Ruhnau KJ, Meissner HP, Lobisch M, Schutte K, Gries FA: Treatment of symptomatic diabetic peripheral neuropathy with the antioxidant alpha-lipoic acid: a 3-week multicenter randomized controlled trial (ALADIN Study). *Diabetologia* 38:1425–1433, 1995

Ziegler D, Low PA, Litchy WJ, Boulton AJM, Vinik AI, Freeman R, Samigullin R, Tritschler H, Munzel U, Maus J, Schutte K, Dick PJ: Efficacy and safety of antioxidant treatment with alpha-lipoic acid over 4 years in diabetic polyneuropathy: the NATHAN 1 Trial. *Diabetes Care* 34:2054–2060, 2011

Ziegler D, Nowak H, Kempler P Vargha P, Low PA: Treatment of symptomatic diabetic polyneuropathy with the antioxidant alpha-lipoic acid: a meta-analysis. *Diabet Med* 21:114–121, 2004

Joshua J. Neumiller, PharmD, CDE, CGP, FASCP, is an Assistant Professor of Pharmacotherapy in the College of Pharmacy, Washington State University, and co-owner of Pharmacy Advocates, LLC, Spokane, WA.

Chapter 4
Alcohol and Diabetes

Marion J. Franz, MS, RD, CDE

Highlights

Metabolism of Alcohol

Effects of Alcohol on Glycemia and Other Metabolic Outcomes

Effects of Alcohol on Diabetes Complications

Alcohol: Triglycerides, HDL Cholesterol, Blood Pressure, and Weight

Guidlines for Consuming Alcohol

Highlights
Alcohol and Diabetes

■ Moderate alcohol consumption (~15–30 g/day; one to two drinks) has minimal acute or long-term effects on blood glucose levels in people with type 1 or type 2 diabetes. Studies on alcohol consumption report a U- or J-shaped association, suggesting benefit from moderate consumption.

■ Moderate consumption of alcohol by people with type 2 diabetes is associated with reduced risk of and mortality from coronary heart disease and lower total mortality rates. The mechanism for this benefit is unclear but is likely related to improvements in insulin sensitivity with consumption of moderate amounts of alcohol.

■ If individuals with diabetes choose to drink alcoholic beverages, daily intake should be limited to an average of up to one drink per day for adult women and up to two drinks per day for adult men and no more than three drinks in any single day for women and no more than four drinks in any single day for men. Insulin or insulin secretagogue users, to prevent hypoglycemia, should consume alcohol with food.

■ There are no data to support recommending alcohol use to people with or without diabetes who do not currently drink. Abstinence is recommended for people with risks related to alcohol consumption. However, for the majority of people with diabetes who choose to consume alcohol in moderation, alcohol consumption does not need to be discouraged.

Alcohol and Diabetes

lcohol consumption in the United States is common. It is estimated that 76% of men and 65% of women consumed alcohol at least once in the last year. A large number of individuals exceed the recommended upper limits of average intake. An estimated 9% of men consumed an average of more than two drinks per day and 4% of women consumed an average of more than one drink per day (Report of the Dietary Guidelines Advisory Committee [DGAC] 2010). Surveys of Kaiser Permanente Northern California adult diabetes patients reported that just over 50% currently consumed alcohol, 22% had never consumed alcohol (abstainers), and 28% were former drinkers (Ahmed 2008). In the Third National Health and Nutrition Examination Survey (NHANES III), adults with diabetes also reported drinking half the amount of alcohol as adults without diabetes (Mackenzie 2006). The lower prevalence of alcohol consumption by people with diabetes may be the result of the higher prevalence of former drinkers among people with diabetes compared with the general population (28 and 15%, respectively) (Ahmed 2006), or alcohol consumption may have been discontinued because of declining health, perceived risk of alcohol on diabetes management, or physician advice to limit alcohol intake. If people with diabetes choose to drink alcoholic beverages, they need to know what effect it can have on blood glucose control and the management of their diabetes and how to drink safely.

The alcohol in beverages is ethanol (ethyl alcohol, C_2H_5OH), which is the intoxicating molecule present in distilled spirits, wine, and beer. It is the byproduct of the oxidation of sugars for energy by yeast enzymes (fermentation). The term "alcohol" will be used in this chapter. One drink is commonly defined as 12 oz regular beer, 8 oz malt liquor, 5 oz wine, or 1.5 oz 80-proof distilled spirits, each of which contains ~15 g alcohol.

The American Diabetes Association (ADA) nutrition recommendations state: "If adults with diabetes choose to drink alcohol, daily intake should be limited to a moderate amount (one drink per day or less for women and two drinks per day or less for men). Abstention from alcohol should be advised for people with a history of alcohol abuse or dependence, women during pregnancy, and people with medical problems such as liver disease, pancreatitis, advanced neuropathy, or severe hypertriglyceridemia" (ADA 2008).

This chapter begins with a summary of the metabolism of alcohol from the 1999 book *American Diabetes Association Guide to Medical Nutrition Therapy of Diabetes* (Franz 1999) and then proceeds with reviews and updates on the evidence for effects of alcohol on glycemia and other metabolic outcomes, its effect on diabetes complications, and summarizes recommendations for the consumption of moderate amounts of alcoholic beverages.

A literature search was conducted using PubMed MEDLINE, and additional articles were identified from reference lists. Search criteria included the following: alcohol research in human subjects with diabetes, English language articles, and publication after the completion of the 1999 chapter on alcohol. The initial search of potentially relevant articles identified 957 articles, of which 934 articles were excluded because titles or abstracts did not meet inclusion criteria. A total of 37 articles were retrieved for more detailed evaluation. Fourteen of these articles are included and 18 were added from the review of reference lists, making a total of 32 articles that met inclusion criteria. A total of 28 primary studies (15 epidemiological/observational studies and 13 clinical trials), 1 meta-analysis, and 3 reviews are included in Tables 4.1 and 4.2. All studies in the meta-analysis and reviews published after publication of the 1999 book (Franz 1999) are included in the tables.

METABOLISM OF ALCOHOL

Alcohol is absorbed by a process of simple diffusion across the gastrointestinal mucosa of the stomach, duodenum, and jejunum and enters the portal circulation. It is one of the few substances that can be readily absorbed through the walls of the stomach into the bloodstream. With the ingestion of food, especially high-fat food, fewer alcohol molecules diffuse from the stomach. Ethanol does not require gastrointestinal digestion and may undergo first pass metabolism by gastric alcohol dehydrogenase (ADH). Adult men have greater gastric ADH activity then adult women; thus, alcohol bioavailability in men is reduced relative to that in women (Baraona 2001).

The primary mechanism by which the body disposes of alcohol is oxidation and use as a fuel source. Alcohol is the only nutrient that does not require insulin to be metabolized. The liver is the major organ for alcohol oxidation. The total quantity of alcohol and the rate of ingestion determine its effect. The liver contains three pathways for ethanol metabolism, each located in a different subcellular compartment: 1) the ADH pathway in the cytoplasm; 2) the microsomal ethanol-oxidizing system (MEOS) located in the endoplasmic reticulum; and 3) catalase, located in the peroxisomes. All three pathways result in the production of acetaldehyde, a highly toxic metabolite (Lieber 1976).

Alcohol is primarily oxidized to acetaldehyde and acetate and then to energy through the ADH pathway (Figure 4.1). Hepatic ADH is the rate-limiting enzyme

Figure 4.1 Alcohol oxidation.

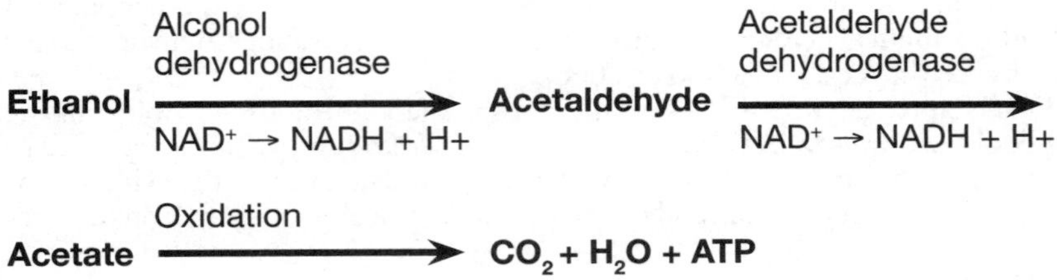

$$\text{Ethanol} \xrightarrow[\text{NAD}^+ \rightarrow \text{NADH} + \text{H}+]{\overset{\text{Alcohol}}{\text{dehydrogenase}}} \text{Acetaldehyde} \xrightarrow[\text{NAD}^+ \rightarrow \text{NADH} + \text{H}+]{\overset{\text{Acetaldehyde}}{\text{dehydrogenase}}}$$

$$\text{Acetate} \xrightarrow{\text{Oxidation}} \text{CO}_2 + \text{H}_2\text{O} + \text{ATP}$$

and determines the action and timing of alcohol metabolism. If the limited number of ADH molecules in hepatocytes are occupied, excess alcohol molecules enter the general circulation and return to the liver when ADH molecules are free to process them. The detoxification rate of ethanol by hepatic ADH is thus limited to a processing rate of ~15 g/h (Goodsell 2006). Thus, longer time periods between ingestion of alcohol are essential so that oxidation can occur in the liver. Additionally, an alcohol-induced increase within the liver cell of the NADH/NAD ratio (NAD, nicotinamide adenine dinucleotide; NADH, reduced NAD) contributes to inhibition of gluconeogenesis. Acetate is released into the bloodstream and completes oxidation in other tissues. Alcohol oxidation is an effective source of energy because it is coupled with the synthesis of adenosine triphosphate.

Alternatively, alcohol may also be metabolized via reactions in the smooth endoplasmic reticulum by the MEOS. The role of the MEOS is small, but may play a more predominant role at intoxicating levels of blood alcohol. Both the MEOS pathway and the smooth endoplasmic reticulum are also involved in the metabolism of many drugs, and this occurrence can potentially lead to adverse drug reactions. Only a small percentage of alcohol is oxidized via the catalase pathway.

Excessive alcohol that the liver cannot metabolize immediately enters the general circulation, where it becomes a part of all body fluids and enters into cells. Alcohol has a special affinity for the brain and quickly reaches the brain cells. At first, this results in a state of euphoria, often accompanied by release of inhibitions. However, longer-term alcohol use has a depressive effect on mental status.

In people with no history of chronic exposure to alcohol, it is estimated that ~75% of alcohol is oxidized by the ADH pathway, whereas 25% involves the MEOS. At high alcohol concentrations and longer duration of intake, as much as 80% of alcohol metabolism can proceed via a non-ADH pathway. Therefore, steady and prolonged alcohol consumption allows drinkers to tolerate larger amounts of alcoholic beverages. In addition to the MEOS pathway, there are increases in the ability of the hepatocytes to synthesize ADH to help clear the circulation of alcohol. As a result, the amount of alcohol that can be cleared in 1 h is doubled in an alcoholic (Lieber 1976).

EFFECTS OF ALCOHOL ON GLYCEMIA AND OTHER METABOLIC OUTCOMES

The 1999 chapter concluded that in short-term studies, in people with type 1 and type 2 diabetes, consumption of moderate amounts of alcohol had no acute postprandial impact on blood glucose and insulin levels in people with either type of diabetes (Franz 1999). However, for individuals with type 1 diabetes, a risk of late-onset hypoglycemia may exist. In individuals with type 2 diabetes, the risk of alcohol-induced acute hypoglycemia was modest (Franz 1999). Table 4.1 summarized studies published after 1999 on alcohol consumption and its effect on glycemia and other metabolic outcomes in people with type 1 and type 2 diabetes.

A large cross-sectional study of adults with diabetes ($n = 38,564$) reported that alcohol consumption was linearly and inversely associated with A1C levels; however, with three or more drinks per day, A1C levels began to increase (Ahmed 2008). Similar findings were reported in NHANES III, in which adults with dia-

Table 4.1 Alcohol Consumption and Its Effect on Glycemia and Other Metabolic Outcomes in Persons with Type 1 and Type 2 Diabetes

	Population/ Duration of Study	Intervention (type of study)	Major Findings	Comments
Rasmussen 1999	Study 1: $n = 12$ untrained adults with diet-treated type 2 diabetes/3 test days; Study 2: $n = 11$ untrained adults with type 2 diabetes/4 test days; blood samples drawn for 4 h after test in both studies	Study 1: On each test day, light meal ingested followed by either: (A) rest, (B) 30 min exercise, or (C) meal with alcohol (0.4 g/kg) and 30 min exercise; Study 2: No meal, subjects (A) resting, (B) alcohol (0.4 g/kg), (C) 30 min exercise, or (D) alcohol and 30 min exercise (crossover trial)	Study 1: A and B: similar glucose response; C: glucose response ↓ slightly; similar insulin responses in A, B, and C; Study 2: Similar glucose responses to all four tests; insulin response ↑ slightly with C and D, but not with B	Author conclusions: moderate exercise with or without moderate alcohol intake does not cause acute hypoglycemia either after a meal or in the fasting state in type 2 diabetes
Umpierrez 2000	$n = 12$ patients with DKA and 8 patients with AKA/on admission followed 24 h	Patients studied on admission and every 4 h during treatment for ketone bodies, lactate and pyruvate, insulin, and counterregulatory hormones (time series)	At admission, with similar β-hydroxybutyrate, patients with DKA had higher glucose (576 vs. 119 mg/dL), lower β-hydroxybutyrate–to–acetoacetate ratio, and lower lactate-to-pyruvate ratio than patients with AKA (all $P < 0.01$); nonsignificant insulin (both ↓) and glucagon levels (both ↑); counterregulatory hormones ↓ at similar rates	
Rasmussen 2001	$n = 8$ diet-treated adults with type 2 diabetes/2 test days; tested twice after overnight fast	After euglycemic period, 200 mL water ingested alone or with alcohol (0.4 g/ kg); hypoglycemia induced (50 mg/dL) with insulin (crossover trial)	Circulating glucose, insulin, catecholamines, cortisol, and growth hormone levels were similar on both study days; alcohol intake ↓ peak glucagon response ($P = 0.038$)	Author conclusions: alcohol does not modify recovery from insulin-induced hypoglycemia

	Population/ Duration of Study	Intervention (type of study)	Major Findings	Comments
Turner 2001	*n* = 6 men with type 1 diabetes/2 test days; 5:00 p.m. to 12:00 noon the next day	Bolus insulin before dinner (6:00 p.m.) and breakfast (8:00 a.m.), basal insulin infusion from 11:00 p.m.; drank wine (0.75 g/kg alcohol) or water at 9:00 p.m. over 90 min (crossover trial)	Nonsignificant evening or overnight glucose levels; in the morning, fasting PP glucose significantly lower after consumption of wine (PP 160 mg/dL with wine vs. 270 mg/dL with water); five subjects required treatment for hypoglycemia, none with water; growth hormone significantly ↓ from midnight to 4:00 a.m. ($P = 0.04$)	Author conclusions: moderate consumption of alcohol in the evening may predispose individuals with type 1 diabetes to hypoglycemia after breakfast the next day
Howard 2004	6 studies: 1 in people with type 1 diabetes and 6 in people with type 2 diabetes; 5–20 adults in each study and subjects served as their own control/not applicable	Effect of alcohol from 1–2 drinks (4 studies) to 5–6 drinks/day (2 studies); alcohol ingested with food (3 studies) or without food (2 studies) and administered intravenously in one study (systematic review)	1 study: ↓ in glucose after alcohol without a meal; 1 study: ↓ in glucose after ethanol infusion during a fast; 4 studies: ingesting small to moderate amounts of alcohol with (3 studies) or without (1 study) had no acute effect on glycemic control	All studies were published between 1974 and 1999, and all except the ethanol infusion study were included in the 1999 text
Cheyne 2004	*n* = 17 subjects with type 1 diabetes (A1C ~8.1%)/4 tests	Effect of euglycemia or mild hypoglycemia (50 mg/ dL) with modest alcohol intoxication (45–50 mg/100 mL) on cognitive and driving performance: (A) euglycemic (80 mg/dL) with placebo; (B) euglycemic with alcohol; (C) hypoglycemic (50 mg/ dL) with placebo; (D) hypoglycemic with alcohol (crossover trial)	B and D: average blood alcohol level 43 mg/dL, associated with ↓ in cognitive performance; C: ↓ in some cognitive performance; D: marked ↓ in all cognitive function tests; only 8 of the 17 patients were aware they were hypoglycemic and only 6 when hypoglycemic and consuming alcohol	Author conclusions: both alcohol and hypoglycemia impair cognitive function and together the effects are additive; the cumulative effect is a concern if patients with type 1 diabetes are driving
van de Wiel 2004	Patients with diabetes/not applicable	Effect of alcohol on metabolism and metabolic outcomes (review article)	Moderate consumption of alcohol associated with limited effects on glycemia, ↑ insulin sensitivity, ↓ risk of atherosclerosis disorders and blood pressure	

Table 4.1 Alcohol Consumption and Its Effect on Glycemia and Other Metabolic Outcomes in Persons with Type 1 and Type 2 Diabetes (*continued*)

	Population/ Duration of Study	Intervention (type of study)	Major Findings	Comments
Richardson 2005	n = 16 free-living patients with type 1 diabetes (A1C 8.1%) who consumed alcohol on a regular basis (<28 oz/ week)/2 tests, each used continuous glucose monitoring systems for 36 h	Patients used continuous glucose monitoring system and ingested either orange juice or vodka and orange juice; with evening meal with same dose of insulin given at meal and before bed (crossover trial)	After alcohol, patients reported more than twice as many hypoglycemic episodes throughout the next 24 h than after placebo (P = 0.02); alcohol consumption resulted in increased risk of hypoglycemia continuing into the next day	
Ahmed 2006	n = 65,996 adults with diabetes in the Kaiser Permanente Northern California Registry/not applicable	Alcohol consumption (average number of drinks/day in the past year) and adherence to self-monitoring of blood glucose, A1C testing, and diabetes medications (determined from electronic record); smoking, diet, and exercise (self-reported) (cross-sectional study)	Gradient of increasing risk for poor adherence with each of the six diabetes self-care behaviors with increasing alcohol consumption, starting with even 1 drink/day	Author conclusions: diabetes health care providers should ask patients about alcohol consumption and be aware that heavy consumption may be a marker for poor self-care behaviors
Mackenzie 2006	Adults with (n = 1,024) and without diabetes who participated in NHANES III/not applicable	Diabetes status, A1C, and 1-month food frequency questionnaires examined in adults with and without diabetes compared to nondrinkers (cross-sectional study)	≥30 drinks/month in people with diabetes: associated with an A1C lower by 1.2% vs. nondrinkers with diabetes (P < 0.001), A1C lower by 0.2% vs. nondrinkers without diabetes (P < 0.001)	

	Population/ Duration of Study	Intervention (type of study)	Major Findings	Comments
Kerr 2007	*n* = 17 subjects with type 1 diabetes/4 tests of 150 min	Influence of mild alcohol intoxication (45–50 mg/dL) on counterregulatory hormone responses to hypoglycemia (50 mg/dL): (A) euglycemic with placebo; (B) euglycemic with alcohol; (C) hypoglycemic with placebo; (D) hypoglycemic with alcohol (crossover trial)	During hypoglycemia, peak growth hormone levels were significantly lower after alcohol vs. placebo ($P <$ 0.001); ↓ insulin sensitivity in both hypoglycemia and euglycemia after alcohol; no differences in other hormone levels	
Shai 2007	*n* = 109 adult patients with type 2 diabetes who abstained from alcohol/3 months	Patients were randomly assigned to drink 150 mL wine (13 g alcohol) or nonalcoholic beer during dinner (RCT	At 3 months, alcohol group FPG ↓ from ~140 to 118 mg/dL compared to control (~137 to 139 mg/dL); alcohol had no significant effect on 2-h PP glucose; patients in alcohol group with higher baseline A1C had greater reductions in FPG ($P < 0.001$	
Bantle 2008	*n* = 18 adults with non–insulin-treated type 2 diabetes/1 meal; 30 days	One-meal inpatient study: wine (24 g alcohol) or grape juice with evening meal; 30-day study: wine (18 g alcohol) or abstinence (crossover trial)	1 meal: alcohol had no acute effect on glucose or insulin; 30 days: alcohol had no effect on total, HDL- or LDL-C; triglycerides; glucose; ↓ fasting insulin ($P = 0.03$)	Author conclusions: because alcohol had no harmful metabolic effect, people with type 2 diabetes should not be discouraged from using alcohol in moderation

Table 4.1 Alcohol Consumption and Its Effect on Glycemia and Other Metabolic Outcomes in Persons with Type 1 and Type 2 Diabetes (*continued*)

	Population/ Duration of Study	Intervention (type of study)	Major Findings	Comments
Ahmed 2008	$n = 38,564$ adults with diabetes in the Kaiser Permanente Northern California Registry/not applicable	Self-reported alcohol consumption and A1C done within 1 year of survey date (cross-sectional study)	A1C: 8.88 (lifetime abstainers), 8.79 (former drinkers), 8.90 (<0.1 drinks/day), 8.71 (0.1–0.9 drink/day), 8.51 (1–1.9 drinks/day), 8.39 (2–2.9 drinks/day), 8.47 (≥3 drinks/day)	Alcohol consumption linearly (*P* < 0.001) and inversely (*P* = 0.001) is associated with A1C, although A1C increased among heaviest drinkers
Kerr 2009	$n = 10$ patients with type 1 diabetes (A1C ~8.0%)/ 2 lunches followed for 4 h	600-kcal lunch with either wine (men 8 units, women 6 units) or alcohol-free wine (crossover trial)	Nonsignificant difference between alcohol and alcohol-free days in glucose, triglycerides, free fatty acids, cortisol, and growth hormone; β-hydroxybutyrate ↓ PP on alcohol-free days vs. ↑ with alcohol (*P* < 0.001); lactate ↑ after meal but with alcohol response was greater (*P* = 0.014)	

AKA, alcoholic ketoacidosis; DKA, diabetic ketoacidosis; HDL-C, HDL cholesterol; LDL-C, LDL cholesterol; PP, postprandial; RCT, randomized controlled trial.

betes who had ≥30 drinks of alcohol per month, compared with nondrinkers, had average A1C levels 1.2% lower than other adults with diabetes (Mackenzie 2006). However, increasing risk for poor adherence to diabetes self-care behaviors with increasing alcohol consumption, starting with individuals who consume one drink per day, has also been reported (Ahmed 2006). Therefore, it is important that health care providers ask people with diabetes about alcohol consumption and encourage moderate and sensible use, shown to have potentially beneficial effects on glycemic control (van de Wiel 2004).

Type 2 Diabetes

Two clinical trials examined the effect of alcohol in individuals with type 2 diabetes (Shai 2007; Bantle 2008). Adults with type 2 diabetes ($n = 109$) who abstained from alcohol were randomly assigned to drink wine (13 g alcohol; ~5 oz) or nonalcoholic beer (controls) each day for 3 months. In individuals drinking wine, fasting plasma glucose (FPG) decreased ~22 mg/dL, but no effect on postprandial glucose levels was observed. In the controls, FPG and postprandial glucose levels did not change. Interestingly, patients in the alcohol group with the higher baseline A1C levels had greater decreases in FPG and reported improvements in their ability to fall asleep (Shai 2007). In the second study, adults with type 2 diabetes drank either wine (24 g alcohol; ~8.5 oz) or grape juice with their evening meal, with no acute effect on glucose or insulin levels. Wine (18 g alcohol; ~6.5 oz) or abstinence was continued for 30 days, with wine having no effect on glucose or lipids but insulin sensitivity improving (Bantle 2008). A systematic review of earlier, small, acute studies also concluded that moderate consumption of alcohol does not acutely impair glycemic control in individuals with type 2 diabetes and may actually result in a small decrease in glucose concentrations (Howard 2004). However, chronic ingestion (>45 g/day) has been shown to cause deterioration in glucose control; the effects from excess alcohol are reversed, however, after abstinence for a number of days.

In individuals with diet-treated type 2 diabetes, meals with or without alcohol were followed by either rest or 30 min of exercise, and the combination of moderate exercise with or without alcohol did not cause hypoglycemia (Rasmussen 1999). In a second study, in people with diet-treated type 2 diabetes, alcohol or water were ingested before insulin-induced hypoglycemia to determine the influence of alcohol on glucose counterregulation and recovery from insulin-induced hypoglycemia. Alcohol had no effect on recovery from hypoglycemia, although it decreased peak glucagon response (Rasmussen 2001).

Type 1 Diabetes

Previous studies reported no acute effect of moderate alcohol intake with a meal on blood glucose levels in people with type 1 diabetes. However, a risk of late-onset hypoglycemia was reported (Franz 1999). Inhibition of gluconeogenesis, reduced hypoglycemia awareness due to cerebral effects of alcohol, and/or impaired counterregulatory responses to hypoglycemia have been reported as possible causes. Five of six men with type 1 diabetes had dinner at 6:00 p.m. followed by drinking wine (70 g alcohol, 20 oz) or water at 9:00 p.m. After drinking wine, treatment for hypoglycemia was required after breakfast; growth hormone was significantly reduced, with no other differences in insulin or other hormone levels (Turner 2001). Similarly, in adults with type 1 diabetes, hypoglycemia (blood glucose 50 mg/dL) resulted in lower peak growth hormone levels compared to placebo; however, this result was also associated with a decrease in insulin sensitivity (Kerr 2007). In a study similar to the Turner study, individuals with type 1 diabetes drank either orange juice or vodka with their evening meal. After drinking alcohol, based on continuous glucose monitoring data, individuals reported more than twice as many hypoglycemic episodes throughout the next 24 h than after drinking orange juice (Richardson 2005).

In people with type 1 diabetes, both mild alcohol intoxication and hypoglycemia (blood glucose ~43 mg/dL) were associated with deterioration in reaction time and other tests of cognitive function, and the total impairment was greater when both were experienced together (Cheyne 2004). The authors emphasize the importance of individuals testing blood glucose levels before driving and not driving when mildly hypoglycemic, even if asymptomatic. Individuals also must be aware that the effects of alcohol and hypoglycemia on cognitive function are additive and significant even after small quantities of alcohol. It is important to completely avoid alcohol when driving.

Elevated total ketone body concentrations are characteristic of both diabetic ketoacidosis (DKA) and alcoholic ketoacidosis (AKA). However, DKA compared to AKA is characterized by a higher glucose concentration and a lower β-hydroxybutyrate–to–acetoacetate and lactate-to-pyruvate ratios. Hormonal profiles are similar with decreased insulin levels and elevated levels of counterregulatory hormones (Umpierrez 2000). Liberal lunchtime ingestion of alcohol by patients with type 1 diabetes compared to placebo resulted in postprandial β-hydroxybutrate levels being elevated with alcohol and suppressed with placebo (Kerr 2009). The authors suggest that "binge" drinking may increase the risk of significant ketosis, especially if insulin administration is erratic. They recommend that patient education materials contain information to highlight these potential problems.

Summary

In people with type 2 diabetes, acute or longer-term moderate consumption of alcoholic beverages appears to have no detrimental effect on glucose control, whereas longer-term consumption of alcohol may actually improve fasting glucose levels and insulin sensitivity. Alcohol consumption also does not influence responses to exercise or hypoglycemia.

In people with type 1 diabetes, moderate consumption of alcohol appears to have minimal, if any, acute effect on glucose levels and insulin needs. However, of concern is the occurrence of late-onset hypoglycemia, likely due to reduced growth hormone levels after alcohol consumption. Thus, it is important that individuals repeatedly self-monitor blood glucose levels after drinking alcoholic beverages to determine if treatment for hypoglycemia is needed. Also of concern is the additive effect of alcohol and hypoglycemia on cognitive function and the need to avoid alcohol when planning to drive.

EFFECTS OF ALCOHOL ON DIABETES COMPLICATIONS

The protective effect of alcohol against coronary heart disease (CHD) in the general population is well established. Over 40 studies in diverse populations have documented a 10–40% reduction in risk associated with one to three drinks per day (Rimm 1999). The mechanisms responsible for the effect of alcohol in individuals without diabetes are reported to be increased HDL cholesterol, decreased platelet aggregation, decreased clotting factors such as fibrinogen, improvement in markers of inflammation and endothelial dysfunction (increased tissue plasminogen activator and decreased plasminogen activator inhibitor 1), and enhanced insulin sensitivity (Tanasescu 2001a; Koppes 2006). Studies on alcohol consumption and diabetes complications are summarized in Table 4.2.

Importantly, in men and women with diabetes, moderate alcohol intake is also associated with a lower risk of CHD (Ajani 2000; Solomon 2000; Tanasescu 2001b; Wakabayashi 2002; Pitsavos 2005), lower mortality risk from CHD (Valmadrid 1999; de Vegt 2002), and lower total mortality risk (Diem 2003). A system-

Table 4.2 Alcohol Consumption and Diabetes Complications

	Population/ Duration of Study	Intervention (type of study)	Major Findings	Comments
Valmadrid 1999	n = 983 older-onset individuals with diabetes in the Wisconsin Epidemiologic Study of Diabetic Retinopathy/12 years follow-up	Patients reported their past-year intake of alcoholic beverages (prospective cohort study)	During 7,004 person-years' follow-up, 198 CHD deaths; CHD mortality rates in never, former, <2 g (<1 drink/week), 2–13 g, and ≥14 g (~1 drink/day)/day: 43.9, 39.5, 25.3, 20.8, and 10.0/1,000 person-years, respectively; RR for former drinkers and <2, 2, and ≥14 g/day: 0.69, 0.54, 0.44, and 0.21, respectively	Alcohol use inversely associated with CHD mortality
Ajani 2000	n = 2,790 with diabetes in the Physicians' Health Study/5.5 years follow-up	Relationship between light to moderate alcohol intake and CHD in men with and without diabetes (prospective cohort study)	During 480,876 person-years' follow-up, 850 CHD deaths (717 in men without diabetes, 133 in men with diabetes); RR in men without diabetes for rarely/never, monthly, weekly, and daily alcohol consumption: 1.00, 1.02, 0.82, and 0.61 (*P* for trend <0.0001); RR in men with diabetes: 1.00, 1.11, 0.67, and 0.42 (*P* for trend = 0.0019)	Light to moderate alcohol consumption is associated with similar risk reduction in CHD among men with and without diabetes
Solomon 2000	n = 5,103 women with type 2 diabetes in the Nurses' Health Study/14 years follow-up	Association between moderate alcohol intake and CHD in women with type 2 diabetes (prospective cohort study)	During 39,092 person-years of follow-up, 194 nonfatal MI and 101 fatal CHD (295 events); RR for CHD compared with non-drinkers with intake of 0.1–4.9 g (<0.5 drinks)/day: 0.74; intake of ≥5 g/day: 0.48 (*P* for trend <0.0001)	Moderate alcohol consumption associated with reduced CHD risk in women with type 2 diabetes
Tanasescu 2001a	Patients with type 2 diabetes/not applicable	Effect of moderate alcohol intake and risk of CHD and possible mechanisms for this association (review article)	Results indicated ↓ risk ranging from 34 to 79%, associated with light to moderate alcohol intake; potential mechanisms include ↑ HDL cholesterol, ↓ coagulation, and ↑ insulin sensitivity	

Table 4.2 Alcohol Consumption and Diabetes Complications (*continued*)

	Population/ Duration of Study	Intervention (type of study)	Major Findings	Comments
Tanas-escu 2001b	n = 2,419 men with type 2 diabetes in the Health Professionals Follow-up Study/10 years	Relationship between alcohol intake and risk of CHD among men with type 2 diabetes (prospective cohort study)	During 11,411 person-years of follow-up, 150 new cases of CHD (81 nonfatal MI and 69 fatal CHD); RR compared to non-drinkers for ≤0.5, 0.5–2, and >2 drinks/day: 0.78, 0.62, and 0.48 (P for trend = 0.03)	
de Vegt 2002	n = 659 with diabetes and impaired fasting glucose in the Hoorn Study/6 years	Association between alcohol and 10-year mortality (prospective cohort study)	People drinking up to 10 g/day had the lowest mortality risk; RR of total mortality for 0, 5, 20, and 45 g alcohol: 1.00, 0.62, 0.97, and 1.05; higher alcohol ↑ risks for mortality	
Waka-bayashi 2002	n = 194 people with type 2 diabetes/not applicable	Subjects divided by average weekly alcohol consumption: nondrinkers, light drinkers (<210 g/week), and heavy drinkers; degree of atherosclerotic progression evaluated using a-PWV; atherosclerosis risks evaluated using risk factors (cross-sectional)	a-PWV lower in light drinkers than non-drinkers and heavy drinkers (P < 0.05); SBP, HDL, triglycerides higher in heavy drinkers than in non-drinkers and light drinkers (all P < 0.05); BMI, A1C, uric acid, fibrinogen, NS different between groups	Light but not heavy drinking had preventive effects on atherosclerosis
Cooper 2002	n = 1,625 participants in the Insulin Resistance and Atherosclerosis Study with measured S_I (45% normal glucose tolerance, 23% impaired glucose tolerance, 22% type 2 diabetes)/not applicable	Tested whether adjustment for S_I attenuated the alcohol consumption and common carotid artery intima-medial thickness J-shaped relationship (cross-sectional)	In comparison to never-drinkers, in normal glucose tolerance status, all levels of alcohol associated with less atherosclerosis; impaired glucose tolerance status had a J-shaped alcohol-atherosclerosis association; in diabetes status, all levels of alcohol consumption associated with more atherosclerosis	Author conclusions: moderate alcohol consumption may increase the risk of atherosclerosis in people with diabetes

	Population/ Duration of Study	Intervention (type of study)	Major Findings	Comments
Diem 2003	n = 287 Swiss patients with type 2 diabetes from the World Health Organization Multinational Study of Vascular Diseases in Diabetes/follow-up of 12.6 years	Examined the effects of alcohol consumption on mortality from CHD and all causes (prospective cohort study)	During follow-up, 70 deaths (21 from CHD); compared to nondrinkers, risk rates of death from CHD for alcohol 1–15, 16–30, and ≥30 g/day: 0.87, 0.00, and 0.37; risk rates of death from all cause: 1.27, 0.36, and 1.66	Moderate alcohol (16–30 g/day) intake associated with ↓ mortality from CHD and all causes; alcohol >30 g/day, tendency towards ↑ all-cause mortality
Howard 2004	n = 9,940 people with diabetes in 6 studies/not applicable	4 studies assessed relationship of alcohol and CHD or death; 2 studies assessed association between alcohol and risk for retinopathy (systematic review)	Each study reported ↓ risk for death due to CHD in association with alcohol use; compared to nondrinkers, moderate drinkers had a 34–55% ↓ incidence of CHD and a 55–79% ↓ in death rate from CHD; one study, no association between alcohol and incidence or progression of diabetic retinopathy; one study, ↑ risk for diabetic retinopathy with heavy alcohol use	All studies related to CHD included in this table and two studies related to retinopathy were published in 1994 and 1984
Avogaro 2004	n = 8 individuals with and 8 without diabetes/ 2 tests of 4 h	Frequently sampled intravenous glucose tolerance tests performed twice after participants sipped 40 g alcohol (vodka) or water (nonrandomized trial)	After alcohol: lactate higher in both groups; free fatty acids ↓ 17% in controls (P = 0.1) and ↓ 23% in people with diabetes (P = 0.007); ↑ S_i in both groups; β-cell response ↓ in people with diabetes regardless of the study	Acute alcohol improves insulin action without affecting β-cell function; may be partly due to inhibitory effect of alcohol on lipolysis
Shai 2004	n = 726 men in the Health Professionals Follow-up Study with type 2 diabetes and who returned blood samples/not applicable	Relationship between alcohol intake and inflammation (cross-sectional)	Alcohol intake associated with lower A1C, markers of inflammation and endothelial dysfunction, and increased HDL and adiponectin	

Table 4.2 Alcohol Consumption and Diabetes Complications (*continued*)

	Population/ Duration of Study	Intervention (type of study)	Major Findings	Comments
Pitsavos 2005	n = 216 hospitalized Greek patients with diabetes and a first event of ACS and 196 people with diabetes without CHD/not applicable	To determine the threshold of alcohol above which the balance of risk and benefit becomes adverse in diabetes; alcohol intake was quantified (cross-sectional)	Alcohol was associated in a J-shaped relationship with risk of ACS, total cholesterol, blood pressure, and smoking (all P < 0.001); low alcohol consumption (<12 g/day) associated with a 47% ↓ in ACS; higher intake (12–24 and >24 g/day) ↑ prevalence by 2.7- and 5.4-fold	Low to moderate alcohol associated with ↓ in ACS in diabetes; higher consumption associated with ↑ in lipids, blood pressure, and risk of ACS
Marfella 2006	n = 115 people with type 2 diabetes who had a first nonfatal MI/1 year	Moderate daily amount of red wine (11 g alcohol) with meals or none (control); echocardiographic parameters of functional cardiac outcome, inflammatory cytokines, and nitrotyrosine measured at baseline and 12 months (RCT)	1-year control compared to alcohol group: ↑ nitrotyrosine, C-reactive protein, tumor necrosis factor-a, interleukin-6, and interleukin-18 (all P < 0.01); other markers of ventricular dys-synchrony also higher in control group	Red wine consumption reduces oxidative stress and proinflammatory cytokines as well as improving cardiac function after MI
Koppes 2006	6 cohort studies of people with type 2 diabetes/ not applicable	Risk of total mortality and/or fatal or incident CHD in alcohol non-consumers and in at least two groups of alcohol consumers (meta-analysis)	Lower risk of mortality and CHD in alcohol consumers than in non-consumers; RR of total mortality in <6 g/day: 0.64; RR of total mortality in 6 to <18 and ≥18 g/day: NS; RR fatal and total CHD lower in all three categories of alcohol consumers, ranging from 0.34 to 0.75	All six studies are included in this table
Bantle 2008	n = 18 adults with non–insulin-treated type 2 diabetes/one meal; 30 days	One-meal inpatient study: wine (24 g alcohol) or grape juice in random order with evening meal; 30-day study: wine (18 g alcohol) or abstinence in random order (randomized crossover trial)	One meal: alcohol had no acute effect on glucose or insulin; 30-day: alcohol had no effect on total, HDL, or LDL cholesterol; triglycerides; glucose; ↓ fasting insulin (P = 0.03)	

	Population/ Duration of Study	Intervention (type of study)	Major Findings	Comments
Beulens 2008	*n* = 1,857 type 1 diabetes patients in the EURODIAB Prospective Complications Study/not applicable	Moderate alcohol consumption and risk of retinopathy (304 cases), neuropathy (660 cases), and nephropathy (157 cases) (cross-sectional)	Alcohol associated with risk of microvascular complications in U-shaped fashion; moderate (30–70 g alcohol/week) had lowest risk of microvascular complications; alcohol not associated with ketoacidosis or hypoglycemia	
Schaller 2010	*n* = 12 men with type 2 diabetes/2 tests	Reference ultrasound measurements of brachial artery, insulin-modified frequently sampled intravenous glucose tolerance test followed by second series of ultrasound measurement with alcohol (40 g) or without alcohol (crossover trial)	Alcohol intake improved insulin sensitivity directly related to blood alcohol levels and acutely increases endothelium-dependent brachial artery vasodilation	
Lee 2010	*n* = 1,239 patients with type 2 diabetes enrolled in the AdRem study (substudy of ADVANCE trial)/5.5 years follow-up	Association between alcohol and diabetic retinopathy and visual acuity; moderate (1–14) and heavy (>14 drinks/weeks) alcohol intake (prospective cohort study)	182 participants had two-step progression of early treatment of diabetes retinopathy, 639 had ↓ in visual acuity; current alcohol compared with none not associated with presence or progression of diabetes retinopathy but was associated with ↑ risk of deterioration of visual acuity (*P* < 0.001)	

ACS, acute coronary syndrome; a-PWV, aortic pulse wave velocity; RCT, randomized controlled trial; S_I, insulin sensitivity; SBP, systolic blood pressure.

atic review demonstrated that among people with diabetes, moderate alcohol consumption is associated with a 34–55% decrease in risk for CHD and a 55–79% decrease in risk for death from CHD (Howard 2004). In a meta-analysis, statistical pooling of studies comparing alcohol consumers to non-consumers showed a reduced relative risk (RR) for incident CHD (RR = 0.57). RR for CHD mortality was reduced in alcohol consumption categories until ≥18 g/day (RR = 0.75), after which it increased. RR for total mortality was lower in the <6 g/day category (RR = 0.64) (Koppes 2006).

In contrast, one study reported that all levels of alcohol consumption in people with diabetes compared to nondrinkers were associated with more atherosclerosis (as measured by high-resolution β-mode ultrasound of carotid arteries). However, in people with normal and impaired glucose tolerance, compared to nondrinkers, alcohol consumption was associated with less atherosclerosis (Cooper 2002).

Researchers have attempted to determine potential mechanisms for the overwhelming association of alcohol with decreased risk for CHD and mortality in people with diabetes. Alcohol intake in the Health Professionals Follow-Up Study of men with type 2 diabetes was associated with increased HDL cholesterol and adiponectin and decreased levels of fibrinogen and other markers of inflammation and endothelial dysfunction (Shai 2004). However, in a cross-sectional study measuring degree of atherosclerotic progression in people with type 2 diabetes, light drinking but not heavy drinking was associated with decreased atherosclerotic progression, but changes in serum HDL cholesterol and plasma fibrinogen levels were not involved in this beneficial effect (Solomon 2000). In two studies, acute alcohol consumption (40 g) improved insulin sensitivity in individuals with and without type 2 diabetes (Avogaro 2004; Schaller 2010). In individuals with type 2 diabetes, alcohol consumption also significantly reduced acute free fatty acid levels (Avogaro 2004) and acutely increased artery vasodilation (Schaller 2010). In a crossover trial, individuals drank wine (18 g alcohol) with meals or abstained for 30 days; consumption of alcohol had no effect on lipids, including HDL cholesterol, or glucose, but did lower fasting serum insulin levels (Bantle 2008). In a year-long study, individuals were randomized to moderate daily wine (11 g alcohol) with meals or none after a first nonfatal myocardial infarction (MI). Compared to the controls, wine consumption significantly reduced oxidative stress markers and proinflammatory cytokines as well as improving cardiac function after MI (Marfella 2006).

Risk of microvascular complications related to alcohol consumption was examined in two studies. In the EURODIAB Prospective Complications Study, in people with type 1 diabetes, moderate alcohol consumption was associated with risk of proliferative retinopathy, neuropathy, and macroalbuminuria in a U-shaped manner. Moderate consumers (30–79 g alcohol/week) had the lowest risk of microvascular complications; alcohol consumption also was not associated with occurrence of ketoacidosis or hypoglycemia (Beulens 2008). In the AdRem Study, in people with type 2 diabetes, moderate alcohol consumption, compared to not drinking at all, was not associated with presence or progression of diabetic retinopathy, but was associated with a higher risk of deterioration of visual acuity—the magnitude increased with increasing amount of alcohol (Lee 2010).

Summary

In people with type 2 diabetes, moderate alcohol consumption is associated with decreased CHD and mortality risks and decreased total mortality. The type of alcoholic beverage does not influence beneficial effects (Valmadrid 1999; Howard 2004; Shai 2004; Koppes 2006). The observed mortality risk reduction related to moderate alcohol consumption in people with type 2 diabetes is largely attributed to the reduced risk of CHD. The most consistent mechanism for the beneficial effects of alcohol is an increase in insulin sensitivity. However, improvements in markers of inflammation and endothelial dysfunction are also reported. Improvements in HDL cholesterol and fibrinogen have been mixed.

In individuals with type 1 diabetes, moderate alcohol consumption is associated with lower risk of microvascular complications. In individuals with type 2 diabetes, moderate alcohol consumption was not associated with retinopathy.

ALCOHOL: TRIGLYCERIDES, HDL CHOLESTEROL, BLOOD PRESSURE, AND WEIGHT

Concern has been expressed that excessive intake of alcohol may result in hypertriglyceridemia, hypertension, and weight gain in individuals with diabetes even though, at moderate levels of consumption, this does not result in higher risk of CHD or total mortality (Koppes 2006). A limited number of studies have examined the effect of alcohol consumption on triglycerides, blood pressure, and weight in people with diabetes. Advice to avoid alcohol is often given to people with diabetes because of the assumption that even moderate amounts of alcohol will raise triglycerides and blood pressure and contribute to weight gain. However, the limited available research does not support this advice.

Triglycerides

In people without diabetes, some evidence exists to suggest that moderate intake of alcohol has no detrimental effects on triglyceride levels, even in people who are hypertriglyceridemic. Two observational studies suggested moderate consumption of alcohol had beneficial effects on triglyceride and HDL cholesterol levels. Analysis of NHANES III data from 8,125 participants revealed that mild-to-moderate alcohol consumption (1–19 drinks of alcohol per month) was associated with a lower prevalence of the metabolic syndrome and was significantly and inversely associated with three of its components—elevated triglycerides, low serum HDL cholesterol, and hyperinsulinemia (Frieberg 2004). In a study of 14,077 British women, women consuming 1–14 drinks of alcohol per week, compared to nondrinkers, had a reduction in CHD associated with the lowest triglyceride levels and highest levels of HDL cholesterol (Nanchahal 2000).

Although excessive alcohol intake, high intake of saturated fatty acids, and elevated glucose concentrations are reported to be the cause of secondary hypertriglyceridemia (especially in people with obesity) (Chait 1972), clinical trials show that the effect of moderate alcohol intake on triglycerides in people with or without hypertriglyceridemia is limited. When two alcoholic drinks or water per day for 2 weeks were consumed by people with fasting triglyceride levels of 200–750 mg/dL or by people with normal triglyceride levels (90 mg/dL), there were no significant differences reported between the effect of alcohol or the effect of water on triglyceride levels. The authors concluded that acute alcohol intake is not an important determinant of triglyceride concentrations in individuals with hypertriglyceridemia (Pownall 1999). In fact, moderate alcohol intake may actually have a beneficial effect on triglyceride levels. In a trial of healthy women, either none, one, or two drinks per day of alcohol were consumed for 8 weeks. Fasting triglyceride levels were significantly reduced by 7.8% after consumption of one drink per day and by 10.3% with two drinks per day. Fasting insulin levels decreased by 19.2% and insulin sensitivity increased by 7.2% (Davies 2002).

Only a few studies conducted in people with diabetes are available. In men with type 2 diabetes, light drinkers (<14 drinks per week) had an average triglyceride level of 115 mg/dL compared to 132 mg/dL in nondrinkers and 170 mg/dL in heavy drinkers (>14 drinks per week). Thus, triglyceride levels were significantly higher in heavy drinkers than in nondrinkers and light drinkers (Wakabayashi 2002). Subjects with type 2 diabetes either consumed wine (6.5 oz) with the evening meal or abstained for 30 days, and alcohol had no effect on triglycerides or total, LDL, or HDL cholesterol (Bantle 2008). Clearly, to answer the question of alcohol and its effects on triglyceride levels, additional clinical trials are needed, especially in individuals with diabetes. However, in individuals with high triglyceride levels (>500 mg/dL), complete abstinence is recommended along with reduced saturated fat intake to reduce the risk of pancreatitis (Miller 2011).

HDL Cholesterol

In an epidemiological study, in subjects without diabetes, 30 g alcohol a day was reported to increase HDL cholesterol by ~4 mg/dL; this, along with other positive biological marker effects, was calculated to lower risk of CHD by ~25% (Rimm 1999). In a study in people with diabetes that included the relationship of alcohol intake and HDL cholesterol, each additional drink per day was also related to increases in HDL cholesterol (~2.0 mg/dL) (Shai 2004). In a year-long study, people with type 2 diabetes ate a Mediterranean diet with either one daily 4 oz glass of wine or no alcoholic beverage; at year-end drinking wine with the Mediterranean diet resulted in a significant increase in HDL cholesterol (34.8 mg/dL) compared to the Mediterranean diet without alcohol (Marfella 2006). However, in a 30-day study, wine (24 g alcohol) with the evening meal or abstinence had no effect on HDL cholesterol (Bantle 2008). Thus, the effect of alcoholic beverages on HDL cholesterol in people with diabetes is unclear.

Hypertension

The 2010 Report of the Dietary Guidelines Advisory Committee concluded that "strong evidence indicates that moderate alcohol consumption does not elevate risk of either hypertension or stroke. It is also well documented that alcohol consumed in excess of moderate causes an increase in blood pressure and stroke" (DGAC Report 2010). There are limited available data on moderate alcohol consumption and hypertension in people with diabetes. In individuals with diabetes, a J-shaped relationship was observed between alcohol intake and blood pressure (Pitsavos 2005), and in another study, moderate drinking compared to no alcoholic beverage had no effect on blood pressure (Marfella 2006).

Weight Gain

The 2010 report of the DGAC also examined the relationship between alcohol intake and weight gain and concluded that "moderate evidence suggests that among free-living populations, moderate drinking is not associated with weight gain. However, heavier consumption over time is associated with weight gain" (DGAC Report 2010). The report does note that regardless of the alcoholic beverage, all contain calories that are not a good source of nutrients and, when consumed beyond an average of two drinks a day, may lead to weight gain. Below this level of consumption, the evidence suggests that individuals who drink in moderation do not gain weight at a faster rate than nondrinkers. Table 4.3 contains a list of alcoholic beverages and their caloric content. No studies examining the effect of alcohol consumption on weight have been done in people with diabetes.

GUIDELINES FOR CONSUMING ALCOHOL

Information regarding benefits and contraindications should be given to individuals with diabetes so that they can make their own decisions regarding consumption of alcoholic beverages. For the majority of people, moderate consumption with food will have minimal, if any, acute or long-term effects on blood glucose levels and may have beneficial effects on insulin sensitivity and create a decreased risk for CHD.

Abstention from alcohol should be advised for individuals who cannot restrict their drinking to moderate levels; children and adolescents; individuals taking prescription or over-the-counter medications that can interact with alcohol; and individuals with medical problems such as liver disease, pancreatitis, advanced neuropathy, or severe hypertriglyceridemia. In addition, alcohol should be avoided by women who are pregnant or nursing or who are unsure if they are pregnant and by individuals who plan to drive, operate machinery, or take part in activities that require attention, skill, or coordination. Risk of unintentional injuries and breast and colon cancer should also be taken into consideration (DGAC Report 2010). No one should drink alcohol before driving.

The data do not support recommending alcohol consumption to individuals with or at risk for diabetes who do not currently drink (ADA 2008), since only observational and small clinical trials documenting the effects of alcohol are available. On the other hand, for many with diabetes, consumption of moderate amounts of alcohol does not need to be discouraged.

Table 4.3 Percentage and Grams of Alcohol and Calories in Alcoholic Beverages

	Standard Serving Size (fluid ounces)	Alcohol %	Alcohol Grams in One Serving	Carbohydrate Grams in One Serving	Calories in One Serving
Distilled spirits (gin, rum, vodka, whiskey), 80 proof	1.5	30	14	0	97
Beer, regular	12	4.6	13	13	146
Beer, light	12	4	11	5	99
Wines	5	9–20 (13 average)	14	2 (average)	123
Cocktails	2–6.5	33 (average)	18 (average)	Varies	124–175
Liqueurs	1.5	20–55	13	20 (varies)	186

If alcohol is consumed, it should be consumed in moderation and only by adults. The *Dietary Guidelines for Americans, 2010*, defines moderate alcohol consumption as *average* daily consumption of up to one drink per day for women and up to two drinks per day for men and no more than three drinks in any single day for women and no more than four drinks in any single day for men (DGAC Report 2010). They also advise to drink alcohol with food to slow alcohol absorption.

The type of alcohol-containing beverage consumed does not make a difference. Because alcohol does not affect blood glucose levels or require insulin to be metabolized, occasional use of alcoholic beverages can be considered an addition to the regular meal plan, and no food should be omitted. If consumed on a regular basis, calories from alcoholic beverages may need to be considered. Although regular beer does contain carbohydrate, because of the risk of hypoglycemia (likely due to reduced gluconeogenesis by alcohol), it is prudent that individuals not count the carbohydrate from alcohol when determining insulin boluses. Light beer may be a better choice. In addition, individuals with diabetes may not realize that wine and distilled spirits contain negligible amounts of carbohydrate.

For people using insulin or insulin secretagogues, alcohol should be consumed with food to prevent hypoglycemia. Evening consumption of alcohol by insulin users may increase the risk of nocturnal and fasting hypoglycemia. Hypoglycemia during the morning after consuming alcohol the evening before can be avoided by awakening at the usual time, eating a usual breakfast, and frequently testing blood glucose levels.

Drinking excessive amounts of alcohol and/or "binge" drinking can increase risk for lactic acidosis, which can be fatal. Although lactic acidosis associated with metformin is rare, patients who routinely drink more than moderate amounts of alcohol or with a history of binges of alcohol intake may not be good candidates for metformin therapy.

For all people with diabetes, meals and snacks should be eaten on time and selected with usual care. Alcohol can have a relaxing effect and may dull judgment. The decision to drink or not drink alcoholic beverages must be made by the individual with diabetes. Individuals should be educated about the effects of alcohol on metabolic parameters and health if they are to make the best decision for their health and well-being.

BIBLIOGRAPHY

Ahmed AT, Karter AJ, Liu J: Alcohol consumption is inversely associated with adherence to diabetes self-care behaviours. *Diabet Med* 23:795–802, 2006

Ahmed AT, Karter AJ, Warton M, Doan JU, Weisner CM: The relationship between alcohol consumption and glycemic control among patients with diabetes: the Kaiser Permanente Northern California Registry. *J Gen Intern Med* 23:275–282, 2008

Ajani UA, Gaziano M, Lotufo PA, Liu S, Hennekens CH, Buring JE, Manson JE: Alcohol consumption and risk of coronary heart disease by diabetes status. *Circulation* 102:500–505, 2000

American Diabetes Association: Nutrition recommendations and interventions for diabetes (Position Statement). *Diabetes Care* 31 (Suppl. 1):S61–S78, 2008

Avogaro A, Watanabe RM, Dall'Arche A, Kreutzenberg SVD, Tiengo A, Pacini G: Acute alcohol consumption improves insulin action without affecting insulin secretion in type 2 diabetic subjects. *Diabetes Care* 27:1369–1374, 2004

Bantle AE, Thomas W, Bantle JP: Metabolic effects of alcohol in the form of wine in persons with type 2 diabetes mellitus. *Metabolism* 57:241–245, 2008

Baraona E, Abittan CS, Dohmen K, Moretti M, Pozzato G, Chayes ZW, Schaefer C, Lieber CS: Gender differences in pharmacokinetics of alcohol. *Alcohol Clin Exp Res* 25:502–507, 2001

Beulens JWJ, Kruidhof JS, Grobbee DE, Chaturvedi N, Fuller JH, Soedamah-Muthu SS: Alcohol consumption and risk of microvascular complications in type 1 diabetes patients: the EURODIAB Prospective Complications Study. *Diabetologia* 51:1631–1638, 2008

Chait A, Mancini M, February AW, Lewis B: Clinical and metabolic study of alcoholic hyperlipidaemia. *Lancet* 2:62–64, 1972

Cheyne EH, Sherwin RS, Lunt MJ, Cavan DA, Thomas PW, Kerr D: Influence of alcohol on cognitive performance during milk hypoglycaemia; implications for type 1 diabetes. *Diabet Med* 21:230–237, 2004

Cooper DE, Goff DC, Bell RA, Zaccaro D, Mayer-Davis EJ, Karter AJ: Is insulin sensitivity a causal intermediate in the relationship between alcohol consumption and carotid atherosclerosis? *Diabetes Care* 25:1425–1431, 2002

Davies MJ, Baer DJ, Judd JT, Brown ED, Campbell WS, Taylor PR: Effects of moderate alcohol intake on fasting insulin and glucose concentrations and insulin sensitivity in postmenopausal women: a randomized controlled trial. *JAMA* 287:2559–2562, 2002

de Vegt F, Dekker JM, Groeneveld WJ, Nipels G, Stehouwer CD, Bouter LM, Heine RJ: Moderate alcohol consumption is associated with lower risk for incident diabetes and mortality: the Hoorn Study. *Diabetes Res Clin Pract* 57:53–60, 2002

Diem P, Deplazes M, Fajfr R, Bearth A, Muller B, Christ ER, Teuscher A: Effects of alcohol consumption on mortality in patients with type 2 diabetes mellitus. *Diabetologia* 46:1581–1585, 2003

Franz MJ: Alcohol and diabetes. In *American Diabetes Association Guide to Medical Nutrition Therapy for Diabetes*. Franz MJ, Bantle JP, Eds. Alexandria, VA, American Diabetes Association, 1999, p. 192–208

Frieberg MS, Cabral HJ, Heeren TC, Vasan RS, Ellison RC: Alcohol consumption and the prevalence of the metabolic syndrome in the U.S. *Diabetes Care* 27:2954–2959, 2004

Goodsell DS: The molecular perspective: alcohol. *Oncologist* 11:1045–1046, 2006

Howard AA, Amsten JH, Gourevitch MN: Effect of alcohol consumption on diabetes mellitus: a systemic review. *Ann Intern Med* 140:211–219, 2004

Kerr D, Cheyne E, Thomas P, Sherwin R: Influence of acute alcohol ingestion on the hormonal responses to modest hypoglycaemia in patients with type 1 diabetes. *Diabet Med* 24:312–316, 2007

Kerr D, Penfold S, Zouwail S, Thomas P, Begley J: The influence of liberal alcohol consumption on glucose metabolism in patients with type 1 diabetes: a pilot study. *Q J Med* 102:169–174, 2009

Koppes LLJ, Dekker JM, Hendriks HFJ, Bouter LM, Heine RJ: Meta-analysis of the relationship between alcohol consumption and coronary heart disease and mortality in type 2 diabetic patients. *Diabetologia* 49:648–652, 2006

Lee CC, Stolk RP, Adler AI, Patel A, Chalmers J, Neal B, Poulter N, Harrap S, Woodward M, Marre M, Grobbee DE, Beulens JW, on behalf of the AdRem project team and ADVANCE management committee: Association between alcohol consumption and diabetic retinopathy and visual acuity: the AdRem Study. *Diabet Med* 27:1130–1137, 2010

Lieber CS: Alcohol and the liver: 1994 update. *Gastroenterology* 106:1085–1105, 1994

Lieber CS: The metabolism of alcohol. *Sci Am* 234:25–33, 1976

Mackenzie T, Brooks B, O'Connor G: Beverage intake, diabetes, and glucose control in America. *Ann Epidemiol* 16:688–691, 2006

Marfella R, Cacciapuoti F, Siniscalchi M, Sasso FC, Marchese F, Cinone F, Musacchio E, Marfella A, Ruggiero L, Chiorazzo G, Liberti D, Chiorazzo G, Nicoletti GF, Saron C, D'Andrea F, Ammendola C, Verza M, Coppola L: Effect of moderate red wine intake on cardiac prognosis after recent myocardial infarction of subjects with type 2 diabetes mellitus. *Diabet Med* 23:974–981, 2006

Miller M, Stone NJ, Ballantyne C, Bittner V, Criqui MH, Ginsberg HN, Goldberg AC, Howard WJ, Jacobson MS, Kris-Etherton PM, Lennie TA, Levi M, Mazzone T, Pennathur S: Triglycerides and cardiovascular disease: a scientific statement from the American Heart Association. *Circulation* 123:2292–2333, 2011

Nanchahal K, Ashton WD, Wood DA: Alcohol consumption, metabolic cardiovascular risk factors and hypertension in women. *Int J Epidemiol* 29:57–64, 2000

Pitsavos C, Makrilakis K, Panagiotakos DB, Chrysohoou C, Ioannidis I, Dimosthenopoulos C, Stefanadis C, Katsilambros N: The J-shape effect of alcohol intake on the risk of developing acute coronary syndromes in diabetic subjects: the CARDIO2000 II Study. *Diabet Med* 22:243–248, 2005

Pownall HJ, Ballantyne CM, Kimball KT, Simpson SL, Yeshurun D, Gotto AM Jr: Effect of moderate alcohol consumption on hypertriglyceridemia. *Arch Intern Med* 159:982–987, 1999

Rasmussen BM, Christiansen C, Rasmussen OW, Hansen C, Hermansen K: Alcohol and postexercise metabolic responses in type 2 diabetes. *Metabolism* 48:597–602, 1999

Rasmussen BM, Orskov L, Schmitz O, Hermansen K: Alcohol and glucose counterregulation among acute insulin-induced hypoglycemia in type 2 diabetic subjects. *Metabolism* 50:451–457, 2001

Report of the Dietary Guidelines Advisory Committee on the Dietary Guidelines for Americans, 2010. Available at: http://www.cnpp.usda.gov/dgas2010-dgacreport.htm

Richardson T, Weiss M, Thomas P, Kerr D: Day after the night before: influence of evening alcohol on risk of hypoglycemia in patients with type 1 diabetes. *Diabetes Care* 28:1801–1802, 2005

Rimm EB, Williams P, Fosher K, Criqui M, Stampfer MJ: Moderate alcohol intake and lower risk of coronary heart disease: meta-analysis of effects on lipids and haemostatic factors. *BMJ* 319:1523–1528, 1999

Schaller G, Kretschmer S, Gouya G, Haider DG, Mittermayer F, Riedl M, Wagner O, Pacini G, Wolzt M, Ludvik B: Alcohol acutely increases vascular reactivity together with insulin sensitivity in type 2 diabetic men. *Exp Clin Endocrinol Diabetes* 118:57–60, 2010

Shai I, Rimm EB, Schulze MB, Rifai N, Stampfer MJ, Hu FB: Moderate alcohol intake and markers of inflammation and endothelial dysfunction among diabetic men. *Diabetologia* 47:1760–1767, 2004

Shai I, Wainstein J, Harman-Boehm I, Raz I, Fraser D, Rudich A, Stampfer MJ: Glycemic effect of moderate alcohol intake among patients with type 2 diabetes: a multicenter, randomized, clinical intervention trial. *Diabetes Care* 30:3011–3016, 2007

Solomon CG, Hu FB, Stampfer MJ, Colditz GA, Speizer FE, Rimm EB, Willett WC, Manson JE: Moderate alcohol consumption and risk of coronary heart disease among women with type 2 diabetes. *Circulation* 102:494–499, 2000

Tanasescu M, Hu FB: Alcohol consumption and risk of coronary heart disease among individuals with type 2 diabetes. *Curr Diab Rep* 1:187–191 2001a

Tanasescu M, Hu FB, Willett WC, Stampfer MJ, Rimm EB: Alcohol consumption and risk of coronary heart disease among men with type 2 diabetes mellitus. *J Am Coll Cardiol* 38:1836–1842, 2001b

Turner BC, Jenkins E, Kerr D, Sherwin RS, Cavan DA: The effect of evening alcohol consumption on next-morning glucose control in type 1 diabetes. *Diabetes Care* 24:1888–1893, 2001

Umpierrez GE, DiGirolamo M, Tuvlin JA, Isaacs SD, Bhoola SM, Kokko JP: Differences in metabolic and hormonal milieu in diabetic- and alcohol-induced ketoacidosis. *J Crit Care* 15:52–59, 2000

Valmadrid CT, Klein R, Moss SE, Klein BE, Cruickshanks KJ: Alcohol intake and the risk of coronary heart disease mortality in persons with older-onset diabetes mellitus. *JAMA* 282:239–246, 1999

van de Wiel A: Diabetes mellitus and alcohol. *Diabetes Metab Res Rev* 20:263–267, 2004

Wakabayashi I, Kobaba-Wakabayashi R, Masuda H: Relation of drinking alcohol to atherosclerotic risk in type 2 diabetes. *Diabetes Care* 25:1223–1228, 2002

Marion J. Franz, MS, RD, CDE, is a Nutrition/Health Consultant at Nutrition Concepts by Franz, Inc., Minneapolis, MN.

Chapter 5
Nutrition Therapy for Adults with Type 1 and Insulin-Requiring Type 2 Diabetes

Alison B. Evert, MS, RD, CDE

Highlights

Insulin Therapy

Nutrition Therapy for Type 1 Diabetes and Insulin-Requiring Type 2 Diabetes

Summary

Highlights
Nutrition Therapy for Adults with Type 1 and Insulin-Requiring Type 2 Diabetes

■ Carbohydrate intake and available insulin are the primary determinants of postprandial glucose levels. Management of carbohydrate intake is therefore a primary strategy for achieving glycemic control.

■ Adjusting prandial insulin doses to match desired carbohydrate intake (using a meal-planning approach such as carbohydrate counting) in people with type 1 diabetes results in improved glycemic control.

■ For individuals using fixed daily insulin doses, carbohydrate intake on a day-to-day basis should be kept consistent with respect to time and amount.

■ Prandial and blood glucose correction insulin-dosing algorithms may help people with type 1 and insulin-requiring type 2 diabetes to achieve glycemic control when using flexible intensive insulin therapy.

■ Timing of prandial insulin dose 15–20 min before initiation of the meal may help to reduce postprandial hyperglycemia.

■ Postprandial hyperglycemia and glucose variability occur frequently in people with diabetes, and this result may convey increased risk of cardiovascular morbidity and mortality. Nutrition therapy interventions may help to reduce postprandial hyperglycemia and reduce glycemic variability.

Nutrition Therapy for Adults with Type 1 and Insulin-Requiring Type 2 Diabetes

Nutrition therapy plays an integral role in the treatment and self-management of type 1 diabetes and insulin-requiring type 2 diabetes. The Centers for Disease Control and Prevention (CDC) estimates that 25.8 million people are affected by diabetes. Out of these people, 12% of adults with diagnosed diabetes (type 1 or type 2) are treated with insulin and an additional 14% take insulin and oral medication(s) (CDC 2011).

For centuries, the only therapeutic option for type 1 diabetes was "starvation diets"; thankfully, this strategy was ultimately short-lived. After 1922, insulin became available and, in the 1980s, the technology for self-monitoring blood glucose (SMBG). However, despite all the advances in the treatment of insulin-requiring diabetes, nutrition therapy continues to be a difficult strategy for individuals to implement. For the individual with type 1 (or type 2) diabetes, learning how to administer an injection of insulin is a skill that is often quickly mastered, whereas mastering the ability to "count carbohydrates" and match insulin to food intake is usually more difficult.

There are two types of normal physiological insulin secretion: continuous basal insulin secretion and incremental prandial insulin secretion, controlling meal-related glucose excursions. People with type 1 and insulin-requiring type 2 diabetes lack both basal and meal-related prandial secretion. Historically, conventional treatment included predetermined or "fixed" insulin doses and following a rigid calorie- and carbohydrate-controlled meal plan based on the insulin regimen. Some people with type 1 and insulin-requiring diabetes still use this method for a variety of reasons, such as age, cost, fewer required injections, lack of access to insulin analogs, personal preference, or prescribing habits of the health care provider.

In the 1990s, the Diabetes Control and Complications Trial (DCCT) showed unequivocally that intensive insulin therapy using multiple daily injections reduced the risk of complications when compared to conventional treatment (DCCT 1993). Improved glycemic control was achieved through an intensive program of multiple daily insulin injections (at least three injections per day) or the use of an insulin pump. Intensive insulin therapy DCCT participants performed SMBG (four times per day) and were taught how to adjust their insulin using treatment algorithms based on glucose test results, food choices, and physical activity. Carbohydrate counting was used as one of the meal-planning approaches and was found to be effective in helping people achieve glycemic control (DCCT 1993).

Outside of the United States, flexible intensive insulin therapy (FIIT) for the management of type 1 diabetes was developed in Düsseldorf in the late 1970s (Mühlhauser 1983). FIIT is now taught as a part of many structured education programs, such as the Dose Adjustment for Normal Eating (DAFNE) course in the United Kingdom and in Australia (DAFNE 2002; Lowe 2008).

Both the DCCT and DAFNE research trials involved frequent follow-up with members of the diabetes team that included registered dietitians (RDs) and nurses to assist the person with diabetes on an ongoing basis to adjust insulin doses (DCCT 1993; DAFNE 2002). The improvements in blood glucose were the result of physiological insulin replacement combined with self-management of insulin dose adjustment in conjunction with a "flexible" meal-planning approach such as carbohydrate counting. Excellent reviews are available to guide insulin initiation and management of insulin therapy to achieve optimal glycemic control; therefore, this topic will not be extensively reviewed here (DeWitt 2003; Mooradian 2006).

The chapter begins with a review of the literature pertaining to insulin dose algorithms, especially as they relate to insulin-to-carbohydrate ratios, timing of prandial insulin doses, and factors contributing to postprandial hyperglycemia. Nutrition therapy using carbohydrate-counting meal-planning approaches is reviewed and incorporates research published after 1 September 2009.

INSULIN THERAPY

Insulin-Dosing Algorithms

Since the advent of basal-bolus insulin therapy and SMBG, there has been interest in developing insulin-dosing algorithms for the self-adjustment of insulin therapy, and a variety of formulas or "rules" have been developed (Skyler 1981; Palerm 2007). Prandial dosing algorithms are commonly referred to as an insulin-to-carbohydrate ratio (ICR), and blood glucose correction algorithms are frequently referred as an insulin sensitivity factor (ISF). Guidelines also exist for estimating basal insulin as a fraction of the total daily dose (TDD) (see Table 5.1 for definitions of basal-bolus insulin terms).

The "1500 rule" for blood glucose correction was an original formula based on informal clinical observations using regular insulin by Davidson and his colleagues in 1982 (Table 5.2) (Davidson 2008). In 1998, Davidson and colleagues developed a formula for the ICR, and in 2008, they published a paper on how their mathematical models for basal-bolus insulin-dosing guidelines in patients with type 1 diabetes were derived from a retrospective controlled study (Davidson 2008). The goal of their analysis was to determine how best to prescribe insulin for use in continuous subcutaneous insulin infusion (CSII) pump therapy in their large endocrine practice. These formulae were statistically correlated and are referred to as the Accurate Insulin Management (AIM) formulae (Davidson 2002; Davidson 2003). The AIM system guidelines are based on the TDD. If the TDD is not available, the AIM system includes an additional formula to estimate TDD based on body weight in pounds (Table 5.2).

In 1990, Howorka and colleagues also developed prandial algorithms (meal-related and correctional insulin doses for blood glucose increases induced by car-

Table 5.1 Basal-Bolus Insulin Therapy Terms

- **Physiological insulin replacement:** The insulin secretion of normally functioning β-cells is mimicked with prandial (mealtime) or "bolus" insulin and long-acting or "basal" insulin.

- **Basal insulin:** Basal insulin represents the level of insulin always present in fasting and postmeal states. Basal insulin suppresses excess gluconeogenesis and the release of free fatty acids and enables the glucose transport in the fasting state. Insulin glargine and detemir are examples of "basal" insulin and are essentially peakless. Neutral protamine Hagedorn (NPH) can also be used as a basal insulin, but it has a pronounced peak. Basal insulin delivery can also be delivered via an insulin pump using either rapid- or short-acting insulin (see examples listed under "Bolus insulin" below). Basal insulin typically represents ~50% of the TDD insulin required each day.

- **Bolus insulin:** Rapid-acting insulin (lispro, aspart, and glulisine) or short-acting insulin (regular) can be used at mealtimes and/or to correct an elevated blood glucose level. In the case of rapid-acting insulin, onset is typically 5–15 min and peak action is at 30–90 min after injection. The duration of rapid-acting insulin is ~4–6 h in most people. This is the "other" 50% of the TDD insulin required each day.

- **Total daily dose (TDD):** TDD is the total number of units taken each day to achieve desirable blood glucose control. This number includes basal insulin plus bolus insulin used to "cover" the carbohydrates consumed at meals and the blood glucose correction needs.

PRANDIAL INSULIN:

- **ICR or carbohydrate factor (CarbF):** This ratio indicates how many grams of carbohydrate are "covered" or "matched" by 1 unit rapid- or short-acting insulin. The ICR is related to an individual's insulin sensitivity and body size. An ICR for an adult with type 1 diabetes is typically 1:10 (1 unit of rapid-acting insulin is needed to "match" 10 g carbohydrate), whereas an obese person might require an ICR of 1:5 (1 unit of rapid-acting insulin to "match" 5 g carbohydrate due to insulin resistance).

GLUCOSE CORRECTION INSULIN:

- **ISF or glucose correction factor (CorrF or CF):** The ISF can be defined as the estimated drop in blood glucose (mg/dL) expected from the administration of 1 unit of rapid- or short-acting insulin. ISF is also related to the individual's insulin sensitivity and body size. A typical ISF for an adult with type 1 diabetes is typically 1:50 mg/dL (1 unit of rapid-acting insulin will drop the blood glucose level 50 mg/dL). However, an overweight/insulin-resistant person may have an ISF of 1:20 mg/dL (1 unit rapid-acting insulin will drop the blood glucose level 20 mg/dL).

---

bohydrate) for personalized adjustment with flexible insulin dosing (Table 5.3) (Howorka 1990). These formulae are still used by some researchers outside the U.S. In an observational study of 35 patients with type 1 diabetes using the Howorka flexible intensive insulin therapy algorithms, the authors concluded that use of these individualized parameters permitted fast and accurate adjustment of insulin doses (Franc 2009). Howorka also proposed additional algorithms for protein/fat in meals low in carbohydrate. However, the protein/fat algorithms have not been extensively studied, and patients are not being taught to use these currently in clinical practice. Another researcher proposed the addition of 1 unit of insulin per 20 g protein (Sachon 2003).

Table 5.2 Insulin Dosing Formula or "Rules"

Formula or rule	Accurate insulin management formula (Davidson 2008)	500 rule and 1800 rule, using rapid-acting insulin (Walsh 2003) 450 rule and 1500 rule, using regular insulin (Walsh 1994)
Prandial insulin Carbohydrate-to-insulin ratio (CIR)/ICR or carbohydrate factor (CarbF)	CIR = 2.8 × BWlb/TDD For example: if TDD = 50 units 2.8 × 180 lbs/50 = 10 CIR = 1:10 1 unit of rapid-acting insulin will "match" 10 g carbohydrate	If using the 500 rule: 500/TDD For example: if the TDD = 50 units 500/50 = 10 CarbF = 1:10 1 unit of rapid-acting insulin will "match" 10 g carbohydrate
Glucose correction insulin Glucose correction factor (CF) or (CorrF)	CF = 1,700/TDD For example: if the TDD = 34 units 1700/34 = 50 mg/dL CF = 1:50 1 unit of rapid-acting insulin will "lower" blood glucose 50 mg/dL	If using the 1800 rule: 1800/TDD For example: if the TDD = 36 units 1800/36 = 50 mg/dL CorrF = 1:50 1 unit rapid-acting insulin will "lower" blood glucose 50 mg/dL
Basal insulin	Basal units/day = 0.47 × TDD	Basal dose/day = 0.50 × TDD
TDD	TDD = 0.24 × BWlb	Five-step process: dose based on process of SMBG, varies based on weight, levels of fitness and stress, and special conditions
Comments	Mathematical models statistically correlated based on data from large endocrine practice (two groups analyzed: well-controlled test group [*n* = 167], A1C ≤7%, on pump >180 days; and control group [*n* = 209], A1C >7%, on pump <180 days) (Davidson 2008)	1500 rule derived from Davidson 2002; 450 rule and 500 rule based on clinical experience (Walsh 1994; Walsh 2003)

Adapted from Davidson 2008; Walsh 2003; and Walsh 1994. BWlb, body weight in pounds.

Other researchers also determined ICR through use of the hyperinsulinemic-euglycemic clamp with a meal challenge to determine a prandial dosing algorithm in people with type 1 diabetes (Bevier 2007). In 1994, based on clinical experience, a carbohydrate factor formula was introduced: a "450 rule" for multiple daily injection and CSII patients (Walsh 1994). An updated carbohydrate factor formula and a glucose correction factor formula were published in the consumer book *Using Insulin* (Table 5.2) (Walsh 2003). The authors have further refined

Table 5.3 Howorka Algorithms for Flexible Insulin Therapy

Insulin sensitivity coefficient K = $\dfrac{\text{current total insulin requirement}}{\text{theoretical (prandial + basal) insulin}}$

Theoretical basal insulin requirement = 0.35 units/kg (body weight)

Theoretical prandial insulin requirement = [average daily carbohydrate (g)/20] × 2.2

Prandial insulin and correction of abnormal blood glucose (BG) values

Insulin requirement for one 20-g carbohydrate portion = 2.2 × K

1 unit extra short-acting insulin BG-lowering effect: ΔBG (mmol/L) = –1.94 × 1/K × 60/kg

BG increase induced by one 20-g carbohydrate portion: ΔBG (mmol/L) = 4.44 × 60/kg
Basal insulin requirement = 0.35 units/kg × K

An additional algorithm for protein/fat was proposed by Howorka (1990) for meals low in carbohydrate: 0.45 units/100-kcal protein or fat × K

Adapted for 20-g carbohydrate portions at mealtime. Blood glucose units are in mmol/L. To convert to mg/dL, multiply mmol/L by 18.

Adapted from Howorka 1990.

their formula after analyzing anonymous consecutive downloads from 1,020 pumps collected during a routine pump software upgrade in 2007 (Walsh 2010).

It should be noted that a majority of these popular ICR and ISF formulae were derived from patient populations using CSII with well-controlled blood glucose levels, not multiple daily injections. The authors of the AIM system recommend use of their formula for patients with type 1 diabetes, noting that only one person with insulin-requiring type 2 diabetes was included in their data analysis (Davidson 2008).

Timing of Prandial Insulin Dose

DeWitt and Hirsch described the term "lag time" in their reviews of outpatient insulin therapy in type 1 and type 2 diabetes (Hirsch 2005a; DeWitt 2003). Lag time is defined as the amount of time that elapses between the prandial insulin injection and a meal; lag time is critical in the control of postprandial hyperglycemia and in later risk of hypoglycemia. Given the pharmacodynamics of insulin analogs, sufficient lag time helps to decrease postprandial hyperglycemia (Rassam 1999). The use of lag time for rapid-acting insulin and improved matching action with carbohydrate absorption explains their clinical advantage (DeWitt 2003). In the pre-analog era, it was recommended to administer regular insulin ~20–30 min before eating a meal. With the introduction of rapid-acting insulin analogs, many physicians recommended injection of the prandial dose just before eating, or even after eating. However, these recommendations are not supported by the insulin action times reported by the insulin manufacturers (Hirsch 2005a). The insulin action times of the currently available rapid-acting insulin analogs are as follows: onset 5–15 min, a peak between 30 to 90 min, and duration of ~4–6 h.

A study designed to determine the most effective timing of rapid-acting insulin analog (Novorapid®) with CSII in children with type 1 diabetes reported that glucose levels 3 h after the meal were lower when the prandial insulin was administered 15 min or immediately before the meal, rather than after the meal (Scaramuzza 2010). Also demonstrated was a significant difference in 1-h postprandial glucose levels, which were significantly higher when the prandial insulin was given after the meal and lowest when the insulin was administered 15 min before the meal. This result occurred even if the blood glucose was in the hypoglycemic range before eating.

Subjects with type 1 diabetes using CSII participated in a crossover study consisting of three treatment arms: delivering rapid-acting insulin analog (glulisine) 20 min before a meal, immediately before the meal, and 20 min after the meal initiation (Cobry 2010). At both 60 and 120 min after meal initiation, the 20-min before-meal insulin arm showed significantly lower glycemic excursions than when the prandial insulin was given immediately before the meal. Glycemic area under the curve was significantly less in the before-meal insulin group than in both the immediately before- or after-meal initiation groups. The authors concluded that although delivering the prandial dose of insulin 20 min before the meal may be inconvenient, it is an important strategy that can result in a reduction of postprandial glucose levels over 180 mg/dL.

Another trial assessed the effect of the rapid-acting insulin analog (aspart) timing on postprandial glucose levels in subjects with type 1 diabetes using CSII when the prandial insulin was administered at 30, 15, or 0 min before mealtime (Luijf 2010). The administration of the prandial insulin 15 min before mealtime resulted in lower postprandial glucose excursions and more time spent in desirable ranges without an increase in hypoglycemia.

Data from these three small studies argue for administration of rapid-acting insulin analogs 15–20 min before the start of the meal. However, larger trials outside the clinical research center are needed to confirm these findings. Tridgell and colleagues proposed progressively longer lag times for rapid-acting prandial and correction dose insulin depending on the degree of hyperglycemia (Tridgell 2010) (see Table 5.4 for lag times for prandial insulin).

When recommending preprandial times, clinical judgment is required in specific patient populations such as young children or the elderly, who do not have predictable food intake (Tridgell 2010). It may be appropriate to give these individuals the dose of prandial insulin during the meal or immediately after the meal to reduce the risk of hypoglycemia. In addition, individuals with delayed gastric emptying may benefit from administration of rapid-acting insulin at the end of the meal or the use of regular insulin 30 min before the start of the meal (see Chapter 18, Nutrition Therapy for Diabetic Gastropathy).

If hypoglycemia is determined before the start of a meal, the individual should treat the low glucose level with a carbohydrate food, inject the prandial insulin, and then eat (Scaramuzza 2010). Others have suggested treating the hypoglycemia and delaying the prandial injection for a brief time (Trigdell 2010). On the basis of clinical experience, the individual could additionally be advised to reduce the prandial insulin dose or instructed to increase carbohydrate food consumed at the meal.

Table 5.4 Recommended Insulin Lag Times for Rapid-Acting Insulin Based on Degree of Preprandial Hyperglycemia

Preprandial Blood Glucose (mg/dL)	Lag Times (min)
80–99	0
100–199	10–20
200–299	20–30
≥300	30–40

Adapted from Tridgell 2010.

Postprandial Glycemic Control and Diabetes Complications

Diabetes management decisions have traditionally been made using fasting and premeal blood glucose measurements as well as A1C test results. This approach has left many people with diabetes with suboptimal glycemic control because of inadequate control of postprandial hyperglycemia. Postprandial glucose excursions and postprandial hyperglycemia occur frequently in people with diabetes, even when A1C may be <7%, and this result may convey increased risk of cardiovascular morbidity and mortality (Ceriello 2005; Home 2005). Advocates of postprandial monitoring propose that it is critical to the establishment of good glycemic control (Hirsch 2005b; Tridgell 2010), whereas others are not convinced that postprandial SMBG is essential (Buse 2003).

Some surrogate measures of vascular pathology, such as endothelial dysfunction, are negatively affected by postprandial hyperglycemia (American Diabetes Association [ADA] 2012; Ceriello 2002). The mechanisms through which postprandial hyperglycemia exerts its effects may be related to the production of free radicals, which in turn can induce endothelial dysfunction and inflammation (Ceriello 2006).

It has been proposed that dysglycemia of patients with diabetes is the sum of the two following disorders: *1*) sustained chronic elevations of glucose and *2*) glycemic variability with its main component of postprandial excursions (Monnier 2003). Glucose variability not only includes upward acute fluctuations (postprandial excursions), but also includes downward changes (i.e., decreases from either baseline or interprandial concentrations to glucose nadirs) and is also associated with activation of oxidative stress, one of the main mechanisms leading to diabetes complications (Brownlee 2006). It is therefore suggested that both glycemic variability and postprandial excursions should be monitored and managed in people with diabetes.

In addition, in people with type 2 diabetes, it was reported that there is a progressive shift in the respective contributions of fasting and postprandial hyperglycemia when patients progress from moderate to high hyperglycemia, with the contribution of postprandial glucose excursions being predominant in patients with moderate diabetes. In addition, the contribution of fasting hyperglycemia increases with worsening diabetes (Monnier 2003). The results of the Monnier study suggest that as the patient gets closer to A1C goals of 7%, more attention must be given to reducing postprandial hyperglycemia. Therefore, effective management of diabetes must also include control of postprandial glucose levels, with current guidelines recommending postprandial blood glucose levels <180 mg/dL (ADA 2012).

Other Diabetes Medications for Treating Postprandial Hyperglycemia

People with type 2 as well as type 1 diabetes may have significant postprandial hyperglycemia because of a rapid influx of glucose from the gut (resulting from increased gastric motility), impaired insulin release, excess hepatic glucose production (from inappropriate elevations in glucagon), and insulin resistance (Sudhir 2002). Nine distinct classes of medications are now available for treatment of diabetes in the U.S. and six specifically affect postprandial hyperglycemia: meglitinides, α-glucosidase inhibitors, incretin mimetics, an amylin analog, dipeptidyl peptidase-4 inhibitors, and insulin. Two of these classes of medications, the incretin mimetics (exenatide and liraglutide) and the amylin analog (pramlintide), in addition to their ability to treat these numerous abnormalities, are also associated with modest weight loss (Garber 2011; Nathan 2009).

NUTRITION THERAPY FOR TYPE 1 DIABETES AND INSULIN-REQUIRING TYPE 2 DIABETES

The ADA published nutrition recommendations and interventions in 2008 (ADA 2008). These recommendations are integrated into their annual standards of medical care and updated as new evidence becomes available (ADA 2012). In addition, in 2008, the Academy of Nutrition and Dietetics (formerly the American Dietetic Association) (Acad Nutr Diet) published evidence-based nutrition practice guidelines (EBNPG) for adults with type 1 and type 2 diabetes in the Acad Nut Diet Evidence Analysis Library (EAL) (Acad Nutr Diet 2008). Subsequently, a review of the research leading to the EBNPG and a summary of the research published after the completion of the EAL (through 1 September 2009) were published (Franz 2010).

To update this chapter, a literature search was conducted using PubMed MEDLINE for research published after 2009 on nutrition therapy for insulin-requiring adult patients. Search criteria included the following: carbohydrate counting, medical nutrition therapy, dietary therapy, healthy eating, nutrition counseling, nutrition education, glycemic index, glycemic load or treatment research in human subjects with type 1 diabetes, and English language articles. Study design preferences were randomized controlled trials, clinical controlled studies, large nonrandomized observational studies, cohort studies, or case-controlled studies. The literature search identified 251 articles. Fifteen articles were retrieved for more detailed evaluation, and two articles were identified from reference lists. Of these, 10 met inclusion criteria and are included in Table 5.5.

Table 5.5 Studies on Nutrition Therapy for Adults with Type 1 Diabetes: Carbohydrate-Counting Meal-Planning Approach

	Population/ Duration of Study	Intervention (type of study)	Major Findings	Comments
Speight 2010	n = 88 adults with type 1 diabetes (DAFNE trial participants)/4 years	Evaluated A1C and QoL 44 months after DAFNE education course (prospective cohort study)	A1C: ↓ from baseline, 9.32 → 8.96 (P < 0.01); QoL: −1.78 vs. −4.27 at baseline (P < 0.0001)	Impact of single education course on glycemic control and QoL remains long term
Rossi 2010	n = 130 adults with type 1 diabetes/6 months	DID (CHO/insulin dose bolus calculator in mobile phone with text messages between patient and physician) vs. control (CHO-counting standard approach) (RCT)	A1C: DID 8.2% → 7.8%, control 8.4% → 7.9% (P = 0.68); DID: 6 h education, control 12 h; DID: less weight gain; DID improved treatment satisfaction and some aspects of QoL	DID at least as effective as traditional CHO counting education
Dias 2010	n = 51 adults with type 1 diabetes/3 months	Evaluated use of CHO counting and insulin dose (1 unit regular/15 g CHO) (clinical trial)	A1C: from baseline 10.40% → 9.52% (P = 0.000); insulin dose: from baseline 0.99 IU/kg → 1.05 (P = 0.003); BMI: from baseline nonsignificant	Used fixed doses of regular insulin, fixed meal plan, did not use SMBG
Ahola 2010	n = 331 adults with type 1 diabetes (average duration 32 years)/one meal randomized for analyses	Patients completed self-administered 3-day food (CHO g)/physical activity/insulin dose/SMBG records (case study)	64% of patients estimated prandial insulin need inappropriately	Estimation of prandial insulin dose not easy, even after long duration of diabetes
Scavone 2010	n = 256 adults with type 1 diabetes/9 months	Group A: multi-disciplinary team taught patients CHO counting (ICR), insulin dose adjustment, and SMBG 6 times/day vs. Group B: control (RCT)	A1C: Group A 7.8% → 7.4%; Group B 7.5% → 7.5% (P < 0.01); hypoglycemic events: 4% vs. 7% (P < 0.05)	Author conclusions: Group A: increases expense and risk of non-compliance (27% of 100 patients did not complete second phase)

Table 5.5 Studies on Nutrition Therapy for Adults with Type 1 Diabetes: Carbohydrate-Counting Meal-Planning Approach (*continued*)

	Population/ Duration of Study	Intervention (type of study)	Major Findings	Comments
Lawton 2011	$n = 30$ adults with type 1 diabetes/6 and 12 months after DAFNE course	Semi-structured interviews of patients in FIIT program (qualitative longitudinal study)	Despite potential of FIIT to increase flexibility, adoption increased diet rigidity	Concerns that FIIT may result in more excessive or unhealthy eating were unfounded
Laurenzi 2011	$n = 61$ adults with type 1 diabetes using CSII/24 weeks	Treatment group (CHO counting [ICR], ISF, SMBG [6 times/ day]) vs. control (estimating premeal insulin in usual way) (RCT)	Treatment vs. control: QoL score ↑ ($P = 0.008$), BMI ↓ ($P = 0.003$), waist circumference ↓ ($P = 0.002$); A1C ↓ (-0.35%, $P = 0.05$)	CHO counting safe and improves QoL, ↓ BMI, waist circumference, and A1C in patients who used CHO counting and CSII
Rankin 2011	$n = 30$ adults with type 1 diabetes/6 and 12 months after DAFNE course	Semi-structured interviews of participants in FIIT program (qualitative longitudinal study)	Patients committed to and wanted to sustain FIIT when patients had stable routines	Follow-up support should encourage patients to identify routines to better integrate FIIT into lives
Casey 2011	$n = 40$ adults with type 1 diabetes/6 and 12 months after course	Semi-structured interviews of participants in DAFNE program (qualitative longitudinal study)	Factors that influence ability to self-manage diabetes over time: embedded knowledge, enduring motivation, continued support, and being empowered	Support at 6 months was found to be crucial for continued motivation
Bao 2011	$n = 28$ adults using CSII with type 1 diabetes/1 week	CHO counting vs. novel food insulin index algorithm to estimate prandial insulin dose (crossover, clinical trial)	Food insulin index algorithm ↓ glucose area under the curve over 3 h (-52%, $P = 0.013$), peak BG (-41%, $P = 0.01$), and improved % of time within normal BG range (31%, $P = 0.001$) compared to CHO counting	Food insulin index algorithm derived from healthy individuals may be a useful tool; currently only 120 foods in food insulin index database

BG, blood glucose; CHO, carbohydrate; DID, Diabetes Interactive Diary (telemedicine system); QoL, quality of life; RCT, randomized controlled trial.

Nutrition Therapy Interventions

Based on the results of the DCCT, ADA recommends intensive insulin therapy for type 1 diabetes, using basal and bolus insulin to reproduce or mimic normal physiological insulin secretion: *1*) use of multiple-dose insulin injections (three to four injections per day of basal and prandial insulin) or insulin pump therapy; *2*) matching prandial insulin-to-carbohydrate intake, premeal blood glucose, and anticipated activity; and *3*) for many people (especially if hypoglycemia is a problem), use of insulin analogs (ADA 2012). The use of basal and prandial insulin replaces insulin in a way that closely approximates normal physiological patterns.

Insulin therapy should be integrated into the individual's usual eating and physical activity pattern; individuals using rapid-acting insulin by injection or insulin pump should adjust the meal and snack insulin doses on the basis of carbohydrate content of the meals and snacks. In individuals using fixed daily doses, carbohydrate intake on a day-to-day basis should be kept consistent with respect to time and amount. For planned exercise, insulin doses can be adjusted; for unplanned exercise, extra carbohydrate may be needed (ADA 2008).

Achieving nutrition-related goals requires a coordinated team effort that includes the person with diabetes and involves the patient in the decision-making process. Because of the complexity of nutrition issues, it is recommended that an RD who is knowledgeable and skilled in implementing nutrition therapy into diabetes management and education be the team member who plays the leading role in providing nutrition therapy (ADA 2012). However, all team members, including physicians and nurses, should be knowledgeable about nutrition therapy and support its implementation (ADA 2008).

The Acad Nutr Diet EBNPG state the following: "Medical nutrition therapy (MNT) plays a crucial role in managing diabetes and reducing the potential complications related to poor glycemic, lipid, and blood pressure control" (Franz 2010; Acad Nutr Diet 2008). Carbohydrate intake and available insulin are the primary determinants of postprandial glucose levels. Therefore, management of carbohydrate intake is the primary strategy for achieving glycemic control. For individuals who adjust mealtime (prandial) insulin or who are on CSII, insulin doses should be adjusted to match carbohydrate intake (ICRs). Comprehensive nutrition education and counseling should be provided that includes instruction on interpretation of blood glucose monitoring patterns and nutrition-related medication management. Specifically, people using "flexible" insulin dosing to manage their diabetes need to understand the relationship and coordination of their basal-bolus insulin plan (insulin action) with the blood glucose–raising effect of their carbohydrate intake.

In people with type 1 (or type 2) diabetes using "fixed" insulin doses, meal and snack carbohydrate intake should be consistently distributed throughout the day on a daily basis, since consistency in carbohydrate has been shown to result in improved glycemic control (Acad Nutr Diet 2008). It is recommended that individuals using "fixed" daily doses of insulin use a carbohydrate-counting meal-planning approach or some other method of quantifying carbohydrate intake to maintain day-to-day consistency, both in the timing and quantity of food intake.

Food Factors Affecting Glycemic Control

There is more to controlling postprandial hyperglycemia than knowing how to "count carbohydrates." Many people with type 1 (and type 2) diabetes struggle to comprehend how their blood glucose levels can dramatically fluctuate on a daily basis despite eating the same number of grams of carbohydrate at meals.

One reason may be a lack of adequate education on how to accurately dose prandial insulin and quantify carbohydrate intake (Boukhors 2003). The CDC reports that only 55.7% of people with diabetes participate in a diabetes self-management education class, suggesting that many people with type 1 (and type 2) are never formally instructed on a meal-planning approach, such as carbohydrate counting, to enable them to accurately quantify their carbohydrate intake (CDC 2011). Consequently, these individuals may either underdose or overdose prandial insulin requirements. Accurate dosing of prandial insulin to actual food (grams of carbohydrate) intake is a key component of basal-bolus insulin therapy.

Another reason may be that in addition to determining the number of grams of carbohydrate consumed at meals, several extrinsic and intrinsic variables may influence the impact of carbohydrates on the postprandial response (ADA 2008). Extrinsic variables that may influence glucose response include macronutrient distribution of the meal, fasting or preprandial blood glucose level, available insulin, antecedent exercise, and degree of insulin resistance.

Intrinsic variables that influence the effect of the carbohydrate-containing foods on blood glucose response include type and source of carbohydrate, the physical form of the food (e.g., whole food versus juice), type of starch (e.g., amylopectin versus amylose), method of food preparation (e.g., baking versus frying), cooking time and amount of heat and moisture used, degree of processing, and ripeness of food (ADA 2008). Individuals can use information from SMBG and continuous glucose sensors to learn how specific foods affect their glycemic control.

Meal-Planning Approaches and Tools

Type 1 diabetes. Meal-planning approaches other than carbohydrate counting, such as the glycemic index, also have been studied. A food insulin index, a physiological basis for ranking foods according to insulin "demand," was developed by a group of researchers in Australia for 120 single foods (Bao 2009). They concluded that the relative insulin demand evoked by mixed meals consumed by lean healthy subjects is best predicted by a physiological index (food insulin index) based on integrating insulin responses to isoenergetic portions of single foods and that eating patterns that provoke less insulin secretion may be helpful in preventing and managing diabetes. In 2011, Bao compared a novel algorithm based on the food insulin index for estimating mealtime insulin dose with carbohydrate counting in adults with type 1 diabetes using CSII (Bao 2011). They concluded that when compared with carbohydrate counting, the food insulin index algorithm improved acute postprandial glycemia in well-controlled subjects with type 1 diabetes. The authors acknowledge that implementation of these findings outside the laboratory setting is not practical at this time, since the food insulin index does not currently appear on food labels and the food insulin index database includes only ~120 foods.

Another group collected data on food intake, physical activity, insulin administration, and blood glucose test results in patients with type 1 diabetes using self-administered questionnaires (Ahola 2010). A total of 64% of the participants inappropriately estimated their prandial insulin, and the authors concluded that optimal prandial insulin dosing is not easy, even after a long duration of diabetes.

Insulin dosing aids such as bolus insulin calculation cards and dosing guides have been developed to assist people with diabetes in reducing potential calculation errors (Anderson 2009; Chiarelli 1990; Kaufman 1999). Bolus calculators with personalized insulin-dosing algorithms can be programmed for use in a wide range of devices, such as personal digital assistants (PDAs), Smartphone applications, or insulin pumps (Gross 2003; Błazik 2010).

The use of a Diabetes Interactive Diary, an automatic carbohydrate/insulin bolus calculator installed on a mobile phone, also using patient-physician communication via text messages, was compared with a standard carbohydrate-counting education program (Rossi 2010). The Diabetes Interactive Diary was as effective as a traditional carbohydrate-counting education program, without an increased risk of hypoglycemia. The authors concluded that use of this type of technology reduces education time while significantly improving treatment satisfaction and several quality-of-life dimensions. These types of adaptive aids are popular with the tech-savvy, but can also be useful for people who have health literacy and numeracy concerns, such as young children or adults who do not possess the ability to perform fairly complex mathematical equations required in intensive insulin therapy plans (Wolff 2009). Use of technology may allow more people with insulin-requiring diabetes to have access to diabetes self-management tools, education, and support.

Type 2 diabetes. Most people with type 2 diabetes will eventually need insulin to achieve target A1C values (Wright 2002). The U.K. Prospective Diabetes Study (UKPDS) showed that β-cell failure is progressive; there is 50% normal β-cell function at diagnosis, with a steady decline after diagnosis (DeWitt 2003; UKPDS 1998). It is also reported that 53% of people with type 2 diabetes initially treated with sulfonylureas require insulin therapy by 6 years, and almost 80% require insulin by 9 years (Turner 1999; Wright 2002).

A small clinical trial examined metabolic control and patient preference in people with type 2 diabetes using conventional "fixed" or flexible insulin therapy (Kloos 2007). The authors concluded that initiation of insulin therapy was safe and effective in both treatment options, but after initially improving glycemic control, neither group achieved A1C levels <7%. After 8 weeks of following both the fixed and flexible insulin plans, the participants stated that they preferred the last therapy they received.

The first randomized study to evaluate intensive basal-bolus analog insulin therapy in people with type 2 diabetes as well as efficacy of carbohydrate counting in this population was conducted in 2008 (Bergenstal 2008). The simple algorithm group was provided with a set dose of prandial insulin to take before meals and compared to a group instructed on carbohydrate counting by an RD who provided an ICR to use for each meal. Prandial and basal insulin levels were adjusted weekly in both groups on the basis of SMBG results from the previous week. A1C levels at the end of study were 6.7% (simple algorithm) and 6.54% (carbohydrate counting). The respective mean A1C changes from baseline to 24 weeks were –1.46 and –1.59% ($P = 0.24$). Both groups used SMBG results to dose insulin. The simple algorithm group participants either consumed fairly consistent amounts of carbohydrates, thus minimizing needed changes in insulin dosing, or learned to modify their carbohydrate intake on the basis of SMBG results.

Factors That May Affect Long-Term Adherence to Basal-Bolus Insulin Regimens

Three studies exploring the food and eating practices of people with type 1 diabetes converted to FIIT as part of the DAFNE course have been published (Lawton 2011; Rankin 2011; Casey 2011). One study reported that adoption of this type of insulin treatment plan can result in greater dietary rigidity over time as opportunities presented for greater dietary freedom are counterbalanced by new challenges and burdens (Lawton 2011). For example, in an effort to simplify food choices for easier carbohydrate estimation, the individual may rely on pre-packaged foods that include nutrition fact information rather than on naturally occurring, unprocessed foods such as fresh fruits and vegetables that do not have food labels. This step could lead to increased consumption of saturated fats and salt. FIIT participants also articulated anxieties about miscalculating carbohydrate amounts and injecting the wrong dose, resulting in the tendency to eat the same things over and over again, limiting intake of new foods or foods with difficult-to-determine carbohydrate content. Some participants purposefully choose low-/no-carbohydrate foods to safely simplify calculations of prandial doses. Despite participation in formal intensive insulin therapy classes, fear of hypoglycemia when matching mealtime insulin to desired food (carbohydrate) intake continues to be a concern for many (Lawton 2011).

Another investigation over 12 months explored participant experiences regarding how they sustain use of FIIT (Rankin 2011). Although patients generally preferred flexible insulin therapy to conventional or "fixed" insulin therapy, the therapy had several constraints. Participants found that they had to make some adjustments to their lives to sustain this method of treatment, such as maintaining a similar weekday schedule on the weekends, adjusting food choices, or by creating food habit routines. The researchers suggested that diabetes education programs need to include interventions or strategies that can help patients successfully convert to FIIT long term.

The third group of researchers interviewed DAFNE program participants and collected information at 6 weeks and 6 and 12 months on how they assimilated course principles over time (Casey 2011). Participants initially (6 weeks) felt support from other participants, for example, by sharing experiences. However, after 6 months, participants began to value support from responsive health care professionals that focused on collaborative decision-making. The authors concluded that there is a need for diabetes educators to clearly communicate and explain to participants that adoption of the FIIT principles takes time (perhaps over 12 months). Support at 6 months appeared to be an important timeframe for participants, since motivation at this point was lowest for many.

People with insulin-requiring diabetes may also diligently perform dose calculations using their individualized algorithms when beginning intensive insulin therapy (Gross 2003). However, adherence to the ongoing determination of the prandial insulin dose may become relaxed as the person with diabetes gains familiarity with the self-adjustment of the insulin. As time passes, there may be the tendency to begin to approximate premeal doses by titrating insulin based on the "standard" or "usual" carbohydrate content of the meal. In addition, many people with insulin-requiring diabetes may actually be hesitant to take on the responsibility of increasing or decreasing their insulin doses on the basis of their carbohydrate intake and premeal blood glucose level (Gross 2003).

SUMMARY

It is important to remember that timing of the insulin dose as well as prandial and correction algorithms are just a starting point when initiating or using insulin therapy plans for individuals with insulin-requiring type 1 or type 2 diabetes. Algorithms for flexible insulin dosing or fixed insulin dose prescriptions will not be effective if the individual self-managing his or her diabetes does not possess a thorough understanding of appropriate actions to implement. Also important is the daily incorporation of the carbohydrate-counting meal-planning approach or another method of accurately quantifying carbohydrate intake. Insulin doses need to be confirmed by one of the cornerstones of diabetes self-management—blood glucose monitoring. Finally, the individual with insulin-requiring diabetes has been shown to benefit from regular interaction with responsive and supportive diabetes health care professionals to effectively optimize blood glucose control to reduce the risk of long-term complications of poorly controlled diabetes.

BIBLIOGRAPHY

Academy of Nutrition and Dietetics: Type 1 and type 2 diabetes evidence-based nutrition practice guidelines for adults, 2008. Available from http://adaevidencelibrary.com/topic.cfm?cat=3253. Accessed 5 June 2011

Ahola AJ, Makimattila S, Saraheimo M, Mikkila V, Forsblom C, Freese R, Groop PH: Many patients with type 1 diabetes estimate their prandial insulin need inappropriately. *J Diabetes* 2:194–202, 2010

American Diabetes Association: Clinical practice recommendations: standards of medical care in diabetes: 2012. *Diabetes Care* 35 (Suppl. 1):S11–S63, 2012

American Diabetes Association: Nutrition recommendations and interventions for diabetes (Position Statement). *Diabetes Care* 31 (Suppl. 1):S61–S78, 2008

Anderson DG: Multiple daily injections in young patients using the ezy-BICC bolus calculation card, compared to mixed insulin and CSII. *Pediatr Diabetes* 10:304–309, 2009

Bao J, de Jong V, Atkinson F, Petocz P, Brand-Miller JC: Food insulin index: physiologic basis for predicting insulin demand evoked by composite. *Am J Clin Nutr* 90:986–992, 2009

Bao J, Gilbertson HR, Gray R, Munns D, Howard G, Petocz P, Colagiuri S, Brand-Miller JC: Improving the estimation of mealtime insulin dose in adults with type 1 diabetes. *Diabetes Care* 34:2146–2151, 2011

Bergenstal RM, Johnson M, Powers MA, Wynne A, Vlajnic A, Hollander P, Rendell M: Adjust to target in type 2 diabetes: comparison of a simple algorithm with carbohydrate counting for adjustment of mealtime insulin glulisine. *Diabetes Care* 31:1305–1310, 2008

Bevier WC, Zisser H, Palerm CC, Finan DA, Seborg DE, Wollizter AO, Jovanovic L: Calculating the insulin to carbohydrate ratio using the hyperglycaemic-euglycaemic clamp: a novel use for a proven technique. *Diabetes Metab Res Rev* 23:472–478, 2007

Błazik M, Pańkowska E: The education of patients in prandial insulin dosing related to the structure of bolus calculators: *Pediatr Endocrinol* 16:301–305, 2010

Boukhors Y, Rabasa-Lhoret R, Langelier H, Soultan M, Lacroix A, Chiasson JL: The use of information technology for the management of intensive insulin therapy in type 1 diabetes mellitus. *Diabetes Metab* 29:619–627, 2003

Brownlee M, Hirsch IB: Glycemic variability: a hemoglobin A1c-independent risk factor for diabetic complications. *JAMA* 295:1707–1708, 2006

Buse JB: Should postprandial glucose be routinely measured and treated to a particular target? No! *Diabetes Care* 26:1615–1618, 2003

Casey D, Murphy K, Lawton J, White FF, Dineen S: A longitudinal qualitative study examining factors impacting on the ability of persons with T1DM to assimilate the Dose Adjustment of Normal Eating (DAFNE) principles into daily living and how these factors change over time. *BMC Public Health* 11:672, 2011

Centers for Disease Control and Prevention: Data and Trends; Preventative Care Services; Diabetes Self-Management Education Classes. Available at http://www.cdc.gov/diabetes/statistics/preventive/fyclass.htm. Accessed 12 June 2011

Centers for Disease Control and Prevention: National Diabetes Fact Sheet, 2011. Available at http://www.cdc.gov/diabetes/pubs/factsheet11.htm. Accessed 12 June 2011

Ceriello A: Postprandial hyperglycemia and diabetes complications: is it time to treat? *Diabetes* 54:208–213, 2005

Ceriello A, Davidson J, Hanefeld M, Leiter L, Monnier L, Owens D, Tajima N, Tuomilehto J, for the International Prandial Regulation (PGR) Study Group: Postprandial hyperglycaemia and cardiovascular complications of diabetes: an update. *Nutr Metab Cardiovas Dis* 16:453–456, 2006

Ceriello A, Taboga C, Tonutti L, Quagliaro L, Piconi L, Bais B, Da Ros R, Motz E: Evidence for independent and cumulative effect of postprandial hypertriglyceridemia and hyperglycemia on endothelial dysfunction and oxidative stress generation: effects of short- and long-term simvastatin treatment. *Circulation* 106:1211–1218, 2002

Chiarelli F, Tumini S, Morgese G, Albisser AM: Controlled study in diabetic children comparing insulin-dosage adjustment by manual and computer algorithms. *Diabetes Care* 13:1080–1084, 1990

Cobry E, McFann K, Messer L, Gage V, VanderWel B, Horton L, Chase PH: Timing of meal insulin boluses to achieve optimal postprandial glycemic control in patients with type 1 diabetes. *Diabetes Technol Tech* 12:173–177, 2010

DAFNE Study Group: Training in flexible, intensive insulin management to enable dietary freedom in people with type 1 diabetes: Dose Adjustment For Normal Eating (DAFNE) randomized controlled trial. *BMJ* 325:746–751, 2002

Davidson PC, Hebblewhite HR, Bode BW, Steed RD, Welch NS, Greenlee MC, Richardson PL, Johnson J: New evidence based guidelines for prescribing insulin by CSII (Abstract). *Diabetes* 51 (Suppl. 2):A128–A129, 2002

Davidson PC, Hebblewhite HR, Bode BW, Steed RD, Welch NS, Greenlee MC, Richardson PL, Johnson J: Statistically based CSII parameters: correction factor, CF (1700 Rule), carbohydrate-to-insulin ratio, CIR (2.8 Rule), and basal-to-total ratio. *Diabetes Technol Ther* 5:237, 2003

Davidson PC, Hebblewhite HR, Steed RD, Bode BW: Analysis of guidelines for basal-bolus insulin dosing: basal insulin, correction factor, and carbohydrate-to-insulin ratio. *Endocr Pract* 14:1095–1101, 2008

DeWitt DE, Hirsch IB: Outpatient insulin therapy in type 1 and type 2 diabetes mellitus: scientific review: *JAMA* 289:2254–2264, 2003

Diabetes Control and Complications Trial Research Group: The effect of intensive treatment of diabetes on the development and progression of long-term complications in insulin-dependent diabetes mellitus. *N Engl J Med* 329:977–986, 1993

Dias VM, Pandini JA, Nunes RR, Sperandei SLM, Portella ES, Cobas RA, Gomes MB: Effect of the carbohydrate counting method on glycemic control in patients with type 1 diabetes. *Diabetol Metab Syndr* 2:54–60, 2010

Franc S, Dardari D, Boucherie B, Riveline JP, Biedzinski M, Petit C, Requeda E, Leurent P, Varroud-Vial M, Hochberg G, Charpentier G: Real-life application and validation of flexible intensive insulin-therapy algorithms in type 1 diabetes patients. *Diabetes Metab* 35:463–468, 2009

Franz MJ, Powers MA, Leontos C, Holmeister LA, Kulkarni K, Monk A, Wedel N, Gradwell E: The evidence for medical nutrition therapy for type 1 and type 2 diabetes in adults. *J Am Diet Assoc* 110:1852–1889, 2010

Garber AJ: Long-acting glucagon-like peptide 1 receptor agonists: A review of their efficacy and tolerability. *Diabetes Care* 34(Suppl 2):S279-S284, 2011

Gross TM, Kayne D, King A, Rother C, Juth S: A bolus calculator is an effective means of controlling postprandial glycemia in patients on insulin pump therapy. *Diabetes Technol Ther* 5:365–369, 2003

Hirsch IB: Insulin analogues. *N Engl J Med* 352:174–183, 2005a

Hirsch IB: Glycemic variability: it's not just about A1c anymore! *Diabetes Technol Ther* 7:780–783, 2005b

Home P: Contributions of basal and postprandial hyperglycemia to micro- and macrovascular complications in people with type 2 diabetes. *Curr Med Res Opin* 21:989–998, 2005

Howorka K, Thoma H, Grillmayr H, Kitzler E: Phases of functional, near-normoglycaemic insulin substitution: what are computers good for in the rehabilitation process in type I (insulin-dependent) diabetes mellitus? *Comput Methods Program Biomed* 32:319–323, 1990

Jovanovič L, Peterson CM: Home blood glucose monitoring. *Compr Ther* 8:10–20, 1982

Kaufman FR, Halvorson M, Carpenter S: Use of a plastic insulin dosage guide to correct blood glucose levels out of the target range and for carbohydrate counting in subjects with type 1 diabetes: *Diabetes Care* 22:1252–1257, 1999

Kloos C, Sämann A, Lehmann T, Braun A, Heckmann B, Müller UA: Flexible intensive versus conventional insulin therapy in insulin-naïve adults with type 2 diabetes: an open-label, randomized, controlled, crossover clinical trial of metabolic control and patient preference. *Diabetes Care* 30:3031–3032, 2007

Laurenzi A, Bolla AM, Panigoni G, Doria V, Uccellatore AC, Peretti E, Saibene A, Galimberti G, Bosi E, Scavini M: Effects of carbohydrate counting on glucose control and quality of life over 24 weeks in adult patients with type 1 diabetes on continuous subcutaneous insulin infusion. *Diabetes Care* 34:823–827, 2011

Lawton J, Rankin D, Cooke DD, Clark M, Elliot J, Heller S, UK NIHR DAFNE Study Group: Dose adjustment for normal eating: a qualitative longitudinal exploration of the food and eating practices of type 1 diabetes patients converted to flexible intensive insulin therapy in the UK. *Diabetes Res Clin Pract* 91:87–93, 2011

Lowe J, Linjawi S, Mensch M, James K, Attia J: Flexible eating and flexible insulin dosing in patients with diabetes: results of an intensive self-management course. *Diabetes Res Clin Pract* 80:439–443, 2008

Luijf YM, van Bon AC, Hoekstra JB, DeVries JH: Premeal injection of rapid-acting insulin reduces postprandial glycemic excursions in type 1 diabetes. *Diabetes Care* 33:2152–2155, 2010

Monnier L, Lapinski H, Colette C: Contributions of fasting and postprandial plasma glucose increments to the overall diurnal hyperglycemia of type 2 diabetic patients: variations with increasing levels of HbA1C. *Diabetes Care* 26:881–885, 2003

Mooradian AD, Bernbaum M, Albert SG: Narrative review: a rational approach to starting insulin therapy. *Ann Intern* 145:125–134, 2006

Mudaliar SR, Lindberg FA, Joyce M, Beerdsen P, Strange P, Lin A, Henry RR: Insulin aspart (B28 Asp-Insulin): a fast-acting analog of human insulin. *Diabetes Care* 22:1501–1506, 1999

Mühlhauser I, Jörgens V, Berger M, Graninger W, Gürlter W, Hornke L: Bicentric evaluation of a teaching and treatment programme for type 1 (insulin-dependent) diabetic patients: improvement of metabolic control and other measures of diabetes care for up to 22 months. *Diabetologia* 25:470–476, 1983

Nathan DM, Buse JB, Davidson MB, Ferrannini E, Holman RR, Sherwin B, Zinman B: Medical management of hyperglycemia in type 2 diabetes: A consensus algorithm for the initiation and adjustment of therapy. *Diabetes Care* 32:193–203, 2009

Palerm CC, Zisser H, Bevier WC, Jovanovic L, Doyle FJ: Prandial insulin dosing using run-to-run control. *Diabetes Care* 30:1131–1136, 2007

Rankin D, Cooke DD, Clark M, Hellert S, Elliott J, Lawton J: How and why do patients with type 1 diabetes sustain their use of flexible intensive insulin therapy? A qualitative longitudinal investigation of patients' self-management practices following attendance at a Dose Adjustment for Normal Eating (DAFNE) course. *Diabet Med* 28:532–538, 2011

Rassam AG, Zeise TM, Burge MR: Optimal administration of lispro insulin in hyperglycemic type 1 diabetes. *Diabetes Care* 22:133–136, 1999

Rossi MC, Nicolucci A, Di Bartolo P, Bruttomesso D, Girelli A, Ampudia FJ, Kerr D, Ceriello A, De la Mayor C, Pellegrini F, Horwitz D, Vespasiani G: Diabetes Interactive Diary: a new telemedicine system enabling flexible diet and insulin therapy while improving quality of life: an open-label, international, multicenter, randomized study. *Diabetes Care* 33:109–115, 2010

Sachon C: Functional insulin therapy. *Rev Prat* 53:1169–1174, 2003

Scaramuzza AE, Iafusco D, Santoro L, Bosetti A, De Palma A, Spiri D, Mameli C, Zuccotti GV: Timing of bolus in children with type 1 diabetes using continuous subcutaneous insulin infusion (TiBoDi Study). *Diabetes Technol Tech* 12:149–152, 2010

Scavone G, Manto A, Pitocco D, Gagliardi L, Caputo S, Mancini L, Zaccardi F, Ghirlanda G: Effect of carbohydrate counting and medical nutritional therapy on glycaemic control in type 1 diabetic subjects: a pilot study. *Diabet Med* 27:477–479, 2010

Skyler JS, Skyler DL, Seigler DE, O'Sullivan MJ: Algorithms for adjustment of insulin dosage by patients who monitor blood glucose. *Diabetes Care* 4:311–318, 1981

Speight J, Amiel SA, Bradley C, Heller S, Oliver L, Roberts S, Rogers H, Taylor C, Thompson G: Long-term biomedical and psychosocial outcomes following DAFNE (Dose Adjustment For Normal Eating) structured education to promote intensive insulin therapy in adults with sub-optimally controlled type 1 diabetes. *Diabetes Res Clin Pract* 89:22–29, 2010

Sudhir R, Mohan V: Postprandial hyperglycemia in patients with type 2 diabetes. *Treat Endocrinol* 1:105–106, 2002

Thomas D, Elliott EJ: Low glycaemic index, or low glycaemic load, diets for diabetes mellitus. *Cochrane Database Syst Rev* CD006296, 2009

Turner RC, Cull CA, Frighi V, Holman RR: Glycemic control with diet, sulfonylurea, metformin, or insulin in patients with type 2 diabetes. *JAMA* 281:2005–2012, 1999

Tridgell DM, Tridgell AH, Hirsch IB: Inpatient management of adults and children with type 1 diabetes. *Endocrinol Metab Clin North Am* 39:595–608, 2010

U.K. Prospective Diabetes Study 24 (UKPDS): A 6-year randomized, controlled trial comparing sulfonylurea, insulin, and metformin therapy in patients with newly diagnosed type 2 diabetes that could not be controlled with diet therapy. *Ann Intern Med* 128:165–175, 1998

Walsh J, Roberts R: *Pumping Insulin.* 2nd ed. San Diego, CA, Torrey Pines Press, 1994

Walsh J, Roberts R, Bailey T: Guidelines for insulin dosing in continuous subcutaneous insulin infusion using new formulas from a retrospective study of individuals with optimal glucose levels. *J Diabetes Sci Technol* 4:1174–1181, 2010

Walsh J, Roberts R, Varma C, Bailey T: *Using Insulin.* San Diego, CA, Torrey Pines Press, 2003

Wolff K, Cavanaugh K, Malone B, Hawk V, Gregory BP, Davis D, Wallston K, Rothman RL: The Diabetes Literacy and Numeracy Education Toolkit (DLNET) materials to facilitate diabetes education and management in patients with low literacy and numeracy skills. *Diabetes Educ* 35:233–245, 2009

Wright A, Burden AC, Paisey RB, Cull CA, Holman RR. UK Prospective Diabetes Study Group: Sulfonylurea inadequacy: efficacy of addition of insulin over 6 years in patients with type 2 diabetes in UK Prospective Diabetes Study (UKPDS 57). *Diabetes Care* 25:330–336, 2002

Alison B. Evert, MS, RD, CDE, is a Diabetes Nutrition Educator and the Coordinator of Diabetes Education Programs at the University of Washington Medical Center, Diabetes Care Center in Seattle, WA.

Chapter 6
Nutrition Therapy for Adults with Type 2 Diabetes

Hope S. Warshaw, MMSc, RD, CDE, BC-ADM

Highlights

Pathophysiology of Type 2 Diabetes

Integration of Nutrition Therapy into Type 2 Diabetes Management

Evidence-Based Nutrition Interventions for Adults with Type 2 Diabetes

Weight-Loss/Maintenance Interventions

Macronutrient Distribution and Food/Eating Patterns

Adjunctive Therapies to Achieve Nutrition Therapy Goals

Summary

Highlights
Nutrition Therapy for
Adults with Type 2 Diabetes

■ Nutrition therapy for adults with type 2 diabetes should be an ongoing process throughout the individual's entire diabetes care plan, including progression of disease and (if prescribed) glucose-lowering medication regimen.

■ Research results from nutrition intervention trials aimed at achieving weight loss and/or glycemic, lipid, and blood pressure goals indicate many eating patterns are successful in managing diabetes, including a macronutrient consumption consistent with the *Dietary Guidelines for Americans, 2010.*

■ For overweight adults with type 2 diabetes, emphasis should be placed on energy reduction within the context of a healthy eating plan and physical activity to achieve a 5–7% weight loss and to minimize weight regain over time. Minimal weight loss that is maintained long term paired with regular physical activity has been shown to decrease the use of medications to control glucose, lipids, and blood pressure.

■ To achieve weight loss, prevent excess weight regain, and/or prevent further weight gain, people must be engaged in a multifaceted program that includes nutrition interventions, physical activity, behavior change, and ongoing support.

■ Physical activity that includes a combination of aerobic and resistance training plays a critical supporting role in weight loss and an even more important role in preventing weight regain. In addition, physical activity, independent of weight loss, decreases insulin resistance and is integral to achieving glucose, lipid, and blood pressure targets over time.

Nutrition Therapy for Adults with Type 2 Diabetes

It is well documented in Chapters 1 and 2 that nutrition therapy based on evidence-based research and the individual goals, needs, and abilities of the client, when implemented appropriately and continuously in adults with type 2 diabetes, contributes to positive clinical outcomes. Clinical goals include glucose, lipid, and blood pressure control to reduce the risks for potential long-term complications of diabetes. This chapter provides an overview of the current understanding of the pathophysiology of type 2 diabetes and the importance of integrating nutrition therapy into the management of type 2 diabetes. Previously published and new evidence for nutrition therapy for type 2 diabetes is reviewed.

PATHOPHYSIOLOGY OF TYPE 2 DIABETES

It is critical that nutrition therapy for adults with type 2 diabetes be considered within the overarching pathophysiology and progression of this disease. Research over the past two decades has greatly broadened and deepened the understanding of this pathophysiology, yet much remains to be elucidated. Evidence demonstrates that the chronic inflammatory response initiated by excess weight in individuals at risk for type 2 diabetes is integrally involved in the development of insulin resistance. The links between obesity and type 2 diabetes that have been identified include proinflammatory cytokines (tumor necrosis factor-α and interleukin-6), insulin resistance, deranged fatty acid metabolism, and cellular processes such as mitochondrial dysfunction and endoplasmic reticulum stress (Eckel 2011). Risk factors for the development of type 2 diabetes beyond family history, genetic predisposition, and excess weight have been identified as visceral adiposity, resulting in abdominal girth and different subtypes of adipose tissue, which negatively affect glucose homeostasis (Eckel 2011).

The inflammatory response to excess weight, insulin resistance, and β-cell failure occurs ~5–10 years before the elevation of glucose above normoglycemia. At the point that type 2 diabetes is diagnosed, it is estimated that people have lost at least 50% of their β-cell function. There continues to be disagreement among researchers about whether this loss is of β-cell mass or function. Subjects in the upper tertile of impaired glucose tolerance before the diagnosis of type 2 diabetes are maximally/near-maximally insulin resistant and have lost over 80% of their β-cell function (DeFronzo 2009). Research also suggests that eight organs are involved in the development and progression of type 2 diabetes. Figure 6.1 illustrates multiple organ development and progression of type 2 diabetes.

INTEGRATION OF NUTRITION THERAPY INTO TYPE 2 DIABETES MANAGEMENT

Nutrition therapy must be integrated holistically into each individual's diabetes care plan. A majority of people with type 2 diabetes are overweight or obese. Moderate weight loss (5–7% of initial weight) achieved by consuming a reduced energy intake coupled with regular physical activity are key goals of therapy. This result is particularly true early in the disease course, when moderate weight loss has the potential to achieve glycemic control and other health improvements in most people, even if this weight loss is partially regained.

Weight-loss studies of more than 1-year duration document that the common trend is to achieve maximal weight loss by 6 months to 1 year. In the ensuing years, people often regain a portion of the lost weight (Franz 2007; Eckel 2011), in the pattern depicted in Figure 6.2. Although the absolute weight loss is minimal, it appears to have initial as well as long-term positive health benefits, which have been described as "legacy" or "memory" effects of this weight loss. In a retrospective cohort study, a weight-loss pattern after the new diagnosis of type 2 diabetes predicted improved glycemic and blood pressure control despite weight regain (Feldstein 2008). It remains difficult for people to retain their maximal weight loss because of many socioeconomic, environmental, and physiological (hormonal changes designed to protect against weight loss) factors. For example,

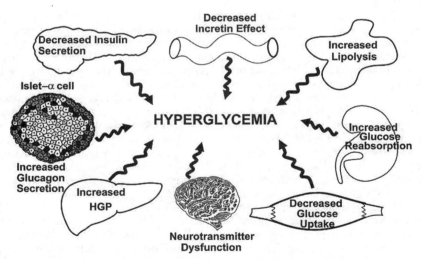

Figure 6.1 Members of the ominous octet: muscle (decreased glucose uptake), adipocyte (increased lipolysis), liver (increased hepatic glucose production [HGP]), β-cells (decreased insulin secretion), gastrointestinal tissues (decreased incretin effect), pancreatic α-cell (increased glucagon secretion), kidney (increased glucose reabsorption), and brain (neurotransmitter dysfunction). Reprinted with permission from DeFronzo 2009.

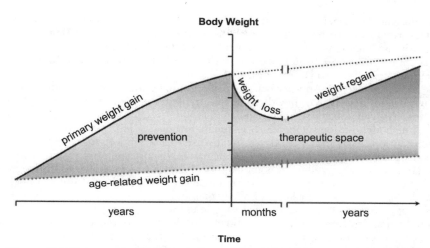

Figure 6.2 Schematic representation of the natural history of obesity. Primary (excess) weight gain occurs usually over years against the background of mild age-related increase in weight in the general population. Intentional weight loss frequently is at least partially successful, but in the vast majority of cases, is followed by weight regain. Weight loss and its maintenance is the therapeutic goal; prevention of primary weight gain is a societal endeavor. Reprinted with permission from Eckel 2011.

compensatory changes in circulating hormones that encourage weight regain after weight loss is achieved with calorie reduction persisted for at least 12 months after weight loss (Sumithran 2011). Furthermore, lack of or insufficient reimbursement for initial and ongoing nutrition therapy remains a challenge for many individuals.

It also is not clear if the benefits from nutrition therapy interventions on glycemia are from the weight loss per se or from a reduced energy intake. In general, glucose levels improve rapidly when energy intake is reduced and before much weight is lost. Over the years, as insulin resistance persists, endogenous insulin supply dwindles, and other physiological dysfunctions occur, weight loss is less likely to be effective in improving glycemic outcomes (Franz 2010; Academy of Nutrition and Dietetics [Acad Nutr Diet] 2008). However, maintaining a healthy weight, an energy-appropriate and nutrient-dense eating pattern, and healthy eating habits remains important throughout the years in patients with type 2 diabetes.

Current algorithms for glucose-lowering medications advise initiating medication to treat insulin resistance/improve insulin sensitivity in tandem with energy reduction and physical activity to achieve a moderate weight loss (ADA 2012; American Association Clinical Endocrinologists/American College Endocrinologists 2009). Today, health care providers have a wide array of glucose-lowering medications from which to choose based on the individual's physiological defects. Several categories of glucose-lowering medications are known to exacerbate weight gain, yet other existing and impending categories are known to positively affect weight loss or be weight neutral because of their modes of action. When choosing medications for the person with type 2 diabetes attempting weight loss, it is optimal to choose from glucose-lowering medications that do not exacerbate weight gain (Eckel 2011). The effects of glucose-lowering medication on weight are listed in Table 6.1. Another benefit of glucose-lowering medications that don't cause weight gain is that they do not cause hypoglycemia or excess hunger, two factors that can affect weight control.

The body of evidence underscores the importance of implementing nutrition interventions early in the course of the disease to achieve weight loss and other clinical outcomes. Figure 6.3 illustrates the natural history and progression of type 2 diabetes. Nutrition education and support have also been shown to minimize weight gain from use of glucose-lowering medications, including insulin (Coppell 2010; Wadden 2011). However, it is likely that multiple glucose-lowering medications or increased dosages of those already in use will be required for the majority of individuals to achieve glycemic control with disease progression. At this juncture, the prevention of further weight gain rather than weight loss becomes an important therapeutic goal (Franz 2010).

In summary, an understanding of the pathophysiology of type 2 diabetes, the available glucose-lowering medication treatments and recommended algorithms, the individual's glucose-lowering medication regimen, and the individual's duration of diabetes and weight control history will assist in determining optimal nutrition therapy.

EVIDENCE-BASED NUTRITION INTERVENTIONS FOR ADULTS WITH TYPE 2 DIABETES

With the primary goals of nutrition therapy in type 2 diabetes being control of glycemia, blood pressure, and lipids to prevent/delay complications of diabetes and with weight loss and/or weight maintenance being primary interventions, an

Table 6.1 Weight Effects of Glucose-Lowering Medications

Medication Class	Weight Effects
GLP-1 analogs	↓
Pramlintide	↓
Metformin	± or ↓
α-Glucosidase inhibitors	±
Dipeptidyl peptidase-4 inhibitors	±
Insulin	↑
Sulfonylureas	↑
Glinides	↑
Thiazolidinediones	↑

Reprinted with permission Eckel 2011.

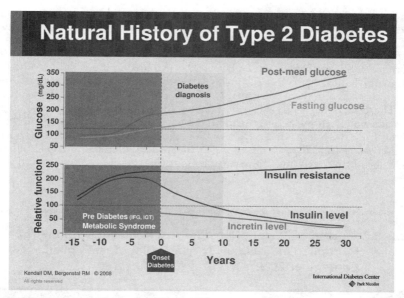

Figure 6.3 Natural History of Type 2 Diabetes. The top line (Insulin resistance) of the bottom half of the figure illustrates the role of insulin resistance as an initial cause of increased insulin production. The line (Insulin level) below it illustrates the body's attempt to keep blood glucose levels normal by increasing insulin production. However, β-cell dysfunction leads, over the course of years, to relative insulin deficiency and the diagnosis of diabetes and eventually to severe insulin deficiency requiring exogenous insulin. The bottom line (Incretin level) illustrates the decrease in incretins that also occurs as type 2 diabetes progresses. The top line (Post-meal glucose) in the top half of the figure illustrates the increase in postprandial blood glucose levels as the first sign of dysglycemia as a result of insufficient insulin production. The line (Fasting glucose) below it illustrates the effects of insulin deficiency on fasting blood glucose levels. Reprinted with permission from the International Diabetes Center at Park Nicollet, Minneapolis, MN. ©2008 International Diabetes Center, Minneapolis, MN. Used with permission.

array of interventions and meal-planning approaches have been investigated. A literature search was conducted using PubMed MEDLINE, and additional articles were identified from reference lists. Search criteria included the following: type 2 diabetes, diet, nutrition, dietary therapy, human subjects with diabetes, and English language articles. In addition, studies on weight management had to be 1 year or longer in duration. Five articles related to weight loss achieved with energy restriction met study criteria and are summarized in Table 6.2. Three studies related to macronutrient distribution, food, or eating pattern variations met study criteria and are summarized in Table 6.3. Four articles related to physical activity in adults with type 2 diabetes met study criteria and are summarized in Table 6.4. Evidence published before September 2009 is included in the tables in "The Evidence for Medical Nutrition Therapy for Type 1 and Type 2 Diabetes in Adults" (Franz 2010) and in the Academy of Nutrition and Dietetics (formerly the American Dietetic Association) (Acad Nutr Diet) Evidence Analysis Library (http://www.adaevidencelibrary.com) (Acad Nutr Diet 2008). Evidence and recommendations from the Report of the Dietary Guidelines Advisory Committee (DGAC) on the *Dietary Guidelines for Americans, 2010*, are also referenced and are publicly available at http://www.nutritionevidencelibrary.gov.

Table 6.2 Studies on Weight Management Achieved with Energy Reduction in Adults with Type 2 Diabetes, Published After September 2009*

	Population/ Duration of Study	Intervention (type of study)	Major Findings	Comments
Kattelmann 2009	*n* = 114 Northern Plains Indians, with type 2 diabetes/6 months	Nutrition education (6 lessons based on Medicine Wheel Model for Nutrition) vs. usual care (RCT)	Nutrition education group lost weight (1.4 kg) and ↓ BMI (1.0) (both *P* ≤ 0.05); usual care no change in weight	Culturally based intervention promoted weight loss
Malpass 2009	*n* = 30 with type 2 diabetes from early ACTID study/ not applicable	Interviews at 6 and 9 months to assess if *1*) efforts to increase PA supported or hindered dietary changes and *2*) if making multiple lifestyle changes was counterproductive or beneficial (cohort study)	Providing nutrition and PA together encourages use of PA to aid in disease management; undertaking multiple lifestyle changes found helpful	Increasing PA can act as a gateway behavior that results in positive effects in other behaviors
Coppell 2010	*n* = 93 adults with type 2 diabetes of average 9 years, A1C >7% despite diabetes medications plus at least two of three: overweight/obese, hypertension, and dyslipidemic/6 months	Intensive nutrition intervention based on EASD recommendations provided by dietitian vs. usual care; both groups continued usual medical care (RCT)	6-month intervention vs. usual care: A1C (−0.4 vs. −0.1%, *P* = 0.007); weight (−1.3 vs. −0.1 kg, *P* = 0.026); BMI (−0.5 vs. −0.1, *P* = 0.026); ↓ saturated fat (−1.9% total energy, *P* = 0.006)	Nutrition therapy effective in diabetes of long duration; support from dietitian and family essential for success

	Population/ Duration of Study	Intervention (type of study)	Major Findings	Comments
Look AHEAD Research Group 2010	$n = 5,145$ over-weight/obese adults with type 2 diabetes /4 years results	4-year changes from ILI (meal replacements or structured food plan, 175 min physical activity/week) vs. control (DSE) on weight, fitness, and cardiovascular disease risk factors (multicenter RCT)	ILI vs. DSE: weight loss (−6.15 vs. −0.88%, $P < 0.001$); treadmill fitness (12.74 vs. 1.96%, $P < 0.001$): A1C (−0.36 vs. −0.09%, $P < 0.001$); systolic BP (−5.33 vs. −2.97 mmHg, $P < 0.001$); diastolic BP (−2.92 vs. −2.48 mmHg, $P = 0.01$); HDL cholesterol (3.67 vs. 1.97 mg/dL, $P < 0.001$); triglyceride (−25.56 vs. −19.75 mg/dL, $P < 0.001$)	Study reports on 4-year interim results in 14-year study to determine effects of early and maintained weight loss on cardio-vascular morbidity and mortality
Andrews 2011	$n = 593$ adults with type 2 diabetes diagnosed within 5–8 months prior in early ACTID study/1 year	Usual care vs. ID only (weight loss goal 5–10% initial weight and maintenance) vs. ID and PA (30 min 5 days/week) (DPAI); treatment changed during first 6 months if fasting plasma glucose or BP elevated or subject symptomatic; during second 6 months, subjects treated to target A1C, BP, and lipids (RCT)	6-month A1C: usual care ↑ from 6.72 to 6.86%; ID improved −0.28% ($P = 0.005$); DPAI −0.33% ($P < 0.001$): differences persisted to 12 months with less use of diabetes medications; improvements in weight, insulin resistance in intervention vs. usual care; BP similar in all groups	

*Studies published before September 2009 are summarized in the Academy of Nutrition and Dietetics Evidence Analysis Library (Franz 2010). BP, blood pressure; EASD, European Association for Study of Diabetes; ID, intensive diet; ILI, intensive lifestyle intervention; PA, physical activity.

A summary of research is presented and arranged into the following topics:

- Weight loss/maintenance interventions
- Macronutrient distribution and food or eating patterns
- Adjunctive therapies to achieve nutrition therapy goals

Several confounding variables must be considered when reviewing nutrition research. It is often challenging to tease out the key factors for positive results in these studies because they frequently combine the use of several interventions, such as energy deficit, diabetes and nutrition education, frequent support, behavior change therapy, and/or physical activity.

Table 6.3 Studies on Macronutrient Distribution and Food/Eating Pattern Variations in Adults with Type 2 Diabetes Published After September 2009

	Population/ Duration of Study	Intervention (type of study)	Major Findings	Comments
Elhayany 2010	n = 194 overweight individuals with type 2 diabetes/1 year	Isocaloric diets: low CHO MED vs. traditional MED vs. 2003 ADA diet (50% CHO, 20% protein, 30% fat); all advised to engage in 30–45 min aerobic activity 3 days/week (RCT)	Mean weight loss: all 8.3 kg (nonsignificant between groups); A1C: ↓ −2.0% in low CHO MED, −1.6% in ADA diet; HDL cholesterol: ↑ (3.9 mg/dL) only in low CHO MED; triglyceride: ↓ in low CHO MED (−115 mg/dL) and traditional MED (−133 m/dL) than in ADA diet (−62 mg/dL); LDL cholesterol: ↓ in low CHO MED 24.8%, traditional MED 20.9%, 13.8% ADA	
He 2010	n = 7,822 women with type 2 diabetes in the Nurses' Health Study/up to 26-year follow-up	Association with whole grains and cereal fiber, bran, and germ in relation to all-cause and cardiovascular disease–specific mortality (cohort study)	853 all-cause, 296 cardiovascular disease deaths; after adjusting for age, the highest vs. lowest fifth of intakes of whole grain, cereal fiber, bran, and germ associated with 16–31% lower all-cause mortality; bran had the strongest association (P for r trend = 0.01)	
Azadbakht 2011	n = 4,431 completers with type 2 diabetes/ 8 weeks for each diet	Isocaloric control diet vs. DASH (crossover RCT)	DASH vs. control: lower weight (P = 0.007) and waist circumference (P = 0.002); fasting plasma glucose ↓ (−29.4 mg/dL, P = 0.04); A1C ↓ (−1.7%, P = 0.04); HDL cholesterol ↑ (P = 0.001); LDL cholesterol ↓ (P = 0.02); systolic BP ↓ (P = 0.02); DBP ↓ (P = 0.04)	DASH diet vs. control: lower in sodium; higher in dairy, fruit, vegetable, and legumes, different fats; not different in calories, macronutrients, and fiber

CHO, carbohydrate; MED, Mediterranean.

WEIGHT-LOSS/MAINTENANCE INTERVENTIONS

Weight-Loss Research

Over the years, numerous randomized weight-loss trials of shorter and longer duration in people with type 2 diabetes have been conducted. In randomized trials of 1-year duration or longer, using a variety of nutrition interventions, approximately half of the studies reported improvement in A1C related to weight loss, whereas about half reported no improvement in A1C despite fairly similar weight losses (Franz 2010). The diet intervention groups in five studies reported improvement in A1C ranging from –0.2 to –0.5%, with body-weight losses ranging from –1.0 to –3.4 kg (Mertz 2000; Hanefeld 2002; Kelley 2002; Miles 2002; Berne 2005). Yet, the nutrition intervention groups in five other studies reported no improvement in A1C, with weight losses ranging from –0.8 to –4.4 kg (Brinkworth 2004; Hollander 1998; Redmon 2003; Redmon 2005; Wolf 2004; Li 2005). The difference in improvements of A1C despite weight loss could be related to the subject's duration of diabetes.

Studies on weight loss/maintenance in type 2 diabetes published after September 2009 are summarized in Table 6.2. Previous studies are summarized in the Acad Nutr Diet Evidence Analysis Library (Franz 2010).

To clarify and determine the role of weight management, several National Institutes of Health (NIH)–funded trials 2 years or longer have and are providing insights and factors for success on weight loss in a population without type 2 diabetes (Sacks 2009) and weight loss in people with type 2 diabetes (Look AHEAD 2007; Look AHEAD 2010).

The Look AHEAD (Action for Health in Diabetes) study is a 14-year multi-center randomized controlled trial (RCT), currently funded through 2014. It is the first trial in type 2 diabetes to assess if weight reduction combined with physical activity can reduce cardiovascular disease morbidity and mortality (Look AHEAD 2007). The study randomized 5,145 overweight or obese individuals with type 2 diabetes to either intensive lifestyle intervention (ILI) or diabetes support and education (DSE) for an average of 6.8 years (Bertoni 2008).

The ILI is modeled after the landmark DPP (DPP Research Group 2002). However, the ILI in Look AHEAD set a more ambitious individual goal of losing ≥7% of initial weight at year 1 (vs. 7% in the DPP) and ≥175 min moderate-intensity physical activity per week (vs. ≥150 min per week in the DPP). Look AHEAD energy consumption goals were as follows: 1,200–1,500 kcal/day (40–50 g fat) for individuals whose initial weight was <250 lb and 1,500–1,800 kcal/day (50–60 g fat) for individuals whose initial weight was >250 lb (Delahanty 2008). The ILI nutrition intervention strategies focused on self-monitoring of food intake by calorie counting with fat gram goals and aggressive use of meal replacements (mainly beverages and bars provided at no charge) during the first 4 months (during months 5–12, participants were encouraged to continue to replace one meal and one snack with a meal replacement) (Wadden 2011). Subjects in the ILI group were seen weekly for the first 6 months and three times per month from 6 months to 1 year, using group and one-on-one contact. During years 2 through 4, ILI subjects were seen at least once a month individually, received follow-up at least monthly, and were invited to group classes and activities to support their

Table 6.4 Studies on Physical Activity in Adults with Type 2 Diabetes Published After September 2009

	Population/ Duration of Study	Intervention (type of study)	Major Findings	Comments
Church 2010; HART-D study	$n = 262$ sedentary adults with type 2 diabetes and A1C $\geq 6.5\%/9$ months	Four groups: *1*) nonexercise control, *2*) resistance training 3 days/ week, *3*) aerobic exercise to expend 12 kcal/ kg/week, *4*) combined aerobic to expend 10 kcal/kg/week and resistance training 3 times per week (RCT)	A1C in group 4 ↓ (-0.34%, $P = 0.03$), nonsignificant change in other three groups vs. control; VO_{2max} improved only in group 4 ($P > 0.05$); group 2 lost -1.4 kg fat mass ($P < 0.05$), -1.7 ($P < 0.05$) vs. control	Although both resistance and aerobic training provide benefits, only combining aerobic and resistance training improved A1C
Lohman 2010	$n = 127$ adults with type 2 diabetes	Nonrandomized design (no control group), use of fitness testing (arm curl and chair stand test) results used by six general practitioners (who received training in motivational interviewing, stages of change, and principles of exercise) to test whether using motivational interviewing in type 2 diabetes to encourage lifestyle, exercise, and home-based self-managed exercise programs changed cardio-respiratory fitness, expressed by VO_{2max}, upper and lower extremities muscle strength, and A1C and HDL cholesterol	Results from 102 (80.3%) participants; VO_{2max} ↑ 2.5% ($P = 0.032$) with ↑ of 33.2% ($P < 0.001$) and 34.1% ($P < 0.001$) for arm curl and chair stand test, respectively. HDL cholesterol ↑ 8.6% ($P < 0.001$), but A1C unchanged ($P = 0.57$) at 6.8%; subjects without cardiovascular disease or pain from function limitation: ↑ VO_{2max} by 5.2% ($P < 0.0001$) and 7.9% ($P = 0.0008$), respectively; waist circumference, BMI, and fasting plasma glucose did not change	
Negri 2010	$n = 59$ adults with type 2 diabetes/4 months (interim visit at 2 months to adjust, if needed, diabetes medications)	Control group (standard lifestyle recommendations) vs. study group (assigned to 3 45-min supervised walking sessions/week and counseling) (RCT)	Study group: metabolic changes not different at 4 months; attending >50% of walking sessions ↓ A1C and ↓ total cholesterol vs. controls; stopping or reduction of glucose-lowering medications in 33% of study subjects vs. 5% controls ($P < 0.05$); change in overall PA correlated with ↓ in body weight ($P = 0.005$)	

	Population/ Duration of Study	Intervention (type of study)	Major Findings	Comments
Umpi-erre 2011	n = 47 RCTs of at least 12 weeks and subjects with type 2 diabetes/not applicable	Evaluated structured exercise training or PA advice to lower A1C vs. control group (systematic review meta-analysis)	A1C: structured exercise training (23 studies) associated with ↓ −0.67%; structured aerobic exercise ↓ −0.73%; structured resistance training ↓ −0.57%; structured aerobic and resistance training combined ↓ −0.51%; PA advice (24 studies) ↓ −0.43%; combined PA and dietary advice ↓ −0.58%; PA advice alone, no A1C change; all vs. control	Structured exercise >150 min/ week ↓ A1C −0.89%, <150 min/ week −0.36%

PA, physical activity.

efforts. The DSE control group members were invited to three group sessions each year.

The 1-year Look AHEAD weight-loss data follow the trend of other weight-loss trials in both people with and without type 2 diabetes. ILI subjects had significant reduction in average body weight loss and improvements in cardiovascular fitness and A1C when compared to DSE subjects. The amount of weight loss at 1 year was also associated with improvements in triglycerides and HDL cholesterol but not LDL cholesterol (Wing 2011). Improvements in most risk factors were greater in individuals who lost 10–15% of their body weight. Of note, the ILI treatment was clinically effective in a diverse study population (Look AHEAD 2007).

Weight-loss strategies associated with a lower BMI in the ILI group at 1 year were regular self-weighing, eating breakfast, and infrequent consumption of fast food (Raynor 2008). Other factors associated with success at 1 year include greater attendance at treatment sessions (~35), exercising a mean of 137 minutes/week, and consuming 361 meal replacements. Greater self-reported physical activity was the strongest correlate of weight loss, followed by treatment attendance and consumption of meal replacements (Wadden 2009).

Longer-term follow-up to the Look AHEAD trial reveals maximal weight lost by the end of year 1, with slow weight regain in the ensuing years (Bertoni 2008; Look AHEAD 2010). This speaks to the physiological, environmental, and other challenges of maintaining weight loss, even when subjects are provided with more frequent than usual, high-quality education and support at no cost. At 4 years, ILI subjects maintained greater weight loss than DSE subjects, with the strongest predictor for weight loss at 4 years being the amount of weight lost at 1 year. Session attendance, physical activity, and lower reported caloric intakes were also important. Older subjects had greater weight loss all 4 years, had a lower self-reported calorie intake, and attended more sessions than younger ILI participants (Wadden 2011). This finding was also documented in the DPP (Wing 2004).

Also of interest is the finding that insulin users lost a similar amount of weight as non–insulin users. This emphasizes the need for ongoing education and support, as people are often started on insulin without the benefit of nutrition counseling advice and strategies. The ILI group also had greater improvements in treadmill fitness, A1C, blood pressure, and lipids (Look AHEAD 2010). In addition, less medication was needed in the ILI group at 4 years to control LDL cholesterol, hypertension, and glucose, which can translate into individual and health care system cost savings.

A trial to determine the effectiveness of nutrition therapy and/or physical activity within the first year of diagnosis of type 2 diabetes in adults was conducted in the United Kingdom (Early Activity in Diabetes [ACTID]) (Andrews 2011). Subjects were randomized to usual care (standard advice), intensive diet advice only (ID), or intensive dietary advice and physical activity intervention (DPAI) (brisk walking most days of the week). The weight loss goal for the ID and DPAI groups was 5–10% of initial body weight. Dietitian visits were scheduled regularly throughout the study, with opportunities for regular reinforcement of visit content with study nurses. At 6 months, A1C in the usual care group had worsened, whereas A1C had improved in the ID and DPAI groups. Differences persisted to 12 months with less use of glucose-lowering medications in the intervention groups. Interestingly, the addition of physical activity to the diet intervention added no benefit. This study adds to the existing database that demonstrates the multiple benefits of providing education and support by dietitians and nurses soon after the diagnosis of type 2 diabetes.

An ancillary study of ACTID was conducted using in-depth interviews to assess if efforts to increase physical activity supported or hindered dietary changes or vice versa, and whether people found making multiple lifestyle changes counterproductive or beneficial (Malpass 2009). Findings suggest that providing intensive diet and physical activity information together encouraged the DPAI subjects to use physical activity strategically to assist in their diabetes self-management. Most subjects found that undertaking multiple lifestyle changes at one time was helpful as opposed to overwhelming. ACTID demonstrates that although adding physical activity to diabetes self-care did not enhance weight loss, it can serve as a gateway behavior that encourages the person to implement additional positive eating and physical activity behaviors.

To determine the effect of nutrition interventions in people with longer-duration diabetes (average duration of 9 years), subjects in New Zealand who were hyperglycemic (A1C >7%) despite being on at least two glucose-lowering medications were studied (Coppell 2010). Participants in the intensive nutrition advice group were seen by the study dietitian within the first month after randomization and then monthly for 5 months, with additional group education and telephonic support being provided. A1C improved without additional medications and weight loss, and positive changes in food choices were seen. This study documents that even in longstanding diabetes, nutrition interventions can be as effective as adding a third medication and adds less cost to health care systems.

The importance of using culturally sensitive nutrition education materials was demonstrated in a population of Northern Plains Indians with type 2 diabetes. The intervention was based on a culturally adapted Medicine Wheel Model for Nutrition (Kattelmann 2009). At 6 months, the group receiving the culturally adapted education lost significant weight and decreased their BMI, whereas the usual care group experienced no significant change in weight or BMI.

In summary, these studies corroborate previously existing research that demonstrates the effectiveness of intensive and ongoing nutrition education and support on clinical outcomes and the reduced need for the use of medications both early in the course of type 2 diabetes and during ensuing years after diagnosis.

Meal Replacements and Structured Meal Plans

Meal replacements and structured meal plans, both used in the Look AHEAD study, are considered nutrition counseling strategies for weight control (Spahn 2010). Using meal replacements reduces the time spent thinking about food choices and preparation and limits exposure to foods that may prompt patients to overeat. Meal replacement also solves problems with underestimating portions. Structured meal plans are detailed meal plans providing the exact foods and portions to consume.

Meal replacement products are prepackaged as soups, bars, entrees, or drinks and provide a defined number of calories and macronutrients. Typically, they are used in programs to replace one or two meals a day to achieve weight loss. However, to maintain the weight loss long term, their use, along with structured meal planning, must be continued indefinitely (American Diabetes Association [ADA] 2008; Spahn 2010). Some brands of meal replacements can be purchased at retail stores, whereas others are only available as part of a comprehensive weight management program.

The use of meal replacements was compared to standard self-selected diet in overweight subjects with type 2 diabetes (Cheskin 2008). However, because of the study duration (1 year) and insufficient resources for follow-up, fewer than half of subjects completed the active phase and only about a quarter of subjects completed the study. A larger proportion of subjects using meal replacements lost $\geq$5% of their initial weight compared with those on self-selected diets; however, significant weight loss occurred in both groups with no significant differences between groups.

At the end of first year of the Look AHEAD trial, greater use of meal replacements (from beverages and bars that were provided at no cost) was reported to be correlated with successful weight loss, but 4-year data did not demonstrate their continued benefit (Wadden 2011). Meal replacements as part of a structured meal plan can be a helpful adjunct for weight loss by helping people achieve early weight loss. This in turn helps people feel successful and increases their self-efficacy. The long-term use and effectiveness of meal replacements in weight loss and prevention of weight regain remains in question.

Behavior-Change Theories in Weight Management

In evaluating most weight-loss studies in people with type 2 diabetes, it is critical to factor in the impact of positive behavior changes and long-term support. Many of the studies detailed in Table 6.1 and other evidence-analysis reviews include as a component of the multifaceted program a range of behavior-change curriculum, along with nutrition and diabetes education and continuous and regular support. Shown to be beneficial is a combination of behavioral theory and cognitive behavior therapy, social cognitive theory, and the transtheoretical model, along with the length of treatment (Spahn 2010). Positive results were noted from the use of cognitive behavior therapy in the Look AHEAD study at 1 year. In a small study in people with type 2 diabetes, cognitive behavior therapy was used as part of an ILI and, at 1 year, showed significant improvements in fasting blood glucose, A1C, and weight as well as improvements in systolic blood pressure and carotid mean media thickness (Kim 2006).

MACRONUTRIENT DISTRIBUTION AND FOOD/EATING PATTERNS

Although numerous research studies have been conducted over the years to determine the ideal macronutrient intake for adults with type 2 diabetes, it is unlikely that one exists (Wheeler 2012; ADA 2008). Chapter 2 provides a review of the research on macronutrients as well as subcomponents, such as dietary fiber and saturated fat. However, the impact of various eating patterns (the composition of the entire caloric intake) on weight loss and other clinical indicators for type 2 diabetes have also been examined.

It is reported that individuals ≥2 years of age in the U.S. eat ~50% of calories as carbohydrate (256 g/day) (U.S. Department of Agriculture 2011). Furthermore, it appears difficult to change carbohydrate intake in the long term. The POUNDS LOST study, a 2-year trial in an overweight and obese free-living population, attempted to have subjects follow one of four eating plans ranging from lower carbohydrate (35%) to higher carbohydrate (65%), with corresponding changes in fat and protein. Despite intensive counseling, subjects did not achieve the macronutrient goals of the group to which they were assigned (Sacks 2009). By the study's end, subjects had reverted to their customary intake of macronutrients, with carbohydrate intake between 43 and 53% of calories.

The nutrient intake of individuals with diabetes is reported to be consistent with the current nutrient intakes of Americans. A sample of the food frequency questionnaires completed by participants in the Look AHEAD trial showed an average carbohydrate intake of 44% of total calories; an average fat intake of 40% of total calories with two-thirds consuming more than 10% of total calories from saturated fat; 20% met the fiber goal, and <50% met the minimum recommendation for servings of fruits, vegetables, dairy foods, and whole grains (Vitolins 2009).

With the interest in lower carbohydrate intakes for people with type 2 diabetes, several studies and meta-analyses have been conducted. Two RCTs found that subjects with diabetes on a low-carbohydrate diet lost more weight at 6 months than individuals on a low-fat diet (Foster 2003; Stern 2004), but at 1 year, weight loss was the same (Stern 2004). In the subjects with diabetes, A1C levels decreased more in the low-carbohydrate group compared to the conventional diet group. However, other 1-year studies comparing differing percentages of carbohydrate have not found significant differences from the amount of carbohydrate on glycemic control A1C and body weight (Davis 2009; Brehm 2009; Wolever 2008; Gardner 2007; Mayer-Davis 2004). A meta-analysis on restricted-carbohydrate diets in people with type 2 diabetes (ranging from 1 to 26 weeks with few long-term studies) also reported that weight loss was similar (Kirk 2008).

In a community-based nutrition intervention trial, overweight individuals with type 2 diabetes followed one of three isocaloric diets: *1*) low-carbohydrate (35%) Mediterranean (LCM), *2*) traditional Mediterranean (TM), and *3*) eating plan reflecting the 2004 ADA nutrition recommendations (ADA) (Elhayany 2010). The TM and ADA eating plans contained 50–55% carbohydrate, 30% fat, and 15–20% protein. Mean weight loss in all subjects was 8.3 kg. Cardiovascular risk factors for all treatment groups improved, but the LCM group experienced significantly greater improvements in several cardiovascular risk factors compared with the ADA or TM eating plans.

The Nurses' Health Study, a comprehensive 26-year epidemiological study, documented the food intake in a large cohort of women, with a subset diagnosed with diabetes. When adjusting for age, intakes of whole grain, cereal fiber, bran, and germ were associated with lower all-cause mortality, but after further adjustment for lifestyle and dietary risk factors, only the association between bran intake and all-cause mortality remained significant (He 2010). Several mechanisms have been suggested to explain the protective effects of whole grains and their components on health, including reduction of serum lipids and blood pressure, improvement of glucose and insulin metabolism, endothelial function, and alleviation of oxidative stress and inflammation. However, this study suggests that bran, a major source of cereal fiber, may be the fiber component of importance.

A study was conducted in Iran in people with type 2 diabetes that compared the use of the Dietary Approaches to Stop Hypertension (DASH) eating plan to a control diet (usual eating habits) for 4 weeks each (Azadbakht 2011). While on the DASH eating plan, subjects experienced significantly more weight loss, a waist circumference decrease, and improvements in glycemia, lipids, and blood pressure. The researchers concluded that the greater benefits from the DASH eating plan could be related to the lower caloric density of the foods, higher intake of dairy foods and legumes, and higher intake of dietary fiber, including naturally occurring plant components such as phytoestrogens and isoflavone.

In summary, the research supports that weight loss and management of diabetes can be achieved with different eating patterns. Therefore, eating patterns based on the guidelines set forth in the *Dietary Guidelines for Americans, 2010* (USDA 2010), can be used to manage diabetes. A reduced energy intake has additional benefits. Within these parameters, an individual's food choices and eating habits should be based on what he or she is able and willing to follow long term and should be culturally relevant.

ADJUNCTIVE THERAPIES TO ACHIEVE NUTRITION THERAPY GOALS

Weight-Loss Medications and Metabolic Surgery

Several adjunctive therapies, such as weight-loss medications and metabolic surgery, can assist people in achieving weight-loss and metabolic goals and have been successfully used in conjunction with multifaceted programs. Weight-loss medications, approved by the U.S. Food and Drug Administration, provide modest weight-loss benefits (>5–10% weight loss) when used in combination with other nutrition interventions and physical activity (ADA 2008) and may provide the greatest benefit for weight-loss maintenance (Franz 2007). Orlistat was offered to ILI subjects as an add-on therapy in the Look AHEAD study. However, in the small percentage of subjects taking orlistat, 6-month weight losses were smaller than in the subjects who declined the drug (Wadden 2009). Generally, people who chose to take orlistat were not achieving weight-loss goals and were not maximally implementing ILI strategies.

Categories of glucose-lowering medications—glucagon-like peptide (GLP)-1 analogs and amylin—both lower glucose and can cause weight loss. People with type 2 diabetes who used exenatide (a GLP-1 analog) for 82 weeks experienced weight loss of –4.0 to –5.3 kg and an A1C decrease of 1.0–1.3% (Riddle 2006; Ratner 2006; Blonde 2006). Additional weight-loss medications as well as additional glucose-lowering agents within existing and new categories are expected in the future.

The ADA currently recommends that metabolic (bariatric) surgery may be considered for adults with BMI >35 kg/m^2 and type 2 diabetes, especially if the diabetes or associated comorbidities are difficult to control with lifestyle and pharmacological therapy (ADA 2012). Bariatric surgery in type 2 diabetes is reviewed in Chapter 19.

Physical Activity

The joint position paper "Exercise and Type 2 Diabetes" covers a wide array of topics related to exercise and type 2 diabetes, including the acute and chronic effects of exercise, the importance of resistance training, pre-exercise evaluation, exercise with long-term complications, and how to assist people in adopting and maintaining physical activity as part of their lifestyle (Colberg 2010). An extensive evidence-based review is included. To be beneficial, exercise must be undertaken regularly using varying types of exercise. It concludes by stating that most people with type 2 diabetes can perform exercise safely as long as certain precautions are taken.

In people with type 2 diabetes, at least 150 min of accumulated moderate-intensity aerobic physical activity per week spread out over at least 3 days with no more than 2 consecutive days without exercise as well as resistance/strength training at least 2 times per week is recommended (Colberg 2010). Individuals who already exercise at moderate intensity may be encouraged to consider increasing the intensity of their exercise to obtain additional benefits in both aerobic fitness and glycemic control (Franz 2010). Physical activity is also important in long-term maintenance of weight loss, an area that is critically important, since weight regain after weight loss is a chronic challenge. Of particular relevance is the Look AHEAD trial, in which 4-year data indicated that greater physical activity is one factor for success in minimizing weight regain (Wadden 2011). Efforts by health care providers to promote physical activity should focus on discussing its importance, developing self-efficacy, and fostering social support from family, friends, and health care providers. In addition, encouraging mild or moderate physical activity can result in maximizing the adoption of a regular physical activity plan (Colberg 2010).

In type 2 diabetes, physical activity paired with nutrition interventions for weight loss has been shown to help people achieve weight control and improve glycemia, blood pressure, and lipids (Franz 2010; ADA 2008). Exercise and physical activity without nutrition intervention have only a modest weight-loss effect. However, increased physical activity, especially if implemented soon after diagnosis of diabetes and independent of weight loss, improves insulin sensitivity, decreases insulin resistance, and reduces cardiovascular risk factors (Colberg 2010). The optimal amount of physical activity to achieve sustained major weight loss is estimated to be 7 h per week of moderate to vigorous intensity and is greater than the amount required to achieve improved glucose control and cardiovascular health (Boule 2001; Colberg 2010). Both aerobic and resistance training improve insulin action, glucose control, and fat oxidation and storage in muscle.

Recent studies combining physical activity and nutrition intervention are summarized in Table 6.4. To better determine the effects of aerobic exercise versus resistance training, adults with type 2 diabetes were randomized to resistance training alone, aerobic training alone, or a combination of the two that was equal to the energy expenditure when each was done separately (Church 2010). Compared to a control group, A1C improved significantly in the aerobic and resistant training group, but not in the groups doing either alone. Although both resistance and aerobic training can offer clinical benefits, to decrease A1C, a combination of aerobic and resistance training appears to be necessary.

The value of a supervised walking program for adults with type 2 diabetes was demonstrated (Negri 2010). Subjects who attended >50% of the walking sessions had positive changes in A1C and total cholesterol, and more glucose-lowering medications were stopped or reduced.

Because supervised physical activity programs are not available to most adults with type 2 diabetes, a study using motivational interviewing to encourage lifestyle exercise and home-based self-managed exercise is of interest (Lohman 2010). VO_{2max} increased along with positive results when testing muscle strength. HDL cholesterol increased significantly, but A1C was unchanged at 6.8%.

A recent systematic review and meta-analysis of RCTs assessed the associations of structured exercise training regimens (aerobic, resistance, or both) and physical activity advice with or without nutrition advice on A1C in people with type 2 diabetes (Umpierre 2011). A1C lowering was observed with structured exercise training and structured aerobic and resistance training combined with nutrition advice. Structured exercise of >150 min/week decreased A1C more than exercise of <150 min/week. Combined physical activity and nutrition advice resulted in a decrease in A1C, whereas physical activity advice alone did not. This extensive systematic review supports recommendations that encourage people to engage in a combination of regular aerobic and resistance training that is >150 min/week. It also reinforces that, to be clinically effective, physical activity needs to be paired with nutrition therapy, especially to achieve weight loss.

SUMMARY

Research on nutrition therapy and/or physical activity interventions in adults with type 2 diabetes provides several key themes. Type 2 diabetes is a progressive disease with a pathophysiology involving numerous organs. Management requires a long-term multifaceted and comprehensive approach that includes nutrition therapy, physical activity combining aerobic and resistance training, and behavioral modification strategies. In addition, as type 2 diabetes progresses, most individuals require an increasing number and higher doses of medications to achieve glucose, lipid, and blood pressure targets to prevent and/or delay chronic complications. Emphasis as early as possible after the diagnosis of type 2 diabetes or prior, if the individual is diagnosed with prediabetes, should encourage the loss of

5–7% of initial body weight with the implementation of an eating plan deficit in energy. Adults with type 2 diabetes can be encouraged to consume a food intake that is nutrient dense and in the macronutrient ranges of 45–65% carbohydrate, 10–20% protein, and 25–35% fat. When counseling individuals to make changes in eating habits and food choices, it should be remembered that people generally do not veer far from their usual lifelong pattern of eating. Food preferences, cultural practices, environmental factors, and, most importantly, the person's willingness and ability to implement a healthy eating plan all need to be considered.

The evolution of our health care system through health care reform (Rice 2011) and the continued development of communication technologies are likely to play a key role in our ability to offer adults with type 2 diabetes the frequent ongoing education and support research has demonstrated they need to achieve clinically meaningful outcomes.

BIBLIOGRAPHY

Academy of Nutrition and Dietetics: Type 1 and type 2 diabetes evidence-based nutrition practice guidelines for adults, 2008. Available from http://www.adaevidencelibrary.com/topic.cfm?=3252. Accessed November 2011

American Association Clinical Endocrinologists/American College Endocrinologists: Consensus panel on type 2 diabetes mellitus: an algorithm for glycemic control. *Endocr Pract* 15:542–559, 2009

American Diabetes Association: Nutrition recommendations and interventions for diabetes (Position Statement). *Diabetes Care* 31 (Suppl. 1):S61–S78, 2008

American Diabetes Association: Standards of medical care in diabetes: 2012. *Diabetes Care* 35 (Suppl. 1):S11–S63, 2012

Andrews RC, Cooper AR, Montgomery AA, Norcross AJ, Peters TJ, Sharp DJ, Jackson N, Fitzsimmons K, Bright J, Coulman K, England CY, Gorton J, McLenaghan A, Paxton E, Polet A, Thompson C, Dayan CM: Diet or diet plus physical activity versus usual care in patients with newly diagnosed type 2 diabetes: the Early ACTID randomized controlled trial. *Lancet* 378:129–139, 2011

Azadbakht L, Pour Fard NR, Karimi M, Baghaei MH, Surkan PJ, Rahimi M, Esmaillzadeh A, Willett WC: Effects of the Dietary Approaches to Stop Hypertension (DASH) eating plan on cardiovascular risks among type 2 diabetic patients. *Diabetes Care* 34:55–57, 2011

Berne C, for the Orlistat Swedish Type 2 Diabetes Study Group: A randomized study of orlistat in combination with a weight management programme in obese patients with type 2 diabetes treated with metformin. *Diabet Med* 22:612–618, 2005

Bertoni AG, Clark JM, Feeney P, Yanovski SZ, Bantle J, Montgomery B, Safford MM, Herman WH, Haffner S; The Look AHEAD Research Group: Suboptimal control of glycemia, blood pressure, and LDL cholesterol in overweight adults with diabetes: the Look AHEAD Study. *J Diabetes Complications* 22:1–9, 2008

Bissett L: Lessons from the Diabetes Prevention Program. *Diabetes Care and Education* 29:23–26, 2008

Blonde L, Klein EJ, Han J, Zhang B, Mac SM, Poon TH, Taylor KL, Trautmann ME, Kim DD, Kendall DM: Interim analysis of the effects of exenatide treatment on A1C, weight and cardiovascular risk factors over 82 weeks in 314 overweight patients with type 2 diabetes. *Diabetes Obes Metab* 8:436–447, 2006

Boule NG, Haddad E, Kenny GP, Wells GA, Sigal RJ: Effects of exercise on glycemic control and body mass in type 2 diabetes mellitus: a meta-analysis of controlled clinical trials. *JAMA* 286:1218–1227, 2001

Brehm BJ, Lattin BL, Summer SS, Boback JA, Gilchrist GM, Jandacek RJ, A'Aessio DA. One-year comparison of a high-monounsaturated fat diet with a high-carbohydrate diet in type 2 diabetes. *Diabetes Care* 32:215–220, 2009

Brinkworth GD, Noakes M, Parker B, Foster P, Clifton PM: Long term effects of advice to consume a high-protein, low-fat diet, rather than a conventional weight-loss diet, in obese adults with type 2 diabetes: 1-year follow-up of a randomized trial. *Diabetologia* 47:1677–1686, 2004

Cheskin LJ, Mitchell AM, Jhaveri AM, Mitola AH, Davis LM, Lewis RA, Yep MA, Lycan TW: Efficacy of a meal replacement versus a standard food-based diet for weight loss in type 2 diabetes. *Diabetes Educ* 3:118–127, 2008

Church TS, Blair SN, Cocreham S, Johannsen N, Johnson W, Kramer K, Mikus CR, Myers V, Nauta M, Rodarte RQ, Sparks L, Thompson A, Earnest CP: Effects of aerobic and resistance training on hemoglobin A1c levels in patients with type 2 diabetes. *JAMA* 304:2253–2263, 2010

Colberg SR, Sigal RJ, Fernhall B, Regensteiner JG, Blissmer BJ, Rubin RR, Chasan-Taber L, Albright AL, Braun B: Exercise and type 2 diabetes. *Diabetes Care* 33:e147–e167, 2010

Coppell KJ, Kataoka M, Williams SM, Chisholm AW, Vorgers SM, Mann JI: Nutritional intervention in patients with type 2 diabetes who are hyperglycaemic despite optimised drug treatment: lifestyle over and above drugs in diabetes (LOADD) study: randomised controlled trial. *Br Med J* 341:c3337, 2010

Davis NJ, Tomuta N, Schechter C, Isasa CR, Segal-Isaacson CJ, Stein D, Zonszein J, Wylie-Rosett J. Comparative study of the effects of a 1-year dietary intervention of a low-carbohydrate diet versus a low-fat diet on weight and glycemic control in type 2 diabetes. *Diabetes Care* 32:1147–1152, 2009

DeFronzo R: From the triumvirate to the ominous octet: a new paradigm for the treatment of type 2 diabetes mellitus. *Diabetes* 58:773–795, 2009

Delahanty LM, Nathan DM: Implications of Diabetes Prevention Program and Look AHEAD clinical trials. *J Am Diet Assoc* 108 (Suppl. 1):S66–S72, 2008

Diabetes Prevention Program Research Group: Reduction in the incidence of type 2 diabetes with lifestyle intervention or metformin. *N Engl J Med* 346:393–403, 2002

Dietary Guidelines Advisory Committee Report on the Dietary Guidelines for Americans, 2010. Available at http://www.cnpp.usda.gov/dgas2010-dgacreport.htm

Eckel RH, Kahn SE, Ferrannini E, Goldfine AB, Nathan DM, Schwartz MW, Smith RJ, Smith SRL: Obesity and type 2 diabetes: what can be unified and what needs to be individualized? *Diabetes Care* 34:1424–1430, 2011

Elhayany A, Lustman A, Abel R, Attal-Singer J, Vinker S: A low carbohydrate Mediterranean diet improves cardiovascular risk factors and diabetes control among overweight patients with type 2 diabetes mellitus: a 1-year prospective randomized intervention study. *Diabetes Obes Metab* 12:204–209, 2010

Feldstein AC, Nichols GA, Smith DH, Stevens VJ, Bachman K, Rosales AG, Perrin N: Weight change in diabetes and glycemic and blood pressure control. *Diabetes Care* 31:1960–1965, 2008

Foster GD, Wyatt HR, Hill JO, McGuckin BG, Brill C, Mohammed BS, Szapary PO, Rader DJ, Edman JS, Klein S: A randomized trial of a low-carbohydrate diet for obesity. *N Engl J Med* 348:2082–2090, 2003

Franz MJ, Powers MA, Leontos C, Holzmeister LA, Kulkarni K, Monk A, Wedel N, Gradwell E: The evidence for medical nutrition therapy for type 1 and type 2 diabetes in adults. *J Am Diet Assoc* 110:1852–1889, 2010

Franz MJ, VanWormer JJ, Crain AL, Boucher JL, Histon T, Caplan W, Bowman JD, Pronk NP: Weight-loss outcomes: a systematic review and meta-analysis of weight-loss clinical trails with a minimum 1-year follow-up. *J Am Diet Assoc* 107:1755–1767, 2007

Gardner C, Kiazand A, Alhassan S, Soowon K, Stafford R, Balise R, Kraemer H, King A: Comparison of the Atkins, Zone, Ornish, and LEARN diets for change in weight and related risk factors among overweight premenopausal women. *JAMA* 297:969–977, 2007

Hanefeld M, Sachse G: The effects of orlistat on body weight and glycaemic control in overweight patients with type 2 diabetes: a randomized, placebo-controlled trial. *Diabetes Obes Metab* 4:415–423, 2002

He M, van Dam RM, Rimm E, Hu FB, Qi L: Whole grain, cereal fiber, bran, and germ intake and the risks of all-cause and CVD-specific mortality among women with type 2 diabetes. *Circulation* 21:2162–2168, 2010

Hollander PA, Elbein SC, Hirsch IB, Kelley D, McGill J, Taylor T, Weiss SR, Crockett SE, Kaplan RA, Comstock J, Lucas CP, Lodewick PA, Canovatchel W, Chung J, Hauptman J: Role of orlistat in the treatment of obese patients with type 2 diabetes. *Diabetes Care* 21:1288–1294, 1998

Kattelmann KK, Bonti K, Ren C: The medicine wheel nutrition intervention: a diabetes education study with the Cheyenne River Sioux tribe. *J Am Diet Assoc* 109:1532–1539, 2009

Kelley DE, Bray GA, Pi-Sunyer FX, Klein S, Hill J, Miles J, Holland P: Clinical efficacy of orlistat therapy in overweight and obese patients with insulin-treated type 2 diabetes: a 1-year randomized controlled trial. *Diabetes Care* 25:1033–1041, 2002

Kim S, Lee S, Kang E, Kange S, Hur K, Lee H, Ahn C, Cha B, Yoo J, Lee HL: Effects of lifestyle modification on metabolic parameters and carotid intima-media thickness in patients with type 2 diabetes. *Metabolism* 55:1053–1059, 2006

Kirk JK, Graves DE, Craven TE, Lipkin EW, Austin M, Margolis KL: Restricted-carbohydrate diet in patients with type 2 diabetes: a meta-analysis. *J Am Diet Assoc* 108:91–100, 2008

Li Z, Hong K, Saltsman P, DeShields S, Bellman M, Thames G, Liu Y, Wang H-J, Elashoff R, Heber D: Long-term efficacy of soy-based meal replacements vs an individualized diet plan in obese type II DM patients: relative effects on weight loss, metabolic parameters, and C-reactive protein. *Eur J Clin Nutr* 59:411–418, 2005

Lohmann H, Siersma V, Olivarius NF: Fitness consultations in routine care of patients with type 2 diabetes in general practice: an 18-month non-randomised intervention study. *BMC Family Practice* 11:83, 2010

Look AHEAD Research Group: Long-term effects of a lifestyle intervention on weight and cardiovascular risk factors in individuals with type 2 diabetes mellitus: four-rear results of the Look AHEAD trial. *Arch Intern Med* 170:1566–1575, 2010

Look AHEAD Research Group, Pi-Sunyer X, Blackburn G, Brancati FL: Reduction in weight and cardiovascular disease risk factors in individuals with type 2 diabetes: one-year results of the Look AHEAD trial. *Diabetes Care* 30:1374–1383, 2007

Malpass A, Andrews R, Turner KM: Patients with type 2 diabetes experiences of making multiple lifestyle changes: a qualitative study. *Patient Educ Couns* 74:258–263, 2009

Mayer-Davis EJ, D'Antonio AM, Smith SM, Kirkner G, Levin MS, Parra-Medina D, Schultz R: Pounds off with empowerment (POWER): a clinical trial of weight management strategies for black and white adults with diabetes who live in medically underserved rural communities. *Am J Public Health* 94:1736–1742, 2004

Mertz JA, Stern JS, Kris-Etherton P, Reusser ME, Morris CD, Hatton DC, Oparil S, Haynes RB, Resnic LM, Pi-Sunyer FX, Clark S, Chester L, McMahon M, Snyder GW, McCarron DA: A randomized trial of improved weight loss with a prepared meal plan in overweight and obese patients: impact on cardiovascular risk reduction. *Arch Intern Med* 160:2150–2158, 2000

Miles JM, Leiter L, Hollander P, Wadden T, Anderson JW, Doyle M, Foreyt J, Aronne L, Klein S: Effect of orlistat in overweight and obese patients with type 2 diabetes treated with metformin. *Diabetes Care* 25:1123–1128, 2002

Negri C, Bacchi E, Morgante S, Soave D, Marques A, Menghini E, Muggeo M, Bonora E, Moghetti P: Supervised walking groups to increase physical activity in type 2 diabetic patients. *Diabetes Care* 33:2333–2335, 2010

Ratner RW, Maggs D, Nielsen LL, Stonehouse AH, Poon T, Zhang B, Bicsak TA, Brodows RG, Kim DD: Long-term effects of exenatide therapy over 82 weeks on glycaemic control and weight in overweight metformin-treated patients with type 2 diabetes. *Diabetes Obes Metab* 8:419–428, 2006

Raynor HA, Jeffery RW, Ruggiero AM, Clark JM, Delahanty LM, the Look AHEAD Research Group: Weight loss strategies associated with body mass index in overweight adults with type 2 diabetes at entry into the Look AHEAD Trial. *Diabetes Care* 31:1299–1304, 2008

Redmon JB, Raatz SK, Reck KP, Swanson JE, Kwong CA, Fan Q, Thomas W, Bantle JP: One-year outcome of a combination of weight loss therapies for subjects with type 2 diabetes: a randomized trial. *Diabetes Care* 26:2505–2511, 2003

Redmon JB, Reck KP, Raatz SK, Swanson JE, Kwong CA, Ji H, Thomas W, Bantle JP: Two-year outcomes of a combination of weight loss therapies for type 2 diabetes. *Diabetes Care* 28:1311–1315, 2005

Rice D, Roberts WL, Collinsworth A, Fleming N: Diabetes and accountable care organizations: an accountable care approach to diabetes management. *Clinical Diabetes* 29:70–72, 2011

Riddle MC, Henry RR, Poon TH, Zhang B, Mac SM, Holcombe JH, Kim DD, Maggs DG: Exenatide elicits sustained glycaemic control and progressive reduction in body weight in patients with type 2 diabetes inadequately controlled by sulphonylureas with or without metformin. *Diabetes Metab Res Rev* 22:483–491, 2006

Sacks FM, Bray GA, Carey VJ, Smith SR, Ryan DH, Anton SD, McManus K, Champagne DM, Bishop LM, Laranjo N, Leboff MS, Rood JC, de Jonge L, Greenway FL, Loria DM, Obarzanek E, Williamson DA: Comparison of weight-loss diets with different compositions of fat, protein, and carbohydrates. *N Engl J Med* 360:859–873, 2009

Spahn JM, Reeves RS, Keim KS, Laquatra I, Kellogg M, Jortberg B, Clark NA: State of the evidence regarding behavior change theories and strategies in nutrition counseling to facilitate health and food behavior change. *J Am Diet Assoc* 110:879–891, 2010

Stern L, Iqbal N, Seshadri P, Chicano KL, Daily DA, McGrory J, Williams M, Gracely EJ, Samaha FF: The effects of low-carbohydrate versus conventional weight loss diets in severely obese adults: one-year follow-up of a randomized trial. *Ann Intern Med* 140:778–785, 2004

Sumithran P, Prendergast LA, Delbridge E, Purcell K, Shulkes A, Kriketos A, Proietto J: Long-term persistence of hormonal adaptations to weight loss. *N Engl J Med* 365:1597–1604, 2011

Umpierre D, Ribeiro PAB, Kramer CK, Leitão CB, Zucatti ATN, Azevedo MJ, Gross JL, Ribeiro JP, Schaan BD: Physical activity advice only or structured exercise training and association with HbA1c levels in type 2 diabetes: a systematic review and meta-analysis. *JAMA* 305:1790–1799, 2011

U.S. Department of Agriculture, Agricultural Research Service, Beltsville Human Nutrition Research Center, Food Surveys Research Group; U.S. Department of Health and Human Services, Centers for Disease Control and Prevention, National Center for Health Statistics: What We Eat in America, NHANES 2007–2008. Available from http://www.ars.usda.gov/SP2UserFiles/Place/12355000/pdf/0708/Table_1_NIN_GEN_07.pdf. Accessed 14 November 2011

U.S. Department of Agriculture, U.S. Department of Health and Human Services: *Dietary Guidelines for Americans, 2010*. 7th ed. Washington, DC, U.S. Government Printing Office, 2010 (www.dietaryguidelines.gov)

Vitolins MZ, Anderson AM, Delahanty L, Raynor H, Miller GD, Mobley C, Reeves R, Yamamoto M, Champagne C, Wing RR, Mayer-Davis E, the Look AHEAD Research Group Action for Health in Diabetes (Look AHEAD) Trial: Baseline evaluation of selected nutrients and food group intake. *J Am Diet Assoc* 109:1367–1375, 2009

Wadden TA, Neiberg RH, Wing RR, Clark JM, Delahanty LM, Hill JO, Krakoff J, Otto A, Ryan DH, Vitolins MZ, The Look AHEAD Research Group: Four-year weight losses in the Look AHEAD study: factors associated with long-term success. *Obesity (Silver Spring)* 19:1987–1998, 2011

Wadden TA, West DS, Neiberg RH, Wing RR, Ryan DH, Johnson KC, Foreyt JP, Hill JO, Trence DL, Vitolins MZ, The Look AHEAD Research Group: One-year weight losses in the Look AHEAD study: factors associated with success. *Obesity* 17:713–722, 2009

Wheeler ML, Dunbar SA, Jaacks LM, Karmally W, Mayer-Davis EJ, Wylie-Rosett J, Yancy Jr WS: Macronutrients, food groups, and eating patterns in the management of diabetes: a systematic review of the literature, 2010. *Diabetes Care* 35:434–445, 2012

Wing RR, Hamman RF, Bray GA, Delahanty L, Edelstein SL, Hill JO, Horton ES, Hoskin MA, Kriska A, Lachin J, Mayer-Davis EJ, Pi-Sunyer X, Regensteiner JG, Venditti B, Wylie-Rosett J, Diabetes Prevention Program Research Group: Achieving weight and activity goals among diabetes prevention program lifestyle participants. *Obes Res* 12:1426–1434, 2004

Wing RR, Lang W, Wadden TA, Safford M, Knowler WC, Bertoni AG, Hill JO, Brancati FL, Peters A, Wagenknecht L, the Look AHEAD Research Group: Benefits of modest weight loss in improving cardiovascular risk factors in overweight and obese individuals with type 2 diabetes. *Diabetes Care* 34:1481–1486, 2011

Wolever TMS, Gibbs AL, Mehling C, Chiasson J-L, Connelly PW, Josse RG, Leiter LA, Maheux P, Rabasa-Lhoret R, Rodger NW, Ryan EA: The Canadian Trial of Carbohydrates in Diabetes (CCD), a 1-y controlled trial of low-glycemic-index dietary carbohydrate in type 2 diabetes: no effect on glycated hemoglobin but reduction in C-reactive protein. *Am J Clin Nutr.* 2008;87:114-125.

Wolf AM, Conaway MR, Crowther JQ, Nadler JL, Oneida B, Bovbjerg VE: Translating lifestyle intervention to practice in obese patients with type 2 diabetes: Improving Control with Activity and Nutrition (ICAN) study. *Diabetes Care* 27:1570–1576, 2004

Hope S. Warshaw, MMSc, RD, BC-ADM, CDE, is a Nutrition/Diabetes Consultant, freelance writer, and Diabetes Educator at Hope Warshaw Associates, LLC, in Alexandria, VA.

Chapter 7
Nutrition Therapy for Youth with Diabetes

GAIL SPIEGEL, MS, RD, CDE

Highlights

Nutrition Therapy Goals and Recommendations for Youth

Nutrition Therapy Interventions

Insulin Regimens

Nutrition Education and Counseling

Management of Type 2 Diabetes in Youth

Summary

Highlights
Nutrition Therapy for
Youth with Diabetes

■ Healthy eating guidelines for children and adolescents with diabetes are the same as guidelines for all children. The *Dietary Guidelines for Americans, 2010,* can be used as a reference for healthy eating.

■ Many children and adolescents with type 1 diabetes are now using physiological insulin replacement therapy (basal/bolus) including multiple daily injections or pump therapy, providing maximum flexibility in eating schedules and food intake.

■ Carbohydrate counting is the most commonly used approach to meal planning for children and adolescents with diabetes. Families and youth are being taught to match insulin to the individual youth's carbohydrate intake.

■ Provision of adequate caloric intake for normal growth and development is an important goal for this population. Height and weight should be recorded on growth charts and evaluated regularly.

■ Type 2 diabetes has become more common in youth with the increasing rates of overweight and obesity in the U.S. and studies have begun to evaluate the best approaches to effectively manage this population.

Nutrition Therapy for Youth with Diabetes

bout 215,000 young people under 20 years of age in the U.S. have diabetes (type 1 or type 2), with most having type 1 diabetes (National Diabetes Education Program 2011). As obesity rates in children continue to increase, type 2 diabetes, which used to be seen primarily in adults over age 45 years, is becoming more common in youth. On the basis of data from 2002 to 2005, the SEARCH for Diabetes in Youth study found that 15,600 youth were newly diagnosed with type 1 diabetes annually and 3,600 were newly diagnosed with type 2 diabetes annually (SEARCH for Diabetes in Youth Study Group 2007).

The 1999 book *American Diabetes Association Guide to Medical Nutrition Therapy for Diabetes* concluded that, "Nutrition therapy for children and adolescents with diabetes has been enhanced by a variety of factors that have guided practitioners toward a more flexible approach to helping patients manage diabetes" (Sharp 1999). This statement continues to be true today. With the availability of more physiological insulins and improved technology, including more advanced insulin pumps and continuous glucose sensors, practitioners have been able to advise youth with diabetes on flexible approaches to managing nutrition therapy and diabetes.

This chapter reviews and updates the recommendations, guidelines, and research on nutrition therapy in children and adolescents with type 1 and type 2 diabetes since the publication of the 1999 book (Sharp 1999). A literature search was conducted using PubMed MEDLINE, and articles were also identified from reference lists. Search criteria included the following: nutrition, nutrition interventions, diet, diet interventions and type 1 and type 2 diabetes in children, carbohydrate counting and type 1 and type 2 diabetes, English language articles, and publication after the publication of the 1999 book. Studies evaluating nutrition intake of children and adolescents with diabetes are listed in Table 7.1, with intervention studies and studies evaluating carbohydrate counting accuracy in this population listed in Table 7.5. Table 7.1 includes 12 studies and Table 7.5 includes 6 studies that met the search criteria. There is limited research published on nutrition interventions in either type 1 or type 2 diabetes in youth to inform practice. Some intervention recommendations for this population are formulated from the Diabetes Control and Complications Trial (DCCT), research on adults, and expert opinion.

NUTRITION THERAPY GOALS AND RECOMMENDATIONS FOR YOUTH

As for adults, nutrition therapy goals for children and adolescents with type 1 and type 2 diabetes include achievement and maintenance of glucose, lipid, and blood pressure goals to prevent or slow the development of chronic complications of diabetes and to prevent and treat acute complications (Silverstein 2005; American Diabetes Association [ADA] 2008b). However, there are goals and recommendations that apply specifically to the youth population and its unique needs. Nutrient recommendations are based on requirements for all healthy children and adolescents because there is no research on the nutrient requirements for children and adolescents with diabetes (Silverstein 2005). Therefore, youth and families of youth with diabetes should be instructed to follow the Dietary Guidelines for Americans, 2010, which outline general nutrition recommendations for all youth ≥2 years of age (Dietary Guidelines Advisory Committee [DGAC] 2010). Those recommendations include 3–10 oz of grains, 1–2.5 cups of fruit, 1.5–4 cups of vegetables, 3–7 oz protein foods, and 2–3 cups of dairy per day depending on age, sex, and activity level.

A literature review (Table 7.1) indicated that children and adolescents with diabetes fail to meet their nutrition goals (Helgeson 2006; Mayer-Davis 2006; Patton 2007; Overby 2007a). They are eating more total and saturated fat than recommended and inadequate amounts of several food groups and nutrients such as fruits, vegetables, and grains (Mayer-Davis 2006; Helgeson 2006; Overby 2007b). The SEARCH for Diabetes in Youth study, the largest study conducted on youth, found that only 6.5% of the cohort (1,697 youth) met ADA recommendations of <10% of energy from saturated fat, and <50% met recommendations for total fat, vitamin E, fiber, fruits, vegetables, and grains (Mayer-Davis 2006).

Calories for Normal Growth and Development

Provision of adequate calories for normal growth and development in children and adolescents with diabetes is a key component of nutrition therapy. Therefore, it is important to monitor growth by measuring height and weight every 3 months and recording it on a Centers for Disease Control and Prevention (CDC) pediatric growth chart (http://www.cdc.gov/growthcharts) (Silverstein 2005). Table 7.2 lists approximate caloric requirements for children and adolescents based on sex, age, and activity level (DGAC 2010). Children do, however, appear to have the inherent ability to select appropriate amounts and type of food to sustain normal growth. Nutrition assessment tools such as 24-h recall, 3-day food records, and food frequency questionnaires can be used in conjunction with a computer nutrient analysis program to determine usual nutrient intake. Once calorie and nutrient needs are established, they can be adjusted to accommodate growth or prevent accelerated weight gain.

At the time of diagnosis, many children and adolescents with type 1 diabetes present with weight loss that must be restored with insulin initiation, hydration, and adequate energy intake. With weight loss or lack of weight gain at diagnosis, youth with diabetes usually require additional calories to promote catch-up growth. Because energy requirements change with age, physical activity, and growth rate, an evaluation of height, weight, BMI, and nutrition plan is recommended at least every year (Kulkarni 1998). Children and adolescents, along with

Table 7.1 Nutrient Intake of Children and Adolescents with Diabetes

	Population/ Duration of Study	Intervention (type of study)	Major Findings	Comments
Cook 2002	n = 61 adolescents (13–16 years) with type 1 or type 2 diabetes from three diabetes clinics/ not applicable	Analysis of 24-h dietary recalls compared to recalls from national sample of adolescents without diabetes (descriptive study)	♂ kcal ~100% RDA, ♀ kcal ~81% of RDA; ♂ exceeded RDA for protein, vitamin A and C, Fe, Ca; ♂ protein 2× RDA; ♀ did not meet recommended daily averages for Ca, cholesterol, and Fe	Author conclusions: diets of adolescents with diabetes and their adolescent counterparts are similar
Wilson 2003	n = 35 adolescents (11–16 years) with type 1 diabetes/not applicable	Analysis of food records/diet history from medical records; compared nutrients of patients using insulin pumps to patients using "traditional" insulin therapy (descriptive study)	Nonsignificant difference between groups in nutrients (kcal, % CHO, protein, fat); average kcal slightly higher for patients using traditional insulin therapy	
Faulkner 2006	n = 50 adolescents with type 1 diabetes, 14 with type 2 diabetes, 53 control subjects (ages 13–19 years)/not applicable	Analysis of 3-day food records (descriptive study)	Non-diabetes ♀ CHO intake ↑, total fat and SFA ↓, than for ♀ with diabetes; ♂ with diabetes had ↑ SFA than non-diabetes ♂ (all $P <$ 0.05)	Author conclusions: overall dietary intake patterns similar to NHANES II data for all groups
Helgeson 2006	n = 132 adolescents with type 1 diabetes, 131 without diabetes (ages 10–14 years)/not applicable	Analysis of 3 24-h recall interviews with participant and one parent (descriptive study)	kcal for ♀ in both groups below recommendations; % of fat kcal ↑ than recommended for people with diabetes; SFA in both groups ↑ than recommended; people with diabetes had ↑ fat and protein % than people without diabetes	

Table 7.1 Nutrient Intake of Children and Adolescents with Diabetes (*continued*)

	Population/ Duration of Study	Intervention (type of study)	Major Findings	Comments
Mayer-Davis 2006	n = 1,697 youth (10–22 years) with type 1 and type 2 diabetes (89% type 1 diabetes, 11% type 2 diabetes)/not applicable	Analysis of food frequency questionnaire (descriptive study)	37–38% of kcal from fat across age and diabetes type; youth with type 2 diabetes consumed less Ca, Mg, and vitamin E than youth with type 1 diabetes (P < 0.01); only 6.5% had <10% of kcal from SFA; <50% met recommendations for total fat, vitamin E, fiber, fruit, vegetables, and grains	Author conclusions: overall, dietary intake in youth with diabetes substantially failed to meet current recommendations
Lodefalk 2006	n = 174 Swedish adolescents with type 1 diabetes and 160 matched control subjects/not applicable	Analysis of food frequency questionnaire and 38 randomly chosen patients completed a prospective 4-day food record (descriptive study)	Diabetes patients ate fruit and fruit juice (P = 0.006) and potatoes, root vegetables, meat, fish, eggs, offal and sugar-free sweets more often than control subjects (P < 0.001 for all); diabetes patients chose more low-fat dairy products (P = 0.001); SFA ↑ more than recommended for type 1 diabetes patients (P < 0.004) and diabetes ♂ consumed more protein than recommended (P = 0.04)	Author conclusions: food habits of adolescents with type 1 diabetes healthier than those of control subjects
Patton 2007	n = 33 children (~5–6 years) with type 1 diabetes and families/not applicable	3-day diet diaries evaluated for dietary adherence and glycemic control (cross-sectional study)	CHO intake ~80% of recommended; kcal ~78% of recommended age levels; <50% met DRI for Ca and only 1 child met 100% of DRI for vitamin B-12; positive association between poor dietary adherence and high BG levels	

	Population/ Duration of Study	Intervention (type of study)	Major Findings	Comments
Overby 2007a	n = 550 Norwegian youth (2–19 years) with type 1 diabetes on intensive therapy/ not applicable	Analysis of precoded 4-day food diaries and relationship of dietary intake to BG control (cross-sectional study)	Fat ↑ and fiber ↓ than recommended (NS); youth with optimal BG had ↓ intake of added sugar (P = 0.004), ↑ fiber (P = 0.01), ↓ sugar-sweetened soft drinks (P = 0.01), and ↑ fruits (NS) and vegetables (P = 0.01)	Author conclusions: optimal BG control associated with eating a recommended diet and not skipping meals
Overby 2007b	n = 177 Norwegian adolescents (12–13 years) with type 1 diabetes and 1,809 control subjects/ not applicable	Analysis of precoded 4-day food diaries (descriptive study)	33–35% kcal from fat and 14–15% SFA, higher than recommended for type 1 diabetes patients and higher than control subjects ($P < 0.001$ for both); fiber, fruit, and vegetable intakes lower compared with recommendations	
Papadaki 2008	n = 41 Greek youth (6–17 years) with type 1 diabetes and 41 matched control subjects/ not applicable	Analysis of 24-h dietary recalls (descriptive study)	% kcal from sucrose ↓ and fiber ↑ in diabetes group compared with control subjects ($P ≤ 0.05$); % kcal from fat, SFA, and sucrose ↑ and CHO and fiber ↓ for both groups than recommended	
Overby 2008	n = 655 Norwegian youth (3–19 years) with type 1 diabetes/not applicable	Analysis of precoded 4-day food diaries and questionnaire (eating, TV, and computer habits questions) from diabetes youth compared to healthy peers (cross-sectional study)	Youth who skip meals have ↑ odds of suboptimal A1C (OR 4.7, P = 0.02), ↑ LDL cholesterol (OR 4.0, $P < 0.001$), being overweight (OR 2.8, P = 0.03), watching TV (OR 3.6, $P < 0.001$), have ↑ intake of added sugar (OR 2.1, P = 0.01), and ↓ intake of fiber (OR 0.2, P = 0.04) than youth not skipping meals	

Table 7.1 Nutrient Intake of Children and Adolescents with Diabetes (*continued*)

	Population/ Duration of Study	Intervention (type of study)	Major Findings	Comments
Bortsov 2011	*n* = 2,176 youth with type 1 diabetes and 365 youth with type 2 diabetes (ages 10–22 years)/not applicable	Evaluating food frequency questionnaire and association of dietary intake, demographics, socioeconomic status, and behavioral and diabetes-related measures (cross-sectional study)	Type 1 diabetes ♂ had ↓ intake of vegetables, fruit, fiber and ↑ intake of soda and SFA than ♀ (*P* < 0.01); African Americans had ↓ dairy and Ca and ↑ soda intake than non-Hispanic white type 1 diabetes individuals (*P* < 0.01); soda consumption was ↑ in type 2 diabetes youth ≥15 years old compared to younger youth (*P* < 0.01); in youth with type 1 diabetes, lower parental education and watching TV for ≥2 h/day was associated with ↓ fruit and fiber intake (*P* < 0.01 for both)	Author conclusions: identified demographic and behavioral correlates may help dietitians focus on groups of youth who have lower adherence to a healthful eating pattern

BG, blood glucose; CHO, carbohydrate; DRI, dietary reference intake; OR, odds ratio; RDA, recommended dietary allowance; SFA, saturated fatty acids.

their families, should be taught meal-planning basics to prevent excess weight gain. Regular physical activity should be encouraged, and children and their families should be taught the proper treatment of hypoglycemia to prevent excess caloric intake and weight gain.

Chronic undertreatment with insulin along with longstanding poor diabetes control often leads to poor growth and weight loss, whereas overtreatment with insulin can lead to excessive weight gain. In addition, impaired linear growth or poor weight gain should raise concern for the development of other related autoimmune diseases such as hypothyroidism and celiac disease and behaviors such as disordered eating behaviors or insulin omission. Evaluation of height and weight on the CDC growth curves at each clinic visit will allow for early recognition of any changes from normal, which then can be evaluated and treated (Silverstein 2005).

Glycemic Goals for Youth with Type 1 and Type 2 Diabetes

Type 1 diabetes. One of the most important goals of nutrition therapy is to help youth and their families achieve glycemic goals. Because of the changing

Table 7.2 Estimated Calorie Needs per Day by Age, Sex, and Physical Activity Level*

| Sex | Age (years) | Physical Activity Level† | | |
		Sedentary	Moderately Active	Active
Child (female and male)	2–3	1,000–1,200‡	1,000–1,400‡	1,000–1,400‡
Female	4–8	1,200–1,400	1,400–1,600	1,400–1,800
	9–13	1,400–1,600	1,600–2,000	1,800–2,200
	14–18	1,800	2,000	2,200
Male	4–8	1,200–1,400	1,400–1,600	1,600–2,000
	9–13	1,600–2,000	1,800–2,200	2,000–2,600
	14–18	2,000–2,400	2,400–2,800	2,800–3,200

*Based on Estimated Energy Requirements (EER) equations, using reference heights (average) and reference weights (healthy) for each age/sex group. For children and adolescents, reference height and weight vary. EER equations are from the Institute of Medicine (2002). Estimated amounts of calories needed to maintain calorie balance for various sex and age groups at three different levels of physical activity are shown. The estimates are rounded to the nearest 200 calories. An individual's calorie needs may be higher or lower than these average estimates.

†Sedentary means a lifestyle that includes only the light physical activity associated with the typical day-to-day life. Moderately active means a lifestyle that includes physical activity equivalent to walking about 1.5–3 miles per day at 3 to 4 miles per hour, in addition the light physical activity associated with typical day-to-day life. Active means a lifestyle that includes physical activity equivalent to walking >3 miles per day at 3–4 miles per hour, in addition to the light physical activity associated with typical day-to-day life.

‡The calorie ranges shown are to accommodate needs of different ages within the group. For children and adolescents, more calories are needed at older ages. Adapted from DGAC 2010.

needs of the developing child, age-specific glycemic goals for youth with type 1 diabetes have been developed (Silverstein 2005) (Table 7.3). These age-specific goals were designed to balance the benefits of improved glycemic control with the child's unique vulnerability to hypoglycemia. Because young children (<6 years old) whose brains are developing are at greater risk for impaired brain development with significant hypoglycemia, their glycemic goals are less stringent. In addition, very young children are not able to independently recognize and treat hypoglycemia. As adolescents approach adulthood, the glycemic goals should approach those of adults.

Despite advances in diabetes management, youth around the U.S. fail to meet A1C goals. Recent research indicates that 17% of youth with type 1 diabetes and 27% of individuals with type 2 diabetes have poor control with A1C ≥9.5% (Petitti 2009). The mean A1C in this multicenter study was 8.2% for youth with type 1 diabetes and 8.0% for youth with type 2 diabetes.

Table 7.3 Plasma Blood Glucose and A1C Goals for Youth with Type 1 Diabetes by Age-Group

Age	Before Meals (mg/dL)	Bedtime Goal (mg/dL)	A1C (%)	Rationale
Toddlers, preschoolers (0–6 years)	100–180	110–200	<8.5	■ Vulnerability to hypoglycemia ■ Insulin sensitivity ■ Unpredictability in food intake and physical activity ■ A lower goal (<8%) is reasonable if it can be achieved without excessive hypoglycemia
School-age (6–12 years)	90–180	100–180	<8	■ Vulnerability to hypoglycemia ■ A lower goal (<7.5%) is reasonable if it can be achieved without excessive hypoglycemia
Adolescents, young adults (13–19 years)	90–130	90–150	<7.5	■ A lower goal (7.0%) is reasonable if it can be achieved without excessive hypoglycemia

Key concepts in setting glycemic goals:
■ Goals should be individualized, and lower goals may be reasonable based on benefit-risk assessment.
■ Blood glucose goals should be modified in children with frequent hypoglycemia or hypoglycemia unawareness.
■ Postprandial blood glucose values should be measured when there is a discrepancy between preprandial blood glucose values and A1C levels to help assess glycemia in individuals on basal/bolus regimens.

From ADA 2012.

Adolescents (13–17 years old) with type 1 diabetes were included in the DCCT, and individuals in the intensive management group were found to have the same improvements in glycemic control and reduced risk of complications as the adults did (DCCT 1993). However, A1C levels were ~1% higher than the adult levels in the study, and adolescents were only able to maintain a mean A1C of 8.1%. They also had a higher incidence of hypoglycemia and gained more weight. The study was conducted before the advent of rapid- and long-acting insulin analogs, and research has demonstrated that these analogs are associated with less hypoglycemia with equal A1C lowering (DeWitt 2003; Rosenstock 2005).

Follow-up of DCCT adolescent participants showed an increase in A1C in individuals in the intensive group (from 8.1 to 8.4%) and a decrease in individuals in the conventional group (from 9.8 to 8.5%) after study end (DCCT/Epidemiology of Diabetes Interventions and Complications [EDIC] 2000), suggesting that it may be difficult to maintain an A1C consistently <8% without the resources of a clinical trial (Silverstein 2005). However, the study did show that intensive diabetes therapy has long-term beneficial effects on health. At 4 years after the close of the DCCT, the adolescents in the intensive treatment group of the DCCT had little further retinopathy, whereas the previously conventionally treated group had progression in an additional 15% of participants (DCCT/EDIC 2000). The previously intensive treatment group also had a 42% reduced risk of any cardiovascular disease (CVD) event compared to the conventionally treated group (DCCT/EDIC 2005). These results supported the recommendation to intensify diabetes management as early as possible (Silverstein 2005).

Type 2 diabetes. Goals of treatment of youth with type 2 diabetes include achieving glycemic control with near-normal fasting blood glucose values (<126 mg/dL) and A1C <7%. Additional goals include ceasing excessive weight gain with normal linear growth, improving CVD risk factors, and improving physical and emotional well-being (ADA 2000).

Reducing Risk of Diabetes Complications in Youth with Type 1 and Type 2 Diabetes

Long-term complications. CVD resulting from atherosclerosis is the leading cause of morbidity and mortality in adults with type 1 diabetes (Vinik 2002; Blendea 2003). The atherosclerotic process begins early in life and high lipid levels during childhood are associated with coronary atherosclerosis in adulthood (McGill 2000; Li 2003; Raitakari 2003). A lipid profile should be performed on prepubertal children with type 1 diabetes >2 years of age after diagnosis of diabetes if the family history of diabetes is positive or unknown. If the family history is known and negative, screening should begin at puberty. All children diagnosed with diabetes at or after puberty should have a fasting lipid profile performed soon after diagnosis. Youth who have borderline or abnormal LDL cholesterol values should have screenings repeated yearly. If LDL values fall within the accepted levels, a lipid profile should be repeated every 5 years based on CVD risk status. For youth with type 2 diabetes, screening should occur at diagnosis regardless of age and repeated every 2 years. All screenings should be conducted after glucose control has been established (ADA 2012).

Table 7.4 lists the lipid goals for LDL, HDL, and triglycerides. The American Academy of Pediatrics Expert Panel on Integrated Guidelines for Cardiovascular Health and Risk Reduction in Children and Adolescents: Summary Report details guidelines for treatment of lipid abnormalities (Expert Panel on Integrated Guidelines for Cardiovascular Health and Risk Reduction in Children and Adolescents: 2011). Nutrition recommendations for normal children and children with hypercholesterolemia, over 2 years of age, include an intake of total fat, which can be safely limited to 30% of total calories; saturated fat intake limited to 7% to 10% of calories; and dietary cholesterol limited to 300 mg/day. The remaining 20% of fat intake should be a combination of monounsaturated and polyunsaturated fats. Intake of *trans* fats should be limited as much as possible.

Acute complications: hypoglycemia and sick-day management. Preventing acute complications with nutrition therapy in children and adolescents is another important goal. Because hypoglycemia is a common acute complication for youth

Table 7.4 Lipid Goals for Children and Adolescents with Type 1 and Type 2 Diabetes

LDL cholesterol*	<100 mg/dL
HDL cholesterol	>35 mg/dL
Triglycerides	<150 mg/dL

*In youth with diabetes, LDL cholesterol ≥130 mg/dL is considered abnormal, 100–120 mg/dL borderline, and <100 mg/dL normal. From ADA 2012 and Silverstein 2005.

using insulin therapy, youth and their families should be taught proper treatment. A general recommendation for the treatment of a hypoglycemic episode in children is the consumption of 15 g (10 g for younger children) of glucose. Glucose is the preferred treatment for hypoglycemia, although any form of carbohydrate that contains glucose may be used (ADA 2008a). Blood glucose should be retested 15 min after treatment with carbohydrate, and an additional 10–15 g carbohydrate should be given as needed until blood glucose returns to the target range. Adding protein to carbohydrate does not affect the glycemic response and does not prevent subsequent hypoglycemia (see Chapter 12).

It is also important to teach concepts related to the prevention of hypoglycemic episodes. Strategies to reduce hypoglycemic episodes may include the adjustment of insulin for varying carbohydrate intake or for changes in physical activity. Youth should be taught to carry a source of carbohydrate with them at all times, and this principle should be reinforced regularly.

Principles of blood glucose management during acute illness, including use of well-tolerated carbohydrate sources in place of usual choices, should be taught at the time of diabetes diagnosis (see Chapter 12).

NUTRITION THERAPY INTERVENTIONS

Food plans for youth must be individualized to meet food preferences, eating schedules, physical activity patterns, and cultural influences. Education on the basic diabetes nutrition concepts and rationale for coordination of the food intake and insulin therapy should begin early after diagnosis and be reviewed regularly to reinforce concepts to improve adherence. Basic concepts of a food plan should be taught to young children in a developmentally appropriate manner, with specific details given to parents, other family members, and caretakers. Older children and adolescents are often capable of understanding the basics of a meal plan, but require parental support and guidance for adherence.

The most widely used method of meal planning for youth with both type 1 and type 2 diabetes is carbohydrate counting. For people who have difficulty with carbohydrate counting, simplified, healthy eating meal-planning guidelines are prescribed. The exchange system of meal planning is infrequently prescribed for children with diabetes, but can be helpful for youth with type 2 diabetes, who need to control portions, carbohydrate, and caloric intake. In the past, meal planning was much less flexible, and children often were prescribed a rigid meal plan to match insulin dosing. Today, the prevailing approach is to match insulin to the child's nutrition (carbohydrate) intake.

Carbohydrate Counting

Carbohydrate counting is a meal-planning method based on the principle that all types of carbohydrate (except fiber) are digested, with the majority being absorbed into the bloodstream as molecules of glucose, and that the total amount of carbohydrate consumed has a greater effect on blood glucose elevations than the specific type consumed. There are two main methods of meal planning using carbohydrate counting: using an insulin-to-carbohydrate ratio to adjust prandial insulin for variable carbohydrate intake (physiological insulin regimen) or following a consistent carbohydrate meal plan when using a fixed insulin regimen.

Which method a child uses will depend on the insulin regimen the child uses and the family's skill level. Some families start with a consistent carbohydrate meal plan and predetermined doses of prandial insulin. Over time, the youth should be transitioned to a basal-bolus insulin regimen (multiple daily injections [MDIs] or an insulin pump).

Adjusting Insulin for Carbohydrate (Insulin-to-Carbohydrate Ratios)

Basal-bolus insulin management mimics normal physiological insulin secretion by giving MDIs of rapid-acting insulin with basal insulin (glargine, detemir) or using an insulin pump. This method allows for variability in appetite and types of meals served. Most children, from toddlers to teens, have variable appetites and benefit from this approach to meal planning. Children using this method do not have to follow a fixed schedule for meals and snacks.

Children using this method of meal planning will have an individualized insulin-to-carbohydrate ratio and blood glucose correction factor for dosing of their rapid-acting insulin, determined by their registered dietitian (RD) or health care provider.

Insulin-to-carbohydrate ratios vary from child to child. For example, a 5-year-old may use an insulin-to-carbohydrate ratio of 1 unit of rapid-acting insulin per 30–45 g carbohydrate, whereas teenagers may use 1 unit for each 5–15 g carbohydrate.

To count carbohydrate amounts accurately, children and their families are taught how to read the "Nutrition Facts" on food labels for total carbohydrate grams. Families should measure or weigh foods periodically to estimate portion sizes and carbohydrate content accurately. There are also many resources available for families to refer to for unlabeled foods. Resources include books, websites, and smartphone applications. Families should have easy access to one of these resources to estimate carbohydrates as accurately as possible. Also, many school districts are making carbohydrate content information available for school breakfast and lunch, making carbohydrate counting in the school setting much easier.

Because accurate carbohydrate counting is essential for accurate insulin dosing, researchers have evaluated carbohydrate counting accuracy in the pediatric population (Table 7.5). Research on children, adolescents, and their parents indicates that these individuals may not be accurate in estimating carbohydrates. In one study, parents of 4- to 12-year-old children overestimated carbohydrate intake of their children by an average of 120% of the nutrition database calculated intake (Mehta 2009). Another study found that adolescents either significantly over- or underestimated carbohydrate content of 23 of 32 individual foods presented as real foods or food models (Bishop 2008). Lastly, a study conducted in the United Kingdom and Australia found that adolescents estimated carbohydrates within 10–15 g of the actual amount for 73% of meals presented (Smart 2010). These authors concluded that adolescents carbohydrate count reasonably accurately, but if accuracy was defined more stringently (within 10 g of the actual amount), then many estimates would have been considered inaccurate. Additional research is needed in this area to help determine the best strategies for helping children, adolescents, and their families improve their carbohydrate-counting skills and accuracy and potentially glycemic control.

Consistent Carbohydrate Meal Plan

On a consistent carbohydrate meal plan with fixed doses of prandial insulin, the child with diabetes should keep his or her carbohydrate intake consistent on a day-to-day basis with respect to time and amount (ADA 2008a; Silverstein 2005). The amount of carbohydrate is individualized to the nutritional needs of the child

Table 7.5 Nutrition Therapy Interventions for Youth with Diabetes

	Population/ Duration of Study	Intervention (type of study)	Major Findings	Comments
Gilbert-son 2001	n = 104 youth with type 1 diabetes (8–13 years)/12 months	A measured CHO exchange diet (set number of exchanges for meals/snacks) vs. a more flexible low-GI dietary regimen (randomized controlled trial)	At 3 and 6 months, non-significant difference in A1C; at 12 months, A1C was improved for the low-GI group vs. the CHO exchange group but no difference in GI value between groups (P < 0.05)	Author conclusions: flexible dietary instruction based on the food pyramid with emphasis on low-GI foods improves A1C
Willi 2004	n = 35 morbidly obese youth (~ 15 years) with type 2 diabetes/ >6 weeks	High-protein, low-fat, low-CHO VLCD/ (retrospective case-control study)	Adherence to the VLCD for >6 weeks decreased A1C (P < 0.005); at 2 years, A1C decrease not sustained; a sustained improvement in BMI compared to control and baseline at 2 years (P < 0.05 for both)	Author conclusions: The ketogenic VLCD is an effective short-term and possibly long-term therapy for pediatric patients with type 2 diabetes

	Population/ Duration of Study	Intervention (type of study)	Major Findings	Comments
Mehta 2009	$n = 67$ youth with type 1 diabetes and their parents/ not applicable	Parents estimated CHO content of children's' meals in 3 diet recalls (cross-sectional)	CHO estimate ~120% of database calculated intake; CHO counting precision ($P = 0.02$) and more frequent blood glucose testing ($P = 0.04$), but not accuracy, associated with lower A1C; A1C 0.8% lower if parents demonstrated precision	
Bishop 2008	$n = 48$ adolescents (12–18 years) with type 1 diabetes/not applicable	Assessed CHO content of 32 foods commonly consumed by youth (descriptive study)	Overestimation of CHO content for 15 of 32 foods ($P < 0.01$ for all); underestimation for 8 of 32 foods ($P < 0.01$ for all); only 23% estimated daily CHOs within 10 g of actual amount	Author conclusions: Adolescents with type 1 diabetes do not accurately count carbohydrates
Smart 2010	$n = 102$ youth (8–18 years) with type 1 diabetes and 110 caregivers/not applicable	Estimated CHO content of 17 standardized meals (descriptive study)	73% of estimates within 10–15 g of actual CHO content; the longer children had been CHO counting the greater the mean percentage error ($r = 0.173$, $P = 0\,0.014$)	Author conclusions: CHO content of meals can be estimated with reasonable accuracy
Koontz 2010	$n = 75$ youth (~13 years) ($n = 41$) with type 1 diabetes and parents ($n = 34$)/ not applicable	PCQ used to assess recognition of CHO, CHO counting in foods and meals, label reading, use of insulin dose correction factors, and insulin-to-CHO ratios (cross-sectional)	↑ PCQ scores correlated with ↓ A1C ($r = -0.29$, $P = 0.01$) and expert assessments ($r = 0.56$, $P < 0.001$); scores higher in parents with college degrees ($P = 0.01$) and in participants with more complex insulin regimens ($P = 0.003$)	Author conclusions: The PCQ is a novel, easily administered instrument to assess knowledge about CHOs and insulin dosing calculations

CHO, carbohydrate; GI, glycemic index; PCQ, PedCarbQuiz; VLCD, very-low-calorie diet.

and his or her usual intake. The amount of prandial insulin (rapid- or short-acting) that the child takes only changes for the blood glucose level. Snacks are often necessary and must be eaten to stay in balance with the peak times of insulin action and with physical activity. Furthermore, depending on the child's age, many children and youth prefer smaller meals with snacks in between. Carbohydrate counting is also used in children with type 2 diabetes who take only oral medication and need to moderate carbohydrate and caloric intake. Sample carbohydrate ranges for meals and snacks based on age and sex are listed in Table 7.6.

Physical Activity

Children with diabetes are encouraged to participate in the same forms of physical activity as children without diabetes (Silverstein 2005). Children and adolescents are encouraged to do ≥60 min of physical activity daily. Most of the ≥60 min a day should be either moderate- or vigorous-intensity aerobic physical activity and should include vigorous-intensity physical activity at least 3 days a week. It is important to encourage youth to participate in physical activities that are appropriate for their age, that are enjoyable, and that offer variety (DGAC 2010). Benefits of exercise in type 1 diabetes include a greater sense of well-being, help with weight control, improved physical fitness, and improved cardiovascular fitness, with lower pulse and blood pressure levels and an improved lipid profile (Wasserman 1994; Austin 1993).

Of hypoglycemic episodes in children, 10–20% are associated with exercise, which is generally of greater than usual intensity, duration, or frequency (Silverstein 2005). To prevent hypoglycemia in type 1 diabetes patients, the following recommendations can be given:

- Blood glucose monitoring before exercise is recommended, with a suggested intake of 15 g carbohydrate (amount may be lower in younger children, e.g., 10 g) for a blood glucose level below target range before exercise.
- For vigorous activity expected to be >30 min, an additional 15 g carbohydrate may be necessary.
- For prolonged vigorous exercise, hourly blood glucose monitoring during the exercise, as well as blood glucose monitoring after completion of exercise, is recommended to guide carbohydrate intake and prospective insulin dose adjustment for recurring exercise events.
- At the onset of a new sports season, frequent blood glucose monitoring during the 1-h post-exercise period should be undertaken to guide insulin dose adjustments.
- In the child or adolescent (particularly if overweight/obese), physical exercise should be encouraged and sedentary activity should be discouraged.

Decreasing insulin dose for planned exercise rather than increasing calories should be the primary approach, when possible, to help prevent excess weight gain. This strategy may be difficult in the young child whose physical activity is more sporadic than planned; therefore, increased carbohydrates will be necessary (Silverstein 2005). Children with diabetes may consume carbohydrate-containing fluids, such as diluted fruit juices or commercial sports drinks, for fluid and carbohydrate replacement during activity.

Hyperglycemia may occur with physical activity for a few reasons. If the child or adolescent is deficient in insulin, resulting from an inadequate insulin regimen or missed injection, then blood glucose will remain elevated during and after exercise. High-intensity exercise may result in hyperglycemia, likely because of higher levels of catecholamine and growth hormone, which may last from 30 to 60 min after exercise (Riddell 2006). Many times, this type of hyperglycemia is followed by hypoglycemia within 1–6 h of the completion of the exercise because of hepatic

Table 7.6 Average Carbohydrate Amount Per Meal for Children with Diabetes

| | Meal Carbohydrate Amounts by Age* | |
	5–12 years old	Teens
Boys	45–60 g carbohydrate at each meal	60–75+ g carbohydrate at each meal
Girls	45–60 g carbohydrate at each meal	45–75 g carbohydrate at each meal

*Carbohydrate amount must be individualized based on caloric needs, preferences, and activity levels. Snacks, if needed, are usually 15–30 g carbohydrate. The child's diabetes health care provider helps determine the amount of carbohydrate that is right for each child at each meal. Adapted from Evert 2006.

glycogen depletion (Silverstein 2005). With prior planning, all children with diabetes should be able to enjoy the many benefits of physical activity. (See Chapter 10 for additional information on exercise, sports, and diabetes.)

INSULIN REGIMENS

In this age-group, the MDI regimen used with the carbohydrate-counting meal-planning approach is very popular and allows for flexibility in eating times and amounts. However, the number of insulin injections required may be a barrier to good control for some. Growing children and adolescents eat meals and snacks throughout the day. To reduce frequency of prandial insulin injections while striving to achieve maximum flexibility with eating, many youth and their caregivers may choose an insulin pump if it is an option financially (Silverstein 2005). Insulin pumps also have features that can improve accuracy of insulin dosing, by potentially reducing dose calculation errors that can be an issue with this age-group. Bolus calculators can determine prandial insulin doses based on the amount of carbohydrate consumed, premeal blood glucose, and active insulin on board. The SEARCH study found that almost half of the 2,753 pediatric patients participating were managed with basal-bolus therapy, including 22% on insulin pump therapy (Paris 2009). Adult support at both home and in school is essential for success with all diabetes management, but especially with pump treatment until the child is able to manage the diabetes independently (Weissberg-Benchell 2003). Pump therapy requires additional training to prepare the child and family for this form of diabetes management, with carbohydrate counting review being an important aspect of the education.

Excellent reviews are available to guide insulin initiation and management of other insulin therapy regimens to achieve optimal glycemic control; therefore, this topic will not be extensively reviewed here (ADA 2009; DeWitt 2003; Silverstein 2005).

NUTRITION EDUCATION AND COUNSELING

Nutrition therapy for children and adolescents with diabetes includes a variety of topics that should be initiated at diagnosis and continued on an ongoing basis. One model for educating families on nutrition therapy for diabetes is to begin with survival skills at diagnosis, with more intensive education at 1 week and continued review at 1 month and 3 months into diagnosis.

It is recommended that nutrition therapy be provided by an RD with expertise in pediatric nutrition and diabetes. Nutrition therapy should be part of the initial team education and requires a series of sessions over the 3 months after diagnosis. Then, the child or adolescent should be seen by an RD at least annually to evaluate height, weight, BMI, and the food plan. Young children require more frequent evaluations (Silverstein 2005).

Age Components of Nutrition Education and Counseling

The challenges of nutrition education for children and adolescents with diabetes are often age-related and require consideration of the specific nutrition and developmental needs of different age-groups. The defining characteristics of different age-groups must be considered when providing nutrition care to children and adolescents. Below is a summary of some of the specific characteristics to consider when working with each age-group.

Toddlers
- Variable appetites
- Eat small, frequent meals
- Prone to food jags/selective eating, resulting in food battles with parents
- Daycare providers need instruction on diabetes management

Preschool/School Age
- More consistent growth and nutrition intake
- Usually eat three meals and snacks between meals
- Begin to be involved in organized sports and physical education class
- School personnel need understanding and training in diabetes management

Adolescents
- Variable schedules/more inconsistency
- Often working and going to school
- Peer influence on food choices
- More responsible for food choices and diabetes self-care
- More likely to miss shots/boluses
- Alcohol use needs to be discussed
- School personnel need understanding and training in diabetes management

Disordered Eating Behaviors/Eating Disorders and Other Age-Related Concerns

Body image and weight management concerns in adolescent females as well as males with diabetes are of particular concern. Eating disorders and disordered eating behaviors are a significant health problem for many children and adolescents. Controversy exists regarding whether there is an increased prevalence of diagnosable eating disorders and disordered eating behaviors in patients with type 1 diabetes compared with people without diabetes, with some studies showing a higher rate in type 1 diabetes patients and others finding the same or lower rates (Young-Hyman 2010). Estimates of diagnosable eating disorders and disordered eating behaviors in adolescent and young adult females with type 1 diabetes range from 3.8 to 27.5% for patients classified as bulimic or having binge eating disorder. When insulin omission is considered purging the estimate goes as high as 38–40%. The presence of diagnosable eating disorders and behavior categorized as subclinical disordered eating behaviors has been associated with increases in retinopathy, neuropathy, transient lipid abnormalities, hospitalizations for diabetic ketoacidosis, and poor short-term metabolic control. Adolescents with diabetes should be screened regularly for insulin omission and eating disorders to prevent the serious medical consequences of very poor glycemic control. Warning signs that may be indicative of an eating disorder in adolescents include lack of adequate weight gain or growth, significant weight loss without illness, suboptimal overall glycemic control, and recurrent diabetic ketoacidosis.

Other issues of concern in adolescents with diabetes include the potential use of alcohol. Adolescents must be instructed on the potential hypoglycemic effects of alcohol and on responsible drinking, should they choose to use alcohol. Adolescents who drive should be instructed on blood glucose monitoring before driving and carrying a source of carbohydrate with them at all times should hypoglycemia occur. Finally, adolescents with diabetes may experiment with alternative eating patterns, such as a vegetarian diet, or they may choose to use nutritional supplements. Practical information on these topics will enable adolescents to make wise choices for their health.

MANAGEMENT OF TYPE 2 DIABETES IN YOUTH

Overweight and obesity are the main reasons for the increased number of youth with type 2 diabetes. The 2005–2006 National Health and Nutrition Examination Survey (NHANES) found that 16–17% of children had BMIs greater than or equal to the 95th percentile for age and sex, about double the numbers of 20 years previously (Ogden 2008). Type 2 diabetes is more common in minority populations, with Asian/Pacific Islanders and American Indian youth having a greater risk of type 2 diabetes than type 1 diabetes. Type 2 diabetes is rare in children younger than 10 years of age, regardless of race or ethnicity. After 10 years of age, type 2 diabetes becomes increasingly common, especially in minority populations, representing 14.9% of newly diagnosed cases of diabetes in non-Hispanic whites, 46.1% in Hispanic youth, 57.8% in African Americans, 69.7% in Asian/Pacific Islanders, and 86.2% in American Indian youth (SEARCH 2007). The SEARCH for Diabetes in Youth study also found that 84% of adolescents with type 2 diabetes had a first-degree relative with diabetes.

The following are proposed strategies for the treatment of asymptomatic and symptomatic children with type 2 diabetes (Bloomgarden 2004):

For asymptomatic children:
- Start with lifestyle intervention approaches to nutrition and exercise.
- Add monotherapy, emphasizing the use of metformin.
- Use combinations of oral medications.
- Add insulin.

For symptomatic children with blood glucose levels >300 mg/dL or when ketoacidosis is present:
- Start with insulin, with subsequent efforts to taper insulin and substitute metformin.
- Lifestyle intervention may be sufficient, although this appears to be applicable in ~10% of patients at the time of presentation.

Treatment with medication may include insulin, metformin, insulin secretagogues, and α-glucosidase inhibitors. Metformin and glimepiride are the only oral agents approved for pediatric use (National Diabetes Education Program 2008). The most recent statistics on medication treatment of youth with type 2 diabetes was published in 2004 and, at that time, approximately one-half of youth with type 2 diabetes treated with medication received insulin and one-half oral agents, most commonly metformin (Bloomgarden 2004). A clinical trial assessing the use of liraglutide, a glucagon-like peptide-1 drug, in pediatric patients is currently underway (National Institutes of Health [NIH] 2011).

Lifestyle Intervention Strategies

Referral to an RD with expertise in weight management of children with diabetes is recommended. Nutrition interventions should be culturally appropriate, sensitive to family resources, and provided to all caregivers. The entire family should be included in the lifestyle intervention, since parents and family members influence the child's food intake and physical activity. Parents are often overweight or obese and may have diabetes as well (ADA 2000).

Families should be counseled to decrease energy intake by focusing on healthy eating and strategies to decrease portion sizes of foods and lower intake of high-energy, fat- and sugar-containing foods. Increasing energy expenditure by increasing daily physical activity is also an important component of treatment. Decreasing sedentary behaviors such as television viewing, computer use, text messaging, and the use of a variety of other electronic devices has been shown to be an effective way to increase daily physical activity in children (ADA 2000). The American Academy of Pediatrics recommends that children limit screen time to ≤2 h per day (Davis 2007). Follow-up should include periodic reevaluation and reinforcement of treatment modalities (ADA 2000).

Although family-based behavioral weight-loss treatments have been found to be effective in improving weight status in children, the impact of family-based lifestyle interventions on weight and metabolic control in youth with type 2 diabetes has not been evaluated (Treatment Options for Type 2 Diabetes in Adolescents and Youth [TODAY] 2010). A large multicenter study to investigate the best approaches to lifestyle intervention and medication management of this population is currently being completed. The TODAY study is a 15-center clinical trial sponsored by NIH. Subjects ages 10–17 years with type 2 diabetes are randomized into one of three treatment arms: metformin; metformin plus rosiglitazone, or metformin plus an intensive lifestyle (weight management) intervention. The much-anticipated results of this study will help provide evidence to inform practitioners about the best approaches to managing this challenging population.

SUMMARY

Today, practitioners working in the field of pediatric diabetes will encounter children with both type 1 and type 2 diabetes. Nutrition guidelines for youth with type 1 diabetes are designed to help them achieve optimal glycemic control with normal growth and development and to prevent the long-term and acute complications of the disease. Healthy eating guidelines are the same as those for all children. The current approach to diabetes and food management is to provide maximum flexibility in food intake and eating schedules by using basal/bolus regimens and matching insulin to the youth's carbohydrate intake.

As children grow and change developmentally, their insulin and nutrition regimens must be monitored and adjusted to meet their individual needs. A visit with an RD with expertise in pediatric diabetes is recommended at least annually, and education of the child and family is an ongoing, continuous process.

As the rates of overweight and obesity have increased, more children and adolescents are being diagnosed with type 2 diabetes, with minority ethnic groups being at highest risk. In addition to the goals to achieve optimal glycemic control and prevent complications of diabetes, nutrition management of type 2 diabetes also focuses on providing lifestyle intervention for the whole family, including nutrition therapy and physical activity to achieve weight loss or prevent excessive weight gain.

Studies indicate that youth with type 1 and type 2 diabetes are not meeting their A1C and nutrition goals and are not accurate in carbohydrate counting. Few studies on nutrition interventions have been conducted in youth with diabetes to guide practice. A large 15-center study on lifestyle intervention for type 2 diabetes in youth has been completed, and the results of this study will help to inform the treatment of this population. Additional research is needed to determine the best nutrition interventions to help youth with diabetes meet their nutrition goals, carbohydrate count more accurately, and achieve optimal metabolic outcomes.

BIBLIOGRAPHY

American Diabetes Association: Diabetes care in the school and day care setting (Position Statement). *Diabetes Care* 32 (Suppl. 1):S68–S72, 2008a

American Diabetes Association: Management of dyslipidemia in children and adolescents with diabetes (Consensus Statement). *Diabetes Care* 26:2194–2197, 2003

American Diabetes Association: *Intensive Diabetes Management.* Alexandria, VA, American Diabetes Association, 2009

American Diabetes Association: Nutrition recommendations and interventions for diabetes (Position Statement). *Diabetes Care* 31 (Suppl. 1):S61–S78, 2008b

American Diabetes Association: Standards of medical care in diabetes: 2012. *Diabetes Care* 35 (Suppl. 1):S11–S63, 2012

American Diabetes Association: Type 2 diabetes in children and adolescents (Consensus Statement). *Diabetes Care* 23:381–389, 2000

Austin A, Warty V, Janosky J, Arslanian S: The relationship of physical fitness to lipid and lipoprotein (a) levels in adolescents with IDDM. *Diabetes Care* 16:421–425, 1993

Bishop FK, Maahs DM, Spiegel G, Owen D, Klingensmith GJ, Bortsov A, Thomas J, Mayer-Davis EJ: The carbohydrate counting in adolescents with type 1 diabetes (CCAT) study. *Diabetes Spectrum* 22:56–62, 2008

Blendea MC, McFarlane SI, Isenovic ER, Gick G, Sowers JR: Heart disease in diabetic patients. *Curr Diab Rep* 3:223–229, 2003

Bloomgarden ZT: Type 2 diabetes in the young: the evolving epidemic. *Diabetes Care* 27:998–1010, 2004

Bortsov A, Liese AD, Bell RA, Dabelea D, D'Agostino RB, Hamman RF, Klingensmith GJ, Lawrence JM, Maahs DM, McKeown R, Marcovina SM, Thomas J, Mayer-Davis EJ: Correlates of dietary intake in youth with diabetes: results from the SEARCH for Diabetes in Youth study. *J Nutr Educ Behav* 43:123–129, 2011

Cook S, Solomon MC, Berry CA: Nutrient intake of adolescents with diabetes. *Diabetes Educ* 28:382–388, 2002

Davis MM, Gance-Cleveland B, Hassink S, Johnson R, Paradis G, Resnicow K: Recommendations for prevention of childhood obesity. *Pediatrics* 120:S229–S253, 2007

DeWitt DE, Hirsch IB: Outpatient insulin therapy in type 1 and 2 diabetes mellitus: scientific review. *JAMA* 289:2254–2264, 2003

Diabetes Control and Complications Trial Research Group: Effect of intensive treatment of diabetes on the development and progression of long-term complications of insulin-dependent diabetes mellitus. *N Eng J Med* 329:977–986, 1993

Diabetes Control and Complications Trial/Epidemiology of Diabetes Interventions and Complications (DCCT/EDIC) Study Research Group: Intensive diabetes treatment and cardiovascular disease in patients with type 1 diabetes. *N Engl J Med* 353:2643–2653, 2005

Diabetes Control and Complications Trial/Epidemiology of Diabetes Interventions and Complications (DCCT/EDIC) Study Research Group: Retinopathy and nephropathy in patients with type 1 diabetes four years after a trial of intensive therapy. *N Engl J Med* 342:381–389, 2000

Diabetes Control and Complications Trial Research Group: Effect of intensive diabetes treatment on the microvascular complications of type 1 diabetes mellitus. *JAMA* 287:2563–2569, 2002

Dietary Guidelines Advisory Committee Report on the Dietary Guidelines for Americans, 2010. Available at http://www.cnpp.usda.gov/dgas2010-dgacreport.htm. Accessed June 2011

Evert A, Gerken S: Children with diabetes: birth to adolescence. *On The Cutting Edge* 7:4–8, 2006

Expert Panel on Integrated Guidelines for Cardiovascular Health and Risk Reduction in Children and Adolescents: Expert Panel on Integrated Guidelines for Cardiovascular Health and Risk Reduction in Children and Adolescents: Summary report. *Pediatrics* 128:S213–S256, 2011

Faulkner MS, Chao WH, Kamath SK, Quinn L, Fritschi C, Maggiore JA, Williams RH, Reynolds RD: Total homocysteine, diet and lipid profiles in type 1 and type 2 diabetic and nondiabetic adolescents. *J Cardovasc Nurs* 21:47–55, 2006

Gilbertson HR, Brand-Miller, JC, Thorburn AW, Evans S, Chondros P, Wether GA: The effect of flexible low glycemic index dietary advice vesus measured carbohydrate exchange diets on glycemic control in children with type 1 diabetes. *Diabetes Care* 24:1137–1143, 2001

Helgeson VS, Viccaro L, Becker D, Escobar O, Siminerio L: Diet of adolescents with and without diabetes. *Diabetes Care* 29:982–987, 2006

Institute of Medicine: *Dietary Reference Intakes for Energy, Carbohydrate, Fiber, Fat, Fatty Acids, Cholesterol, Protein, and Amino Acids.* Washington, DC, The National Academies Press, 2002

Koontz MB, Cuttler L, Palmert MR, O'Riordan M, Borawski EA, McConnell J, Kern EO: Development and validation of a questionnaire to assess carbohydrate and insulin-dosing knowledge in youth with type 1 diabetes. *Diabetes Care* 33:457–462, 2010

Kulkarni K, Castle G, Gregory R, Holmes A, Leontos C, Powers M, Snetselaar L, Spett P, Wylie-Rosett J, for the Diabetes Care and Education Dietetic Practice Group: Nutrition practice guidelines for type 1 diabetes mellitus positively affect dietitian practices and patient outcomes. *J Am Diet Assoc* 98:62–70, 1998

Li S, Chen W, Srinivasa SR, Bond MG, Tang R, Urbina EM, Berenson GS: Childhood cardiovascular risk factors and carotid vascular changes in adulthood: the Bogalusa Heart Study. *JAMA* 290:2271–2276, 2003

Lodefalk M, Aman J: Food habits, energy and nutrient intake in adolescents with type 1 diabetes mellitus. *Diabet Med* 23:1225–1232, 2006

Mayer-Davis EJ, Nichols M, Liese AD, Bell RA, Dabelea DM, Johansen JM, Pihoker C, Rodriguez BL, Thomas J, Williams D: Dietary intake among youth with diabetes: the SEARCH for Diabetes in Youth Study. *J Am Diet Assoc* 106:689–697, 2006

McGill HC Jr, McMahon CA, Zieske AW, Sloop GD, Walcott JV, Troxclair DA, Malcolm GT, Tracy RD, Oalmann MC, Strong JP: Associations of coronary heart disease risk factors with intermediate lesion of atherosclerosis in youth: the Pathobiological Determinants of Atherosclerosis in Youth (PDAY) Research Group: *Arterioscler Throm Vasc Biol* 20:1998–2004, 2000

Mehta SN, Quinn N, Volkening LK, Laffel LM: Impact of carbohydrate counting on glycemic control in children with type 1 diabetes. *Diabetes Care* 32:1014–1016, 2009

National Diabetes Education Program: The Facts about Diabetes: A Leading Cause of Death in the U.S., 2011. Available at http://ndep.nih.gov/diabetes-facts/index.aspx. Accessed June 2011

National Diabetes Education Program: Overview of diabetes in children and adolescents: a fact sheet from the National Diabetes Education Program, 2008. Available at http://ndep.nih.gov/media/Youth_FactSheet.pdf. Accessed May 2011

National Institutes of Health: Safety of liraglutide in pediatric patients with type 2 diabetes, 2011. Available at http://clinicaltrials.gov. Accessed June 2011

Ogden CL, Carroll MD, Flegal KM: High body mass index for age among US children and adolescents, 2003–2006. *JAMA* 299:2401–2405, 2008

Overby NC, Flaaten V, Veierod MB, BergstadI, Margeirdottir HD, Dahl-Jorgensen K, Andersen LF: Children and adolescents with type 1 diabetes eat a more atherosclerosis-prone diet than healthy control subjects. *Diabetologia* 50:307–316, 2007b

Overby NC, Margeirsdottir HD, Brunborg C, Andersen LF, Dahl-Jorgensen K: The influence of dietary intake and meal pattern on blood glucose control in children and adolescents using intensive insulin treatment. *Diabetologia* 50:2044–2051, 2007a

Overby NC, Margeirsdottir HD, Brunborg C, Dahl-Jorgensen K, Andersen LF, Norwegian Study Group for Childhood Diabetes: Sweets, snacking habits, and skipping meals in children and adolescents on intensive insulin treatment. *Pediatr Diabetes* 9:393–400, 2008

Papadaki A, Linardakis M, Codrington C, Kafatos A: Nutritional intake of children and adolescents with insulin-dependent diabetes mellitus in Crete, Greece. *Ann Nutr Metab* 52:308–314, 2008

Paris CA, Iperatore G, Klingensmith G, Petitti D, Rodriguez B, Anderson AM, Schwartz D, Standiford DA, Pihoker C: Predictors of insulin regimens and impact on outcomes in youth with type 1 diabetes: the SEARCH for Diabetes in Youth study. *J Pediatr* 155:183–189, 2009

Patton SR, Dolan LM, Powers SW: Dietary adherence and associated glycemic control in families of young children with type 1 diabetes. *J Am Diet Assoc* 107:46–52, 2007

Petitti DB, Klingensmith GJ, Bell, RA, Andrews JS, Dabalea D, Impratore G, Marcovina S, Pihoker C, Standiford D, Waitzfelder B, Mayer-Davis E: Glycemic control in youth with diabetes: the SEARCH for Diabetes in Youth study. *J Pediatr* 155:668–672, 2009

Raitakari OT, Juonala M, Kahonen M, Taittonen L, Laitinen T, Maki-Torkko N, Jarvisalo M, Uhari M, Jokinen E, Ronnemaa T, Akerblom, HK, Vikari JSA: Cardiovascular risk factors in childhood and carotid artery intima-media thickness in adulthood: the Cardiovascular Risk in Young Finns Study. *JAMA* 290:2277–2283, 2003

Riddell MC, Iscoe KE: Physical activity, sport and pediatric diabetes. *Pediatr Diabetes* 7:60–70, 2006

Rosenstock J, Dailey G, Masi-Benedetti M, Tritsche A, Lin Z, Salzman A: Reduced hypoglycemia risk with insulin glargine: a meta-analysis comparing insulin glargine with human NPH insulin in type 2 diabetes. *Diabetes Care* 28:950–955, 2005

SEARCH for Diabetes in Youth Study Group: Incidence of diabetes in youth in the United States. *JAMA* 297:2716–2724, 2007

Sharp A: Nutrition therapy for children and adolescents with diabetes. In *American Diabetes Association Guide to Medical Nutrition Therapy for Diabetes*. Franz MJ, Bantle JP, Eds. Alexandria VA, American Diabetes Association, 1999, p. 211–228

Silverstein J, Klingensmith G, Copeland K, Plotnich L, Kaufman F, Laffel L, Deeb L, Grey M, Anderson B, Holzmeister LA, Clark N: Care of children and adolescents with type 1 diabetes: a statement of the American Diabetes Association. *Diabetes Care* 28:186–212, 2005

Smart CE, Ross K, Edge JA, King BR, McElduff P, Collins CE: Can children with type 1 diabetes and their caregivers estimate the carbohydrate content of meals and snacks? *Diabet Med* 27:348–353, 2010

The Today Study Group: Design of a family-based lifestyle intervention for youth with type 2 diabetes: the TODAY study. *Int J Obes* 34:217–232, 2010

Vinik A, Flemmer M: Diabetes and macrovascular disease. *J Diabetes Complications* 16:235–245, 2002

Wasserman DH, Zinman B: Exercise in individuals with IDDM. *Diabetes Care* 17:924–937, 1994

Weissberg-Benchell J, Antisdel-Lomaglio J, Seshadri R: Insulin pump therapy: a meta-analysis. *Diabetes Care* 26:1079–1087, 2003

Willi SN, Martin K, Datko FM, Brant BP: Treatment of type 2 diabetes in childhood using a very-low-calorie diet. *Diabetes Care* 27:348–353, 2004

Wilson MA, Smith CB: Nutrient intake, glycemic control, and body mass index in adolescents using continuous subcutaneous insulin infusion and those using traditional insulin therapy. *Diabetes Educ* 29:230–238, 2003

Young-Hyman DL, Davis CL: Disordered eating behavior in individuals with diabetes. *Diabetes Care* 33:683–689, 2010

Gail Spiegel, MS, RD, CDE, is a Senior Instructor and Manager of Nutrition Services at the Barbara Davis Center for Childhood Diabetes Pediatric Clinic, University of Colorado, Anschutz Medical Campus, Aurora, CO.

Chapter 8
Nutrition Therapy for Older Adults with Diabetes

Kathleen Stanley, MSEd, RD, CDE, BC-ADM

Highlights
Nutrition Therapy for
Older Adults with Diabetes

■ The population of individuals over the age of 65 years is expected to increase in the future. In the older population, prevalence of diabetes is estimated to be ~33%.

■ Diagnosis of diabetes in the older adult may be delayed or missed because of the lack of recommended standards for routine screening in the elderly population, physiological changes due to aging, and lack of common symptoms being reported by the individual.

■ Comorbid conditions, changes in cognition and memory, physical limitations, and the presence of additional chronic illnesses complicate the older person's ability to learn about diabetes care and to comply with therapeutic recommendations.

■ Nutrition therapy for the older adult with diabetes should include meeting the Dietary Reference Intakes for age for nutrients, evaluating fluid intake, avoiding significant weight loss, and being sensitive to individual preferences and longstanding food habits while advocating good nutrition.

■ Life expectancy and quality of life need to be considered in developing glycemic and nutrition goals for the home or a health care facility setting.

Nutrition Therapy for Older Adults with Diabetes

It has been predicted that, by the year 2030, approximately one-fifth of all Americans will be 65 years of age or older. Additionally, the group of individuals aged ≥80 years is one of the fastest-growing population groups in the U.S. (Gambert 2006). This increase in the aged population compared to past demographics is due to many factors, including aging individuals from the "baby boom" period, improved medical care overall, and better living conditions in the U.S. compared to past generations. It is difficult to grasp the complexity of the impact this new growth of older adults (for the purpose of this chapter, individuals >65 years of age) will have on medical care in the U.S. Advances in technology, economic status, and evolving new medical delivery systems already contribute significant changes to health care delivery. These issues will have a significant impact on consumers and the entire health care delivery system.

The latest census numbers should serve as an alert to all health care professionals to prepare for the future. Health care professionals must contemplate strategies to manage multiple medical conditions of the aged, especially chronic diseases, and for longer lengths of time because of the new longevity expectations. The demand for care will challenge currently available resources and systems. Chronic diseases known to be common in the older population include heart disease, diabetes, cancer, and respiratory and circulatory diseases and should be targeted in future plans for health care delivery systems and institutions.

The 2010 U.S. census estimated 26.9% of adults age ≥65 years have diabetes already, or roughly 11 million. Additionally, individuals with prediabetes were estimated at 50% of adults 65 years or older (Centers for Disease Control and Prevention 2011). Costs of treating diabetes are high in the U.S. and will grow with more individuals being diagnosed. The environment in which an individual performs daily self-care for diabetes is not limited to just the home in the older population, creating further challenges for health care delivery.

There is a higher incidence of hospitalizations for older adults with diabetes, which further increases financial burden. Hospitalized patients with diabetes also have a higher risk of death (Gambert 2006). Prevalence of diagnosed diabetes in older adults in nursing homes is expectedly high, but differences exist with respect to actual numbers. In a review of the literature, one conservative estimate reports ~33% of nursing home residents have diabetes (Garcia 2011).

DIABETES IN THE OLDER ADULT

Age-related physiological changes, treatment of other chronic disease, changes in body composition, and reduced physical activity contribute to the higher incidence of diabetes in the older adults versus younger adults (McLaughlin 1999). Type 1 diabetes comprises ~5–10% of the adult population diagnosed with diabetes, whereas type 2 diabetes comprises 85–90% (National Diabetes Information Clearinghouse 2011). Specific rates are not readily available of type 1 and type 2 diabetes from recent census data for regions within the U.S. for the older adult subset aged ≥65 years. It is however accurate to state that type 2 diabetes remains the dominant form of diabetes in older adults, despite not knowing the exact percentage of incidence. Insulin resistance combined with age-related decreasing insulin production is considered to be the most common etiology of type 2 diabetes in older adults (Gambert 2006; Mooradian 1999).

The clinical presentation of type 2 diabetes in the older adult is often different than in a younger adult, potentially causing a delay in diagnosis. Typical symptoms of excess thirst, fatigue, and weight changes may not be reported by older adults. The delay in reporting thirst in the presence of hyperglycemia can be due to subtle physiological changes, including decreased response to thirst, as part of the normal aging process. Urine diagnostic lab work may also be difficult to interpret because of changes in the glucose renal threshold, which are higher with advanced age (Terrio 2009). Fatigue is a common complaint in this population and does not usually warrant concern. The older adult likely sees fatigue as a natural consequence of aging and therefore does not report this as a health concern.

Older adults do not frequently check their weight, so a weight change as a symptom of diabetes is not always detected by the individual. Weight changes are not perceived as unusual to many older adults. Overweight older adults as well as underweight adults age 60–79 years of age are thought to be at risk for developing diabetes compared to normal-weight individuals (Sairenchi 2008; Odegard 2007). Other diabetes risk factors of the younger adult still apply to the older adult, such as ethnicity, family history, and history of gestational diabetes. Additionally, older individuals with hypertension or dyslipidemia are also at higher risk of developing diabetes (Kanaya 2005; American Diabetes Association [ADA] 2012). Because of costs, seniors may choose to see their specialists for specific conditions and may not pursue regular visits to their primary care providers, where health screenings are more likely to occur.

At present, there are no recommendations for practitioners to change the frequency of performing routine medical (glucose or A1C) screening of older adults for diabetes. In general, screening for diabetes is recommended at least at 3-year intervals for adults over 45 years of age (ADA 2012), but screening frequency intervals specific to the older adult in advanced years are not addressed. In the future, as the older population continues to expand, new screening criteria may need to be explored for diagnosis of diabetes. To conclude, there are several physiological factors and barriers contributing to delayed diagnosis of diabetes in older adults. Once diagnosed, the older adult with diabetes is thought to be more vulnerable to chronic complications (compared to younger adults) in incidence and at a more accelerated rate (Mooradian 1999). Clinicians in primary care and diabetes care may need to plan for additional time for diabetes management assessment, since the individual will likely have more than one health condition to address during the visit. Symptoms of hyperglycemia, such as reports of increased urination from an older adult, may have several possible causes aside from diabetes, including age-related urinary incontinence, urinary tract infections, improper use of prescribed medications, and other genito-urinary problems.

Older adults have a variety of health concerns and complaints due to physical changes and managing chronic conditions. Common physical struggles associated with aging include changes in vision, hearing, mobility, dexterity, and cognitive changes (Suhl 2006; Kocurek 2009). Chronic disease management for more than one condition presents treatment challenges for the individual, such as polypharmacy, difficulties with activities of daily living, health care system navigation, and financial burdens. Older adults may also be dealing with loss of a spouse, loss of friends, changes in independence and living conditions, financial instability, and loss of identity, which affect their ability to provide self-care. Because diabetes management is primarily daily self-care, health care professionals need to be sensitive to the variety of issues possibly obstructing care. Health care professionals need to consider the unique needs of this population for clinical assessment, treatment, education, and continued medical care.

Challenges for health care professionals treating or counseling older adults will encompass establishing realistic clinical target goals and treatment plans. Educational strategies will also need to be modified for the older adult to achieve expected outcomes. Diabetes education is known to benefit adults in terms of clinical outcomes; however, there is a lack of long-term studies specific to the older population for obvious reasons. Despite the lack of evidence in the literature specific to older adults, education is key to self-care as a management strategy. Education must address the abilities of the patient to carry out normal activities of daily living along with diabetes care.

Typical self-care tasks using syringes, lancet devices, home blood glucose monitoring devices, and measuring cups can be formidable to the older adult with poor vision and/or dexterity issues. Adaptive tools such as magnifiers, insulin pens, medication reminder aids, and adaptive equipment for the kitchen are available. Instructional methods may need to be modified because of the visual or cognitive changes in this population (American Association of Diabetes Educators [AADE] 2009). An occupational therapist can be a resource for health care and lifestyle aids for independent living.

Once diagnosed, a comprehensive assessment should take place. The older adult's health care team/provider will need to be informed of the patient's ability to perform other self-care tasks such as physical activity, home blood glucose monitoring, medication administration, and other personal health care activities. An integrated treatment plan with collaboration of a multidisciplinary health care team including the patient and his or her caregivers may be the best strategy to achieve desirable outcomes.

REVIEW OF EXISTING DIABETES NUTRITION RECOMMENDATIONS FOR OLDER ADULTS

A literature search was conducted using PubMed MEDLINE. Search criteria included the following: human subjects with diabetes, older adults, elderly, nutrition, nutrition therapy, nutrition intervention, diet, dietary therapy, English language articles, and published after 1998. No articles related to diabetes nutrition interventions in older adults were found. In general, nutrition recommendations are based on the knowledge of the professional and clinical judgment rather than study outcomes.

NUTRITION THERAPY FOR OLDER ADULTS WITH DIABETES

The Academy of Nutrition and Dietetics (Acad Nutr Diet) supports individualized, comprehensive, and coordinated nutrition care for all ages. Along with meeting the nutrition needs of the older adult, self-sufficiency and quality of life need to be addressed when developing nutrition recommendations for the older adult (Acad Nutr Diet 2005). Because of the diversity of the U.S. population in regard to ethnicity, religion, and culture, health care professionals need to be sensitive to individual preferences and longstanding food habits while advocating good nutrition. Good nutrition throughout the lifespan is one of the key elements responsible for successful aging, along with genetic factors, physical activity, and abstinence from tobacco products. Change of food habits may be threatening or daunting to older adults. To aid acceptance of new recommendations, the health care professional should initially explain the purposes and benefits of making food and eating modifications. A sound nutrition therapy plan should be developed that supports the individual's personal, social, and cultural needs along with respecting his or her vision of quality of life (Acad Nutr Diet 2005).

The health care professional providing nutrition care as part of diabetes education will need to take into account a variety of potential nutrition-risk issues along with diabetes management. Table 8.1 summarizes barriers related to implementation of nutrition therapy for diabetes self-management in the older adult with diabetes. These issues will need to be examined and incorporated into the nutrition therapy plan for diabetes. Additional resources and counseling time may be needed to create a comprehensive and realistic plan. As part of a multidisciplinary care team, the registered dietitian (RD) has the opportunity to help the older adult with diabetes succeed in meeting his or her diabetes treatment goals.

Access to nutrition therapy can be a barrier to self-care for older adults living with diabetes because of availability of qualified health care professionals, transportation issues, financial concerns, and lack of referral for services. Goals of nutrition therapy for diabetes are to lessen the risks of chronic complications and reduce symptoms of hypoglycemia and hyperglycemia. As part of a comprehensive medical treatment plan for diabetes, individualized MNT delivered by an RD should be pursued because of the unique needs of the population.

First and foremost, the nutrient needs of the older person with diabetes should be met when developing a nutritionally adequate meal plan. The Dietary Reference Intake for older adults specifies nutrient needs for ages 51–70 years as well as needs above the age of 70 years and is readily available online as a reference for health care professionals to use (Institute of Medicine [IOM] 2011). At present, vitamin D, vitamin B_6, chromium, and iron (women only) intakes differ for individuals over 70 years of age compared to younger adults. Dietary fiber recommendations are also different, with the recommended amount decreasing for

Table 8.1 Barriers to Implementing Nutrition Therapy for Diabetes Self-Management in the Older Adult with Diabetes

Barriers	Nutrition Care Issues	Suggested Interventions
Dementia	Skipping meals and irregular schedule	■ Meal delivery services ■ Timed reminders/establishing meal cues ■ Group meals ■ Basal-bolus insulin regimens ■ Meal/medication assistance from caregivers
	Poor food preparation skills	■ Meal delivery services ■ Appropriate convenient food choices ■ Menus and recipes using simple food preparation techniques
Physical impairments	Swallowing disorders	■ Referral to speech pathologist ■ Dysphagia diet modifications ■ Give insulin after meal rather than before because of extended meal time
	Inability to self-feed	■ Decrease frequency of monitoring because of physical challenges ■ Adaptive equipment ■ Referral to occupational therapist ■ Caregiver need/caregiver education
	Limited ability to cook/lack of interest in cooking	■ Meal delivery services ■ Group meals ■ Batch cooking and planned-over strategies ■ Suitable convenience foods ■ Simplified menu requiring minimal preparation
Depression	Altered food intake (more or less than required needs)	■ Screening/treatment for depression ■ Increase socialization ■ Address food behaviors and coping strategies for boredom ■ Make food interesting ■ Make meal setting attractive (bright placements, listen to music while eating, simple centerpieces on table) ■ Make simple-to-prepare meals
Financial barriers	Inadequate nutritional intake	■ Suggest multivitamin/mineral supplements ■ Recommend nutrient-dense food choices ■ Referral to SNAP* ■ Referral to social services ■ Referral to food banks ■ Referral for medical assistance programs ■ Decrease frequency of home blood glucose monitoring ■ Budget shopping strategies (buy produce in season; non-animal protein sources; use of senior discounts; use of coupons, etc.)

Table 8.1 Barriers to Implementing Nutrition Therapy for Diabetes Self-Management in the Older Adult with Diabetes (*continued*)

Barriers	Nutrition Care Issues	Suggested Interventions
Multiple medical conditions (for example, cancer, acute and chronic illnesses)	Drug/nutrient interactions, restricted diet plan, multiple diagnosis on problem list	■ Individualized nutritional counseling ■ Referral to case manager or social services agencies ■ Collaborate with interdisciplinary care team approach to develop care plan ■ Determine realistic target blood glucose range ■ Consider supplement usage or nutrition support when indicated ■ Relaxation of dietary restrictions

*Supplemental Nutrition Assistance Program (SNAP) special rules for the elderly or disabled are available at http://www.fns.usda.gov/snap/applicant_recipients/eligibility.htm#Special

adults ≥51 years of age compared to younger adults. In terms of macronutrients, carbohydrate and protein recommendations are the same throughout adulthood, but there are no specific fat-intake guidelines for older adults (IOM 2011).

Weight management is also important, specifically avoiding unintentional weight loss in the older adult, which has shown to increase morbidity and mortality (Suhl 2006). This result is different when comparing the weight management strategies for a younger adult with diabetes. In fact, recommendations focus on maintaining a reasonable weight, rather than using standard ideal weight charts or formulas in this population. Weight loss and caloric restriction (deficit to estimated metabolic needs) are not encouraged in the older adult with diabetes and should only be considered and implemented with caution (Suhl 2006; Terrio 2009; Odegard 2007; Johnson 2008; AADE 2009).

DIABETES NUTRITION THERAPY FOR ELDERLY IN HEALTH CARE FACILITIES

In addition to a home nutrition plan, the RD is an invaluable resource for diabetes care of the elderly in health care facilities. Older adults have a higher frequency of admission than younger adult with or without diabetes (Gambert 2006). Sudden changes in medication regimens from hospital plan to a home regimen, or to long-term care facilities, are all too common at discharge because of changes in health status and recovery needs. The nutrition plan made for hospitalization may need modification to be coordinated with the new regimen. Education is difficult to execute because of the patient's availability and distraction with the discharge process. This is especially true for the older adult, who can have significant or multiple educational barriers. Education at these times is challenging to both instructor and patient and does not always result in positive lifestyle changes or clinical outcomes; therefore, a plan for follow-up should be constructed.

Diabetes care guidelines are limited for long-term care facilities, rehabilitation facilities, group homes, and other elder care facilities (elder day cares) due to the diversity of environments and populations served. These facilities face unique challenges in managing diabetes, such as complex medical needs of the individual, education of licensed and non-licensed caregivers, multiple nutritional restrictions, and developing practical and effective care guidelines suitable for their resources. Strategies should also be available to address a decline in health (including physical limitations and mental) status of individuals. Advanced directives must be followed for end-of-life care. Consultation with the patient (if possible), family, and caregivers, and all health care providers, including palliative care professionals, will help determine appropriate treatment plans, including modified diabetes meal plans and treatment goals (Haas 2006) (see Chapter 11 for a more thorough discussion of nutrition therapy for long-term care in patients with diabetes).

PRACTICE-BASED DIABETES NUTRITION THERAPY INTERVENTIONS

Current nutrition therapy interventions for adults with diabetes are reviewed in Chapters 2, 5, and 6. However, there are unique nutritional needs of the older adult to consider, and they are summarized below.

Assessment of Nutritional Intake

- Food intake and variety of foods decline as age advances (Niedert 2004; Johnson 2008), with lower-income adults consuming even less.
- Cognitive and physical barriers may prevent problems with food acquisition, food preparation, and recall of intake (Alzheimer's Association 2004; American Geriatric Society 2011; Niedert 2004).
- Alcohol abuse incidence increases with age (Blow 2003).
- Changes in gastrointestinal tract function may impair intake (Niedert 2004).

Physiological Changes in Aging

- Gastrointestinal disturbances occur from gastroparesis, gastroesophageal reflux disease (GERD), lactase deficiency, inadequate fluid and fiber intake, and laxative abuse.
- Dentition changes result in painful chewing, restricted diet, and inadequate fiber.
- Swallowing difficulties are due to age-related motility changes, xerostomia, and poor oral health.
- Taste and appetite changes are related to lack of variety in diet, lack of activity/social stimulation, drug/nutrient interactions, poor oral health, depression, and dementia.

Macronutrient Needs

- For better accuracy, use formulas that include age of the patient.

- Review lab data for risk of anemia, albumin deficiency, and electrolyte abnormalities in older adults (Niedert 2004).
- No specific adjustments based on advanced age are needed for carbohydrate, protein, and fat needs for older adult with diabetes.
- Fluid imbalance is more common because of decreased thirst sensitivity and availability of fluids, putting individuals at higher risk of hyperglycemia hyperosmolar nonketotic syndrome (Niedert 2004; Natow 1986) and dehydration.

Outcome Evaluation

- Individual may be a poor historian; consider tools to collect information (such as meter memory data, grocery store itemized receipts, and written diaries).
- Focus on short-term goals and minimize time between appointments.

SUMMARY

Providing health care in the future to the expanding geriatric population in the U.S. presents opportunities for all health care professionals to learn more about the special needs of this population. There is a lack of current recommendations for diabetes care for individuals over the age of 65 years, both in terms of therapeutic goals and nutrition goals. Therefore, practice-based diabetes nutrition therapy interventions for the older adult with diabetes should be individualized once glycemic and other medical treatment goals are established and communicated. Glycemic goals should take into consideration the overall health of the person and quality-of-life aspects. Nutrition therapy for this stage of the lifespan is more complex than for the younger adult with diabetes during the assessment, education, and continuum of care phases. There may be multiple nutrition restrictions because of other health care problems, lifestyle issues, financial barriers, and the ability of the person to perform daily-living activities as well as diabetes self-care.

When developing an appropriate diabetes meal plan, there are minor differences for the older adult to consider compared to the younger adult. Likely, there are more lifestyle issues to address to implement a realistic plan. An important goal of nutrition therapy in regard to diabetes is to minimize hypo- and hyperglycemia and meet individualized glycemic goals. Glycemic targets may be liberalized compared to younger adults because of quality of life and life expectancy and to accommodate additional necessary nutritional plan modifications. One key difference is that weight loss for overweight individuals is not necessarily recommended in older adults with diabetes. Other elements of the meal plan that may be modified to meet the needs of the individual are meal frequency, snack frequency, use of meal supplements, food texture and consistency, and additional restrictions because of other health conditions. The health care professional should work closely with the patient, caregivers, and other members of the health care team at reasonable short-term intervals for optimal treatment outcomes when dealing with the older adult with diabetes.

BIBLIOGRAPHY

Academy of Nutrition and Dietetics: Position paper of the American Dietetic Association: Nutrition across the spectrum of aging. *J Am Diet Assoc* 105:616–633, 2005

Alzheimer's Association, South Central Wisconsin Chapter: Planning guide for dementia care at home: a reference tool for care managers. Document number PDE-3195 (part 7), 2004

American Association of Clinical Endocrinologists: Medical guidelines for clinical practice for developing a diabetes mellitus comprehensive care plan. *Endocr Pract* 17 (Suppl. 2):1–53, 2011

American Association of Diabetes Educators: Special considerations in the management and education of older persons with diabetes. *Diabetes Educ* 35:60S–63S, 2009

American Diabetes Association: Standards of medical care in diabetes: 2012. *Diabetes Care* 35 (Suppl. 1):S11–S63, 2012

American Geriatric Society: Aging in the know: nutrition, 2011. Available at www.healthinaging.org/agingintheknow/chapters_print_ch_trial.asp?ch=28. Accessed 1 November 2011

Blow FC, Barry KL: Use and misuse of alcohol among older women, 2003. Available at http://pubs.niaaa.nih.gov/publications/arh26-4/308-315.htm. Accessed 1 November 2011

Centers for Disease Control and Prevention: National Diabetes Fact Sheet: National Estimates and General Information on Diabetes and Prediabetes in the United States, 2011. Atlanta, GA, U.S. Department of Health and Human Services, Centers for Disease Control and Prevention, 2011

Gambert SR, Pinkstaff S: Emerging epidemic: diabetes in older adults: demography, economic impact, and pathophysiology. *Diabetes Spectrum* 19:221–228, 2006

Garcia TJ, Brown SA: Diabetes management in the nursing home: a systematic review of the literature. *Diabetes Educ* 37:167–187, 2011

Haas LB: Caring for community-dwelling older adults with diabetes: perspectives from health care providers and caregivers. *Diabetes Spectrum* 19:240–244, 2006

Institute of Medicine, Food and Nutrition Board: *Dietary Reference Intakes (DRIs), 2011*. Available from http://www.nap.edu. Accessed 1 November 2011

Johnson MA, Park S, Penn D, McClellan JW, Brown K, Adler A: Nutrition education issues for older adults. *The Forum for Family and Consumer Issues* 13, 2008. Available at http://ncsu.edu/ffci/publications/2008/v13-n3-2008-winter/index-v13-n3-winter-2008.php. Accessed 1 November 2011

Kanaya AM, Wassel Fyr CL, deRekeneire N, Shorr RL, Schwartz AV, Goodpaster BH, Newman AB, Harris T, Barrett-Connor E: Predicting the development of diabetes in older adults. *Diabetes Care* 28:404–408, 2005

Kocurek B: Promoting medication adherence in older adults…and the rest of us. *Diabetes Spectrum* 22:80–84, 2009

McLaughlin S: Nutrition therapy for the older adult with diabetes. In *American Diabetes Association Guide to Medical Nutrition Therapy for Diabetes.* Franz MJ, Bantle JP, Eds. Alexandria, VA, American Diabetes Association, 1999, p. 249–274

Mooradian AD, McLaughlin S, Boyer CC, Winter J: Diabetes care for older adults. *Diabetes Spectrum* 12:70–77, 1999

National Diabetes Information Clearinghouse: *National Diabetes Statistics, 2011.* Available at http://diabetes.niddk.nih.gov/dm/pubs/statistics. Accessed 1 November 2011

Natow AB, Heslin JA: *Nutritional Care of the Older Adult.* New York, MacMillian, 1986

Niedert KC, Dorner B: *Nutrition Care of the Older Adult.* 2nd ed. Chicago, American Dietetic Association, 2004

Odegard PS, Setter SM, Neumiller JJ: Considerations for the pharmaceutical treatment of diabetes in older adults. *Diabetes Spectrum* 20:239–247, 2007

Sairenchi T, Iso H, Fujiko I, Fukasawa N, Ota H, Muto T: Underweight as a predictor of diabetes in older adults. *Diabetes Care* 31:583–584, 2008

Suhl E, Bunsignore P: Diabetes self-management education for older adults: general principles and practical application. *Diabetes Spectrum* 19:234–240, 2006

Terrio L: Self-sufficient diabetes management: maintaining independence in older adults. *On the Cutting Edge* 30:14–10, 2009

Kathleen Stanley, MSEd, RD, CDE, BC-ADM, is the Diabetes Program Coordinator at Central Baptist Hospital, Lexington, KY.

Chapter 9
Nutrition Therapy for Pregnancy, Lactation, and Diabetes

Diane M. Reader, RD, CDE

Highlights
Nutrition Therapy for
Pregnancy, Lactation, and Diabetes

■ For women with type 1 or type 2 diabetes, near-normal glucose control is recommended at least 3 months before conception and throughout the pregnancy; this is achieved with a balance of nutrition therapy, glucose monitoring, and medications.

■ For women who develop gestational diabetes, nutrition therapy plus glucose monitoring, and insulin when indicated, has been shown to reduce the complications of pregnancy associated with diabetes.

■ The nutrition recommendations for weight gain, macronutrients, and vitamin and mineral supplementation for all pregnant women also apply to women with diabetes during pregnancy.

■ Because women with a history of gestational diabetes have a sevenfold increased risk of developing type 2 diabetes within 10 years, all women with gestational diabetes should be screened postpartum and counseled regarding diabetes prevention: 150 min exercise per week and weight reduction of at least 5%, if overweight (see Chapter 25).

■ Breastfeeding is recommended for the infants of women with diabetes if possible.

Nutrition Therapy for Pregnancy, Lactation, and Diabetes

The multifaceted nutritional status of the mother during pregnancy is crucial for healthy fetal development. Inadequate calorie intake, as well as excessive calorie intake, will affect fetal growth and the lifelong health of the infant. Consuming the recommended amount of macronutrients and micronutrients during pregnancy provides for healthy development of all fetal organs and tissues. In addition to a well-balanced eating pattern, women with diabetes during pregnancy must use food planning, with glucose monitoring and appropriate dosing of medication, to achieve excellent glucose control. Achieving these important outcomes is enhanced when the mother has the support of an experienced team of health care professionals who understand diabetes and pregnancy, which includes a registered dietitian (RD).

The following three evidence-based practice guidelines/reports are used for this chapter: the Academy of Nutrition and Dietetics (formerly the American Dietetic Association) (Acad Nutr Diet) evidence-based nutrition practice guidelines for gestational diabetes mellitus (GDM), first developed in 1998 and updated in 2001 and 2008 (Acad Nutr Diet 2008); the American Diabetes Association (ADA) consensus statement "Managing Preexisting Diabetes for Pregnancy" (Kitzmiller 2008a); and the proceedings from the Fifth International Workshop-Conference on Gestational Diabetes Mellitus (Metzger 2007).

MULTIDISCIPLINARY TEAM FOR SUCCESSFUL PREGNANCY OUTCOMES

Before discussing nutrition therapy recommendations and the research supporting them, the first question that needs to be asked is whether medical nutrition therapy (MNT) implemented by RDs is important in a pregnancy complicated by diabetes. The RD is the only professional in the health care team trained to thoroughly assess a complex nutrient intake within the socioeconomic, cultural, and individual lifestyle characteristics of each patient. This information is then used to diagnose nutrition problems and to collaborate with the patient to create a food plan that will provide a healthy well-balanced foundation for intensive glucose interventions.

The ADA's *Managing Preexisting Diabetes and Pregnancy* (ADA-MPDP) begins with the following recommendation: "Whenever possible, organize multidisciplinary patient-centered team care for women with preexisting diabetes in preparation for pregnancy and continue multidisciplinary team care throughout pregnancy and postpartum" (Kitzmiller 2008a). Models of care with a responsible patient at the center of the management team have had the best success. Successful diabetes management depends on the person with diabetes making daily choices and decisions based on diabetes self-management education and data from monitoring glucose, food, activity, and medications. Pregnancy profoundly affects all aspects of the management of diabetes.

The Fifth International Workshop-Conference summary and recommendations state the following: "MNT is the cornerstone of treatment for GDM and…. MNT is best prescribed by a registered dietitian or qualified individual with experience in the management of GDM" (Metzger 2007). The Acad Nutr Diet evidence-based nutrition practice guidelines for GDM state the following: "Research indicates that MNT results in improved maternal and neonatal outcomes, especially when diagnosed and treated early" (Acad Nutr Diet 2008).

NUTRITION THERAPY FOR DIABETES AND PREGNANCY

To update nutrition therapy for pregnancy complicated by diabetes, a literature search was conducted using PubMed MEDLINE, and additional articles were identified from references and bibliographies. Search criteria included the following: published after 2008, gestational diabetes, preexisting diabetes, and nutrition therapy. The initial search produced 87 articles on the topic of nutrition, gestational diabetes, and pregestational diabetes; 83 were excluded because titles or abstracts did not meet inclusion criteria. Eight articles either from the initial search or identified from reference lists met inclusion criteria and are included in Table 9.1.

Table 9.1 Nutrition Therapy for GDM and Preexisting Diabetes (Studies Published After 2008*)

	Population/ Duration of Study	Intervention (type of study)	Major Findings	Comments
Moses 2009	63 women diagnosed with GDM/followed during pregnancy	Low-GI or conventional high-fiber, low-sugar diet; if women using high-fiber diet needed insulin, changed to low-GI diet (RCT)	Low GI (48): half needed insulin (29 vs. 59%), with no compromise of obstetric or fetal outcomes; high GI (56), if changed to low GI (50), half (9/19) did not need insulin	3-day food record used to calculate GI

	Population/ Duration of Study	Intervention (type of study)	Major Findings	Comments
Perichart-Perera 2009	n = 49 pregnant women with type 2 diabetes; 39 women with GDM; 47 control group selected from medical charts/followed during pregnancy	Individualized MNT every 2 weeks (moderate CHO intake, ↓ kcal, blood glucose testing 6 times per day, 2 days/week) vs. control group with usual care (1 group nutrition session and <5% had glucose meter) (quasi-experimental design)	MNT: ↓ risk of pre-eclampsia; 5.7 vs. 68.2% hospitalizations due to hyperglycemia; no neonatal deaths; low birth weight was ↓ in GDM; ↓ neonatal intensive care unit admissions in type 2 diabetes pregnancy	Average kilocalorie count during intervention was ~1,500 per day (47% CHO); ↓ hospitalization supports MNT as a cost-effective way to reduce health care expenditures
Salmen-haara 2010	n = 3,613 pregnant women (174 [4.7%] with GDM) from the Type 1 Diabetes Prediction and Prevention Study study/not applicable	Self-administered, semiquantitative food frequency questionnaire (validated) used to compare diet and weight gain in women with GDM to non-GDM (cross-sectional study)	GDM women: higher weight at beginning of pregnancy, but gained less during pregnancy (9.4 vs. 12.6 kg); ate more milk and cereal products, vegetables, and meat and ↓ intake of sugars and saturated fat vs. non-GDM	Women with GDM modified eating habits with healthier food choices; advice received was effective
Collier 2011	n = 9 focus groups with women who had GDM and 7 groups with women who had pregestational diabetes/not applicable	Barriers to glycemic control before, during, and after pregnancy explored and knowledge, attitudes, and behaviors described (cross-sectional study)	Five main barriers: financial and difficulty accessing care; maintaining a healthy diet and exercising; communication difficulties; lack of social support; and barriers related to diabetes care	Low rates of pregnancy planning in both groups
Grant 2011	n = 47 ethnically diverse pregnant women with GDM or impaired glucose tolerance in pregnancy/28 weeks' gestation until delivery	Low-GI (49) diet vs. control diet (GI 58); both received $20 of nonperishable study foods and glucose monitoring strips (RCT)	Glycemic control improved on both diets; nonsignificant changes in fasting or postprandial glucose; more postprandial glucose levels were in target range on low-GI diet (58 vs. 49%)	Pilot study; low-GI diet was feasible and acceptable

Table 9.1 Nutrition Therapy for GDM and Preexisting Diabetes (Studies Published After 2008*) (*continued*)

	Population/ Duration of Study	Intervention (type of study)	Major Findings	Comments
Ferrara 2011	*n* = 197 women with GDM/after GDM diagnosis to 12 months postpartum	Prenatal/postpartum Diabetes Prevention Program intervention delivered by telephone vs. usual care (RCT)	Intervention group: 37.5 vs. 21.4% (NS) women reached postpartum weight goal	Intervention more successful in women who did not exceed the guidelines for gestational weight gain
Kase 2011	*n* = 90 women with GDM and 63 with pregestational diabetes/not applicable	Review of database to describe the frequency of excessive GWG and its impact on adverse pregnancy outcomes (retrospective cohort study)	42.5% had excessive GWG (no difference between groups), and it was not associated with increased rate of adverse perinatal outcomes for either group	
Louie 2011	*n* = 99 women with GDM/followed during pregnancy	Low GI (~50) vs. a high-fiber moderate-GI (~60) diet (randomized clinical trial)	At birth, birth weight, macrosomia, insulin treatment, or adverse pregnancy outcomes nonsignificant between groups	Both diets produced similar pregnancy outcomes

*Studies published before 2008 are available from the Academy of Nutrition and Dietetics 2008.
CHO, carbohydrate; GWG, gestational weight gain; RCT, randomized controlled trial.

Nutrition therapy during a pregnancy with diabetes strives to achieve three important goals (Acad Nutr Diet 2008; Kitzmiller 2008a):

1. Minimize blood glucose excursions and maintain glucose values within target goal ranges before and after meals.
2. Provide a calorie intake that is neither inadequate nor excessive and will achieve an appropriate for gestational weight gain without maternal ketosis.
3. Ensure adequate, and safe, nutrients for maternal and fetal health.

All three outcomes must be achieved, not just one or two. For example, if glucose values are in target, but the woman is losing weight and under-eating to achieve glycemic control, action needs to be taken to correct the low energy intake and still provide for glucose control. A more common scenario is that of a woman following a nutrient-dense, calorie-appropriate food plan, but glucose levels are out of target, indicating the need for medication or a medication dose adjustment.

GLUCOSE CONTROL DURING PREGNANCY

Excellent glycemic control has been shown in numerous clinical trials to be associated with improved maternal and neonatal outcomes in type 1 diabetes, type 2 diabetes, and GDM (Kitzmiller 2008a; Acad Nutr Diet 2008). Recently, a large international trial was designed to clarify the associations between various levels of glucose intolerance during pregnancy and maternal, fetal, and neonatal outcomes among women of different cultural and ethnic groups. The Hyperglycemia and Adverse Pregnancy Outcome (HAPO) trial included over 25,000 women from nine countries over a period of 7 years. The results demonstrated that risk of adverse outcomes continuously increased as a function of maternal glycemia, even within ranges previously considered normal (HAPO 2008). The results were independent of age, BMI, and family history of diabetes. The associations did not differ between centers. Using the HAPO study results, an international study group convened and recommended new diagnostic criteria for GDM that are "outcome-based" (International Association of Diabetes and Pregnancy Study Groups 2010). Diabetes medical communities around the world are considering adopting these recommendations; at the time of this publication, universal agreement on the diagnosis of GDM has not yet occurred.

MNT for GDM has been shown to be effective in a number of clinical trials. In these trials, nutrition therapy when provided by an RD, along with glucose monitoring and a protocol for when to add pharmacological therapy, were shown to improve outcomes compared to routine care. In a landmark study in Australia, 1,000 women with GDM were randomly assigned to receive nutrition advice, blood glucose monitoring, and insulin therapy as needed (intervention group) or routine care. A total of 92% of the women in the intervention group saw a dietitian compared to 10% in the routine care group. The rate of serious perinatal complications (defined as death, shoulder dystocia, bone fracture, and nerve palsy) among the infants in the intervention group was 1% compared to 4% in routine care ($P = 0.01$) and maternal health–related quality of life improved in the intervention group as well (Crowther 2005). In a second study, implementation of nutrition practice guidelines for GDM compared to usual nutrition care resulted in fewer women being treated with insulin (24.6 vs. 31.7%, respectively; $P = 0.05$) and a smaller proportion of A1C values above normal at delivery (8.1 vs. 13.6%, respectively; $P = 0.25$) (Reader 2006). A third trial involved 1,889 women with mild GDM (i.e., an abnormal result on an oral glucose tolerance test but a fasting glucose <95 mg/dL) who received either formal nutritional counseling, along with insulin if required, or usual prenatal care. Treatment with MNT compared to usual care significantly reduced mean birth weight, frequency of large-for-gestational-age infants, shoulder dystocia, cesarean delivery, and hypertensive disorders (Landon 2009).

Glucose Monitoring During Pregnancy

The A1C test is the gold standard for measuring glycemic control in people with diabetes who are not pregnant. The A1C is still an important measure during a pregnancy complicated with preexisting diabetes, but self-monitoring of blood glucose, with food records, serves as the primary guide (Kitzmiller 2008a). Because a pregnancy is only 9 months long, waiting for the 2- to 3-month results from an

A1C test misses important days and weeks to achieve tight glycemic control. The goal is to achieve near-normal glycemia during pregnancy. Continuous glucose monitoring may be a supplemental tool to self-monitoring of blood glucose for selected patients with type 1 diabetes, especially patients with hypoglycemia unawareness (Kitzmiller 2008a). With the capabilities of continuous glucose monitoring, we now have a better understanding of normal glycemia during pregnancy (Yogev 2004). Table 9.2 compares normal glucose and glucose targets from various consensus statements and practice guidelines.

The frequency of glucose monitoring usually increases during pregnancy to four to seven times per day: before and after meals and at bedtime or 3:00 a.m. Throughout the entire pregnancy complicated by diabetes, the combination of self-monitoring of glucose results with a detailed food record for at least 1 week before each clinic visit provides key information to make therapy adjustments.

Nutrition Therapy for Glucose Control During Pregnancy

It is well known that carbohydrate intake is the major nutrient that affects glucose control, especially postprandial levels. Monitoring carbohydrate remains the key strategy in achieving glycemic control (ADA 2012). Guidelines for carbohydrate intake for preexisting diabetes and GDM are discussed below.

Carbohydrate guidelines for preexisting diabetes. The amount and distribution of calories and carbohydrates are individualized and based on the woman's food preferences, blood glucose records, and physical activity level. Prandial or mealtime insulin must match the amount of mealtime carbohydrate to keep glucose levels in the target range before and after eating. Many women use insulin-to-carbohydrate ratios to determine mealtime insulin. Insulin requirements increase substantially during pregnancy; therefore, the insulin-to-carbohydrate ratio will change frequently during the second half of the pregnancy.

Table 9.2 Glucose Goals for GDM and Preexisting Type 1 or Type 2 Diabetes and Pregnancy Compared to Normal Pregnancy

GDM	Preprandial ≤95 mg/dL (5.3 mmol/L) and EITHER 1-h postmeal ≤140 mg/dL (7.8 mmol/L) OR 2-h postmeal ≤120 mg/dL (6.7 mmol/L)
Preexisting type 1 or type 2 diabetes*	Premeal, bedtime, and overnight glucose: 60–99 mg/dL (3.3–5.5 mmol/L) Peak postprandial glucose: 100–129 mg/dL (5.5–7.2 mmol/L) A1C <6.0%
Normal	Preprandial ~75 mg/dL (4.1 mmol/L) 1-h postmeal 105 mg/dL (5.8 mmol/L) Peak postprandial glucose 110 mg/dL (6.1 mmol/L)

*If goals can be achieved without excessive hypoglycemia. From ADA 2012 and Yogev 2004.

It is recommended that pregnant women with diabetes be instructed to estimate the quantity of carbohydrate per serving and meal/snack and to select the type of carbohydrate that will contribute to postprandial glucose control (Kitzmiller 2008a). This step includes emphasis on consistent timing of meals and snacks on a daily basis to minimize hypoglycemia and in proper relation to insulin doses to prevent hyperglycemia.

Carbohydrate guidelines for GDM. The food plan is the primary, and often the only, therapeutic strategy for managing GDM. Two recent clinical trials reported earlier in the chapter used the food plan with glucose monitoring to establish glycemic control in >90% of the study participants (Crowther 2005; Landon 2009).

The carbohydrate consumed affects postprandial blood glucose levels; therefore, the food plan for GDM focuses on total amount, type, and distribution of carbohydrate. Women randomized to the MNT program, which included a moderate intake of carbohydrate (40–45% of total energy), a reduction in energy intake, glucose monitoring, and education, compared to the control group, had a lower risk of preeclampsia, fewer maternal hospitalizations, and fewer neonatal deaths in both women with GDM and pregnant women with type 2 diabetes (Perichart-Perera 2009).

The total carbohydrate intake for women with GDM is recommended to be on the lower side of the range (~45% of energy) to prevent hyperglycemia (Acad Nutr Diet 2008). It is suggested that carbohydrate intake be divided into three small-to-moderate meals with two to four snacks. An initial food plan would suggest the following carbohydrate ranges for each meal and snack:

Breakfast: 15–45 g carbohydrate
Lunch and dinner: 45–75 g carbohydrate at each meal
Snacks: 15–45 g carbohydrate

The range of carbohydrate for meals and snacks needs be individualized based on the nutrition requirements of the woman and based on results of blood glucose monitoring. The food plan for the pregnant woman should not be more restrictive than it has to be. As pregnancy progresses and insulin requirements change, the food plan may need to be reevaluated. The most difficult blood glucose level to manage is the postbreakfast value, because of the insulin resistance associated with higher hormone levels seen in the early morning hours. Therefore, the recommendation is to restrict carbohydrate at breakfast time to 15–45 g. Breakfast cereals are often discouraged, since the total amount of carbohydrate in a serving may be >45 g, and postmeal blood glucose levels are higher than with other food choices. In addition to highly processed breakfast cereals, sweet drinks, fast foods, and pizza are frequently found to raise postmeal levels higher than less processed, higher-fiber foods with the same amount of total carbohydrate.

The glycemic index (GI) may help explain why some foods produce higher postmeal glucose levels. A study using the GI to manage postmeal glucose levels in GDM reported that GI use was effective at reducing the number of women who advance to insulin therapy (Moses 2009). However, the criterion to initiate insulin therapy was stringent: only one glucose value out of target was needed to begin insulin therapy. There were no differences in infant outcomes. In another trial, a low-GI diet (GI = 47) was compared to a control diet or a high-fiber moderate-GI diet (GI = 53), and there were no differences in key pregnancy outcomes—infant birth weight, birth weight centile, and ponderal index (Louie 2011). Both diets were equally effective. A pilot study comparing a low-GI diet (GI = 49) to a control diet (GI = 58) also found glycemic control improved in both study groups. However, more postprandial levels were in target on the low-GI diet (Grant 2011). An eating plan including foods with a low GI may improve postmeal glucose readings; however, the first nutrition therapy intervention is to control the total amount and distribution of carbohydrate (ADA 2008).

As women with GDM learn about controlling their carbohydrate intake to manage their blood glucose levels, they may unintentionally cut back on nutrient-rich carbohydrates such as fruit, milk, and starches (such as whole grains). RDs, diabetes educators, and health care providers should review the food record and analyze the number of servings of fruit, milk or dairy, and starchy foods to ensure adequate intake. It is a common practice to shift milk and fruit to snack time so that a more normal portion of starch can be consumed during meals. Eating a healthy eating pattern is a challenge. In focus groups of women who had diabetes during a recent pregnancy, five main barriers to glycemic control were identified. Difficulties in eating a healthy diet and exercising was a primary barrier; other barriers were related to financial status, lack of support, communication, and diabetes (Collier 2011).

Pharmacological Therapy and Pregnancy

When optimal blood glucose levels have not been maintained with nutrition therapy and/or the rate of fetal growth is excessive, the clinician should recommend initiating pharmacological therapy for women with GDM (Acad Nutr Diet 2008). Research indicates that pharmacological therapy, such as the use of insulin, insulin analogs, and glyburide, improves glycemic control and reduces the incidence of poor maternal and neonatal outcomes (Conway 2004). Metformin is used by some clinicians for the management of GDM. However, there is little research on this topic (Rowan 2011).

Women with preexisting diabetes will experience dramatic changes in insulin requirements throughout the pregnancy because of the changes in hormone levels. For women with type 1 diabetes, insulin sensitivity increases at 10–14 weeks' gestation, and subsequently insulin requirements drop. After this time, insulin requirements will continue to gradually rise until the last few weeks of pregnancy. Women with type 2 diabetes and oral medications are usually converted to insulin therapy before conception or very early in the pregnancy, knowing that insulin will be needed to achieve glucose control. The insulin requirements during pregnancy will depend on the individual's degree of insulin resistance, weight, and the carbohydrate content of the food plan. The book *Managing Preexisting Diabetes and Pregnancy* (Kitzmiller 2008b) provides more information on starting insulin, selecting insulin regimens, and expected total amounts of insulin based on weeks of gestation.

WEIGHT GAIN DURING PREGNANCY

The topic of weight gain during pregnancy has been debated and researched extensively for >50 years. In 1990, the Institute of Medicine published, for the first time, weight gain guidelines based on the woman's prepregnancy BMI (IOM 1990). In 2009, the weight gain guidelines were updated (IOM 2009). One significant change in the new guidelines is the use of the World Health Organization BMI categories (Table 9.3). Recommended weight gain ranges for pregnancy for all BMI categories remained the same, except for obese women. The 2009 guidelines provide a range of 11–20 lb for the obese woman; previously, the guideline was simply stated 15 lb.

A key recommendation to all health care professionals is to identify women at risk for excessive gestational weight gain early in their pregnancy and intervene to control weight gain. The Acad Nutr Diet GDM guidelines recommend that the clinician should assess BMI because it is a better indicator of maternal nutrition status than weight alone. At the first prenatal visit, BMI should be assessed, based on actual or estimated prepregnancy weight, as a baseline to determine the recommended weight gain goal. The ADA-MPDP recommends assessment of pregravid BMI and then target individual weight gain at a lower range of the IOM recommendation according to BMI to prevent excess maternal weight gain and postpartum weight retention. The added emphasis on the lower range of the weight gain target is because of the common problem of excessive gestational weight gain. In the IOM 1990 report, research indicated that only ~30% of women with BMI values in the normal weight, overweight, and obese categories gained weight within the recommended ranges. Approximately 46% of normal and obese women and 59% of overweight women gained weight in excess of the recommendations. The IOM 2009 report states that these statistics have changed very little.

Table 9.3 Weight Gain Guidelines for Pregnancy Based on Prepregnancy BMI

Prepregnancy BMI	Total Weight Gain		Rates of Weight Gain* 2nd and 3rd Trimester	
	Range in kilograms	Range in pounds	Mean (range) in kilograms per week	Mean (range) in pounds per week
Underweight (<18.5 kg/m²)	12.5–18	28–40	0.51 (0.44–0.58)	1 (1–1.3)
Normal weight (18.5–24.9 kg/m²)	11.5–16	25–35	0.42 (0.35–0.50)	1 (0.8–1)
Overweight (25.0–29.9 kg/m²)	7–11.5	15–25	0.28 (0.23–0.33)	0.6 (0.5–0.7)
Obese (≥30.0 kg/m²)	5–9	11–20	0.22 (0.77–0.27)	0.5 (0.4–0.6)
Twin gestation Normal BMI Overweight Obese	17–25 14–23 11–19	37–54 31–50 25–42		

*Calculations assume a 0.5–2.2 kg (1.1–4.4 lb) weight gain in the first trimester. From Institute of Medicine 2009.

The Fifth International Workshop-Conference on GDM states "plotting weekly body weights on a weight gain grid specific to BMI classification is encouraged to facilitate recognition of inadequate or excessive weight gain." The diagnosis and treatment of GDM will likely influence changes in weight status, as was highlighted in a study comparing women with GDM to women without GDM (Salmenhaara 2010). The women with GDM had a higher BMI at the beginning of pregnancy, but they gained less weight during pregnancy than women without GDM. The women with GDM ate a nutrient-dense food plan consuming more milk, cereal products, vegetables, and meat than the control group; overall, their diets were higher in vitamins A and D, folate, and iron.

Excessive gestational weight gain has been associated with fatter babies; however, in a review of women with GDM, excessive gestational weight gain was not associated with adverse perinatal outcomes (Kase 2011). Excessive gestational weight gain was also associated with higher postpartum weight retention, which of course may lead to the development of type 2 diabetes.

An emerging area of research is focused on first-trimester lifestyle interventions to control weight gain and also to prevent the development of GDM.

Energy Intake for Pregnancy

Adequate calories are necessary to provide for fetal growth and appropriate weight gain and to avoid ketonemia either from ketoacidosis or accelerated starvation ketosis in all pregnant women (Kitzmiller 2008a; Acad Nutr Diet 2008). Low or inadequate weight gain during pregnancy is associated with increased risk of preterm delivery, regardless of prepregnancy BMI levels. Weight loss is not recommended during pregnancy.

The Dietary Reference Intakes (DRIs) are used to determine the estimated energy requirements (EERs) in pregnancy, which are based on age, height, weight, and physical activity level (IOM 2002). The EERs for pregnancy are as follows:

First trimester: Adult EER + 0 kcal
Second trimester: Adult EER + 160 kcal (8 kcal/week × 20 week) + 180 kcal
Third trimester: Adult EER + 272 kcal (8 kcal/week × 34 week) + 180 kcal

The 8 kcal per week represents the change in total energy expenditure due to pregnancy; the 180 kcal is the mean energy deposition during pregnancy. In general, there is no need to increase calories in the first trimester. During the second and third trimesters, calories increase ~340–450 per day. The actual calorie intake varies widely; therefore, calorie calculations are used as a guide, not as a rule. Table 9.4 provides an example of the EER calculated for a 30-year-old woman with a BMI of 25 kg/m^2 and an estimated calorie requirement during the second and third trimesters.

Assessment of fetal growth pattern and maternal weight gain, with assessment of BMI and physical activity level, is recommended for pregnant women with preexisting diabetes (Kitzmiller 2008a). For normal-weight and underweight women with GDM, caloric intake is assessed by weight gain and avoidance of starvation ketosis. Overweight and obese women should be encouraged to modify energy intake slightly to slow weight gain. A calorie intake of ~70% of the DRI is considered acceptable without causing maternal or fetal compromise or ketonuria (Acad Nutr Diet 2008). Urine ketone testing is recommended for women with

GDM who have insufficient calorie and/or carbohydrate intake and/or weight loss. Two studies reported a positive association with ketonemia and ketonuria and poor metabolic control during a diabetic pregnancy, with a lower IQ in offspring (Rizzo 1991; Rizzo 1995).

NUTRIENT NEEDS DURING PREGNANCY

The nutrition recommendations for macronutrients, vitamin, and mineral supplementation that apply to all pregnant women also pertain to women with diabetes during pregnancy. All practice guidelines and consensus statements use the DRI recommendations from the Institute of Medicine (IOM 2002).

Carbohydrate Recommendations

The Recommended Dietary Allowance (RDA) for carbohydrate in pregnant women ages 19–50 years is a minimum of 175 g/day. This amount of carbohydrate provides the fetal brain with glucose (~33 g/day) as a fuel, as well as supplying the glucose fuel requirement for the mother's brain, independent of lipid-derived fuel. The acceptable macronutrient distribution range (AMDR) for carbohydrate is 45–65% (IOM 2002).

Protein Recommendations

The RDA for protein in the nonpregnant woman is 0.8 g/kg/day or 46 g/day. Protein requirements increase to 1.1 g/kg/day or 25 g extra per day for a singleton gestation and 50 g extra for twin pregnancies (IOM 2002). The AMDR for protein is 10–35%. Research is limited regarding protein intake in women with diabetes and pregnancy.

Fat Recommendations

Dietary fat provides energy and essential fatty acids and aids in the absorption of fat-soluble vitamins. The AMDR for total fat is set for 20–35% of energy. Saturated and monounsaturated fatty acids can be synthesized; polyunsaturated fats cannot be synthesized and therefore intake is essential in the mother and fetus.

Table 9.4 Example of EERs Before and During Pregnancy for 30-Year-Old Women with BMIs of 25 kg/m² (65 inches [1.65 meters] and 150 lb [68.0 kg])

Physical activity level	Nonpregnant and First Trimester EER (kcal/day)	Second Trimester EER + 340 kcal*	Third Trimester EER + 450 kcal*
Sedentary	1,982	2,300	2,450
Low active	2,202	2,500	2,650
Active	2,477	2,800	2,950

*Calorie value rounded to nearest 50. Adapted from Kitzmiller 2008b.

The daily requirement for linoleic acid is 13 g and for α-linolenic acid is 1.4 g from sources such as soybean, corn, and safflower oils (IOM 2002). In particular, saturated fat intake should be <10% of energy intake or less than one-third of total fat intake. Trans fats should be avoided. Research is also limited regarding fat intake in pregnancy.

Vitamin and Mineral Recommendations

Adequate calcium, iron, folate, vitamin D, and magnesium intakes are especially important in pregnancy. Table 9.5 lists DRIs in pregnancy. If usual dietary intake does not meet the DRIs for pregnant women, the clinician should encourage vitamin and mineral supplementation to prevent nutritional deficiencies. Both the Acad Nutr Diet GDM guidelines and ADA-MPDP state to consume folate at 600 mg/day in the preconception and the prenatal periods through supplementation or fortified food sources.

Safe and Healthy Eating Recommendations

Safe and healthy eating recommendations for all pregnant women also apply to women with diabetes during pregnancy. The U.S. Department of Agriculture has created a website for pregnancy called "Health & Nutrition for Pregnant & Breastfeeding Women" at *www.choosemyplate.gov/pregnancy-breastfeeding.html*. This is an interactive website that creates an individualized food plan for each woman based on her age, weight, activity level, and weeks of gestation. A general guideline of the number of servings for each food group is listed in Table 9.6.

Fiber and whole grains. Although there is limited research in the area of fiber and pregnancy, patients should be encouraged to have a high-fiber intake, using whole grains, fruits, and vegetables (Kitzmiller 2008a).

Nonnutritive sweeteners. The U.S. Food and Drug Administration (FDA) approved five nonnutritive sweeteners—saccharin, aspartame, acesulfame K, sucralose, and neotame—for all people, including pregnant women. If pregnant women choose to consume products containing nonnutritive sweeteners, the clinician should inform them that only FDA-approved nonnutritive sweeteners should be consumed and that moderation is encouraged. Research in this area is extremely limited. The Acad Nutr Diet GDM position statement on a healthy pregnancy states that "use of products that are classified as Generally Recognized As Safe (GRAS) are acceptable during pregnancy in moderation" (Acad Nutr Diet 2008). Stevia has recently received GRAS status; however, there is little specific research on the use of stevia during pregnancy.

Alcohol. No amount of alcohol consumption can be considered safe during pregnancy. Alcohol use during pregnancy increases the risk of alcohol-related birth defects, including growth deficiencies, facial abnormalities, central nervous system impairment, behavioral disorders, and impaired intellectual development (Centers for Disease Control and Prevention [CDC] 2005).

Mercury-contaminated fish. The FDA has recommended that pregnant women and women of childbearing age avoid eating shark, swordfish, jack mack-

Table 9.5 DRIs per Day for Pregnant and Lactating Women

	Pregnant Woman 14–18 years	Pregnant Woman 19–50 years	Lactating Woman 14–18 years	Lactating Woman 19–50 years
Protein (g)	+25	+25	+25	+25
Vitamin A (mg)	750	770	1,200	770
Vitamin D (mg)	5	5	5	5
Vitamin K (mg)	75	90	75	90
Vitamin C (mg)	80	85	115	120
Thiamin (mg)	1.4	1.4	1.4	1.4
Riboflavin (mg)	1.4	1.4	1.6	1.6
Niacin (mg)	18	18	17	17
Vitamin B6 (mg)	1.9	1.9	2.0	2.0
Folate (mg)	600	600	500	500
Vitamin B12 (mg)	2.6	2.6	2.8	2.8
Calcium (mg)	1,300	1,000	1,300	1,000
Phosphorus (mg)	1,250	700	1,250	700
Magnesium (mg)	400	360	360	320
Iron (mg)	27	27	10	9
Zinc (mg)	12	11	13	12
Iodine (mg)	220	220	290	290
Selenium (mg)	60	60	70	70

Adapted from Trumbo 2002.

Table 9.6 Sample Dietary Guidelines for Normal Pregnancy

Total calories	First Trimester: 1,800	Second Trimester: 2,200	Third Trimester: 2,400	Examples
Grains	6 servings	7 servings	8 servings	1 slice bread; ½ cup potato, rice, pasta
Vegetables	2½ cups	3 cups	3 cups	Carrots, broccoli, onion 2 cups greens = 1 cup
Fruits	1½ cups	2 cups	2 cups	Whole fruit, juice
Milk	3 cups	3 cups	3 cups	Milk, yogurt, cheese
Meat and beans	5 oz	6 oz	6½ oz	½ cup beans = 1-oz serving of meat
Extras	290 calories	360 calories	410 calories	May come from higher-calorie, higher-fat foods or additional food groups
Fats and oils	6 tsp	7 tsp	8 tsp	Oil, butter, nuts

These guidelines are for a pregnant woman who is of normal weight and who exercises <30 min/week. They show the recommended daily food intake. Adapted from American College of Obstetricians and Gynecologists 2010.

erel, and tilefish. These fish often contain high levels of methyl-mercury, a potent human neurotoxin that readily crosses the placenta and has the potential to damage the fetal nervous system (Evans 2002). Women should consult their local health department for further fish advisories in their area.

Listeriosis. Listeria is a type of bacteria found in soil, water, and sometimes plants. Although it is all around our environment, most *Listeria* infections in people are from eating contaminated food. This infection can be passed to an unborn baby through the placenta, even if the mother is not showing signs of illness, and can lead to premature delivery, miscarriage, stillbirth, and other serious health problems (CDC 2011). Approximately one-third of all listeriosis cases involve pregnant women. Pregnant women are advised to avoid the following:

- All deli meats, hot dogs, or luncheon meats, unless reheated until steaming hot
- Soft cheeses (such as feta, Brie, Camembert, blue-veined), queso blanco, or queso fresco
- Refrigerated patés or meat spreads
- Refrigerated smoked seafood, unless cooked
- Raw or unpasteurized milk

PHYSICAL ACTIVITY FOR PREGNANCY AND DIABETES

Physical activity is always an important component of a healthy lifestyle and should continue during pregnancy unless there is a reason to discontinue. Guidelines for successfully incorporating physical activity and maintaining glycemic control are the same as for a nonpregnant woman.

Acad Nutr Diet GDM guidelines recommend 30 min of moderate physical activity 3 days per week (Acad Nutr Diet 2008). The Fifth International Workshop-Conference on GDM recommendations state the following: "Planned physical activity of 30 minutes/day is recommended for all individuals capable of participating….Regular aerobic exercise with proper warm-up and cool-down has been shown to lower fasting and postprandial glucose concentrations in several small studies of previously sedentary individuals with GDM" (Metzger 2007).

The ADA-MPDP consensus statement repeats the recommendations above and highlights the importance of monitoring glucose closely around the times of exercise, considering adjustments in carbohydrate and insulin requirements and maintaining good hydration before, during, and after exercise. Women should also be instructed to monitor the intensity of physical activity and to choose activities that will avoid the supine position and minimize the risk of loss of balance and fetal trauma (Kitzmiller 2008a).

POSTPARTUM TOPICS

With the birth of the infant, the mother with diabetes will face new challenges. Her focus and attention will shift from self-care to caring for her baby. Postpartum care and education should begin before her hospital discharge. A universal recommendation is to encourage the new mother to lose pounds gained during pregnancy and return to her preconception weight, or lower if previously overweight or obese. Women who received a Diabetes Prevention Program type of telephone intervention after being diagnosed with GDM and continuing to 12 months postpartum were more likely to reach postpartum weight goals and breastfeed than women who received usual care (Ferrara 2011).

Glucose Assessment and Management

Women with type 1 diabetes will need less insulin immediately after delivery, and women with type 2 diabetes will need less insulin or may return to oral agent therapy with nutrition therapy. Frequent glucose monitoring may be necessary for a few days to determine new insulin doses.

All women who had GDM during their pregnancy are advised to have glucose levels evaluated 6–12 weeks postpartum with a 75-g oral glucose tolerance test. Many centers encourage women to continue home glucose monitoring a few times a week and to bring that data to their first postpartum appointment. Women with GDM are at increased risk for developing diabetes in the next 10 years. The good news is that diabetes can be prevented or its onset delayed with lifestyle interventions of weight reduction and physical activity, as was shown in the Diabetes Prevention Program and other prevention trials. Chapter 25 outlines diabetes prevention recommendations.

Lactation

A PubMed MEDLINE literature search was also conducted for articles on lactation and diabetes. A total of 43 articles were found and 7 are included in Table 9.7. The beneficial effects of breastfeeding are well documented; all diabetes, nutrition, and pregnancy-related medical professional groups encourage women to breastfeed. The report of the Fifth International Workshop-Conference on GDM states "all women should be actively encouraged to exclusively breastfeed to the greatest extent possible during the first year of life" (Metzger 2007). Breastfeeding has been associated with decreasing the woman's risk of becoming overweight later in life and developing metabolic syndrome and type 2 diabetes (Gunderson 2012; Stuebe 2005). There is also evidence that long-term breastfeeding can have protective effects against the development of type 1 diabetes in individuals who were breastfed (Rosenbauer 2007).

Even though breastfeeding is recommended, in one study, women with type 1 diabetes were less likely to plan to breastfeed (66.7%) compared with women with type 2 diabetes and GDM (80 and 95.5%, respectively) (Soltani 2009). This study did not seek to determine the specific predictors of breastfeeding intention, but suggests that health care professionals support women with preexisting diabetes to make an informed, healthy choice. Other research of women with type 1 diabetes found a positive correlation between breastfeeding and higher education, full-term vaginal delivery, nonsmoking, and previous experience with breastfeeding (Sparud-Lundin 2011; Sorkio 2010; Stage 2006). Another benefit of breastfeeding was found in a study of women with GDM who breastfed in the delivery room; those infants had a lower rate of postpartum hypoglycemia (Chertok 2009). Also compared with exclusively or mostly formula feeding, exclusive and mostly breastfeeding by women with GDM was associated with improved fasting glucose and

Table 9.7 Relationship of Lactation and Mothers' Diabetes

	Population/ Duration of Study	Intervention (type of study)	Major Findings	Comments
Chertok 2009	*n* = 84 infants born to women with GDM at >37 weeks/not applicable	Glycemic levels of infants (*n* = 44) breastfed in delivery room (within 30 min of delivery) vs. those who were not (*n* = 40) (observational study)	Infants breastfed had lower rate of borderline hypoglycemia than those not breastfed (10 vs. 28%) and a higher mean blood glucose (57 vs. 51 mg/dL)	Early breastfeeding may facilitate glycemic stability
Soltani 2009	*n* = 94 pregnant women (with GDM [68], type 1 diabetes [15], and type 2 diabetes [11])	Identification of breastfeeding behaviors by questionnaire and maternal chart records (retrospective observational study)	At 2 weeks postpartum, more GDM women breastfed; at 1 week to 4 months, BMI was negatively associated with breastfeeding; at 6 months, socioeconomic status predicted breastfeeding (all *P* < 0.05)	Understanding influencers may help develop appropriate interventions to increase breastfeeding
Gunderson 2010	*n* = 704 women in the CARDIA study, examined at 7, 10, 15, and 20 years after baseline (620 non-GDM, 84 GDM/not applicable	Assessment of the association between lactation duration and incidence of MetS (prospective observational study)	Increased lactation duration associated with lower incidence of MetS in both groups; in women lactating >9 months, the incidence of MetS was 9.2 (non-GDM) vs. 8.5 (GDM) per 1,000 person-years	Higher rate of MetS in GDM compared to non-GDM (22.1 cases vs. 10.8 per 1,000 person-years)
Ferrara 2011	*n* = 197 women with GDM/after GDM diagnosis to 12 months postpartum	Prenatal/postpartum Diabetes Prevention Program intervention delivered by telephone vs. usual care (randomized controlled trial)	Intervention group had a higher likelihood (but NS) to partially or exclusively breastfeed, 62.7 vs. 47.7% (*P* = 0.09)	
Sparud-Lundin 2011	*n* = 108 mothers with type 1 diabetes matched with 104 mothers, no diabetes/not applicable	Identification of predictive factors for initiation and maintenance of breastfeeding (prospective observational study)	Mothers with diabetes less likely to breastfeed children at 2 and 6 months; type 1 diabetes not an independent predictive factor; higher education and breastfeeding at discharge were predictive of breastfeeding at 2 months	In addition, delivery at >37 weeks and early breastfeeding predicted breastfeeding at 6 months

	Population/ Duration of Study	Intervention (type of study)	Major Findings	Comments
Sorkio 2010	n = 1,096 children born to women with type 1 diabetes and 1,064 to women with no diabetes (mothers in TRIGR trial)/not applicable	Examination of breastfeeding patterns among mothers with/without type 1 diabetes (prospective observational study)	>90% of infants of both groups of mothers initially breastfed; maternal diabetes not associated with shorter breastfeeding	Shorter duration of breastfeeding related to more frequent cesarean sections, earlier delivery, young age, and education
Gunderson 2012	n = 522 women in the SWIFT study diagnosed with GDM/not applicable	Examined the association between breastfeeding intensity and maternal fasting blood glucose and fasting insulin (cross-sectional study)	Exclusive and mostly breastfeeding vs. exclusive and mostly formula feeding groups had lower fasting blood glucose and fasting insulin (all $P < 0.05$) at 6–9 weeks postpartum and lower prevalence of diabetes or prediabetes ($P = 0.02$)	Lactation may reduce diabetes risk after GDM pregnancy

CARDIA, Coronary Artery Risk Development in Young Adults; MetS, metabolic syndrome; SWIFT, Study of Women, Infant Feeding, and Type 2 Diabetes; TRIGR, Trial to Reduce Insulin-Dependent Diabetes Mellitus in the Genetically at Risk.

lower insulin levels at 6–9 weeks postpartum, which may reduce diabetes risk after GDM pregnancy (Gunderson 2012).

It is generally advisable for lactating women to maintain a total energy intake of at least 1,800 kcal/day. This step may allow for a slow weight loss of 0.5–1.0 kg/month and can usually meet the energy and nutrient requirements for lactation. Overweight women may lose up to 2 kg/month without affecting milk volume (Reader 2004). During lactation, 210 g/day carbohydrate and 1.1 g/kg/day protein (or an additional 25 g/day) are recommended to supply these nutrients for maternal needs and adequate milk secretion (IOM 2002).

SUMMARY

The primary goals of nutrition therapy for diabetes during pregnancy are excellent glycemic control, appropriate weight gain, and a nutrient-rich eating pattern. To achieve these goals takes a motivated woman and a health care team, including an RD, collaborating regularly and reviewing food, glucose, and medication records, in addition to monitoring weight changes and other measures of fetal growth.

BIBLIOGRAPHY

Academy of Nutrition and Dietetics: Gestational diabetes mellitus (GDM) evidence-based nutrition practice guidelines, 2008. Available from http://www.adaevidencelibrary.com/topic.cfm?cat=1399. Accessed October 2011

American College of Obstetricians and Gynecologists: *Your Pregnancy and Childbirth: Month by Month.* 5th ed. Washington, DC, American College of Obstetricians and Gynecologists, 2010

American Diabetes Association: Nutrition recommendations and interventions for diabetes (Position Statement). *Diabetes Care* 31 (Suppl. 1):S61–S78, 2008

American Diabetes Association: Standards of medical care in diabetes: 2012. *Diabetes Care* 35 (Suppl. 1):S11–S63, 2012

Centers for Disease Control and Prevention: Listeriosis (*Listeria*) and pregnancy. Available at http://www.cdc.gov/ncbddd/pregnancy_gateway/infections-Listeria.html. Accessed 28 October 2011

Centers for Disease Control and Prevention: Notice to readers: Surgeon General's advisory on alcohol use in pregnancy. *MMWR* 54:229, 2005

Chertok IRA, Raz I, Shoham I, Haddad H, Wiznitzer A: Effects of early breastfeeding on neonatal glucose levels of term infants born to women with gestational diabetes. *J Hum Nutr Diet* 22:166–169, 2009

Collier SA, Mulholland C, Williams J, Mersereau P, Turay K, Prue C: A qualitative study of perceived barriers to management of diabetes among women with a history of diabetes during pregnancy. *J Womens Health* 20:1333–1339, 2011

Conway DL, Gonzales O, Skiver D: Use of glyburide for the treatment of gestational diabetes: the San Antonio experience. *J Matern Fetal Neonatal Med* 15:51–55, 2004

Crowther CA, Hiller JE, Moss JR, McPhee AJ, Jeffries WS, Robinseon JS, for the Australian Carbohydrate Intolerance Study in Pregnant Women (ACHOIS) Trial Group: Effect of treatment of gestational diabetes mellitus on pregnancy outcomes. *N Engl J Med* 352:2477–2486, 2005

Evans EC: The FDA recommendations on fish intake during pregnancy. *J Obstet Gynecol Neonatal Nurs* 31:715–720, 2002

Ferrara A, Hedderson MM, Albright CL, Ehrlich SF, Quesenberry CP, Peng T, Feng J, Ching J, Crites Y: A pregnancy and postpartum lifestyle intervention in women with gestational diabetes mellitus reduces diabetes risk factors. *Diabetes Care* 34:1519–1525, 2011

Grant SM, Wolever TMS, O'Connor DL, Nisenbaum R, Josse RG: Effect of a low glycaemic index diet on blood glucose in women with gestational hyperglycaemia. *Diabetes Res Clin Pract* 91:15–22, 2011

Gunderson EP, Hedderson MM, Chiang V, Crites Y, Walton D, Azevedo RA, Fox G, Elmasian C, Young S, Salvador N, Lum M, Quesenberry CP, Lo JC, Sternfeld B, Ferrara A, Selby JV: Lactation intensity and postpartum maternal glucose tolerance and insulin resistance in women with recent GDM: the SWIFT cohort. *Diabetes Care* 35:50–56, 2012

Gunderson EP, Jacobs DR, Chiang V, Lewis CE, Feng J, Quesenberry CP, Sidney S: Duration of lactation and incidence of the metabolic syndrome in women of reproductive age according to gestational diabetes status: a 20-year prospective study in CARDIA. *Diabetes* 59:495–504, 2010

HAPO Study Cooperative Research Group, Metzger BE, Lowe LP, Dyer AR, Trimble ER, Chaovarindr U, Coustan DR, Hadden DR, McCance M, Hod HD, McIntyre JJ, Oaats B, Persson MS, Rogers MS, Sacks DA: Hyperglycemia and adverse pregnancy outcomes. *N Engl J Med* 358:1991–2002, 2008

Institute of Medicine: *Dietary Reference Intakes: Energy, Carbohydrates, Fiber, Fat, Fatty Acids, Cholesterol, Protein, and Amino Acids*. Washington DC, National Academies Press, 2002

Institute of Medicine: *Nutrition During Pregnancy*. Washington, DC, National Academy Press, 1990

Institute of Medicine: *Weight Gain During Pregnancy: Reexamining the Guidelines*. Washington, DC, National Academy Press, 2009

International Association of Diabetes and Pregnancy Study Groups Consensus Panel: International Association of Diabetes and Pregnancy Study Groups recommendations on the diagnosis and classification of hyperglycemia in pregnancy. *Diabetes Care* 33:676–682, 2010

Kase BA, Cormier CM, Costantine MM, Hutchinson M, Ramin SM, Saade GR, Monga M, Blackwell SC: Excessive gestational weight gain in women with gestational and pregestational diabetes. *Am J Perinatol* 28:761–766, 2011

Kitzmiller JL, Block JM, Brown FM, Catalano PM, Conway DL, Coustan DR, Gunderson EP, Herman WH, Hoffman LD, Inturrist M, Jovanovic LB, Kjos SI, Knopp RH, Montoro MN, Ogata ES, Paramsothy P, Reader DM, Rosenn BM, Thomas AM, Kirkman MS: Managing preexisting diabetes for pregnancy, summary of evidence and consensus recommendations for care. *Diabetes Care* 31:1060–1079, 2008a

Kitzmiller JL, Jovanovic L, Brown F, Coustan D, Reader DM: *Managing Preexisting Diabetes and Pregnancy: Technical Reviews and Consensus Recommendations for Care*. Alexandria, VA, American Diabetes Association, 2008b

Landon MG, Spong CY, Thom E, Carpenter MW, Ramin SM, Casey B, Wapner RJ, Varner MW, Rouse DJ, Thorp JM Jr, Sciscione A, Catalano P, Harper M, Saade G, Lain KY, Sorokin Y, Peaceman AM, Tolosa JE, Anderson GB, Eunice Kennedy Shriver National Institute of Child Health and Human Development Maternal-Fetal Medicine Units Network: A multicenter, randomized trial of treatment for mild gestational diabetes. *N Engl J Med* 361:1339–1348, 2009

Louie JC, Markovic TP, Perera N, Foote D, Petocz P, Ross GP, Brand-Miller JC: Randomized controlled trial investigating the effects of a low-glycemic index diet on pregnancy outcomes in gestational diabetes mellitus. *Diabetes Care* 34:2341–2346, 2011

Metzger BE, Buchanan TA, Coustan DR: Summary and recommendations of the Fifth International Workshop-Conference on Gestational Diabetes Mellitus. *Diabetes Care* 30 (Suppl. 2):S251–S260, 2007

Moses RG, Barker M, Winter M, Petocz P, Brand-Miller JC: Can a low-glycemic index diet reduce the need for insulin in gestational diabetes mellitus? A randomized trial. *Diabetes Care* 32:996–1000, 2009

Perichart-Perera O, Balas-Nakash M, Parr-Covarrubias A, Rodriguez-Cano A, Ramirez-Torres A, Ortega-Gonzalez C, Vadillo-Ortega F: A medical nutrition therapy program improves perinatal outcomes in Mexican pregnant women with gestational diabetes and type 2 diabetes mellitus. *Diabetes Educ* 35:1004–1013, 2009

Reader D, Franz MJ: Lactation, diabetes, and nutrition recommendations. *Curr Diab Rep* 4:370–376, 2004

Reader D, Splett P, Gunderson EP, for the Diabetes Care and Education Dietetic Practice Group: Impact of gestational diabetes nutrition practice guidelines implemented by registered dietitians on pregnancy outcomes. *J Am Diet Assoc* 106:1426–1433, 2006

Rizzo T, Dooley SL, Metzger BE: Prenatal and perinatal influences on long-term psychomotor development in offspring of diabetic mothers. *Am J Obstet Gynecol* 173:1753–1758, 1995

Rizzo T, Metzger BE, Burns WJ: Correlations between antepartum maternal metabolism and child intelligence. *N Engl J Med* 325:911–916, 1991

Rosenbauer J, Herzig P, Kaiser P, Giani G: Early nutrition and risk of diabetes mellitus: a nationwide case-control study in preschool children. *Exp Clin Endocrinol Diabetes* 115:502–508, 2007

Rowan JA, Rush EC, Obolonkin V, Battin M, Wouldes T, Hague WM: Metformin in gestational diabetes: the offspring follow-up (MiG TOFU). *Diabetes Care* 34:2279–2284, 2011

Salmenhaara M, Uusitalo L, Uusitalo U, Kronberg-Kippila C, Sinkko H, Ahonen A, Veijola R, Knip M, Virtanen SM: Diet and weight gain characteristics of pregnant women with gestational diabetes. *Eur J Clin Nutr* 64:1433–1440, 2010

Soltani H, Arden M: Factors associated with breastfeeding up to 6 months postpartum in mothers with diabetes. *J Obstet Gynecol Neonatal Nurs* 38:586–594, 2009

Sorkio S, Cuthbertson D, Barlund S, Reunanen A, Nucci AM, Berseth CL, Koski K, Ormisson A, Savilahti E, Uusitalo U, Ludvigsson J, Becker DJ, Dupre J, Krischer JP, Knip M, Akerblom HK, Virtanen SM; TRIGR Study group:

Breastfeeding patterns of mothers with type 1 diabetes: results from an infant feeding trial. *Diabetes Metab Res Rev* 26:206–211, 2010

Sparud-Lundin C, Wennergren M, Elfvin A, Berg M: Breastfeeding in women with type 1 diabetes. *Diabetes Care* 34:296–301, 2011

Stage E, Norgard H, Damm P, Mathiesen E: Long-term breastfeeding in women with type 1 diabetes. *Diabetes Care* 29:771–774, 2006

Stuebe AM, Rich-Edwards JW, Willett WC, Manson JE, Michels KB: Duration of lactation and incidence of type 2 diabetes. *JAMA* 294:2601–2610, 2005

Trumbo P, Schlicker S, Yates AA, Poos M: Dietary reference intakes for energy, carbohydrate, fiber, fat, fatty acids, cholesterol, protein and amino acids. *J Am Diet Assoc* 102:1621–1630, 2002

Yogev, Y, Ben-Haroush A, Chen R, Rosenn B, Hod M, Langer O: Diurnal glycemic profile in obese and normal weight non-diabetic pregnant women. *Am J Ob Gyn* 191:949–953, 2004

Diane M. Reader, RD, CDE, is Manager of Professional Education at the International Diabetes Center at Park Nicollet, Minneapolis, MN.

Chapter 10
Diabetes Nutrition Therapy for Sports and Exercise

Carla Cox, PhD, RD, CDE, CSSD

Highlights

Review of the Impact of Exercise on Fuel Utilization

Review of Existing Sports Nutrition Recommendations

Diabetes Sports/Exercise Nutrition and Insulin Recommendations

Translation of Evidence into Nutrition Therapy Interventions for Sports or Exercise

Summary

Highlights
Diabetes Nutrition Therapy for Sports and Exercise

■ Understanding physiological responses to exercise and nutrient needs of the athlete/exerciser is critical when counseling people with diabetes.

■ Nutrition recommendations for the athlete with diabetes are the same as recommendations for people without diabetes, including adequate energy intake, carbohydrate, protein, fat, and fluids in relationship to the intensity and duration of activity.

■ The most common problem during and after exercise in individuals with type 1 diabetes is hypoglycemia, which must be treated with carbohydrate in addition to that prescribed for exercise. However, high-intensity exercise and competition stress may result in hyperglycemia after exercise.

■ Checking blood glucose frequently before, during, and up to 72 h after exercise is recommended to help determine insulin dosing and additional carbohydrate intake, above the general exercise requirements, for hypoglycemia.

■ Reducing basal or bolus insulin before, during, and after activity may help to ensure a reduction in risk of hypoglycemia and reduce the need for carbohydrates above that required for the activity itself. If insulin cannot be adjusted, additional carbohydrate may be needed.

■ Hypoglycemia during exercise may occur in individuals with type 2 diabetes on insulin secretagogues and/or insulin and must be treated with additional carbohydrate.

Diabetes Nutrition Therapy for Sports and Exercise

To understand nutrition recommendations for diabetes with regard to exercise and sports, knowledge of the physiology of exercise and its impact on fuel use is important. Nutrition recommendations for exercise are the same for individuals with diabetes as for individuals without diabetes. However, the impact of exercise/sports on reduction of blood glucose values in people with diabetes may require a change in the carbohydrate recommendations for the individual to prevent hypoglycemia. And conversely, blood glucose levels above normal must also be incorporated into carbohydrate planning at the onset of exercise. The basic pharmacokinetics of insulin must also be understood for insulin-requiring patients to determine possible strategies for changes in bolus or basal insulin delivery and/or carbohydrate consumption. The reader is referred to company websites for insulin pharmacokinetics, as well as other publications (Scheiner 2011; Colberg 2009).

This chapter begins with a brief description of the physiological changes that occur in everyone during exercise, followed by a summary of nutrition recommendations for exercise and nutrition recommendations for individuals with diabetes. Although multiple case studies have been reported for accomplished athletes with type 1 diabetes, there is a dearth of evidence-based research on specific nutritional needs of the athlete with type 1 or type 2 diabetes.

REVIEW OF THE IMPACT OF EXERCISE ON FUEL UTILIZATION

Fuel utilization and blood glucose response during exercise depend on the sympathetic nervous system and endocrine systems. As the muscle contracts, there is an increase in glucose uptake by the skeletal muscle, which is usually compensated for by an increase in glycogenolysis and gluconeogenesis and mobilization of free fatty acids and amino acids for fuel (American College of Sports Medicine [ACSM] 2010). At the onset of exercise, and with increasing intensity of exercise, the body relies more predominately on carbohydrate for fuel, as long as carbohydrate is available from the liver and muscle stores. As exercise increases in duration, and glycogen stores are depleted, the individual depends on gluconeogenesis and mobilization of fat and amino acids for energy.

Insulin helps to regulate glucose uptake by the skeletal muscle during rest, which is compromised in individuals with type 2 (but not type 1) diabetes. During exercise, an alternate non–insulin-mediated pathway results in glucose uptake by the skeletal muscle. In the individual with type 2 diabetes, the uptake of glucose may be greater than the body's ability to compensate via glycogenolysis and gluconeogenesis, which can potentially lead to hypoglycemia. Because of the blood glucose–lowering ability of exercise, in individuals who are using exogenous insulin, dosing of insulin must be reduced to prevent low blood glucose levels during exercise. The hypoglycemic impact of exercise can be realized for up to 72 h after a session of exercise, since physical activity increases muscle sensitivity to insulin to facilitate repletion of glycogen stores. The exception to the rule is with very-high-intensity exercise, which increases the production of catecholamines, resulting in immediate hyperglycemia.

REVIEW OF EXISTING SPORTS NUTRITION RECOMMENDATIONS

Energy Needs

Athletes need to consume adequate energy to fuel sport and maintain body weight. Low energy intakes can result in a myriad of consequences, including loss of lean body mass, alternations in hormonal regulation of the menstrual cycle, fatigue, and prolonged recovery (ACSM 2009a). To determine energy needs, both direct and indirect measurement can be used; however, these are often impractical and, with the former, rarely available. Therefore, prediction equations are often used to determine baseline energy requirements. Examples include the Mifflin and Cunningham equations (Table 10.1) (Dunford 2006). A predicted metabolic rate can be determined and metabolic equivalents for activity factors (Table 10.2) (Dunford 2006) added to arrive at an approximation of energy needs for the athlete. Figure 10.1 is an example of energy requirements for a 59-kg (130-lb) female athlete. It is critical to keep in mind this is a starting point, with modifications based on food and exercise records, seasonal alterations in sport, individual response to exercise, and scheduled weight checks.

Carbohydrate

Although the majority of the fuel used in endurance exercise is fat, the limiting factor in performance is carbohydrate supply. Carbohydrate is stored in limited supply in the liver (110 g; 440 calories) and muscle (500 g; 2000 calories) (Wilmore 2008). It has been consistently demonstrated that ingestion of carbohydrate during exercise of >60 min duration is critical to performance and that the longer

---

Table 10.1 Prediction Equations for Resting Metabolic Rate (Background Energy Requirements)

Equation	Females	Males
Mifflin	$-161 + 10\,W + 6.25\,H - 5\,A$	$5 + 10\,W + 6.25\,H - 5\,A$
Cunningham	$500 + 22 \times$ fat-free mass (kg)*	$500 + 22 \times$ fat-free mass (kg)*

W, weight in kilograms; H, height in centimeters; A, age in years. *Determined by body composition assessment such as hydrostatic weighing or skinfold calipers as examples. Adapted from Dunford 2006.

Table 10.2. Metabolic Equivalents for Activity

Activity	Metabolic Equivalents
Very high intensity, short duration	3.0–6.0
Intermittent high-intensity	6.0–10.0
Endurance	5.5–18.0
Weight- and body-focused	4.0–6.0
Low endurance, precision skill	4.5–5.0
Miscellaneous—walking	2.0–5.0
Very light activity	1.1–1.9

Adapted from Dunford 2006.

the duration of sport and the higher the intensity of the exercise, the greater the carbohydrate need (Jeukendrup 2000). Daily carbohydrate recommendations for endurance sports range from 6 to 10 g/kg body weight or more for the ultra-endurance athlete. For most non-endurance sports (figure skating, golf, gymnastics), 5–8 g daily carbohydrate per kilogram body weight per day is recommended.

Figure 10.1 Example of Using the Mifflin Equation and Metabolic Equivalents to Determine Energy Needs

Female athlete:
59 kg (130 lb)
165 cm (5'5")
26 years old

Sleep: 8 h/day
Exercise:
    1 h running moderate intensity
    1.5 h biking moderate intensity
    13.5 h light activity (studying, walking around campus, fixing meals)

Mifflin equation to calculate basic energy needs at rest:
$$-161 + 10 (59) + 6.25 (165) - 5 \times 26 = 1{,}330 \text{ kcal/24 h of no activity}$$
$$\text{OR}$$
$$55.43 \text{ kcal/h}$$

Calculating total energy needs:
55.43×7 MET $\times 1$ h for running = 388 kcal
55.43×7 MET $\times 1.5$ h for biking = 582 kcal
55.43×1.5 MET $\times 13.5$ h light activity = 1,122 kcal
55.43×1 MET $\times 8$ h of sleeping = 443 kcal

2,535 kcal needed for that day of activity

This is equal to 360–585 g carbohydrate (1,440–2,340 calories) per day for a 160-lb (73-kg) individual.

Thirty seconds of a high-intensity anaerobic sport may result in a 25–35% reduction in total muscle glycogen stores (ACSM 2009a). As with endurance sports, this reduction may also have implications for higher carbohydrate intake due to the continuous cycle of depletion and restoration of stored glycogen, particularly when the sport requires multiple high-intensity bouts of activity (ice hockey, wrestling tournaments).

Protein

Protein contributes ~5% of energy needs during endurance sports. It is also essential for maintenance and repair of muscle tissue (Dunford 2006). Protein recommendations for athletes range from 1.2 to 1.7 g/kg body weight/day, with the upper recommended limit for protein being 3.0 g/kg body weight, beyond which additional protein has not been demonstrated to be beneficial (Dunford 2006; Tipton 2004). This result translates to a total protein intake per day for a 73-kg (160-lb) individual of 87–124 g (348–495 kcal from protein), with a maximum of 218 g (872 kcal). Some data support ranges of 0.9–2.5 g/kg body weight/day of habitual protein intake as adequate for whole-body protein synthesis and breakdown during the fasted state, with no difference in the timing of protein intake before, during, or after exercise (Rodriguez 2007). However, clear consensus on optimal timing and quantity of protein during and immediately after exercise has not been established. The source of protein, for example, whey versus casein, does not appear to be the critical issue (Tipton 2011), and generally protein needs are met by most athletes. Vegetarian athletes may need an additional 10% over general recommendations because of the lack of bioavailability of non-animal protein (Institute of Medicine 1989).

Fat

Fat intake is essential, and recommendations vary from 1.0 g fat/kg body weight to using a range of 20–35% of total energy (ACSM 2009a; Dunford 2006). Dietary fat provides energy and essential nutrients. Recommendations have been made for equal contributions from saturated, polyunsaturated, and monounsaturated fat, making sure the essential fatty acids α-linolenic and α-linoleic are present. Individuals with diabetes and people with coronary disease should minimize saturated fat and *trans* fatty acid consumption (Franz 2010). High-fat diets to enhance performance are not supported in the literature. In fact, data suggest a reduction in endurance performance with higher-fat diets, possibly due to impairment of glycogenolysis during a time when muscle requirements are high (Burke 2007; Dunford 2006).

Fluids

Fluid intake is critical, and requirements are based on individual variation in sweat rate and changes in ambient temperature and altitude. Practicing fluid ingestion during training is critical. The use of fluid fuel (sports drink with 6–8% carbohydrate) is often suggested during sports, to provide appropriate carbohydrate intake while helping to maintain hydration. Higher concentrations of carbohydrate can change palatability and delay gastric emptying and intestinal absorption. Thirst should drive intake; however, it is often ignored. Checking weight before and after exercise and calculating fluid lost (including fluid ingested during the exercise session) will provide insight into individual hydration schedules. For each pound (0.5 kg) of body weight lost, a minimum of 16–24 oz (450–675 mL) of fluid should be ingested for recovery. Checking urine color is also a recommended method to help determine level of hydration, with the goal of a light yellow or straw color (Armstrong 1994).

Micronutrients

There are no clear recommendations for vitamin and mineral supplements for endurance athletes. Some research has suggested increased needs for vitamins C and E for endurance sports, but this is not consistent. A daily dietary intake from 100 to 1,000 mg/day vitamin C for athletes who consistently participate in prolonged strenuous exercise has been recommended (ACSM 2009a).

Iron is critical for the delivery of oxygen to the working muscle. Iron depletion is common in athletes, especially females. Frank iron deficiency as well as low stored iron (ferritin) may impair endurance performance. Dietary intakes of greater than the recommended daily intake (18 mg women, 8 mg men) are advised for endurance athletes (ACSM 2009a). Athletes at risk for iron deficiency, such as long-duration runners, menstruating women, adolescents, and vegetarians, should be screened for iron deficiency periodically. Iron supplementation should be recommended when a deficiency is noted via a standard laboratory test such as serum ferritin.

Nutrient Timing

Nutrient timing is important to maximize training and competition. Daily ingestion of carbohydrate to maintain glycogen stores is recommended, with a potential advantage of ingesting high amounts of carbohydrate (70% of dietary intake) 5–7 days before an endurance competition (Kerksick 2008). There is additional evidence that ingestion of protein with carbohydrate 3–4 h before exercise at a ratio of 1–2 g carbohydrate/kg body weight and 0.15–0.25 g protein/kg body weight stimulates greater strength gains than ingesting carbohydrate alone (Kerksick 2008). There is some discussion in the literature regarding fat and carbohydrate cycling (periodization) during training, but the quality of performance does not appear to improve with higher fat versus higher carbohydrate intakes, or macronutrient cycling (Burke 2007).

Meal timing is important in preparation for both training and competition, with carbohydrate recommendations of 0.7–1.1 g/kg body weight per hour prior to exercise (ACSM 2009; Jeukendrup 2000). Some studies demonstrate up to 90 g carbohydrate per hour of high-intensity endurance activity, if different forms of carbohydrate are provided (fructose, glucose) versus glucose alone (Currell 2008). A limiting factor to carbohydrate use appears to be the osmolarity of the fluid. Solutions with high concentrations of carbohydrate (>8%) may cause water to move from the blood back to the intestine, delaying absorption. The consistency of the carbohydrate does not appear to affect use, whether liquids, gels, or solids.

During recovery, consumption of carbohydrates within 30 min of completion of the event or high-level training is recommended. Replenishment of carbohydrate with 1.0–1.5 g carbohydrate per kilogram body weight every 2 h up to 6 h is recommended, particularly when a practice or event occurs on a subsequent day (ACSM 2009b). This is easily accomplished by eating a 4-oz bagel and a banana or 16 oz chocolate milk (nonfat or low-fat) and an orange. Or an individual can choose from a wide variety of recovery supplements available on the market. Protein (~8 g) may be advantageous after an event or high-intensity workout, but the research remains less consistent than that for carbohydrate consumption. Availability of exogenous protein is important for endurance as well as strength in trained athletes; however, amount and timing of protein intake has not been fully elucidated to maximize positive net muscle protein balance (Tipton 2011).

DIABETES SPORTS/EXERCISE NUTRITION AND INSULIN RECOMMENDATIONS

Contraction of the skeletal muscle enhances the uptake of glucose into the skeletal muscle cell through both insulin-mediated (increased production and translocation of GLUT4 transporters) as well as non–insulin-mediated glucose transport. In the individual without diabetes, insulin production is reduced with the onset of exercise. This reduction prevents hypoglycemia during exercise and beyond, both due to reduction in insulin-mediated glucose transport, but also a lack of suppression of glycolysis by the liver (Camacho 2005). However, in the diabetic state, this regulation of glucose by insulin is compromised in type 2 diabetes and absent in type 1 diabetes and can result in hypoglycemia in individuals on either insulin injections or pumps or insulin secretagogues. Therefore, the enhanced glucose uptake requires forward thinking with regard to insulin at a meal before exercise or dosing with additional carbohydrates during activity to prevent hypoglycemia. Further complicating glucose regulation in the athlete with diabetes is the effect of energy for sports and insulin timing during excitement (Friday night football) or high-intensity exercise (including stop-start sports such as ice hockey and basketball) on stress hormones (glucagon, epinephrine, norepinephrine, and cortisol), which drive hepatic glucose production and result in hyperglycemia. In the person without diabetes, the pancreas compensates for the rise in blood glucose, but in the individual with compromised insulin production, this natural adjustment is not available. Herein resides the pivotal challenge in delivering insulin and appropriate nutrition strategies during exercise by individuals with diabetes. The reader is directed to several excellent resources for a detailed description of exercise in relation to diabetes (Regensteiner 2009; Hawley 2008, ACSM 2010).

A literature search was conducted to determine the evidence for carbohydrate and insulin adjustments for exercise in individuals with type 1 and type 2 diabetes using PubMed MEDLINE. Additional articles were identified from reference lists. Search criteria for diabetes-specific research included the following: nutrition, exercise, and diabetes (978 articles); diabetic athlete (40); diabetes, nutrition, and sport (111); children, diabetes, nutrition, and exercise (127); type 2 diabetes, nutrition, and exercise (481); type 1 diabetes and exercise (69); and limited to English language and humans, as of April 2011.

The evidence for carbohydrate and insulin adjustments before and during activity to prevent hypoglycemia in adults and in children and adolescents with type 1 diabetes is summarized in Table 10.3 for adults (10 articles) and in Table 10.4 for children and adolescents (3 articles). The evidence for nutrition for individuals with type 2 diabetes during exercise is summarized in Table 10.5 (only 1 article met search criteria).

Type 1 Diabetes

In the individual with type 1 diabetes, factors that may influence blood glucose levels during exercise include the following: insulin administration site, ambient temperature, duration and intensity of the activity (Guelfi 2005), training status for the specific sport, insulin and glycemic level before exercise (Chokkalingam 2007; Riddell 2006), and recent episodes of hypoglycemia (Hornsby 2005; Galas-

Table 10.3 Evidence for Carbohydrate and Insulin Adjustments Before and During Activity/Exercise to Prevent Hypoglycemia in Adults with Type 1 Diabetes

	Population/ Duration of Study	Intervention (type of study)	Major Findings	Comments
Soo 1996	$n = 8$ male and 1 female with type 1 diabetes/ 3 tests of 45 min	Oral glucose (30 g) vs. bread (30 g) vs. no CHO tested before rest or 45 min of moderate exercise; no insulin given before exercise; early morning (crossover study)	Wide range of subject responses; glucose resulted in greater BG rise than bread, little to no CHO may be required by some subjects during exercise	Study was done in the morning without morning insulin; small sample size
Hernandez 2000	$n = 1$ woman and 6 men with type 1 diabetes/5 tests × 16 h	Five isocaloric snacks (water, whole milk, skim milk, sports drink [CHO and electrolytes], sports drink [CHO, fat, and protein]) were tested before, during, and after 1 h of exercise in late afternoon after usual lunch and insulin dose to prevent LOPEH (randomized crossover trial)	Some form of CHO must be ingested before exercise to prevent LOPEH; sports drinks, skim milk, and whole milk can be used; however, the sports drink that contained CHO, fat, and protein caused sustained hyperglycemia	Treated with ultralente and regular insulin; small sample size
Rabasa-Lhoret 2001	$n = 8$ men with type 1 diabetes/3 trials of 30–60 min	Exercise of 25, 50, and 75% VO_{2max} for 30–60 min after meal of 75 g CHO and 600 kcal to determine insulin dose ↓; pre-meal insulin adjusted by reduction of 0, 50, and 75% (randomized crossover trial)	Full-meal insulin dose associated with ↑ risk of hypoglycemia; the higher the intensity, the greater the ↓ needed to prevent hypoglycemia	Treated with ultralente and lispro insulins; table of recommendations available

Table 10.3 Evidence for Carbohydrate and Insulin Adjustments Before and During Activity/Exercise to Prevent Hypoglycemia in Adults with Type 1 Diabetes (*continued*)

	Population/ Duration of Study	Intervention (type of study)	Major Findings	Comments
Frances-cato 2004	*n* = 12 individuals with type 1 diabetes and 12 controls/4 trials of 1 h	CHO needed to prevent hypoglycemia during moderate exercise at different morning times; rate of glucose oxidation calculated by indirect calorimetry throughout exercise (clinical trials)	Time elapsed from last insulin dose is not a factor in risk of hypoglycemia during exercise when a proportional amount of CHO is ingested	Treated with regular insulin
Grimm 2004	*n* = 67 individuals with type 1 diabetes/4 tests	Four groups: *1)* 10–20 g CHO/h activity, *2)* 10–20 g CHO and ↓ insulin dose by 10%, *3)* ↓ insulin dose by 10% without CHO intake, *4)* no change in insulin dose or added CHO (clinical trial)	Amount of CHO consumed during exercise correlated with the BG 2 h after exercise (*P* < 0.01); no correlation was found with insulin reduction	Treated with NPH and rapid-acting insulin
Lormeau 2005	*n* = 15 individuals with type 1 diabetes/4 days and 8 scuba dives	Strict protocol of insulin adjustment, BG targets, and CHO consumption used to develop guidelines for scuba diving (descriptive study)	25 g CHO protected BG from ↓ of >50 mg/dL during the dive (30 min) in addition to insulin adjustments; table established based on data from the dives	Goal BG before dive 200 mg/dL; table with algorithms available
Guelfi 2005	*n* = 7 individuals with type 1 diabetes/30 min	Moderate- vs. high-intensity exercise (descriptive study)	Glucose remained higher after high-intensity than moderate-intensity exercise; both resulted in decline	Less CHO may be required for high-intensity vs. moderate-intensity exercise without insulin adjustments

	Population/ Duration of Study	Intervention (type of study)	Major Findings	Comments
Chokka-lingam 2007	*n* = 8 men with type 1 diabetes/at rest (2 h) and during 45 min of cycling × 2	Indirect calorimetry, insulin glucose clamps, and thigh muscle biopsies used to determine whole-body energy and muscle metabolism during moderate exercise at differing insulin infusions (descriptive study)	Differing insulin concentrations resulted in similar energy expenditures and muscle glycogen utilization; a substantial ↑ in exogenous glucose use in the high insulin trial vs. low trial to prevent hypoglycemia and a ↓ in lipolysis in the high insulin group	Six men on basal bolus subcutaneous insulin and 2 on twice/day premixed insulin injections; average A1C 7.9%
Jenni 2008	*n* = 7 physically active men with type 1 diabetes/120 min cycling × 2	Magnetic resonance spectroscopy, indirect calorimetry, stable isotopes, counterregulatory hormones measured to determine systemic fuel metabolism in normal or hyperglycemic state (randomized crossover study)	Euglycemia: substrate oxidation similar to individuals without diabetes; Hyperglycemia: fuel metabolism dominated by CHO oxidation but did not spare intramyocellular glycogen	Treated with subcutaneous insulin infusion; small sample size
Murillo 2010	*n* = 14 male runners with type 1 diabetes/2 half marathons, initially and 1 year later	Strategies used and changed over the year between half marathons (descriptive study of within-subject comparisons)	1 year: less insulin reduction and greater CHO consumption than usual guidelines resulted in less hypoglycemia	Treated with insulin analogs

BG, blood glucose; CHO, carbohydrate; LOPEH, late-onset post-exercise hypoglycemia.

setti 2003; Davis 2000) along with both chronic and acute nutrient intake. Fuel metabolism is also affected during exercise in euglycemic versus hyperglycemic status in individuals with type 1 diabetes (Jenni 2008). During hyperglycemia due to inadequate insulin availability, glucose production is accelerated, glucose utilization is impaired, and lipolysis is excessive. During hyperinsulinemia and hypoglycemia, glucose production is impaired and glucose utilization is accelerated with a reduction in lipolysis.

The term "think like a pancreas" becomes clear when acknowledging all the variables that make dosing carbohydrate and insulin a day-to-day challenge in sports and exercise. However, reliability and repeatability of blood glucose response to prolonged exercise within subjects has been demonstrated in adolescents with type 1 diabetes using standardized conditions (Temple 1995). But it

Table 10.4 Evidence for Carbohydrate and Insulin Adjustments Before and During Activity/Exercise to Prevent Hypoglycemia in Children and Adolescents with Type 1 Diabetes

	Population/ Duration of Study	Intervention (type of study)	Major Findings	Comments
Temple 1995	*n* = 9 adolescent boys with type 1 diabetes/6 × 10 min sessions of exercise × 2 sessions over 5–17 days	Intermittent vs. continuous exercise; exercise started 1 h after breakfast; BG values every 10 min (clinical trial)	Intra-subject BG responses to moderate-intensity exercise were reliable and repeatable when meal, exercise, and insulin regimens kept constant	Small sample size
Diabetes Research in Children Network Study Group 2006	*n* = 49 children, 8–17 years, with type 1 diabetes on insulin pump therapy/4–15 min treadmill cycles with 3–5 min rest periods × 2	Day 1 basal insulin was stopped during exercise; day 2 basal insulin was continued during exercise (clinical trial)	Hypoglycemia <70 mg/dL less frequent when insulin was discontinued; hyperglycemia 45 min after exercise more common when insulin discontinued	Treated with insulin pump therapy and rapid-acting insulin
McMahon 2006	*n* = 5 males and 4 female adolescents with type 1 diabetes/45 min of exercise at 95% lactate threshold × 2	Amount of glucose required to prevent hypoglycemia after rest or on exercise days tested by glucose infusion rates (clinical trial)	Glucose requirements immediately after and 7–11 h after exercise were elevated, implicating a biphasic pattern of increased glucose requirements	Intravenous insulin was used to mimic usual insulin doses; small sample size

BG, blood glucose.

Table 10.5 Nutrition Studies in Exercising Individuals with Type 2 Diabetes

	Population/Duration of Study	Intervention (type of study)	Major Findings	Comments
Gualano 2011	*n* = 25 men and women with type 2 diabetes, not taking exogenous insulin/12 weeks	Creatine (5 g/day) vs. placebo during exercise training program (randomized placebo-controlled trial)	Creatine supplementation combined with an exercise program improved glycemic control (*P* = 0.004)	One study with small sample size

takes commitment of the athlete with diabetes to determine, often by trial and error, what works for his or her individual athletic endeavor. Frequent blood glucose monitoring during training and during exercise/sports is critical to understanding the individual's own response to exercise and to determine insulin and carbohydrate strategies to maximize performance and safety.

Adults with type 1 diabetes. Carbohydrate use during moderate cycling was determined to be ~1 g carbohydrate/kg body weight in a 1-h study of cyclists with type 1 diabetes exercising at moderate intensity, after usual dose of regular insulin during morning exercise (Francescato 2004). This result closely matches the carbohydrate oxidation of 0.95 g/kg body weight for the athlete/exerciser without diabetes cycling over the same duration (Pfeiffer 2011). Intra-subject blood glucose response during a 45-min session of cycling in a small group of subjects with type 1 diabetes was not significantly different when glucose was provided in either liquid or solid form (Soo 1996). There was, however, a significant inter-subject variability in response to the same carbohydrate load. Trial and error can lead to a plan that prevents hypoglycemia without excess carbohydrate ingestion, which has the potential to lead to weight gain (Younk 2011). A good starting point would be 1 g carbohydrate per minute of exercise of moderate to high intensity.

A 4-second maximal sprint every 2 min during 30 min of cycling decreased the risk of hypoglycemia (Guelfi 2005), reducing the need for additional carbohydrate ingestion. This carried over to the 60-min recovery period as well. This strategy may be appropriate when inadequate carbohydrate is available to treat hypoglycemia during a workout or when the individual is using exercise as a weight-loss strategy.

In a study of scuba divers with type 1 diabetes, hypoglycemic events were prevented using a strict protocol, including elevated glycemic goals of 200–250 mg/dL before immersion. Using an algorithm based on the study, 25 g carbohydrate were determined to prevent blood glucose levels from decreasing more than 50 mg/dL (Lormeau 2005). It is important to note, this study once again is focused on hypoglycemia prevention, rather than specifically nourishing the athlete for exercise.

A recent study compared insulin dosing and carbohydrate ingestion strategies used by runners with type 1 diabetes in two consecutive years of running the same half marathon. All participants were using insulin analogs. In both events, basal insulin rates were reduced (18.3% in year 1 and 14.2% in year 2). During the second year, carbohydrate intake during activity was increased from ~49 to ~59 g). Glycemic excursions were reduced during the second year with the higher carbohydrate intake and less insulin reduction (Murillo 2010).

Whole milk, a sports drink with carbohydrate and electrolytes, or a sports drink with carbohydrate, fat, and protein but not skim milk attenuated late-onset post-exercise hypoglycemia in adults on ultralente or biosynthetic long-acting insulin and regular insulin after a late-afternoon 1-h session of exercise (Hernandez 2000). The drinks were isocaloric and based on individual energy expenditure; however, the concentration of carbohydrate varied from 28 to 145 g carbohydrate per serving.

Alterations in basal and bolus insulin doses to prevent hypoglycemia have been studied extensively (Toni 2006; Devlin 2000; Rabasa-Lhoret 2001) and many recommendations have been provided (Toni 2006). It is important to note which types of insulin were being used during these studies, since older studies reflect intermediate- and short-acting insulin, which are more difficult to titrate for sports and result in an increased need to compensate by carbohydrate intake. With the availability of rapid-acting insulin and insulin pumps, dosing insulin appropriately for sport has the potential to minimize hypoglycemia and reduce the necessity of ingesting excess carbohydrate above the physiological need for the sport (Riddell 2009). In addition, continuous glucose monitoring systems indicate direction and rate of change of blood glucose, helping to determine the amount of carbohydrate necessary to prevent hypoglycemia and minimizing over- or under-treatment (Cauza 2005). It must be noted that hypoglycemic response from counterregulatory hormones may be suppressed in individuals with diabetes during hypoglycemic episodes, requiring exogenous carbohydrate rescue (Camacho 2005).

Individuals with type 1 diabetes who participate in sports should be aware of the impact of intensity and duration of exercise on blood glucose response. Generally, 1 g carbohydrate per minute of exercise is an appropriate initial strategy to minimize risk of hypoglycemia and maximize exercise safety. Frequent blood glucose monitoring during exercise and over the duration of training is critical to understanding the individual's own response to exercise and to determine carbohydrate and insulin strategies to maximize performance and safety.

Youth with type 1 diabetes. It has been demonstrated that adolescents with type 1 diabetes who exercise improve muscle strength, cardiorespiratory endurance, lipid profiles, amount of lean body mass, psychosocial well-being, and glucose regulation (Riddell 2006; Mosher 1998). As with adults, the challenge to exercise is balancing exercise duration and intensity with insulin dosing and carbohydrate ingestion.

Energy intake should be determined based on the child's appetite and monitored regularly using growth charts from the Centers for Disease Control and Prevention (Silverstein 2005). Decreasing insulin dosing for planned exercise rather than increasing carbohydrates (and therefore calories) should be encouraged.

Total carbohydrate use during heavy exercise can be as high as 1.0–1.5 g/kg body weight per hour of activity in adolescents with and without diabetes (Riddell 2000; Robertson 2008). For example, in a 75-kg (165-lb) high school football player, this amount can translate to 75–113 g carbohydrate per hour of exercise. Table 10.6 lists grams of carbohydrate required per 30 min of specific activities (Riddell 2006). An increase in carbohydrate intake before and during exercise in children and adolescents with type 1 diabetes was prescribed based on body mass and activity using exercise exchanges (1 exercise exchange equals 100 kcal and 15 g carbohydrate) (Riddell 1999). Energy expenditure was determined for various activities and body mass, with an estimate of 60% of energy expenditure for carbohydrates. For example, a 20-kg child would need 15 g carbohydrate (1 exercise exchange) for each 30 min of basketball. However, this information is based on assumptions that have not been proven experimentally (Perkins 2006). But these assumptions may provide a starting place when working with the athlete to discover his or her carbohydrate prescription.

Regardless of the carbohydrate recommendation, insulin dosing must also be considered. In a study of youth with diabetes, 45 min of moderate exercise during the morning hours resulted in nocturnal hypoglycemia in 9 of 10 participants who maintained normal insulin doses (Admon 2005). Hypoglycemia is not restricted to children with lower pre-exercise levels of glycemia (Riddell 1999), and late-onset post-exercise hypoglycemia is common (Riddel 1999; Admon 2005). Nocturnal hypoglycemia may be more prevalent when exercise occurs in the afternoon (McMahon 2007). Reduction in overnight basal insulin, in addition to 15–30 g carbohydrate in the evening after a more active day, may attenuate nocturnal hypoglycemia. Blood glucose testing in the middle of the night is also recommended to determine the adequacy of the preventative treatment.

Spontaneous exercise is frequent in children and adolescents. Checking blood glucose levels and having carbohydrate-rich snacks available at all times provides information and safety for periods of unplanned exercise. Low-level activities have little impact on blood glucose levels (Hopkins 2004), and intermittent activity may help to maintain more stable blood glucose levels than activities of longer duration and moderate intensity (Guelfi 2005). Intermittent high-intensity exercise is less likely to result in a decline in blood glucose values during exercise as well as

Table 10.6 Grams of Carbohydrate Required per 30 Min of Specific Activities Based on the Approximate Body Weight of the Child

Activity	Body Mass (kg)		
	~20	~40	~60
	Carbohydrates (g) for every 30 min of activity		
Basketball (game)	15	30	45
Cross-country skiing	11	23	30
Cycling, 10 km/h	7	11	18
Cycling, 15 km/h	10	18	30
Figure skating	18	30	45
Ice hockey (ice time)	23	45	90
Running, 8 km/h	23	30	45
Running, 12 km/h	15	30	45
Soccer	8	18	30
Swimming, 30 m/min	11	23	30
Swimming, breast stroke	8	15	23
Tennis	10	18	30
Walking, 4 km/h	8	11	15
Walking, 6 km/h	11	15	18

Projected carbohydrate requirements without adjustments of basal or bolus insulin and the assumption that 60% of the predicted energy expenditure is provided by carbohydrate. Adapted from Riddell 2006.

after exercise. The effect on blood glucose levels has been speculated to be related to the higher levels of catecholamine and growth hormone levels with intense exercise. High-intensity exercise, such as running sprints or a wrestling match, may result in hyperglycemia that may last from 30 to 60 min after exercise (Riddell 2006). In addition, competition stress may also raise blood glucose values above predicted levels. This increase is due to the catecholamine response to stress, increasing lipolysis, impaired glucose tolerance, and glucose production. Although bolus insulin can be used to attenuate the hyperglycemia resulting from the competition-related stress hormone responses, it must be used cautiously, since late-onset hypoglycemia may occur. And finally, for children on insulin pump therapy, an alternative to constant carbohydrate feeding during spontaneous activity is reducing or suspending basal rates (Diabetes Research in Children Network Study Group 2006).

General carbohydrate recommendations for active children with diabetes may be the same as those for the general population: 8–10 g/kg body weight for prolonged exercise (Riddell 2006; Petrie 2004). Carbohydrate intake should match carbohydrate expenditure during activity (Riddell 1999), although this may be impractical. Glucose ingestion to match carbohydrate use has been shown to reduce the rate of hypoglycemia without insulin adjustments (Riddell 1999). Carbohydrate was estimated at 0.5–1.5 g/kg body weight per hour of training. For example, a 55-kg (121-lb) tennis player needing 0.9 g carbohydrate/kg body weight/h would require 50 g carbohydrate per hour of activity. That carbohydrate could be consumed in a variety of ways, including but not limited to sports drinks, juice, or fruit. Variation in carbohydrate prescription was based on timing of insulin administration before exercise.

Carbohydrate should also be consumed during activity >60 min to nourish the individual as well as to assist in the prevention of hypoglycemia. There is a large inter-subject variability in carbohydrate use, so customized guidelines are necessary. Through trial and error, carbohydrate intake to maximize blood glucose control may be implemented with some level of predictability.

Hypoglycemia during exercise should be treated with 30–45 g carbohydrate (Rachmiel 2007). Nocturnal hypoglycemia can be avoided with higher nighttime blood glucose goals (>130 mg/dL), reduction in basal rate (25% for 12 h), and a larger-than-normal bedtime snack that contains carbohydrates (Rachmiel 2007).

Protein requirements for active children with type 1 diabetes have not been determined and at this time should follow recommendations for active children without diabetes (Petrie 2004).

Children should stay hydrated during sports. Hyperglycemia will increase fluid requirements above normal levels. Weighing the athlete before and after activity will help the individual, coach, or parent to determine adequate fluid replacement strategies, keeping in mind the amount ingested during the sport. Three cups of fluid is recommended for 1 lb of weight lost. To prevent dehydration, a general recommendation is for 0.5–1 liter per hour (2–4 cups) for vigorous physical activity above that required during non-exercise times (Petrie 2004). Heat and hyperglycemia will increase also fluid requirements; a general recommendation is 0.5–1 liter per hour of activity.

Key points for children include the following:

- Because of the unpredictable nature of exercise, frequent monitoring of blood glucose before, during, and up to 12 h after sports should be done to guide insulin dosing and additional carbohydrate supplementation.
- Blood glucose monitoring before exercise is recommended with an intake of 10–15 g carbohydrate for physical activity when blood glucose is below individually determined goals (generally 100 mg/dL).
- Carbohydrate should be consumed during activity of >30 min to nourish the body as well as to help prevent hypoglycemia.
- Children should stay hydrated during sports.

Adults with Type 2 Diabetes

Most adults with type 2 diabetes are inactive. Physical activity is a treatment strategy for both type 2 diabetes and prediabetes. Both resistance and aerobic exercise has resulted in improved blood glucose control, with a mean decrease in A1C of 0.6% (Sanz 2010). Several studies have demonstrated a greater beneficial impact from a combination program of strength and aerobic exercise (Sigal 2007; Church 2010). Increased muscle mass in response to resistance training and improvement in insulin use from aerobic exercise contribute to improvements in blood glucose management. Improvement from combination training may be related to increased duration of activity and caloric use rather than the unique contribution of each activity (ACSM 2010).

As exercise intensity increases, there is an increased reliance on carbohydrate for fuel. In individuals with type 2 diabetes, muscle contraction enhances glucose transport from the blood into the skeletal muscle at a greater rate than hepatic glucose production, generally resulting in a reduction in blood glucose values. The exception to this is, during short high-intensity sessions of exercise, catecholamines can elevate blood glucose values during and up to several hours after exercise (ACSM 2010).

Exercise stimulates muscle cell GLUT4 receptor activity, increasing the effectiveness of endogenous and exogenous insulin. In addition, non–insulin-mediated glucose transport is also activated with exercise. Unlike the individual with type 1 diabetes, most individuals with type 2 diabetes do not suffer from exercise or post-exercise hypoglycemia, reducing or eliminating the need for supplementary carbohydrate for exercise. In a study using aerobic, strength, or a combination of modes of exercise, there were no hypoglycemic events requiring assistance during the 22-week trial (Sigal 2007). Most individuals will not need carbohydrate for exercise lasting <1 h (ACSM 2010).

Nutrition recommendations for type 2 diabetes in exercise have not been established. However, general recommendations for exercise/sports are appropriate, with an added focus of nutrition for other metabolic disturbances that may co-occur, such as hypertriglyceridemia, hypertension, and obesity (American Diabetes Association 2008). Physical activity of moderate intensity for 150–250 min/week added to calorie restriction provides a modest additional reduction in weight loss to diet alone. This benefit becomes less pronounced as energy restriction is intensified and more profound as activity becomes extreme, such as that found in military training (ACSM 2009b).

Hypoglycemia during exercise is a concern for individuals with type 2 diabetes on insulin and/or insulin secretagogues. The overall rate of hypoglycemia for individuals with type 2 diabetes taking insulin is 10-fold lower than that for individuals with type 1 diabetes, and rates are even lower for patients on oral agents (Church 2010). The majority of individuals with type 2 diabetes are overweight, making supplemental carbohydrate for exercise expenditure counterproductive. Therefore, adjusting medication rather than increasing carbohydrate intake during exercise of <60 min is preferable. If hypoglycemia does occur, 15–20 g carbohydrate should be ingested, such as a sports drink that contains ~15 g carbohydrate per 240 mL (8 oz). Blood glucose should be rechecked in 15 min and treatment repeated if hypoglycemia persists (Nyenwe 2011).

A recent trial with creatine supplementation combined with an exercise program resulted in improved metabolic control in type 2 diabetic patients. In addition, subjects improved strength over the placebo group. Aerobic capacity was not significantly different (Gualano 2011). Further research in this area should clarify recommendations for creatine use in the individual with type 2 diabetes.

TRANSLATION OF EVIDENCE INTO NUTRITION THERAPY INTERVENTIONS FOR SPORTS OR EXERCISE

There is no published research to determine the best eating pattern for the athlete or exerciser with diabetes. The available research has focused on the appropriate dose of carbohydrate to prevent hypoglycemia with or without insulin alterations. Because of the lack of evidence to the contrary, the food plan for the individual with diabetes for sports/exercise does not differ from the food plan for the individual without diabetes.

The recent evidence demonstrates that the protocol to prevent low blood glucose levels can be evidence-based and predictable but is unique for each individual. Carbohydrate recommendations are not dissimilar to individuals without diabetes and should match carbohydrate expenditure during the event. Prediction, such as the Mifflin and Cunningham equations (Dunford 2006), can be used to provide recommendations, but serious athletes might consider the use of metabolic measurement to determine their individual needs. This measurement would include the use of a metabolic chart to determine respiratory quotient (RQ) at rest and during exercise. Using this approach, carbohydrate and fat fuel use can be determined for different intensities of exercise. This system is only practical for a few types of exercises, including running and cycling, and availability is generally limited.

SUMMARY

It is important to recognize the value of fueling the individual for exercise and physical activity, not merely normalizing blood glucose values. Energy requirements will be different for the athlete and the occasional exerciser with diabetes. Individual needs for prevention of hypoglycemia can best be determined by frequent monitoring of blood glucose levels and will vary depending on the type and duration of activity. Matching carbohydrate intake with carbohydrate expenditure as well as adjustments in diabetes medications will minimize risk of hypoglycemia after exercise. Awareness of changes in insulin sensitivity and non–insulin-mediated glucose transport after exercise are important to minimize excess carbohydrate ingestion beyond physiological need, as well as to reduce anxiety and fear of hypoglycemia with exercise. Athletes and occasional exercisers who are not achieving personal performance goals may benefit from referral to a registered dietitian specializing in both diabetes and sports nutrition.

BIBLIOGRAPHY

Admon G, Weinstein Y, Falk B, Weintrob N, Benzaquen H, Otan R, Fayman G, Zigel L, Constantini V, Phillip M: Exercise with and without an insulin pump among children and adolescents with type 1 diabetes mellitus. *Pediatrics* 116:348–355, 2005

American College of Sports Medicine: Appropriate physical activity intervention strategies for weight loss and prevention of weight regain for adults: position stand. *Med Sci Sports Exerc* 41:459–471, 2009b

American College of Sports Medicine: Exercise and type 2 diabetes: a joint position statement of the American Diabetes Association and the American College of Sports Medicine. *Med Sci Sports Exerc* 42:2282–2303, 2010

American College of Sports Medicine: Nutrition and athletic performance: a joint position statement of the American Dietetic Association, Dietitians of Canada and American College of Sports Medicine. *Med Sci Sports Exerc* 41:709–731, 2009a

American Diabetes Association: Nutrition recommendations and interventions for diabetes (Position Statement). *Diabetes Care* 31 (Suppl. 1):S61–S78, 2008

Armstrong LE, Maresh CM, Castellani JW, Bergeron MF, Kenefick RW, LaGasse KE, Riebe D: Urinary indices of hydration status. *Int J Sport Nut* 4:265–279, 1994

Burd NA, Tang JE, Moore DR, Phillips SM: Exercise training and protein metabolism: influences of contraction, protein intake and sex-based differences. *J Appl Physiol* 106:1692–1701, 2009

Burke L: *Practical Sports Nutrition*. Chicago, IL, Human Kinetics, 2007

Camacho RC, Galassetti P, Davis SN, Wasserman DH: Glucoregulation during and after exercise in health and insulin-dependent diabetes. *Exerc Sport Sci Rev* 33:17–23, 2005

Cauza E, Hanusch-Enserer U, Strasser B, Ludvik B, Kostner K, Dunky A, Haber P: Continuous glucose monitoring in diabetic long distance runners. *Int J Sports Med* 26:774–780, 2005

Chokkalingam K, Tsintzas K, Norton L, Jewell K, Macdonald IA, Mansell IA: Exercise under hyperinsulinaemic conditions increases whole-body glucose disposal without affecting muscle glycogen utilization in type 1 diabetes. *Diabetologia* 50:414–421, 2007

Church TS, Blair SN, Cocreham S, Johannsen N, Johnson W, Kramer K, Mikus CR, Myers V, Nauta M, Rodarte RQ, Sparks L, Thompson A, Earnest CP: Effects of aerobic and resistance training on hemoglobin A$_{1c}$ levels in patients with type 2 diabetes: a randomized controlled trial. *JAMA* 304:2253–2262, 2010

Colberg SR: *Diabetic Athlete's Handbook: Your Guide to Peak Performance*. Champaign, IL, Human Kinetics, 2009

Currell K, Jeukendrup AE: Superior endurance performance with ingestion of multiple transportable carbohydrates. *Med Sci Sports Exerc* 40:275–281, 2008

Davis S, Galassetti P, Wasserman D, Tate D: Effects of antecedent hypoglycemia on subsequent counterregulatory responses to exercise. *Diabetes* 49:73–81, 2000

Devlin JT: Exercise therapy in diabetes. In *Medical Management of Diabetes Mellitus*. Leahy JL, Clark NG, Cefalu WT, Eds. New York, Marcel Dekker, 2000

Diabetes Research in Children Network Study Group: Prevention of hypoglycemia during exercise in children with type 1 diabetes by suspending basal insulin. *Diabetes Care* 29:2200–2204, 2006

Dunford M (Ed.): *Sports Nutrition: A Practice Manual for Professionals*. 4th ed. Chicago, IL, American Dietetic Association, 2006

Francescato MP, Geat M, Fusi S, Stupar G, Noacco C, Cattin L: Carbohydrate requirement and insulin concentration during moderate exercise in type 1 diabetic patients. *Metabolism* 53:1126–1130, 2004

Franz MJ, Powers MA, Leontos C, Holmeister LA, Kulkarni K, Monk A, Wedel N, Gradwell E: The evidence for medical nutrition therapy for type 1 and type 2 diabetes in adults. *J Am Diet Assoc* 110:1852–1889, 2010

Galassetti P, Tate D, Neill R, Morrey S, Wasserman D, Davis S: Effect of antecedent hypoglycemia on counterregulatory responses to subsequent euglycemic exercise in type 1 diabetes. *Diabetes* 52:1761–1769, 2003

Grimm JJ, Ybarra J, Berne C, Muchnick S, Golay: A new table for prevention of hypoglycaemia during physical activity in type 1 diabetic patients. *Diabetes Metab* 30:465–470, 2004

Gualano B, De Salles Painneli V, Roschel H, Artioli GG, Neves M, De Sa Pinto AL, Rossi Da Silva ME, Cunha MR, Otaduy MCG, Da Costa Leite C, Ferreira JC, Pereira RM, Brum PC, Bonfa E, Lancha AH: Creatine in type 2 diabetes: a randomized, double-blind, placebo-controlled trial. *Med Sci Sports Exerc* 43:770–778, 2011

Guelfi K, Jones T, Fournier P: The decline in blood glucose levels is less with intermittent high-intensity compared with moderate exercise in individuals with type 1 diabetes. *Diabetes Care* 28:1289–1294, 2005

Hawley JA, Zierath JR (Eds.): *Physical Activity and Type 2 Diabetes*. Champaign, IL, Human Kinetics, 2008

Hernandez JM, Moccia T, Fluckey JD, Ulbrecht JS, Farrell PA: Fluid snacks to help persons with type 1 diabetes avoid late onset postexercise hypoglycemia. *Med Sci Sports Exerc* 32:904–910, 2000

Hopkins D: Exercise-induced and other daytime hypoglycaemic events in patients with diabetes: prevention and treatment. *Diabetes Res Clin Pract* 65:S35–S39, 2004

Hornsby WG, Chetlin RD: Management of competitive athletes with diabetes. *Diabetes Spectrum* 18:102–107, 2005

Institute of Medicine: *Recommended Dietary Allowances*. 10th ed. Washington, DC, National Academy Press, 1989

Jenni S, Oetliker C, Allemann S, Ith M, Tappy L, Wuerth S, Egger A, Boesch C, Schneiter PH, Diem P, Christ E, Stettler C: Fuel metabolism during exercise in euglycaemia and hyperglycaemia in patients with type 1 diabetes mellitus: a prospective single-blinded randomized crossover trial. *Diabetologia* 51:1457–1465, 2008

Jeukendrup A, Jentjens R: Oxidation of carbohydrate feedings during prolonged exercise: current thoughts, guidelines and directions for future research. *Sports Med* 29:407–424, 2000

Kerksick C, Harvey T, Stout J, Campbell B, Wilborn C, Kreider R, Kalman D, Ziegenfuss T, Lopez H, Landis J, Ivy J, Antonio J: International Society of Sports Nutrition position stand: nutrient timing. *J Int Soc Sports Nutr* 5:17, 2008

Lormeau B, Sola A, Tabah A, Chiheb S, Dufaitre L, Thurniger O, Bresson R, Lormeau C, Attali JR, Velensi P: Blood glucose changes and adjustments of diet and insulin doses in type 1 diabetic patients during scuba diving (for a change in French regulations). *Diabetes Metab* 31:144–151, 2005

McMahon SK, Ferreira LD, Ratnam N, Davey RJ, Youngs LM, Davis EA, Fournier PA, Jones TW: Glucose requirements to maintain euglycemia after moderate-intensity afternoon exercise in adolescents with type 1 diabetes are increased in a biphasic manner. *J Clin Endocrinol Metab* 92:963–968, 2007

Mosher PE, Nash MS, Perry AC, LaPerriere AR, Goldberg RB: Aerobic circuit exercise training: effect on adolescents with well controlled insulin-dependent diabetes mellitus. *Arch Phys Med Rehabil* 79:652–657, 1998

Murillo S, Brugnara L, Novials A: One year follow-up in a group of half-marathon runners with type-1 diabetes treated with insulin analogues. *J Sports Med Phys Fitness* 50:506–510, 2010

Nyenwe EA, Jerkins TW, Umpierrez GE, Kitabchi AE: Management of type 2 diabetes: evolving strategies for the treatment of patients with type 2 diabetes. *Metabolism* 60:1–23, 2011

Perkins BA, Riddell MC: Type 1 diabetes and exercise: using the insulin pump to maximum advantage. *Can J Diabetes* 30:72–79, 2006

Petrie HJ, Stover EA, Horswill CA: Nutritional concerns for the child and adolescent competitor. *Nutrition* 20:620–631, 2004

Pfeiffer B, Stellingwerff T, Zaltas E, Hodgson A, Jeukendrup A: Carbohydrate oxidation from a drink during running compared with cycling exercise. *Med Sci Sports Exerc* 43:327–334, 2011

Rabasa-Lhoret R, Bourque J, Ducros F, Chaisson J: Guidelines for premeal insulin dose reduction for postprandial exercise of different intensities and durations in type 1 diabetic subjects treated intensively with a basal-bolus insulin regimen (ultralente-lispro). *Diabetes Care* 24:625–630, 2001

Rachmiel M, Buccino J, Daneman D: Exercise and type 1 diabetes mellitus in youth; review and recommendations. *Ped Endocrinol Rev* 5:656–665, 2007

Regensteiner JG, Reusch JEB, Stewart KJ, Veves A (Eds.): *Diabetes and Exercise.* New York, Humana Press, 2009

Riddell MC, Bar-Or O, Ayub BV, Calvert RE, Heigenhauser GJF: Glucose ingestion matched with total carbohydrate utilization attenuates hypoglycemia during exercise in adolescents with IDDM. *Int J Sport Nut* 9:24–34, 1999

Riddell MC, Bar-Or O, Hollidge-Horvat M, Schwarcz HP, Heigenhauser GJ: Glucose ingestion and substrate utilization during exercise in boys with IDDM. *J Appl Physiol* 88:1239–1246, 2000

Riddell MC, Iscoe KE: Physical activity, sport and pediatric diabetes. *Pediatr Diabetes* 7:60–70, 2006

Riddell MC, Perkins BA: Exercise and glucose metabolism in persons with diabetes mellitus: perspectives on the role for continuous glucose monitoring. *J Diabetes Sci Technol* 3:914–923, 2009

Riddell MC, Perkins BA: Type 1 diabetes and vigorous exercise: applications of exercise physiology to patient management. *Can J Diabetes* 30:63–71, 2006

Robertson K, Adolfsson P, Riddell M, Scheiner G, Hanas R: ISPAD clinical practice consensus guidelines 2006–2007: exercise in children and adolescents with diabetes. *Pediatr Diabetes* 9:65–77, 2008

Rodriguez NR, Vislocky LM, Gaine PC: Dietary protein, endurance exercise, and human skeletal-muscle protein turnover. *Curr Opin Clin Nutr Metab Care* 10:40–45, 2007

Sanz C, Gautier J-F, Hanaire H: Physical exercise for the prevention and treatment of type 2 diabetes. *Diabetes Metab* 36:346–351, 2010

Scheiner G: *Think Like a Pancreas: A Practical Guide to Managing Diabetes with Insulin.* 2nd ed. Philadelphia, PA, Da Capo Press, 2011

Sigal RJ, Kenny GP, Boule NG, Wells GA, Prud'homme D, Fortier M, Reid RD, Tulloch H, Coyle D, Phillips P, Jennings A, Jaffey J: Effects of aerobic training, resistance training, or both on glycemic control in type 2 diabetes. *Ann Intern Med* 147:357–369, 2007

Silverstein J, Klingensmith G, Copeland K, Plotnick L, Kaufman F, Laffel L, Deeb L, Grey M, Anderson B, Holzmeister L, Clark N: Care of the children and adolescents with type 1 diabetes: a statement of the American Diabetes Association. *Diabetes Care* 28:186–212, 2005

Soo K, Furler S, Samaras K, Jenkins A, Campbell L, Chisholm D: Glycemic responses to exercise in IDDM after simple and complex carbohydrate supplementation. *Diabetes Care* 19:575–579, 1996

Temple MY, Bar-Or O, Riddell: The reliability and repeatability of the blood glucose response to prolonged exercise in adolescent boys with IDDM. *Diabetes Care* 18:326–332, 1995

Tipton KD: Protein nutrition and exercise: what's the latest? *Scan's Pulse* 30:1–5, 2011

Tipton KD, Wolfe RR: Protein and amino acids for athletes. *J Sports Sci* 22:65–79, 2004

Toni S, Reali MF, Barni F, Lenzi L, Festini F: Managing insulin therapy during exercise in type 1 diabetes mellitus. *Acta Biomed* 77 (Suppl. 1):34–40, 2006

Wilmore JH, Costill DL, Kenney WL: *Physiology of Sport and Exercise*. Chicago, IL, Human Kinetics, 2008

Younk LM, Mikeladze M, Tate D, Davis SN: Exercise-related hypoglycemia in diabetes mellitus. *Expert Rev Endocrinol Metab* 6: 93–108, 2011

Carla Cox, PhD, RD, CDE, CSSD, is a Diabetes Educator and Sports Dietitian at Western Montana Clinic and St. Patrick Hospital and Health Sciences Center, Missoula, MT.

Chapter 11

Nutrition Therapy for the Hospitalized and Long-Term Care Patient with Diabetes

Carrie S. Swift, MS, RD, BC-ADM, CDE

Highlights
Hospital Care

■ Care of patients with diabetes during and after hospitalization is improved by implementation of nutrition therapy, provided by registered dietitians knowledgeable in glycemic control.

■ An interdisciplinary team approach to providing nutrition care for hospitalized patients and timely specific discharge planning is important to optimize outcomes.

■ Evidence does not support the use of the "no concentrated sweets" or "no sugar" diets in the hospital setting; there is also not an "ADA diet." Foods that contain sucrose may be incorporated into a consistent carbohydrate meal plan.

■ Consistent carbohydrate meal plans are the accepted standard for hospitalized patients with diabetes, whether eating regular food or on a progression diet (clear liquid, full liquid, etc.).

■ Inadequate nutrition intake is common in hospitalized patients. Less restrictive diets, room service "on demand" meal delivery, and offering food choices to meet personal, cultural, or religious food preferences have been implemented in the hospital setting to improve oral intake and enhance patient satisfaction.

Hospital Care

Hospital care for patients with diabetes has a significant health and economic impact in the U.S. Data from the Agency for Healthcare Research and Quality (AHRQ) on hospital use by patients with diabetes indicated that approximately one in five hospitalizations in 2008 were related to diabetes (Fraze 2010). Patients with diabetes as the primary or secondary diagnosis in the medical record incurred over 7.7 million hospital stays and $83 billion in inpatient care costs, comprising 23% of the total hospital costs in the U.S. in 2008. Additionally, hospitalizations were more frequent and the average length of stay was longer and more costly for individuals with diabetes.

Hyperglycemia in hospitalized patients without a diagnosis of diabetes is also common. It may occur during acute illness in patients with previously normal glucose tolerance and is often referred to as stress hyperglycemia (Clement 2004). Administration of pharmacological agents, such as glucocorticoids or vasopressors, may also contribute to hospital-related hyperglycemia. The incidence and cost of in-hospital hyperglycemia is difficult to identify and quantify, but is likely quite substantial. Observational data unequivocally links hyperglycemia to poor outcomes in hospitalized patients with or without diagnosed diabetes (Moghissi 2009). Evidence emerged in the late 1990s and early 2000s from cohort and interventional studies indicating that intensive treatment of hyperglycemia improved hospital outcomes in critically ill patients. Improving glycemic control during hospitalization became a significant topic for enhancing outcomes in hospitalized patients.

The recommendations discussed in this chapter apply to hospitalized patients with known diabetes, previously unrecognized diabetes discovered during the hospital stay, and hospital-related hyperglycemia that reverts to normal after discharge. A brief summary of the early evidence regarding inpatient glycemic control is reviewed first, followed by current evidence and implications of glycemic targets on medical and nutrition care of hospitalized patients. Nutrition therapy and the role of the registered dietitian (RD) as part of the interdisciplinary team will also be reviewed.

EVIDENCE FOR IMPROVED INPATIENT GLYCEMIC CONTROL

Diabetes and hyperglycemia have been associated with poor medical outcomes in hospitalized patients. Hyperglycemia itself has been linked to infection, negative effects on the cardiovascular system, increased risk of thrombosis, inflammation, blood pressure changes, central nervous system injury, and endothelial cell dysfunction (Clement 2004; Garber 2004). Regardless of the cause, treatment of hyperglycemia improves outcomes. Inpatient management of hyperglycemia has become a quality indicator for hospital care, although optimal blood glucose targets remain controversial. On the basis of observational and several early randomized controlled trials (RCTs), intensive glycemic control was recommended in critical care settings (Malmberg 1995; Van den Berghe 2001; Furnary 2003). This recommendation led the American Diabetes Association (ADA) to add recommendations for treatment of hyperglycemia in hospitalized patients to their standards of medical care in 2005 (ADA 2005), and both the American College of Endocrinology and ADA endorsed tight glycemic control in critical care units. Because of the lack of evidence to support specific blood glucose targets in the non–critical care hospital setting, glycemic target recommendations were similar to those for outpatients, with upper limits for blood glucose preprandial of <110 mg/dL and peak postprandial of <180 mg/dL. For critical care patients (e.g., surgical intensive care), ≤110 mg/dL was recommended at all times (Garber 2004; Clement 2004).

While hyperglycemia is associated with increased morbidity and mortality during critical illness, recent RCTs reported inconsistent outcomes and identified an increased risk of severe hypoglycemia with tight glucose control in these patients. The Diabetes Mellitus Insulin-Glucose Infusion in Acute Myocardial Infarction (DIGAMI) study demonstrated improved outcomes in diabetes patients seen in 16 Swedish hospitals (*n* = 620) with acute myocardial infarction, initially treated with insulin-glucose infusion followed by long-term subcutaneous insulin; mortality rates were reduced in the group receiving insulin infusion treatment, from 28 to 19% at 1 year (Malmberg 1995) and at an average of 3.4 years by 11% (from 44 to 33%) (Malmberg 1997). The DIGAMI 2 study attempted to determine if the decrease in mortality was due to te initial insulin infusion or the long-term subcutaneous insulin treatment in the same patient population. The results did not support the findings of the DIGAMI study, since no significant differences were seen between the intensive group and the control group (Malmberg 2005).

The largest study to date, Normoglycemia in Intensive Care Evaluation—Survival Using Glucose Algorithm Regulation (NICE-SUGAR), examined the effect of intensive glucose control on outcomes in over 6,000 critically ill patients in a multicenter, multinational RCT (Finfer 2009). At 90 days, the mortality rate was significantly higher in the intensively treated group than in the conventional group (27.5% death rate vs. 24.9%, respectively [*P* = 0.02]). In addition, severe hypoglycemia occurred more frequently in the intensively treated group (6.8 vs. 0.5% [*P* < 0.0001]) (Finfer 2009).

In a meta-analysis reviewing 26 RCTs (*n* = 13,567), including NICE-SUGAR, the authors concluded that widespread adoption of intensive insulin therapy for critically ill patients should not be recommended (Griesdale 2009). It was noted, however, that protocols and blood glucose targets for "usual care" varied among studies. If study protocols included a usual care group (control group) with lower blood glucose targets, there may be less benefit seen between the intensive insulin treatment group and control group than if higher targets were used. Yet, because of these more recent findings, blood glucose targets in the critical care setting have become less stringent to decrease the potential of adverse outcomes related to hypoglycemia (Moghissi 2009).

Insulin Therapy in Critical Care

Insulin therapy is the preferred method to achieve glycemic control in the hospital setting for the majority of clinical situations. Intravenous (IV) insulin infusion is the treatment of choice for most critical care patients, with initiation at a threshold of 180 mg/dL. After the insulin infusion has been started, blood glucose should be maintained between 140 and 180 mg/dL (Moghissi 2009). Although evidence to support lower glycemic targets is equivocal, more intensive glycemic control may be appropriate for some patients in the critical care setting. Use of an insulin infusion protocol that minimizes glycemic excursions and hypoglycemia is recommended. IV insulin protocols take into account the current blood glucose level, rate of glycemic change, and current insulin infusion rate to determine subsequent adjustments (Clement 2004). Initially, blood glucose monitoring is performed at least hourly; however, once the blood glucose is stable, monitoring may be decreased to every 2 h. Transition to subcutaneous insulin generally occurs once a patient starts eating meals or is transferred to a non–critical care unit. Subcutaneous insulin should be initiated between 1 and 4 h before discontinuation of the IV insulin to prevent hyperglycemia. The transition from IV insulin to subcutaneous insulin can be problematic. Though guidelines are available, an effective, safe transition regimen has not been validated (Moghissi 2009).

Insulin Therapy in Non–Critical Care

While hyperglycemia is common among general medical and surgical patients, and adverse outcomes are known to occur with hyperglycemia, no prospective RCTs have been conducted to determine optimal glycemic targets or to examine the effects of intensive glycemic control in non–critical care settings. On the basis of clinical experience, glycemic goals of <140 mg/dL premeal and random blood glucose <180 mg/dL are recommended in non–critical care units "as long as these targets can be safely achieved" when using these glycemic goals (Moghissi 2009). To avoid hypoglycemia, insulin regimens should be reassessed if blood glucose falls below 100 mg/dL. If blood glucose <70 mg/dL occurs, the regimen should be modified, unless the issue contributing to the hypoglycemia is easily identified and correctable.

Scheduled subcutaneous insulin dosing is the preferred method to achieve and maintain blood glucose control in non–critical care hospital patients. Scheduled insulin doses should be based on basal and nutrition requirements. The nutritional insulin is the amount of insulin necessary to cover enteral or parenteral nutrition, IV dextrose, snacks, or nutrition supplements as appropriate, not just discrete meals. The sole use of supplemental "sliding-scale" insulin is not recommended; it is ineffective and can be potentially dangerous, especially for patients with type 1 diabetes (Moghissi 2009; Clement 2004). Subcutaneous insulin protocols and hypoglycemia protocols should be in place to minimize adverse events. For patients who are eating, blood glucose monitoring is generally performed before each meal to determine if a correction dose needs to be added to the nutritional insulin dose. Correction doses, unlike traditional sliding-scale doses, are used to treat hyperglycemia that occurs even with administration of basal and nutritional insulin. If correction doses are frequently required to get blood glucose back to target, the scheduled insulin for the following day should be increased to accommodate the higher insulin needs.

Oral diabetes medications have a limited role in acute care. Because of potential contraindications that may develop during a hospital stay, such as renal insufficiency, need for imaging with contrast die, or hemodynamic shifts, metformin should only be used with caution (Moghissi 2009; Clement 2004). Injectable non-insulin therapies such as exenatide, pramlintide, and liraglutide have limitations similar to oral diabetes medications.

NUTRITION THERAPY IN THE HOSPITAL SETTING

To determine what evidence is available for nutrition therapy for hospitalized and long-term care patients with diabetes, a PubMed MEDLINE literature search was conducted, and additional articles were identified from references. Search criteria included the following: glycemic control in hospitalized, nonpregnant adults with diabetes; hospital-related hyperglycemia; English language articles; nutrition and diet during hospitalization; and published after 1 January 2000. The initial search resulted in 849 potentially relevant articles; review of article titles and study subjects led to the exclusion of all but 43 articles. Abstract review narrowed the articles meeting the inclusion criteria to three (RCTs); two articles were added from references (one observational study and one nonrandomized clinical trial), for a total of five articles. Selected articles are summarized in Table 11.1.

Currently, expert consensus is the basis for nutrition recommendations for hospitalized patients with diabetes and stress hyperglycemia. Experts agree that nutrition therapy is an essential component of diabetes management and therefore should be incorporated into the medical treatment plan for hospitalized patients (Boucher 2007). Medical nutrition therapy as defined by the Academy of Nutrition and Dietetics (formerly the American Dietetic Association) includes an assessment of nutrition status and the provision of nutrition intervention such as diet modification, counseling, or specialized nutrition therapy (Lacey 2003). Whereas medical nutrition therapy provided by an RD knowledgeable in glycemic control is a critical component of care, the broader term "nutrition therapy" is used in this discussion to include other aspects of nutrition care during hospitalization. Glycemic control is the primary goal of nutrition therapy for hospitalized patients with diabetes; however, additional nutrition therapy goals follow (ADA 2012; American Dietetic Association 2010; Boucher 2007; Swift 2005):

- Achieve and maintain optimal blood glucose, lipids, and blood pressure to promote recovery from illness, surgery, and disease.
- Integrate nutrition therapy in the treatment of diabetes complications, including hypertension, cardiovascular disease, dyslipidemia, and nephropathy.
- Provide adequate calories to meet metabolic requirements.
- Improve health through nutritious foods.
- Allow for individual food preferences based on personal, cultural, ethnic, and religious beliefs.
- Develop an appropriate discharge plan for self-management training and follow-up care.

System changes to improve glycemic control have been initiated in many facilities, but even with these positive changes, implementing diabetes nutrition therapy in the hospital setting remains challenging. Barriers to adequate nutrition

Table 11.1 Summary of Selected Studies Regarding Nutrition Therapy for Hospitalized Patients with Diabetes

	Population/ Duration of Study	Intervention (type of study)	Major Findings	Comments
McCowen 2000	$n = 40$ adult inpatients requiring TPN/5 days	Hypocaloric TPN with 1,000 kcal and 70 g PRO vs. TPN to target 25 kcal/kg and 1.5 g/kg PRO (RCT)	No difference in hyperglycemia, average BG, or infection rates between the two groups at 5 days	1.5 g/kg PRO offered benefit in nutrition status because of positive nitrogen balance compared to hypocaloric regimen
Tariq 2001	$n = 28$ skilled nursing facility residents with type 2 diabetes/6 months	Regular diet vs. no concentrated sweets (nonrandomized clinical trial)	3 months: nonsignificant difference in mean BG, BMI, albumin; 3 and 6 months: nonsignificant difference in A1C	Diabetes medications were increased in both groups
Mesejo 2003	$n = 50$ intensive care unit patients with stress hyperglycemia or diabetes (blood glucose ≥ 160 mg/dL) receiving EN/5 days	Diabetes-specific high-PRO EN formula vs. standard high-PRO EN formula (RCT)	Improvements in BG and less insulin required for BG control in diabetes-specific high-PRO formula compared to standard high-PRO formula	Improved glycemic control did not alter critical care length of stay or mortality; nonsignificant difference between groups after 14 days
León-Sanz 2005	$n = 63$ inpatients with type 2 diabetes and either head and neck cancer surgery or neurological disorders requiring EN via nasogastric tube/13 days	High-CHO EN formula vs. diabetes-specific EN formula (RCT)	Mean BG increased at 7 days in the high-CHO group, but nonsignificant difference between groups in BG or lipids at 13 days	Increased diarrhea, with lower incidence of nausea in high-CHO formula group
Modic 2011	$n = 434$ inpatients with type 1 or type 2 insulin-requiring diabetes from a large tertiary care hospital/4 days	Meal consumption data collected for 4 days in subjects receiving MD-determined diet order or CHO-controlled diet available from self-select menu (observational)	Average daily meals were insufficient for CHO (43–46% of recommendation), PRO (36–38 g/day), and energy (37–39%) compared to estimated needs; nonsignificant difference in intake by day, age, or sex	Primarily older adult patients; average length of stay was 3.7 days; 54% of patients were obese (BMI ≥ 30 kg/m^2)

CHO, carbohydrate; EN, enteral nutrition; PRO, protein.

intake in acute care include the following: poor appetite; medical conditions causing difficulty or inability to eat; NPO (nothing by mouth) status; increased nutrient and calorie needs from catabolic stress; foods differing from usual eating patterns; missed or delayed meals because of surgery, procedures, or tests; timing of meal delivery; and food preferences not being met (McMahon 1996; Swift 2005; Boucher 2007).

It is not surprising given the barriers to adequate nutrition intake that malnutrition is common in acute care. The actual prevalence of malnutrition in hospitals is unknown because of varied criteria used to define malnutrition and lack of standardization in methods (Stratton 2003). An observational study examined meal consumption patterns of hospitalized patients with type 1 or type 2 diabetes receiving subcutaneous insulin and indicated insufficient caloric and macronutrient intake compared to macronutrient needs in hospitalized patients (Modic 2011).

Patients who are unable to meet their nutrition needs through regular foods may need oral nutrition supplements or nutrition support (parenteral or enteral nutrition). A critical component of implementing nutrition therapy is a screening process to identify nutritionally at-risk patients who need a more comprehensive nutrition assessment. The nutrition assessment is then used to develop an appropriate nutrition care plan. Collaboration between RDs and other team members will help ensure that the nutrition care plan and the medical treatment plan work in coordination (Boucher 2007).

Consistent Carbohydrate Meal Planning

What comprises an optimal eating pattern for hospitalized patients with diabetes is yet to be determined. The consistent carbohydrate meal-planning system has become the accepted standard, since carbohydrate intake is the primary nutrition influence on blood glucose. Consistent carbohydrate meal plans are used in the hospital setting to allow a practical method of serving food to patients with diabetes while improving metabolic control (ADA 2008). Specific calorie levels are not used, but rather the carbohydrate content of meals and snacks is kept consistent from day to day. The amount of total carbohydrate is the primary focus rather than the source of carbohydrate. While it is recommended that the majority of carbohydrate in the meal plan should come from whole grains, fruit, legumes, vegetables, and low-fat milk and yogurt, foods containing sucrose may also be included. While diet prescriptions for an "ADA diet" may still surface in some facilities, this is an obsolete term that should no longer be used. With the increasing implementation of electronic medical records and computerized physician order entry, diet orders are starting to more closely reflect actual meal service practices.

Room service "on demand" meal delivery has been implemented in many acute care facilities to improve nutrition intake and increase patient satisfaction during the hospital stay. This system necessitates good communication among patients and family members, meal service representatives, and nursing staff to ensure accurate mealtime insulin dosing. If all staff involved with meal preparation, meal delivery, recording food intake, and administering mealtime insulin fully understand the system, there is potential to improve coordination of meal delivery timing with blood glucose monitoring and insulin administration for patients on insulin. Ongoing education, overseen by an RD, regarding the meal delivery system and consistent carbohydrate meal planning should be in place for all staff members involved.

It is important that nursing staff understand that the amount of carbohydrate eaten, rather than sugar content, or percentage of the total meal eaten is the largest determinant of postprandial blood glucose. Many hospitals continue to monitor only the percent of the meal eaten, which may under- or overestimate the actual carbohydrate consumed. For patients with poor appetite, administering the mealtime insulin immediately after a meal is eaten may yield the most accurate insulin dose. With appropriate training, nursing assistants and meal service representatives can play a key role in increasing accuracy of carbohydrate estimation. "Teachable moments" for patients and family members also occur during tray setup when information can be shared about carbohydrate content of menu items and/or snacks with patients and family members. Guidelines should also address patient and family member involvement in their own care, such as blood glucose monitoring, how to report carbohydrate intake to staff members, and how to substitute food brought in from outside the hospital appropriately. It is important for all staff members involved to understand various diet orders and what foods are included. If the staff members feel comfortable with carbohydrate counting and the rationale behind the meal plans, they are more likely to offer support and glycemic goals are more likely to be achieved (Swift 2005).

RDs play an important role in insulin and hypoglycemia protocol development and revision to ensure processes are in place for coordination between nutrition services and nursing staff. It is necessary for interdisciplinary members of the health care team to work together to achieve glycemic targets. A team approach to discharge planning is also critical to ensure that appropriate nutrition and diabetes management continues after the patient leaves the hospital (Boucher 2007; Swift 2005; ADA 2003).

Progression from Clear Liquid to Regular Texture

Noncaloric or sugar-free liquid diets are not appropriate for hospitalized patients with diabetes or stress hyperglycemia. Energy from carbohydrates is necessary to meet increased glucose requirements during illness or recovery from surgery. Clear liquid and full liquid diets should provide ~200 g carbohydrate, spread throughout the day in meals and snack(s). Progression to solid foods should occur as quickly as tolerated.

Nutrition Support

Patients with compromised nutrition status, unable to meet nutrition requirements through oral intake, may require parenteral or enteral nutrition support. Once it is decided that nutrition support is required, the most advantageous route for nutrient delivery needs to be determined. Hyperglycemia is a common side effect of both enteral and parenteral nutrition in hospitalized patients with or without previously diagnosed diabetes. Overfeeding should be avoided with use of these therapies, since it exacerbates hyperglycemia (ADA 2003; Clement 2004).

Parenteral nutrition. Total parenteral nutrition (TPN) contributes to hyperglycemia because of several factors: the rate of the dextrose infusion, severity of illness, and age (Clement 2004). Approximately 77% of patients with previously diagnosed diabetes will require insulin for glycemic control during TPN (Clement 2004). Insulin needs are frequently higher in patients receiving TPN versus enteral nutrition, since the beneficial effect of incretin hormones is absent when the gut is bypassed for feeding (McKnight 2008). The goal during use of TPN is to sustain the patient nutritionally, while not worsening glycemic control, when an enteral nutrition route is not possible (McMahon 1996). Insulin may be included in the parenteral solution to cover the amount of dextrose delivered, although this method may take days to determine the appropriate insulin dose. Separate insulin infusion therapy is a preferred method to more quickly achieve and adequately maintain glycemic control during TPN, since it allows for more frequent, as needed insulin adjustments (Campbell 2004). If basal insulin is given subcutaneously, sudden discontinuation of TPN contributes to the high risk of hypoglycemia (Clement 2004).

The best parenteral nutrition delivery strategies to minimize hyperglycemia have not yet been determined. Lipids may be added to TPN to decrease dextrose content but should not exceed 0.11 g/kg/h (McCowen 2004). Using a deliberate underfeeding strategy to minimize hyperglycemia in patients receiving TPN has been explored as a means of improving glycemic control. An RCT in adult patients determined that provision of TPN at caloric goal (25 kcal/kg) was not associated with more hyperglycemia or infections than a deliberate underfeeding strategy (McCowen 2000).

Enteral Nutrition. Enteral nutrition is the preferred route for nutrition support when possible. Advantages over parenteral nutrition include a more physiological route, the trophic effect on gastrointestinal cells, prevention of central line–related complications, and lower cost (McMahon 1996). Diabetes-specific enteral formulas have been developed with nutrient composition designed to better manage glycemic control. These formulas generally contain ingredients such as fructose, fiber, and monounsaturated fatty acids with lower carbohydrate content than standard enteral formulas.

Glycemic control was evaluated in hospitalized patients with type 2 diabetes receiving enteral nutrition therapy comparing a diabetes-specific (low-carbohydrate/high–monounsaturated fat) formula to a standard (high-carbohydrate) formula. After an average 13 days of receiving the enteral formulas via nasogastric tube, no significant differences were found in lipids or glycemic control between the groups (León-Sanz 2005). A RCT conducted in critical care patients with stress hyperglycemia and diabetes compared a standard high-protein enteral formula to a disease-specific high-protein enteral formula. Improvements were seen in plasma and capillary blood glucose and amount of insulin required for glucose control, although no significant differences were found in critical care length of stay, mechanical ventilation, or mortality between groups after 14 days (Mesejo 2003). Evidence for improved glycemic control using diabetes-specific formulas in place of standard formulas for hospitalized patients remains inconclusive. Preventing overfeeding, providing adequate insulin, and close monitoring are key considerations for glycemic control when providing enteral nutrition.

Glycemic management options when initiating enteral feeding depend on multiple factors, including diabetes medication regimen before admission (e.g., oral diabetes medications or insulin), admitting diagnosis, stress level, and whether feeding will be intermittent or continuous (Charney 2004; Boucher 2007). One suggested approach for patients with type 1 and insulin-requiring type 2 diabetes is to correlate usual insulin doses with the rate of the enteral feeding. For example, if the enteral feeding is 30% of usual intake, then 30% of the usual insulin may be administered, and insulin should be increased with the feeding as needed. Illness and current blood glucose levels should also be taken into account in determining insulin dosing (Charney 2004; Boucher 2007). In non–critical care units, subcutaneous short-acting insulin every 4–6 h is a common insulin therapy regimen during continuous enteral feeding. Glycemic control was examined in hospitalized patients with type 2 diabetes receiving *1*) enteral nutrition therapy using scheduled basal insulin (glargine) and correction dosing or *2*) sliding-scale insulin only. Glycemic control was similar in the group receiving sliding-scale insulin compared to the scheduled basal insulin group, although 48% of the sliding-scale insulin patients required the addition of intermediate-acting insulin to achieve the glycemic target of <160 mg/dL (Korytkowski 2009).

FUTURE AREAS FOR DIABETES NUTRITION THERAPY IN HOSPITALS

Whereas many nutrition recommendations have been made regarding improvement of glycemic control in hospitals, little evidence is available. Research concerning meal consumption and comparison of consistent carbohydrate to other meal-planning options would be of interest in determining an optimal eating pattern for hospitalized patients with diabetes. Some have advocated for use of regular diets with carbohydrate counting in acute care, especially with older patients, to aid in meeting nutrient requirements. Further exploration of a less restrictive diet approach compared to a traditional consistent-carbohydrate approach and the effect on glycemic control would help acute care facilities determine if a more flexible meal-planning approach is right for their facility. Research on the effect of room service meal delivery on patient satisfaction, improvement in nutrition status, and achieving glycemic control would also be of interest in determining the best possible hospital meal systems.

Nutrition support presents unique challenges in preventing hyperglycemia in hospitalized patients with and without diagnosed diabetes. The effects of various parenteral and enteral nutrition formulas and feeding strategies may be significant factors in glycemic control for patients receiving these therapies and deserve further exploration.

Overcoming system barriers to realize seamless coordination between departments provides ongoing challenges. Encouraging teamwork, open communication, and ongoing staff education is essential for successful implementation of initiatives. RDs play a key role on interdisciplinary teams developing, implementing, and providing input for ongoing evaluation of system changes for optimization of glycemic control for hospitalized patients with diabetes.

Highlights
Long-Term Care

■ Long-term care residents with diabetes should be offered a regular, unrestricted menu with consistent amounts of carbohydrate offered at meals and snacks.

■ Long-term care facilities serving younger patients with diabetes (e.g., physical rehabilitation facilities) will need to offer regular diets with consistent carbohydrate, larger portions, and lower fat content than is recommended for older residents.

Long-Term Care

DIABETES NUTRITION THERAPY IN LONG-TERM CARE

Long-term care (LTC) encompasses facilities that provide services for individuals with chronic conditions, who need physical assistance, or who have functional limitations. These facilities may include physical rehabilitation, assisted living, skilled nursing, group homes, or hospice care. Reasons for admission vary, from long-term stays because of cognitive decline requiring assistance in activities of daily living to short-term stays for physical rehabilitation. Medical treatment goals differ with the expected outcome, whether it is discharge home or living out life expectancy in an LTC setting. The goals for care and treatment shift away from acute care to long-term management and lifestyle goals. Admitting diagnosis and medical treatment goals should be taken into consideration when developing a nutrition care plan for patients with diabetes in the LTC setting (American Dietetic Association 2010).

It is estimated that 25% of LTC nursing facility residents have diagnosed diabetes (Travis 2004; Resnick 2008). Many older adults with diabetes requiring LTC have multiple comorbidities and diabetes-related complications. Effective diabetes and nutrition management for these residents is complex. Key nutrition concerns in LTC residents with diabetes include malnutrition, weight loss, poor wound healing, hypoglycemia, and dehydration.

Delivery of diabetes nutrition interventions is challenging in the LTC setting. The key goals of LTC (improvement in quality of life and maintaining health) may conflict at times when it comes to nutrition therapy strategies. Additional barriers to diabetes management and nutrition therapy in LTC facilities may include inadequate staffing, lack of dedicated resources, physical or cognitive limitations of residents in performing self-management skills, lack of diabetes management guidelines or protocols, and lack of awareness of current nutrition therapy and diabetes management practices. Overcoming barriers requires an interdisciplinary team approach to provide individualized care. This team approach is necessary to incorporate the nutrition care plan into the diabetes management plan for residents with diabetes (ADA 2003; American Dietetic Association 2010).

LTC initiatives have begun to change the environment from institutionalized care to a more home or community emphasis with personal care. Improving quality of care and quality of life has been the driving force behind the changes. Increased awareness for the need to liberalize diets to enhance enjoyment of food, allow for personal food preferences, and improve the dining experience has been a part of these culture change initiatives. Unfortunately, practices for ordering therapeutic diets have lagged behind these initiatives. Although there is increasing support for liberalized diets, especially for older adults in LTC, restrictive, therapeutic diets continue to be ordered (Feldman 2009). The Academy of Nutrition and Dietetics position is that "the quality of life and nutritional status of older adults residing in health care communities (LTC) can be enhanced by individualization to less restrictive diets" (American Dietetic Association 2010). Therapeutic diets are designed to improve health, but unintentional consequences may include decreased variety and flavor of foods offered to residents with diabetes because of additional restrictions to meet therapeutic requirements. This scenario may lead to weight loss and undernutrition, which is the opposite of the desired outcome. Potential benefits of less restrictive diets include increased quality of life, higher satisfaction with meals, improved nutrition status, and enhanced enjoyment of eating (American Dietetic Association 2010). The benefits gained from liberalized diets outweigh the risks for many LTC residents with diabetes.

LTC residents with diabetes should be offered a regular, unrestricted menu with consistent amounts of carbohydrate offered at meals and snacks (ADA 2008; American Dietetic Association 2010). Recommendations are supported from a study conducted in LTC residents with type 2 diabetes who received a "no concentrated sweets" diet or a regular diet. No change in A1C in either group was seen at 6 months (Tariq 2001). Calorie and fat restriction are not appropriate in the older adult population, since adequate nutrition intake is a prime concern. Small portions of dessert are generally offered to all residents, which allows for consistency in carbohydrate intake for people with diabetes. Facilities serving younger patients with diabetes, such as physical rehabilitation centers, should offer regular diets with consistent carbohydrate, with larger portions and lower fat content than is recommended for older residents. Individualization for older or younger patients may be required to meet unique nutrition needs.

Ongoing education overseen by an RD regarding liberalized diets with the focus on total carbohydrate rather than avoidance of sucrose-containing foods should be provided to staff, family members, and residents. Communication of nutrition goals and how sucrose-containing foods fit into the plan will help minimize misunderstanding about residents receiving the "wrong diet." Many older residents with longstanding diabetes have difficulty shifting the focus away from sucrose to total carbohydrate because of previous experience with more sucrose-restrictive meal plans and may need extra encouragement.

SUMMARY

There are many challenges and barriers to providing diabetes nutrition therapy in the LTC setting. Ensuring adequate nutrition intake to prevent malnutrition is a key consideration, especially in the older adult LTC population. Use of liberalized diets in the LTC setting should be encouraged. Offering a regular, consistent carbohydrate diet to residents with diabetes is recommended. The RD, residents themselves, family members, and other LTC staff members all play key roles in meeting the nutrition therapy and diabetes management goals for LTC residents with diabetes. Additional research is needed to determine optimal nutrition therapy and glycemic control strategies in this population.

BIBLIOGRAPHY

American Diabetes Association: Nutrition recommendations and interventions for diabetes. *Diabetes Care* 31 (Suppl. 1):S61–S78, 2008

American Diabetes Association: Standards of medical care in diabetes: 2012. *Diabetes Care* 35 (Suppl. 1):S11–S63, 2012

American Diabetes Association: Standards of medical care in diabetes—2005. *Diabetes Care* 28 (Suppl. 1):S4–S36, 2005

American Dietetic Association: Individualized nutrition approaches for older adults in health care communities (Position Statement). *J Am Diet Assoc* 110:1549–1555, 2010

Boucher JL, Swift CS, Franz MJ, Kulkarni K, Schafer RG, Pritchett E, Clark NG: Inpatient management of diabetes and hyperglycemia: implications for nutrition practice and the food and nutrition professional. *J Am Diet Assoc* 107:105–111, 2007

Campbell K, Braithwaite S: Hospital management of hyperglycemia. *Clinical Diabetes* 22:2:81–88, 2004

Clement S, Braithwaite SS, Magee MF, Ahmann A, Smith EP, Schafer RG, Hirsch IB, on Behalf of the Diabetes in Hospitals Writing Committee: Management of diabetes and hyperglycemia in hospitals (Technical Review). *Diabetes Care* 27:553–591, 2004

Charney P, Hertzler SR: Management of blood glucose and diabetes in the critically ill patient receiving enteral feeding. *Nutr Clin Pract* 19:129–136, 2004

Feldman SM, Rosen R, Destasio J: Status of diabetes management in the nursing home setting in 2008: a retrospective chart review and epidemiology study of the diabetic nursing home residents and nursing home initiatives in diabetes management. *J Am Med Dir Assoc* 10:354–360, 2009

Finfer S, Chittock DR, Su SY, Blair D, Foster D, Dhingra V, Bellomo R, Cook D, Dodek P, Henderson WR, Hébert PC, Heritier S, Heyland DK, McArthur C, McDonald E, Mitchell I, Myburgh JA, Norton R, Potter J, Robinson BG, Ronco JJ (NICE-SUGAR Study Investigators): Intensive versus conventional glucose control in critically ill patients. *N Engl J Med* 360:1283–1297, 2009

Fraze TK, Jiang HJ, Burgess J: Hospital stays for patients with diabetes, 2008. HCUP Statistical Brief #93. Agency for Healthcare Research and Quality, Rockville, MD, 2010. Available at http://www.hcup-us.ahrq.gov/reports/statbriefs/sb93.pdf. Accessed November 2011

Furnary AP, Gao G, Grunkemeier GL, Wu Y, Zerr KJ, Bookin SO, Floten HS, Starr A: Continuous insulin infusion reduces mortality in patients with diabetes undergoing coronary artery bypass grafting. *J Thorac Cardiovasc Surg* 125:1007–1021, 2003

Garber AL, Moghissi ES, Bransome ED Jr, Clark NG, Clement S, Coban RH, Furnary AP, Hirsch IB, Levy P, Roberts R, Van den Berghe G, Zamudio V (American College of Endocrinology Task Force on Inpatient Diabetes and Metabolic Control): American College of Endocrinology position statement on inpatient diabetes and metabolic control. *Endocr Pract* 10:77–82, 2004

Griesdale DE, de Souza RJ, van Dam RM, Heyland DK, Cook DJ, Malhotra A, Dhaliwal R, Henderson WR, Chittock DR, Finfer S, Talmor D: Intensive insulin therapy and mortality among critically ill patients: a meta-analysis including NICE-SUGAR study data. *CMAJ* 180:821–827, 2009

Korytkowski MT, Salata RJ, Koerbel GL, Selzer F, Karslioglu E, Idriss AM, Lee KW, Moser AJ, Toledo FS: Insulin therapy and glycemic control in hospitalized patients with diabetes during enteral nutrition therapy: a randomized controlled clinical trial. *Diabetes Care* 32:594–596, 2009

Lacey K, Pritchett E: Nutrition care process and model: ADA adopts road map to quality care and outcomes management. *J Am Diet Assoc* 103:1061–1072, 2003

León-Sanz M, Garcia-Luna PP, Sanz-Paris A (for the Abbott Study Cooperative Group): Glycemic and lipid control in hospitalized type 2 diabetic patients: evaluation of 2 enteral nutrition formulas (low carbohydrate-high monoun-saturated fat vs. high carbohydrate). *J Parenter Enteral Nutr* 29:21–29, 2005

Malmberg K: Prospective randomized study of intensive insulin treatment on long-term survival after acute myocardial infarction in patients with diabetes mellitus. *BMJ* 314:1512–1515, 1997

Malmberg K, Rydén L, Efendic S, Herlitz J, Nicol P, Waldenström A, Wedel H, Welin: Randomized trial of insulin-glucose infusion followed by subcutaneous insulin treatment in diabetic patients with acute myocardial infarction (DIGAMI study): effects on mortality at 1 year. *J Am Coll Cardiol* 26:57–65, 1995

Malmberg K, Rydén L, Wedel H (DIGAMI 2 Investigators): Intense metabolic control by means of insulin in patients with diabetes mellitus and acute myo-cardial infarction (DIGAMI 2): effects on mortality and morbidity. *Eur Heart J* 26:650–661, 2005

McCowen KC, Bistrian BR: Hyperglycemia and nutrition support: theory and practice. *Nutr Clin Pract* 19:235–244, 2004

McCowen KC, Friel C, Sternberg J, Chan S, Forse RA, Burke P, Bistrian BR: Hypocaloric total parenteral nutrition: effectiveness in prevention of hyper-glycemia and infections complications: a randomized clinical trial. *Crit Care Med* 28:3606–3611, 2000

McKnight KA, Carter L: From trays to tube feedings: overcoming the challenges of hospital nutrition and glycemic control. *Diabetes Spectrum* 21:233–240, 2008

McMahon MM, Rizza RA: Nutrition support in hospitalized patients with diabe-tes mellitus. *Mayo Clin Proc* 71:587–594, 1996

Mesejo A, Acosta JA, Ortega C, Vila J, Fernandez M, Ferreres J, Sanchis JC, Lopez F: Comparison of a high-protein disease specific enteral formula with a high-protein enteral formula in hyperglycemic critically ill patients. *Clin Nutr* 22:295–305, 2003

Modic MB, Kozak A, Siedlecki SL, Nowak D, Parella D, Morris MP: Do we know what our patients with diabetes are eating in the hospital? *Diabetes Spectrum* 24:100–106, 2011

Moghissi ES, Korytkowski MT, DiNardo M, Einhorn D, Hellman R, Hirsch IB, Inzucchi SE, Ismail-Beigi F, Kirkman MS, Umpierrez GE: American Association of Clinical Endocrinologists and American Diabetes Association consensus statement on inpatient glycemic control. *Endocr Pract* 15:1–17, 2009

Resnick H, Heineman J, Stone R, Shorr R: Diabetes in U.S. nursing homes: 2004. *Diabetes Care* 31:287–288, 2008

Stratton RJ, Green CJ, Elia M: *Disease-Related Malnutrition: An Evidence-Based Approach to Treatment*. Cambridge, MA, CABI Publishing, 2003

Swift CS, Boucher JL: Nutrition care for hospitalized individuals with diabetes. *Diabetes Spectrum* 18:34–38, 2005

Tariq SH, Karcic E, Thomas DR, Thomson K, Philpot C, Chapel DL, Morley JE: The use of a no-concentrated-sweets diet in the management of type 2 diabetes in nursing homes. *J Am Diet Assoc* 101:1463–1466, 2001

Travis S, Buchanan R, Wang S, Kim M: Analyses of nursing home residents with diabetes at admission. *J Am Med Dir Assoc* 5:320–327, 2004

Van den Berghe G, Wouters P, Weekers F, VerWaest C, Bruyninckx F, Schetz M, Vlasselaers D, Ferdinande P, Lauwers P, Boullion R: Intensive insulin therapy in critically ill patients. *N Engl J Med* 345:1359–1367, 2001

Carrie S. Swift, MS, RD, BC-ADM, CDE, is a Diabetes Educator at Kadlec Medical Center in Richland, WA.

Chapter 12
Nutrition Therapy for Diabetes: Hypoglycemia and Sick Days

Janine Freeman, RD, CDE

Highlights
Hypoglycemia

■ Medication-induced hypoglycemia can be effectively treated orally with glucose tablets, 15–20 g, or with any carbohydrate-containing foods or beverages. There is insufficient evidence to recommend a specific dose of other types of carbohydrate-containing foods and beverages for treatment of hypoglycemia.

■ The response to treatment of hypoglycemia should be apparent in 15–20 min; plasma glucose should be tested again in ~60 min, as additional treatment may be necessary.

■ The addition of protein and/or fat to meals or snacks appears to have a minimal effect on preventing subsequent hypoglycemia.

Hypoglycemia

Evidence from the Diabetes Control and Complications Trial (DCCT) and other landmark diabetes trials highlights the benefits of optimal glycemic control in preventing microvascular complications of diabetes, resulting in the targeting of more aggressive glycemic goals (DCCT 1993). Treatment-induced hypoglycemia has become the limiting factor in attaining glycemic goals (Cryer 2009a; Cryer 2011). Individuals with type 1 diabetes average two episodes of symptomatic hypoglycemia per week and one episode of severe hypoglycemia per year (Cryer 2009b). The incidence of hypoglycemia is relatively low in type 2 diabetes early in the course of the disease, even when treated with insulin, but approaches that in type 1 diabetes as glycemic defenses become compromised with longer duration and progression of type 2 diabetes (Cryer 2009b; U.K. Hypoglycaemia Study Group 2007). Death due to hypoglycemia is estimated at a rate of 2–4% in individuals with type 1 diabetes, and recent evidence suggests that hypoglycemia can also be fatal in type 2 diabetes (Cryer 2009b; Gerstein 2008). Safety concerns associated with hypoglycemia highlight the importance that the entire diabetes health care team be exceedingly familiar with the risks, treatment, and prevention of hypoglycemia.

This chapter discusses the importance of training individuals treated with insulin or insulin secretagogues in the recognition, treatment, and prevention of hypoglycemia; reviews the recommendations from the 1999 book *American Diabetes Association Guide to Medical Nutrition Therapy for Diabetes* (see the chapter "Nutrition Therapy for Type 1 Diabetes" for information on hypoglycemia) (Kulkarni 1999) and the 2008 American Diabetes Association (ADA) nutrition recommendations (ADA 2008); updates the evidence for the treatment and prevention of hypoglycemia in people with diabetes; and summarizes recommendations for the treatment and prevention of hypoglycemia.

A literature search was conducted using PubMed MEDLINE to identify studies related to treatment of hypoglycemia in diabetes, the effect of protein and fat on postprandial glycemia, and snacks for the prevention of nocturnal hypoglycemia in diabetes published in 1999 or later. Recent publications were also identified from reference lists. Only one new study on the treatment for hypoglycemia was found and is summarized in Table 12.1. Five studies on type of bedtime snack for prevention of nocturnal hypoglycemia events were found and are summarized in Table 12.2.

Table 12.1 Type of Carbohydrate Treatment for Hypoglycemic Events in People with Diabetes

	Population/ Duration of Study	Intervention (type of study)	Major Findings	Comments
Husband 2010	*n* = 33 children and adolescents with type 1 diabetes/15 min after treatment	Treated five hypoglycemic events with *1)* glucose tablets, *2)* sucrose (Skittles), or *3)* fructose (Fruit to Go) (crossover study)	Nonsignificant difference between sucrose and glucose, but less effectiveness with fructose (*P* < 0.001)	

TREATMENT-INDUCED HYPOGLYCEMIA

Hypoglycemia is the result of treatment with insulin or insulin secretagogues. All individuals treated with medications that raise insulin levels are at risk for hypoglycemia. These medications include insulin, sulfonylureas, and glinides (e.g., nateglinide or repaglinide). All individuals at risk for hypoglycemia need to be taught about the recognition, treatment, and prevention of hypoglycemia. Individuals should become concerned about potential hypoglycemia when blood glucose monitoring results are ≤70 mg/dL (≤3.9 mmol/L) or rapidly falling (Cryer 2009a). Symptoms of hypoglycemia (Table 12.3) may or may not be present at the time and in some cases are not able to be communicated, as in very young children. Symptoms are often unique to individuals; therefore, individuals at risk should observe their usual physiological responses to hypoglycemia to alert them to monitor and treat promptly.

Treatment of Hypoglycemia

Recommendations for treatment of hypoglycemia from the 1999 book *American Diabetes Association Guide to Medical Nutrition Therapy for Diabetes* were based on a few studies comparing treatment of hypoglycemia with various types and amounts of carbohydrate sources typically used (Slama 1990; Brodows 1984). Results showed somewhat slower or less response during treatment with orange juice and milk compared with other forms or doses of carbohydrate. A summary of the recommendations included treating hypoglycemia with 15 g carbohydrate, followed by monitoring blood glucose after 15 min to determine if additional carbohydrate was needed. No specific form of carbohydrate was recommended, although glucose tablets were determined to be more convenient, premeasured, and non-spoilable.

The ADA 2008 nutrition recommendations stated that "ingestion of 15–20 g glucose is the preferred treatment for hypoglycemia, although any form of carbohydrate that contains glucose may be used. The response to treatment of hypoglycemia should be apparent in 10–20 min; however, plasma glucose should be tested again in ~60 min, as additional treatment may be necessary" (ADA 2008).

Table 12.2 Type of Bedtime Snack for Prevention of Nocturnal Hypoglycemic Events in People with Diabetes

	Population/ Duration of Study	Intervention (type of study)	Major Findings	Comments
Kalergis 2003	*n* = 15 adults with type 1 diabetes treated with lispro at meals and NPH at bedtime/50 nights	Four bedtime snacks: *1*) placebo, *2*) standard (cheese sandwich), *3*) high protein (½ sandwich + protein powder, *4*) raw cornstarch + ½ sandwich (randomized crossover study)	HS BGs >180 mg/dL had no hypoglycemia in absence of HS snack; high protein and standard snack both prevented nocturnal hypoglycemia; no benefit with cornstarch snack	Use of NPH at bedtime compared with long-acting insulin or CSII may affect need for bedtime snack; snack of only carbohydrate was not used
Raju 2006	*n* = 21 adults with type 1 diabetes on CSII or multiple daily injections with insulin analogs/5 nights	Five bedtime snacks: *1*) no snack, *2*) CS (26 g carbohydrate, 11 g protein, 6 g fat), *3*) CS plus acarbose, *4*) 1½ Extend Bars, *5*) terbutaline (randomized crossover trial)	CS, CS + acarbose, or Extend Bar did not ↓ nocturnal hypoglycemia; average morning glucose similar with snacks vs. no snack; CS and Extend Bar appeared to delay nocturnal hypoglycemia	Authors concluded that conventional bedtime snacks and uncooked cornstarch do not prevent nocturnal hypoglycemia in type 1 diabetes
Wilson 2008	*n* = 10 adolescents with type 1 diabetes/12 days	Low-fat vs. high-fat bedtime snack (RCT)	Frequency of hypoglycemia between high- and low-fat bedtime snack nonsignificant	Authors concluded that increasing fat in bedtime snack had no impact on risk of nocturnal hypoglycemia
Lodefalk 2008	*n* = 7 adolescents with type 1 diabetes treated with preprandial rapid-acting insulin/2 days	Low-fat (2 g) vs. high-fat (38 g) meals with equal protein content (RCT)	Plasma glucose area under the curve was larger for 2 h after low-fat meal; difference in time-to-peak glucose nonsignificant	Authors concluded that preprandial insulin may need adjustment to fat content of the meal
Papakonstantinou 2010	*n* = 23 obese adults with type 2 diabetes on metformin/2 days	Two meals of equal carbohydrate and calories: *1*) high protein (30%) and low fat (19%) vs. *2*) low protein (15%) and high fat (34%) (randomized crossover study)	Glucose and insulin responses nonsignificant	Authors concluded that manipulating protein-to-fat ratio in meals does not affect postprandial blood glucose or insulin responses in obese people with type 2 diabetes

CS, conventional snack; CSII, continuous subcutaneous insulin infusion; HS BG, blood glucose at bedtime; RCT, randomized controlled trial.

Table 12.3 Symptoms of Hypoglycemia in People with Diabetes

Neurogenic (Autonomic)	Neuroglycopenic
Palpitations	Cognitive impairments
Tremor	Behavior changes
Anxiety	Psychomotor
Sweating	Seizure
Hunger	Coma
Parasthesias	

Adapted from Cryer 2009b.

Although 15–20 g glucose has been shown to be effective in treating hypoglycemia, the quality of evidence to support the dose-response relationship of other types of carbohydrate-containing foods or beverages at this time is low (Cryer 2009b). Earlier studies in hypoglycemia treatment demonstrated that 20 g carbohydrate as milk or orange juice had a minimal effect on glycemia compared to an equal amount of glucose (Brodows 1984). In a recent study, treatment of hypoglycemia with sucrose and glucose gave similar glycemic responses in children with type 1 diabetes, whereas fructose was less effective (Husband 2010). The glycemic effect of a particular type and amount of carbohydrate food or beverage depends on several factors including blood glucose level, time action of available insulin or insulin secretagogues used, and intensity of antecedent exercise (Clarke 2009). Treatment of hypoglycemia with either liquid or solid foods has similar gastric-emptying rates (Schvarcz 1993). Hypoglycemic episodes caused by rapid-acting insulin secretagogues or insulin analogs cause a brief period of hypoglycemia compared to those caused by longer-acting insulin analogs or sulfonylureas. The latter may require repeated feedings or glucose infusion (Cryer 2009a). Frequent monitoring of blood glucose levels after self-treating an episode of hypoglycemia can provide feedback regarding a person's individual response to the type and amount of carbohydrate-containing treatment.

Current recommendations include the use of glucose tablets or carbohydrate-containing foods or beverages to effectively treat hypoglycemia. A commonly recommended dose of glucose is 15–20 g. When blood glucose levels are ~50–60 mg/dL (2.7 mmol/L), treatment with 15 g glucose can be expected to raise blood glucose levels ~50 mg/dL (2.7 mmol/L) (Cryer 1994; Wiethop 1993). If self-monitoring of blood glucose ~15–20 min after treatment shows continued hypoglycemia, the treatment should be repeated. The glycemic response to oral glucose is transient, usually lasting <2 h in insulin-induced hypoglycemia (Cryer 2009a; Cryer 2009b). In the setting of continued hyperinsulinemia, as in episodes caused by a long-acting insulin analog, the duration of the hypoglycemic episode may outlast the initial treatment. A more substantial snack or meal is generally advised shortly after blood glucose levels return to normal to prevent recurrent hypoglycemia (Cryer 2009a). If a meal is not consumed within ~1 h, blood glucose levels should be monitored again in ~60 min, since additional treatment may be necessary (ADA 2008).

Protein should not be used in the treatment of hypoglycemia as studies have shown that protein has minimal acute effects on blood glucose levels (Gray 1996;

Gannon 2001; Papakonstantinou 2010; ADA 2008). Protein also stimulates insulin secretion in type 2 diabetes (Franz 2000; Gannon 2001). Although studies have shown that fat may delay the postprandial glycemic response to a meal (Lodefalk 2008), no published studies were identified that evaluated the addition of fat to the treatment of hypoglycemia.

Glucagon administration is necessary for treatment of hypoglycemia when a person is unwilling or unable to take carbohydrate orally. Caregivers or family members of all individuals at significant risk of severe hypoglycemia should be instructed in administration of glucagon (ADA 2012). The usual dose is injection of 1.0 mg for adults and 150 mg for children, repeating if necessary (Cryer 2009a). Glucagon injection is less useful in type 2 diabetes because it stimulates insulin secretion and glycogenolysis (Cryer 2003) and in people with depleted glycogen stores as in prolonged fasting, alcohol bingeing, or recurrent episodes of hypoglycemia (Boyle 2007; Cryer 2009a).

Prevention of Hypoglycemia

Preventing hypoglycemia rather than reacting to it can help avoid serious adverse effects of recurrent episodes of hypoglycemia. Prevention of hypoglycemia should be discussed in every contact with patients treated with insulin or insulin secretagogues. See Table 12.4 for risk factors for hypoglycemia in diabetes (Cryer 2009b).

Very young children and the elderly are especially vulnerable to hypoglycemia. Children <6 years of age may not exhibit the classic counterregulatory responses to hypoglycemia and are unable to communicate symptoms they are experiencing, making the risk of hypoglycemia the highest in this age-group (Clarke 2009; ADA 2005). Variations in activity and food intake in young children and the elderly increase the risk of hypoglycemia, frequently resulting in liberalization of glucose targets in these age-groups (ADA 2012; ADA 2005).

Insulin or Insulin Secretagogues

Choosing an appropriate insulin regimen and providing training on the effects of the dose and timing of individual insulin regimen or insulin secretagogue can help prevent hypoglycemia. Frequent glucose monitoring before and after meals is imperative to learn the best timing and dosage of prandial insulin and ingestion

---

Table 12.4 Risk Factors for Hypoglycemia

■ Insulin or insulin secretagogue doses are excessive, ill-timed, or of the wrong type.
■ Glucose delivery is decreased (delayed, reduced, or missed meals).
■ Endogenous glucose production is decreased (e.g., after alcohol ingestion).
■ Glucose utilization is increased (e.g., during and after exercise).
■ Sensitivity to insulin is increased (e.g., after weight loss or improved glycemic control and in the middle of the night).
■ There is a history of hypoglycemia unawareness, severe hypoglycemia, or recent hypoglycemia.
■ Aggressive glycemic therapy

Adapted from Cryer 2009b.

of the meal. Insulin dosage adjustments based on the premeal blood glucose value and carbohydrate counting may reduce the risk of subsequent hypoglycemia. Theoretically, the use of a rapid-acting insulin analog rather than regular insulin before meals should reduce the likelihood of hypoglycemia before the next meal (Cryer 2003). Evidence shows that the use of long-acting basal insulin analogs can reduce the incidence of overall, symptomatic, and nocturnal hypoglycemia in type 1 and type 2 diabetes, and the use of rapid-acting prandial insulin analogs can reduce nocturnal hypoglycemia in type 1 diabetes (Cryer 2009b; Deiss 2007; Hirsch 2005). Care in prescribing long-acting insulin secretagogues, particularly in the elderly, is important to help prevent severe and prolonged hypoglycemia in this population (Cryer 2009a).

Meal and Snack Composition and Timing

Delayed, missed, or inadequate meals or snacks can increase the risk of hypoglycemia, based on the type of insulin regimen or use of insulin secretagogues. Insulin regimens (e.g., insulin pump therapy and multiple daily injections) that use rapid-acting and long-acting insulin analogs generally do not require snacks, dependent on frequent self-glucose testing. The effects of various bedtime snacks on frequency of hypoglycemia in adults with type 1 diabetes were studied, and it was concluded that the need for a bedtime snack depended on evening glucose level. In this study, a bedtime snack was necessary for evening glucose levels <180 mg/dL to prevent hypoglycemia (Kalergis 2003). A study in adults with type 1 diabetes demonstrated that typical bedtime snacks increase plasma glucose levels only through the first half of the night (Raju 2006).

The addition of protein to snacks is not considered necessary to prevent subsequent hypoglycemia. This is based on a study that compared a snack of bread to bread plus meat and showed similar peak glucose levels and time to subsequent hypoglycemia (Gray 1996). Studies have not provided evidence that protein slows or changes the peak postprandial glucose response (ADA 2008). Although clinicians have frequently suggested that the addition of dietary fat to a snack or meal may slow and then prolong the glycemic response, there is little or no evidence to support this. Several small studies in both type 1 and type 2 diabetes have shown little or no effect in glycemic response by adding fat to a meal (Gentilcore 2006; Thomsen 2003; Lodefalk 2008). Providing children with type 1 diabetes a bedtime snack with either low or high fat also did not affect the frequency of nocturnal hypoglycemia (Wilson 2008). Therefore, in acute studies, with a limited number of subjects, the addition of fat and/or protein to meals or snacks appears to have minimal effect on preventing subsequent hypoglycemia. Consuming snacks comprised of carbohydrate and protein/fat for the purpose of preventing hypoglycemia may result in unnecessary calories and subsequent weight gain. Snacks should be individualized and in monitoring a person's own glycemic response to a snack or meal, it may be determined that additional protein and/or fat would provide needed calories and satiety without the glycemic effect from additional carbohydrate.

Data from earlier small studies suggested that the addition of uncooked cornstarch to the evening snack may help prevent nocturnal hypoglycemia in type 1 diabetes (Kaufman 1995; Kaufman 1996; Axelsen 1999). More recent studies have not supported this, with authors suggesting that study design and the use of newer insulin analogs may be contributing factors (Kalergis 2003; Raju 2006).

Alcohol Consumption

Consumption of alcohol by individuals with type 1 diabetes has been shown to result in late-onset hypoglycemia (Richardson 2005; Kerr 2007), likely due to inhibition of gluconeogenesis and decreased growth hormone levels after alcohol consumption (Kerr 2007; Cryer 2003). For hypoglycemia prevention, individuals using insulin or insulin secretagogues should consume food when drinking alcoholic beverages (ADA 2008). Self-monitoring of blood glucose should be performed frequently after alcohol ingestion to identify and treat hypoglycemia and to determine if additional carbohydrate or reduction in insulin is necessary to prevent nocturnal hypoglycemia. Complete avoidance of alcohol when driving must be emphasized. See Chapter 4 for more information on alcohol and diabetes.

Exercise and Physical Activity

The risk of hypoglycemia as a result of exercise is an ongoing problem, particularly for people with type 1 diabetes. The incidence of hypoglycemia during or after exercise appears to depend on pre-exercise blood glucose levels (Tsalikian 2005). Reviews of the literature showed that moderate-intensity exercise in type 1 diabetes increases the risk of hypoglycemia, both during and for up to 31 h after exercise (Guelfi 2007). The risk of hypoglycemia during and after exercise is further increased after repeated episodes of low- to moderate-intensity exercise (Sandoval 2004) and by antecedent hypoglycemia (Robertson 2009; Galassetti 2003) because of an attenuated counterregulatory response. Late-afternoon exercise has been shown to double the risk of nocturnal hypoglycemia in children with type 1 diabetes (Diabetes Research in Children Network 2005).

Many variables affect the risk of exercise-induced hypoglycemia, making it imperative that individuals, particularly with type 1 diabetes, learn to self-adjust insulin doses or consume carbohydrate based on self-testing of glucose results performed before, during, and after exercise. Limited evidence exists to suggest a specific type and amount of carbohydrate to prevent exercise-induced hypoglycemia. For planned physical activity, a reduction of premeal insulin at the meal before the time of exercise is recommended, based on the intensity and duration of the activity (Rachmiel 2007). For unplanned activity and when insulin has not been adjusted, extra carbohydrate should be consumed after completion of the activity (Franz 2010). Bedtime glucose targets should be increased on days of afternoon or evening activity and evening insulin adjusted (Diabetes Research in Children Network 2005; Rachmiel 2007). A carbohydrate snack should be ingested if pre-exercise glucose levels are <100 mg/dL (Franz 2010). Frequent self-testing of blood glucose will help guide treatment. Continuous glucose monitoring (CGM) is particularly helpful for determining the extent of late-onset hypoglycemia. See Chapter 10 on exercise.

Hypoglycemia Unawareness

Glucose counterregulation, the mechanism that normally prevents or corrects hypoglycemia, is compromised in people with type 1 diabetes and advanced insulin-deficient type 2 diabetes, resulting in the loss of the warning symptoms of developing hypoglycemia. Lack of insulin secretion, absent glucagon response, and decreased epinephrine response are the factors that contribute to the decreased autonomic response to hypoglycemia (Cryer 2009a). Evidence shows that hypoglycemia unawareness can be reversed by raising glucose targets to strictly avoid any episodes of hypoglycemia for at least 2–3 weeks (Cryer 2009a; Cryer 2011).

Glucose Monitoring

Frequent self-monitoring of blood glucose, supplemented in some instances by CGM, should be used to make informed decisions on treatment modifications that will reduce the risk of hypoglycemia. CGM is useful for individuals at high risk for severe hypoglycemia in identifying patterns of unrecognized hypoglycemia by monitoring glucose levels throughout the day and night and providing alerts when glucose levels fall below a designated level (Buckingham 2008). Although CGM is useful for identifying glucose trends, self-testing of blood glucose should be used to confirm hypoglycemia and recovery from hypoglycemia. Results from CGM systems represent a lag between interstitial and blood glucose levels, particularly when glucose levels are changing rapidly (Buckingham 2008). Ideally, self-monitoring of blood glucose should be performed any time hypoglycemia is suspected and always before engaging in any critical activities such as driving (Cryer 2009a). Incidences of hypoglycemia, symptoms, and circumstances surrounding the event should be recorded and discussed with a health care professional. Individuals at risk for hypoglycemia should be trained in pattern management skills and empowered to problem-solve and make management decisions to avoid hypoglycemia. Planning ahead by making insulin adjustments for activities that increase the risk of hypoglycemia is preferable to adding additional snacks that may add unwanted calories. Glycemic goals should be individualized and reevaluated as diabetes progresses based on risk of hypoglycemia.

SUMMARY OF RECOMMENDATIONS FOR HYPOGLYCEMIA

All individuals taking insulin or insulin secretagogues should be instructed in the identification, treatment, and prevention of hypoglycemia. The current recommendation is based on available evidence: promptly treat episodes of hypoglycemia with glucose tablets or other carbohydrate-containing foods or beverages, confirm blood glucose value in 15–20 min and re-treat if indicated, and then self-test glucose in ~60 min to determine if additional carbohydrate is needed. The commonly recommended dose is 15–20 g glucose (amount may be less in younger children, 10 g for example). Future studies need to systematically investigate the effectiveness of various doses and types of carbohydrate, particularly in more contemporary diabetes treatment. Safety guidelines to prevent hypoglycemia are an ongoing and important part of self-management training for all individuals treated with insulin or insulin secretagogues. These include frequent glucose monitoring, timing of meals/snacks in coordination with insulin or insulin secretagogues, appropriate adjustment in insulin dose or carbohydrate intake, and ingesting food with alcoholic beverages.

Current studies do not support the need for adding protein or fat to carbohydrate at meals or snacks to prevent subsequent hypoglycemia. Studies investigating various types and amounts of bedtime snacks with individuals using insulin pump therapy or multiple daily insulin injections with rapid-acting and long-acting insulin analogs may provide more insight into the effectiveness of bedtime snacks in preventing nocturnal hypoglycemia. Adjustment of the insulin dose/regimen or use of alternatives to insulin secretagogues is preferable to recommending changes in food habits to prevent hypoglycemia. Frequent self-monitoring of glucose and interpretation of glucose patterns can help people on multiple daily injections or insulin pump therapy determine their individual responses to changes in food habits, activities, and events that increase their risk of hypoglycemia. Frequent self-monitoring can also help patients, along with their diabetes team, adjust therapy to help reduce the risk of future hypoglycemic events.

Highlights
Sick Days

■ Hyperglycemia is a frequent result of acute illness and increases the risk of diabetic ketoacidosis (DKA) in ketosis-prone individuals. Insulin and oral diabetes medications should be continued and sometimes increased during illness. Frequent monitoring of glucose and urine or blood ketones in ketosis-prone individuals will guide therapy during illness.

■ All individuals with diabetes should be taught what to expect during illness, how to adjust their treatment plan, and how to prevent life-threatening conditions including DKA and hyperosmolar nonketotic state.

Sick Days

Blood glucose levels during acute illness are often increased because of elevated counterregulatory hormones that promote gluconeogenesis and insulin resistance, despite a diminished appetite and/or nausea/vomiting, that often result in decreased ingestion of food and fluids (Brink 2009). The stress of illness, surgery, or trauma often aggravates glycemic control to the extent that DKA or nonketotic hyperosmolar state result, life-threatening conditions that require immediate medical care to prevent complications and death. Dehydration occurs because of decreased fluid intake, polyuria, vomiting, diarrhea, and evaporative losses from fever. Marked hyperglycemia requires adjustment of the treatment plan and, if accompanied by ketosis, vomiting, or change in consciousness, immediate interaction with the diabetes care team (ADA 2012). All individuals with diabetes need specific, written sick-day guidelines provided by their diabetes care team.

This section discusses the acute complications that can occur as a result of illness in people with diabetes and reviews the recommendations for monitoring and treating acute illness from the 1999 book *American Diabetes Association Guide to Medical Nutrition Therapy for Diabetes* (Kulkarni 1999) and the 2008 American Diabetes Association nutrition recommendations (ADA 2008).

A literature search was conducted on PubMed MEDLINE to identify any studies related to sick-day management in diabetes published in 1999 or later. No updated research was found. Evidence for the treatment of sick days in people with diabetes is discussed and recommendations are summarized.

MANAGEMENT OF DIABETES DURING SICK DAYS

Monitoring

Any illness leading to deterioration of glycemic control needs more frequent monitoring of blood glucose and urine or blood ketones in ketosis-prone individuals. The stress of illness may cause increased release of counterregulatory hormones, resulting in increased insulin needs. However, in very young children, counterregulatory responses may not be well developed, resulting in hypoglycemia from decreased calories and excess insulin action. Frequent self-monitoring of glucose will help determine how to proceed. Ketones must be monitored no matter what the blood glucose level is, since starvation ketosis can occur without elevated glucose levels if oral intake is poor (ADA 2005).

Insulin

Insulin or oral diabetes medications need to be continued and sometimes increased during acute illness, regardless of whether the individual is able to eat. Effects of illness on insulin requirements are variable, with hyperglycemia occurring most commonly in adolescents and adults when increased insulin needs due to the illness exceed available insulin. Hypoglycemia is more likely to occur in young children when reduced food intake is accompanied by excess insulin (ADA 2005). Many illnesses, especially those associated with fever, tend to cause higher levels of stress hormones, resulting in hyperglycemia, whereas illnesses associated with vomiting and diarrhea may occasionally lower blood glucose levels because of decreased food intake, poor absorption, and a slower emptying of the stomach. Insulin requirements sometimes increase during the incubation period of an infection for a few days before clinical onset of the illness and may persist for a few days after the illness has abated (Brink 2009). Frequent monitoring during this time will determine the appropriate therapy. Individuals treated with oral diabetes medications or nutrition therapy alone may temporarily require insulin during illness. Guidelines for calculating extra insulin needs on sick days for children and adolescents are available from the International Society for Pediatric and Adolescent Diabetes (ISPAD) Clinical Practice Consensus Guidelines 2009 (Brink 2009). Acute illnesses associated with hyperglycemia and/or ketosis require additional doses of short- or rapid-acting insulin to prevent DKA or a temporary increase in the basal rate. The dose will depend on the blood glucose levels and severity of ketosis.

Carbohydrate and Fluids

Consuming carbohydrate, especially if plasma glucose is <100 mg/dL (5.5 mmol/L), and drinking adequate amounts of fluids are important during acute illness (ADA 2008). Sugar- and electrolyte-containing fluids such as sports drinks provide hydration, glucose, and electrolytes. Consumption of carbohydrate-containing fluids can prevent hypoglycemia in ketosis-prone individuals when starvation ketosis without hyperglycemia indicates poor oral intake. Nutrition recommendations include ingestion of 150–200 g carbohydrate daily (45–50 g every 3–4 h) for adults to prevent starvation ketosis (Kulkarni 1999; ADA 2008). If regular foods are not tolerated, liquids or soft carbohydrate-containing foods such as regular soft drinks, sports drinks, gelatin, and soups should be consumed. See Table 12.5 for a list of the carbohydrate content of common beverages and soft foods.

Table 12.5. Foods and Beverages Equal to ~15 g Carbohydrate

Sports drinks, 8 oz	Ice cream, ½ cup
Regular soft drinks, 6 oz	Cooked cereals, ½ cup
Gelatin, regular-flavored, ½ cup	Applesauce, ½ cup
Soups, broth-based, 1 cup	Toast, 1 slice
Juices, 4 oz or ½ cup	Saltine crackers, 6
Popsicle, 1	

Prevention of DKA

DKA occurs as a result of inadequate insulin; therefore, all ketosis-prone individuals should be instructed not to omit insulin during illness. Insulin correction factors along with basal insulin will usually need to be adjusted to correct hyperglycemia. All individuals with diabetes and their families/caregivers should be taught sick-day management. During illness, people are less likely to perform self-care tasks, particularly the recommended frequency of glucose and ketone monitoring. The diabetes care team should provide to families/caretakers of ketosis-prone individuals specific written instructions on glucose and ketone monitoring, insulin adjustment, carbohydrate and fluid consumption, and when to contact the diabetes care team in an emergency (Brink 2009).

SUMMARY OF RECOMMENDATIONS FOR SICK DAYS

Diabetes management during acute illness includes more frequent blood glucose monitoring (supplemented in some cases by CGM), adjustment of insulin and/or oral diabetes medications, drinking adequate amounts of fluids, and ingesting carbohydrate, especially if blood glucose levels are <100 mg/dL (5.5 mmol/L). In adults, 150–200 g carbohydrate daily (45–50 g every 3–4 h) should be sufficient to prevent starvation ketosis. Written sick-day guidelines should be provided by the diabetes care team to all individuals with ketosis-prone diabetes.

BIBLIOGRAPHY

American Diabetes Association: Care of children and adolescents with type 1 diabetes. *Diabetes Care* 28:186–212, 2005

American Diabetes Association: Nutrition recommendations and interventions for diabetes. *Diabetes Care* 31 (Suppl. 1):S70–S73, 2008

American Diabetes Association: Standards of medical care in diabetes: 2012. *Diabetes Care* 35 (Suppl. 1):S11–S63, 2012

Axelsen M, Wesslau C, Lönnroth P, Arvidsson Lenner R, Smith U: Bedtime uncooked cornstarch supplement prevents nocturnal hypoglycaemia in intensively treated type 1 diabetes subjects. *J Intern Med* 245:229–236, 1999

Boyle PJ, Zrebiec J: Management of diabetes-related hypoglycemia. *Southern Med J* 100:183–194, 2007

Brink, S, Laffel L, Likitmaskul S, Liu L, Maguire AM, Olsen B, Silink M, Hanas R: Sick day management in children and adolescents with diabetes (ISPAD Clinical Practice Consensus Guidelines 2009). *Pediatr Diabetes* 10:146–153, 2009

Brodows RG, Williams C, Amatruda JM: Treatment of insulin reactions in diabetics. *JAMA* 252:3378–3381, 1984

Buckingham B: Clinical overview of continuous glucose monitoring. *J Diabetes Sci Technol* 2:300–306, 2008

Clarke W, Jones T, Rewers A, Dunger D, Klingensmith GJ: Assessment and management of hypoglycemia in children and adolescents with diabetes (ISPAD Clinical Practice Consensus Guidelines 2009 Compendium). *Pediatr Diabetes* 10 (Suppl. 12):134–145, 2009

Cryer PE: Elimination of hypoglycemia from the lives of people affected by diabetes. *Diabetes* 60:24–27, 2011

Cryer PE: Hypoglycemia (Technical Review). *Diabetes Care* 17:734–755, 1994

Cryer PE: Hypoglycemia in diabetes. *Diabetes Care* 26:1902–1912, 2003

Cryer PE: *Hypoglycemia in Diabetes: Pathophysiology, Prevalence, and Prevention*. Alexandria, VA, American Diabetes Association, 2009a

Cryer PE, Axelrod L, Grossman A, Heller SR, Montori VM, Seaquist ER, Service FJ: Evaluation and management of adult hypoglycemic disorders: an endocrine society clinical practice guideline. *J Clin Endocrinol Metab* 94:709–728, 2009b

Deiss D, Kordonouri O, Hartmann R, Hopfenmuller W, Lupke K, Danne T: Treatment with insulin glargine reduces asymptomatic hypoglycemia detected by continuous subcutaneous glucose monitoring in children and adolescents with type 1 diabetes. *Pediatr Diabetes* 8:157-62, 2007

Diabetes Control and Complications Trial Research Group: Effect of intensive diabetes treatment on the development and progression of long-term complications in insulin-dependent diabetes mellitus: Diabetes Control and Complications Trial. *N Engl J Med* 329:977–986, 1993

Diabetes Research in Children Network (DirecNet) Study Group: Impact of exercise on overnight glycemic control in children with type 1 diabetes mellitus. *J Pediatr* 147:528–534, 2005

Franz MJ: Protein controversies in diabetes. *Diabetes Spectrum* 13:132–141, 2000

Franz MJ, Powers MA, Leontos C, Holzmeister LA, Kulkarni D, Monk A, Wedel N, Gradwell E: The evidence for medical nutrition therapy for type 1 and type 2 diabetes in adults. *J Am Diet Assoc* 110:1852–1889, 2010

Galassetti P, Tate D, Neill RA, Morrey S, Wasserman DH, Davis SN: Effect of antecedent hypoglycemia on counterregulatory responses to subsequent euglycemic exercise in type 1 diabetes. *Diabetes* 52:1761–1769, 2003

Gannon MC, Nuttall JA, Damberg G, Gupta V, Nuttall FQ: Effect of protein ingestion on the glucose appearance rate in people with type 2 diabetes. *J Clin Endocrinol Metab* 86:1040-1047, 2001

Gentilcore D, Chaikomin R, Jones KL: Effects of fat on gastric emptying of and the glycemic, insulin, and incretin responses to a carbohydrate meal in type 2 diabetes. *Am J Clin Nutr* 91:2062–2067, 2006

Gerstein JC, Miller ME, Byington RP, Goff DC Jr, Bigger JT, Buse JB, Cushman WC, Genuth S, Ismail-Beigi F, Grimm RH Jr, Probstfield JL, Simons-Morton DG, Friedewald WT: Effects of intensive glucose lowering in type 2 diabetes:

the Action to Control Cardiovascular Risk in Diabetes Study Group. *N Engl J Med* 358:2545–2559, 2008

Gray RO, Butler PC, Beers TR, Kryshak EJ, Rizza RA: Comparison of the ability of bread versus bread plus meat to treat and prevent subsequent hypoglycemia in patients with insulin-dependent diabetes mellitus. *J Clin Endocrinol Metab* 81:1508–1511, 1996

Guelfi KJ, Jones TW, Fournier PA: New insights into managing risk of hypogly-caemia associated with intermittent high-intensity exercise in individuals with type 1 diabetes mellitus: implications for existing guidelines. *Sports Med* 37:937–946, 2007

Hirsch IB, Bode BW, Garg S, Lane WS, Sussman A, Hu P, Santiago OM, Kolac-zynski JW; Insulin Aspart CSII/MDI Comparison Study Group: Continuous subcutaneous insulin infusion (CSII) of insulin aspart versus multiple daily injection of insulin aspart/insulin glargine in type 1 diabetic patients previ-ously treated with CSII. *Diabetes Care* 28:533–538, 2005

Husband AC, Crawford S, McCoy LA, Pacaud D: The effectiveness of glucose, sucrose, and fructose in treating hypoglycemia in children with type 1 diabe-tes. *Pediatr Diabetes* 11:154–158, 2010

Kalergis M, Schiffrin A, Gougeon R, Jones PJ, Yale J: Impact of bedtime snack composition on prevention of nocturnal hypoglycemia in adults with type 1 diabetes undergoing intensive insulin management using lispro insulin before meals. *Diabetes Care* 26:9–15, 2003

Kaufman FR, Devgan S: Use of uncooked cornstarch to avert nocturnal hypogly-cemia in children and adolescents with type I diabetes. *J Diabetes Complications* 10:84–87, 1996

Kaufman FR, Halvorson M, Kaufman ND. A randomized, blinded trial of uncooked cornstarch to diminish nocturnal hypoglycemia at diabetes camp. *Diabetes Res Clin Pract* 30:205–209, 1995

Kerr D, Cheyne E, Thomas P, Sherwin R: Influence of acute alcohol ingestion on the hormonal responses to modest hypoglycaemia in patients with type 1 dia-betes. *Diabet Med* 24:312–316, 2007

Kulkarni K, Franz MJ: Nutrition therapy for type 1 diabetes. In *American Diabetes Association Guide to Medical Nutrition Therapy for Diabetes.* Franz MJ, Bantle JP, Eds. Alexandria, VA, American Diabetes Association, 1999, p. 35–36

Lodefalk M, Aman J, Bang P: Effects of fat supplementation on glycaemic response and gastric emptying in adolescents with type 1 diabetes. *Diabet Med* 25:1030–1035, 2008

Papakonstantinou E, Triantafillidou D, Panagiotakos DB, Iraklianous S, Berdanier CD, Zampelas A: A high protein low fat meal does not influence glucose and insulin responses in obese individuals with or without type 2 diabetes. *J Hum Nutr Diet* 23:183–189, 2010

Rachmiel M, Buccino J, Daneman D: Exercise and type 1 diabetes mellitus in youth: review and recommendations. *Pediatr Endocrinol Rev* 5:656–665, 2007

Raju B, Arbelaez A, Breckenridge SM, Cryer PE: Nocturnal hypoglycemia in type 1 diabetes: an assessment of preventive bedtime treatments. *J Clin Endocrinol Metab* 91:2087–2092, 2006

Richardson T, Weiss M, Thomas P, Kerr D: Day after the night before: influence of evening alcohol on risk of hypoglycemia in patients with type 1 diabetes. *Diabetes Care* 28:1801–1802, 2005

Robertson K, Adolfsson P, Riddell M, Scheiner G, Hanas R: Exercise in children and adolescents with diabetes (ISPAD Clinical Practice Consensus Guidelines 2009 Compendium). *Pediatr Diabetes* 10 (Suppl. 12):154–168, 2009

Sandoval DA, Guy DL, Richardson MA, Ertl AC, Davis SN: Effects of low and moderate antecedent exercise on counterregulatory responses to subsequent hypoglycemia in type 1 diabetes. *Diabetes* 53:1798–1806, 2004

Schvarcz E, Palmer M, Aman J, Lindkvist B, Beckman K-W: Hypoglycemia increases the gastric emptying rate in patients with type 1 diabetes mellitus. *Diabet Med* 10:660–663, 1993

Slama G, Traynard P-Y, Desplanque N, Pudar H, Dhunputh I, Letanoux M, Bornet FRJ, Tchobroutsky G: The search for the optimized treatment of hypoglycemia: carbohydrates in tablets, solution, or gel in the correction of insulin reactions. *Arch Intern Med* 150:589–593, 1990

Thomsen C, Storm H, Holst JJ, Hermansen K: Differential effects of saturated and monounsaturated fats on postprandial lipemia and glucagon-like peptide 1 responses in patients with type 2 diabetes. *Am J Clin Nutr* 77:605–611, 2003

Tsalikian E, Mauras N, Beck RW, Tamborlane WV, Janz KF, Chase HP, Wysocki T, Weinzimer SA, Buckingham BA, Kollman C, Xing D, Ruedy KJ, Diabetes Research in Children Network Direcnet Study Group: Impact of exercise on overnight glycemic control in children with type 1 diabetes mellitus. *J Pediatr* 147:528–534, 2005

U.K. Hypoglycaemia Study Group: Risk of hypoglycaemia in types 1 and 2 diabetes: effects of treatment modalities and their duration. *Diabetologia* 50:1140–1147, 2007

Wiethop BV, Cryer PE: Alanine and terbutaline in the treatment of hypoglycemia in IDDM. *Diabetes Care* 16:1131–1136, 1993

Wilson D, Chase HP, Kollman C, Xing D, Caswell K, Tansey M, Fox L, Weinzimer S, Beck R, Ruedy K, Tamborlane W, Diabetes Research in Children Network (DirecNet) Study Group: Low fat vs. high fat bedtime snacks in children and adolescents with type 1 diabetes. *Pediatr Diabetes* 9:320–325, 2008

Janine Freeman, RD, CDE, is a Diabetes Nutrition Consultant in Atlanta, GA.

Chapter 13
Nutrition Therapy for Diabetes and Lipid Disorders

Wahida Karmally, DrPH, RD, CDE, CLS, and
Jacqueline Santora Zimmerman, MS, RD

Highlights

Evidence for Nutrition Recommendations for Disorders of Lipid Metabolism in People with Diabetes

Nutrition Recommendations for Disorders of Lipid Metabolism in Diabetes

Highlights
Nutrition Therapy for Diabetes and Lipid Disorders

■ Dyslipidemia in diabetes is a cluster of lipid and lipoprotein abnormalities that are known to be metabolically related and atherogenic. Type 2 diabetes is considered a cardiovascular disease risk equivalent.

■ An eating pattern that is designed both to lower glucose and improve lipid patterns and regular physical activity are cornerstones in managing lipid disorders in diabetes.

■ The goal of nutrition therapy, while maintaining the pleasure of eating with a healthy eating pattern, should focus on major strategies: reduction of saturated fatty acids and *trans* fatty acids and cholesterol intake; the use of stanols/sterols, omega-3 fatty acids, nuts, and foods containing soluble fiber; and weight loss, if indicated, to achieve a lipid and lipoprotein profile that reduces the risk for vascular disease.

■ Evidence-based nutrition recommendations for diabetes and lipid disorders are provided by the Academy of Nutrition and Dietetics (formerly the American Dietetic Association), the American Diabetes Association, and the U.S. Department of Agriculture (USDA) Dietary Guidelines for Americans, 2010, committee (USDA DGAC 2010).

Nutrition Therapy for Diabetes and Lipid Disorders

Diabetes mellitus increases the risk for atherosclerotic vascular disease. Diabetes is associated with a three- to fourfold increase in risk of coronary artery disease and is the leading cause of death in individuals with diabetes who are over the age of 35 years. Diabetes alone affects ~26 million individuals in the U.S., and >60% of these individuals are at higher risk for cardiovascular disease (CVD). Additionally, 65% of people with diabetes die from a CVD event. Studies have shown that up to 60% of adults with diabetes have hypertension and nearly all have one or more lipid abnormalities (American Diabetes Association [ADA] 2012). Approximately 34% of adults in the U.S. population meet the criteria for metabolic syndrome (Ervin 2009).

People with diabetes are considered to have the equivalent CVD risk as people with preexisting CVD and no diabetes (Buse 2007). A significant proportion of this increased risk is associated with the presence of well-characterized risk factors for CVD such as dyslipidemia, hypertension, inflammation, smoking, and obesity. Patients with diabetes, particularly those with type 2 diabetes, have abnormalities of plasma lipids and lipoprotein concentrations that are less commonly present in people who do not have diabetes (Packard 2003). Patients with type 1 diabetes can also have a dyslipidemic pattern (Vergès 2009). The consequences of dyslipidemia in the development of CVD in type 1 diabetes are not fully understood. A common abnormal lipid problem in patients with diabetes, as a result of an overproduction of very-low-density lipoprotein (VLDL) cholesterol, is an elevation of VLDL cholesterol, a reduction in HDL cholesterol, and an LDL fraction that contains a greater proportion of small, dense LDL particles and increased postprandial lipemia (Adiels 2008; Vergès 2009). These abnormalities have been shown to be metabolically related and very atherogenic (Taskinen 2005). The prevalence of dyslipidemia in patients with diabetes is high worldwide (Grant 2002; Massing 2003; Pyörälä 2004).

All adults with diabetes are candidates for progressively aggressive therapy. The primary goal of therapy for individuals without overt CVD, as recommended by the ADA, is LDL cholesterol of <100 mg/dL and, in individuals with overt CVD, a lower LDL cholesterol goal of <70 mg/dL, based on evidence from clinical trials (ADA 2012). The desirable goal for triglyceride levels is <150 mg/dL and HDL cholesterol to >40 mg/dL in men and >50 mg/dL in women.

An eating pattern that is designed both to lower glucose and alter lipid patterns and regular physical activity are cornerstones in the management of lipid disorders. Nutrition interventions lasting ≥1 year, such as Mediterranean-style eating patterns (Ciccarone 2003; Diakoumopoulou 2005), reduced A1C, blood pressure, and body weight and improved serum lipid profile, all of which reduce the risk for developing CVD in both type 1 and type 2 diabetes patients (Academy of Nutrition and Dietetics [Acad Nutr Diet] 2008). In a study of 571 individuals with type 1 diabetes, high total and saturated fat intake was reported to be associated with increased coronary disease (Snell-Bergeon 2009). Higher fat intake was associated with worse glycemic control, higher total cholesterol (TC) and LDL cholesterol, adiposity, and hypertension.

This chapter will include an update on published studies that were not previously included in the recommendations by the ADA (2008) or Franz and colleagues (2010) for nutrition therapy interventions for the prevention and treatment of CVD in diabetes. To update the recommendations, a literature search was conducted using PubMed MEDLINE, and additional articles were identified from reference lists. Search criteria included the following: research in human subjects with diabetes, English language, and published after the references cited by Franz and colleagues (2010). References for effects of food sources on lipids include earlier studies. Search terms included the following: nutrition or diet therapy for CVD, lipids, cholesterol, fiber, soy, carbohydrates, protein, fatty acids, monounsaturated fatty acids (MUFAs), polyunsaturated fatty acids (PUFAs) (including omega-3 fatty acids), saturated fatty acids (SFAs), *trans* fatty acids (TFAs), stanols/sterols, and Mediterranean eating pattern. Studies identifying nutrition therapy interventions for the prevention and treatment of CVD in people with diabetes are summarized in Table 13.1. Most of the evidence published before July 2009 is included in the tables in the article "The Evidence for Medical Nutrition Therapy for Type 1 and Type 2 Diabetes in Adults" (Franz 2010) and the Acad Nutr Diet Evidence Analysis Library (Acad Nutr Diet 2008). Evidence from the Report of the Dietary Guidelines Advisory Committee (DGAC) on the Dietary Guidelines for Americans, 2010 (U.S. Department of Agriculture, Nutrition Evidence Library [USDA NEL] 2010), is also referenced and is publicly available at http:www.nutritionevidencelibrary.gov.

EVIDENCE FOR NUTRITION RECOMMENDATIONS FOR DISORDERS OF LIPID METABOLISM IN PEOPLE WITH DIABETES

In individuals with diabetes, lifestyle management that includes nutrition therapy and physical activity are integral to improving glycemic control and CVD risk factors (Buse 2007; Bruckert 2011). The common coexistence of hyperlipidemia and hypertension in people with diabetes (Chapter 14) mandates effective management of both conditions. Nutrition therapy and physical activity, in addition to behavioral interventions to help sustain improved lifestyles, are successful approaches in managing diabetes and lowering risk for CVD (Franz 2010). The goal of nutrition therapy for lipid disorders introduced in Chapter 2, while maintaining the pleasure of eating with a healthy eating pattern, should focus on the following major strategies: reducing SFAs and TFAs and cholesterol intake; using stanols/sterols, omega-3 fatty acids, nuts, and foods containing soluble fiber; and weight loss, if indicated, to achieve a lipid and lipoprotein profile that reduces the risk for vascular disease (ADA 2012). The Dietary Approaches to Stop Hypertension (DASH) (Azadbakht 2011; Liese 2011) and Mediterranean-style eating patterns (Cadario 2011) and increased physical activity also need to be considered.

Table 13.1 Studies on Nutrition Therapy and Lipid Outcomes Published During and After 2007

	Population/ Duration of Study	Intervention (type of study)	Major Findings	Comments
Carbohydrate				
Haimoto 2009	n = 33 adults with type 2 diabetes and A1C >9%/6 months	Effect of lower-CHO diet (30% CHO, 44% fat, 20% protein, 1,852 kcal) (clinical trial)	Compared to baseline, HDL ↑ 8 mg/dL (P = 0.008), LDL ↓ 14 mg/dL (P = 0.036), A1C ↓ 3.5% (P = 0.008)	No comparison group
De Natale 2009	n = 18 adults with type 2 diabetes on diet alone (n = 13) or diet plus metformin (n = 5)/4 weeks	Plant-based HC (52%)/HF (28 g/1,000 kcal)/low-GI (58%) vs. plant-based LC (45%), high-MUFA (23%)/high-GI (88%) (randomized crossover trial)	HC, HF vs. high MUFA: ↓ TC −7.8 mg/dL, ↓ LDL cholesterol −7.7 mg/dL, ↓ HDL cholesterol −3.1 mg/dL, ↑ HDL TG 17.8 mg/dL (all P < 0.05); NS TG; after HC, HF test meal, ↓ in incremental area under the curve for plasma glucose, plasma insulin, TG, and chylomicrons (all P < 0.05)	HC, HF diet was based on legumes, vegetables, fruits, and whole cereals
Total Fat and SFAs				
Snell-Bergeon 2009	n = 571 with type 1 diabetes and 696 control subjects without diabetes) (Coronary Artery Calcification in Type 1 [CACT1] study)/NA	Examined diet and CHD risk factors; FFQ completed at baseline (cross-sectional study)	% kcal from fat, SFAs, MUFAs positively correlated with TC, LDL, non-HDL, apoB (P < 0.001 for all), and A1C (P < 0.05); % kcal from *trans* fat positively correlated with LDL and apoB (P < 0.001); kcal from PUFAs positively correlated with LDL (P < 0.05); % kcal from CHO negatively correlated with TC, LDL, HDL, non-HDL, A1C, and apoB (P < 0.05); HDL negatively correlated with TG, non-HDL, and apoB and positively correlated with GI (P < 0.05 for all)	Author conclusions: adults with type 1 diabetes consume greater than recommended amounts of total fat and SFAs; fat intake is associated with CHD risk factors

Table 13.1 Studies on Nutrition Therapy and Lipid Outcomes Published During and After 2007 (*continued*)

	Population/ Duration of Study	Intervention (type of study)	Major Findings	Comments
Protein				
Pipe 2009 (soy protein)	*n* = 29 adults with type 2 diabetes/ two 57-day periods	Daily supplementation of usual diet with 40 g soy protein isolate and 88 mg soy isoflavones vs. 40 g milk protein isolate without soy isoflavones (crossover RCT)	Soy protein group decreased LDL (*P* = 0.04) and ratio of LDL to HDL (*P* = 0.020) vs. milk protein group	
Wycherley 2010	*n* = 59 adults with type 2 diabetes/16 weeks	Four energy-restricted diets (~1,400 kcal women, ~1,700 kcal for men): *1*) standard diet (53% CHO, 26% fat, 19% protein) vs. *2*) high-protein diet (43% CHO, 22% fat, 33% protein) vs. *3*) standard diet + resistance training 3 days/week vs. *4*) high-protein diet + resistance training 3 days/week (RCT)	NS differences between groups; in all groups, reductions in TC, TG, and LDL cholesterol (*P* < 0.001 for all)	Focus of study was weight loss and changes in body composition
Pearce 2011	*n* = 65 adults with type 2 diabetes or impaired glucose tolerance/12 weeks	Hypoenergenetic (1,400 kcal) diets: HPHchol (590 mg CHO, included two eggs/day) vs. HPLchol) (213 mg CHO, replaced eggs with 100 g animal protein); both 40% CHO, 30% protein, 30% fat (RCT)	HDL ↑ on HPHchol (0.8 mg/dL) and ↓ HPLchol (−2.7 mg/ dL), *P* < 0.05); all lost weight and ↓ TC, TG, and A1C (*P* < 0.001 for all); FBG and fasting insulin also ↓ in all (*P* < 0.01 for both); no change in LDL	Controlled feeding study; authors note plasma folate and lutein ↑ more on HPHchol (*P* < 0.05)

	Population/ Duration of Study	Intervention (type of study)	Major Findings	Comments
MUFAs				
Strychar 2009	*n* = 30 adults with type 1 diabetes/6 months	Two eucaloric diets, SFA and fiber: higher CHO (54–57%)/lower fat (27–30%; 10% from MUFAs) vs. lower CHO (43–46%)/higher fat (37–40%, 20% from MUFAs) (RCT)	6 months: NS differences in TC, LDL cholesterol, HDL cholesterol, TG, or A1C	Lower-CHO/ higher-fat group 2% weight increase (2.4 kg) (*P* < 0.05)
Omega-3 Fatty Acids				
Kabir 2007	*n* = 27 postmenopausal women with type 2 diabetes and without hypertriglyceridemia/8 weeks	Treatment: 3 g/ day fish oil capsules (1.08 g EPA, 0.72 g DHA) vs. control: 3 g/ day paraffin oil capsules (RCT)	Fish oil group: 12% lower TG and ratio of TG to HDL (*P* < 0.03 for both); NS changes in TC, LDL, HDL, or glycemic measures	In fish oil group, some inflammation-related genes were significantly reduced in subcutaneous adipose tissue
Mostad 2008	*n* = 27 normotriglyceridemic adults with type 2 diabetes not treated with insulin/9 weeks	Supplementation of usual diet with fish oil (5.9 g/day total omega-3 fatty acids, 1.8 g 20:5 omega-3, 3.0 g 22:6 omega-3) vs. placebo of corn oil (8.5 g/day 18:2 omega-6 FA) (RCT)	Fish oil vs. control: VLDL size difference (median −15 vs. +0.6%, *P* = 0.001); large VLDL particles (−99 vs. −4.1%, *P* = 0.041); small HDL (−12 vs. +10%, *P* = 0.051); NS effect on oxidized LDL	Statins used by 2 subjects in fish oil group and 2 subjects in control group
Hartweg 2008	*n* = 23 RCTs (1,075 subjects with type 2 diabetes)/NA	Effect of omega-3 PUFAs on lipid profile, glycemic control, and vascular outcomes; mean dose of omega-3 used in trials was 3.5 g/day (8.9 weeks) (Cochrane Review: systematic review and meta-analysis)	Omega-3 PUFAs: TG ↓ 39.9 mg/dL (*P* < 0.00001); VLDL ↓ −2.7 mg/dL (*P* = 0.04); LDL ↑ 4.3 mg/dL (*P* = 0.05); NS, TC, HDL, A1C, FBG, fasting insulin, or body weight	Fixed-effect meta-analysis conducted

Table 13.1 Studies on Nutrition Therapy and Lipid Outcomes Published During and After 2007 (*continued*)

	Population/ Duration of Study	Intervention (type of study)	Major Findings	Comments
Hartweg 2009	*n* = 24 trials from 1966 to 2008 (1,533 subjects with type 2 diabetes)/NA	Examined impact of marine-derived omega-3 PUFAs on lipid, glycemic, and hematological risk using pooled data from RCTs (average daily intake of omega-3 PUFAs ~2.4 g over 24 weeks for 7 studies added 2007–2008) (systematic review and meta-analysis)	TG ↓ with omega-3 PUFA supplementation by 7% vs. control ($P < 0.0001$); LDL ↑ by 3% vs. control ($P = 0.006$); omega-3 PUFA supplementation NS changes in A1C	30 studies included in review; 24 studies pooled for meta-analysis; includes Kabir 2007 and Mostad 2008
Belalcazar 2010	*n* = 2,397 adults with type 2 diabetes, Look AHEAD participants/baseline + 1 year	FFQ analyzed for mO-3FA intake based on eight FFQ line items asking about consumption of seafood (prospective cohort/cross-sectional study)	Baseline: mean mO-3FA intake 162 mg/day; inversely associated with TG ($P < 0.001$) and associated with trend for higher HDL ($P = 0.05$); 1 year: mO-3FA intake and fried fish intake decreased ($P = 0.001$)	Authors' note 1,000 mg/day mO-3FA recommended for people with diabetes; associations seen despite low levels of intake mO-3FA in participants
McEwen 2010	*n* = 23 studies examining omega-3 fatty acids in diabetes and/or CVD/NA	Review assessing role of omega-3 FA on lipid profile, CVD mortality, and platelet function (review article)	omega-3 FAs ↓ TG, TC, LDL, and VLDL and mildly raise HDL	Articles included in review addressed diabetes, CVD, and omega-3 FA intake
Rudkowska 2010	Review examining impact of fish oil supplementation on adults with type 2 diabetes/NA	Review including several meta-analyses examining effect of fish oil on blood glucose, inflammation, blood pressure, and CVD events (review article)	omega-3 PUFA supplementation ↓ TG by 25–30%, ↑ LDL by 5–10%, and HDL by 1–3%; moderate intake of omega-3 PUFAs does not adversely affect insulin resistance and may lower risk factors for CVD	Inclusion/exclusion criteria not specified

	Population/ Duration of Study	Intervention (type of study)	Major Findings	Comments
Saravanan 2010	Review examining mO-3FA and high-risk patients (including type 2 diabetes)/NA	Effect of mO-3FA in patients with CVD, ventricular or atrial arrhythmia, sudden cardiac death, heart failure, atherosclerosis, stroke, dyslipidemia, diabetes, hypertension (review article)	omega-3 PUFAs consistently shown to ↓ TG (2–4 g/day omega-3 PUFAs lower TG by ~30%); no adverse effects on glycemic control seen	Author conclusions: omega-3 PUFAs may significantly reduce CVD risk in people with type 2 diabetes
Nuts				
Jenkins 2008b	Review examining nut consumption in type 2 diabetes/NA	Possible benefit of nuts in type 2 diabetes (review article)	Frequent nut consumption associated with ↓ risk of diabetes and CVD; in people with diabetes, nuts have potential to ↓ CHD risk, may ↓ postprandial glycemia but not A1C levels	Author conclusions: incorporation of nuts may improve overall nutritional quality of eating pattern
Ma 2010	$n = 21$ adults with type 2 diabetes/ two 8-week periods, 8-week washout period	Control: ad libitum diet Intervention: 56 g/day unroasted, shelled walnuts isocalorically substituted for foods in ad libitum diet vs. control ad libitum diet (RCT)	NS CVD measures between groups; walnuts, baseline to 8 week, ↓ in TC (–9.7 mg/dL, $P < 0.01$) and LDL (–7.7 mg/dL, $P < 0.001$), ↑ in FBG (10.0 mg/dL, $P < 0.04$); endothelial function improved after walnut diet vs. control diet (2.2 vs. 1.2%; $P = 0.04$)	
Kendall 2010	$n = 8$ trials in subjects with metabolic syndrome or type 2 diabetes/ NA	Effect of nut consumption in patients with metabolic syndrome or type 2 diabetes (review article)	In patients with type 2 diabetes, nuts may have a moderate beneficial effect on lipid profile (↓ TC, LDL, and TG and ↑ HDL) and glycemic control	Author conclusions: adding nuts to a healthy diet can benefit people with metabolic syndrome or type 2 diabetes and may lower risk of CHD
Berryman 2011	Review of intervention studies with almonds/NA	LDL reduction capability of almonds; possible mechanisms for this effect (review article)	Almonds consistently ↓ LDL in healthy subjects, hypercholesterolemic subjects, and individuals with diabetes	Included epidemiologic studies, pooled and meta-analyses, and clinical trials

Table 13.1 Studies on Nutrition Therapy and Lipid Outcomes Published During and After 2007 (*continued*)

	Population/ Duration of Study	Intervention (type of study)	Major Findings	Comments
Jenkins 2011	*n* = 117 adults with type 2 diabetes/3 months	Substitution of 475 kcal/2,000-kcal diet with: *1)* full portion (75 g/day) mixed nuts (raw almonds, pistachios, walnuts, pecans, hazelnuts, peanuts, cashews, macadamias) vs. *2)* half portion mixed nuts, half portion muffin (similar protein content as nuts) vs. *3)* full portion muffins (RCT)	Full portion nuts vs. muffins: ↓ in TC (–9.3 mg/dL, *P* < 0.001); LDL (–8.5 mg/dL, *P* < 0.001) and TC:HDL ratio (–0.23, *P* = 0.006); NS differences HDL, TG	Kilocalories from MUFAs in nuts same as kilocalories from CHO in muffins
Li 2011	*n* = 20 Chinese adults with type 2 diabetes and mild hyperlipidemia/12 weeks (two 4-week diet periods, 2-week washout)	Control diet (NCEP step II diet) vs. almond diet (NCEP step II diet plus almonds [~60 g/day]) replacing 20% total calories; isocaloric diets (crossover RCT)	Almond diet ↓ TC by 6.0% (*P* = 0.0025); LDL by 11.6% (*P* = 0.0117); LDL:HDL ratio by 9.7% (*P* = 0.0128); plasma apoB by 15.6% (*P* = 0.0046); apo B:apoA-1 ratio by 17.4% (*P* = 0.0084); fasting insulin by 4.1% (*P* = 0.0184); FBG by 0.8% (*P* = 0.0238)	Counseling provided during run-in and washout periods
Plant Stanols/Sterols				
Hallikainen 2008	*n* = 22 adults with type 1 diabetes/12 weeks	Intervention (2 g/day of plant stanol esters [1.66 g sitostanol, 0.38 g campestanol]) in vegetable oil–based spread vs. control (vegetable oil–based spread without plant stanol esters) (RCT)	TC and LDL ↓ in intervention group by 4.9 and 6.9% from baseline and by 10.8 and 16.1% in controls, respectively (*P* < 0.05 for all); NS changes in HDL or TG	All subjects followed usual diet

	Population/ Duration of Study	Intervention (type of study)	Major Findings	Comments
Baker 2009	*n* = 5 RCTs (parallel or crossover) that reported efficacy data in patients with type 2 diabetes (148 subjects total)/NA	Examined effect of plant sterols or stanols on lipid parameters; four evaluated sterol-fortified margarines and one study evaluated sterol-fortified granola bars (systematic review and meta-analysis)	Plant sterol/stanol doses ranging from 1.6 to 3 g/day ↓ TC and LDL, −10.3 mg/dL and −12.2 mg/dL, respectively; HDL NS trend to improvement; no beneficial effect on TG	Majority of studies were crossover trials
Hallikainen 2011	*n* = 24 adults with type 1 diabetes on statin therapy/4 weeks	Intervention (3 g/day of plant stanol esters in vegetable oil–based spread) vs. control (vegetable oil–based spread without plant stanol esters) (RCT)	Intervention group: ↓ TC (7.8%), LDL (14.8%), and non-HDL cholesterol (12.2%) (*P* = 0.05 for all); no effect on HDL or TG	Authors note: "plant stanol esters lower LDL cholesterol level in statin-treated patients with type 1 diabetes by interfering with the absorption and synthesis of cholesterol"
Soluble Fiber				
Liatis 2009	*n* = 41 adults with type 2 diabetes, LDL cholesterol >130 mg/dL/3 weeks	Daily supplementation of usual diet with β-glucan–enriched bread (four slices providing 3 g/day β-glucan) vs. control bread (0 g β-glucan) (RCT)	β-Glucan group ↓ LDL by 15.8% (25.5 mg/dL) vs. 2.7% (4.3 mg/dL) (*P* = 0.009); TC by 12.8% (31.0 mg/dL) vs. 1.9% (4.7 mg/dL), (*P* = 0.006) and non-HDL by 15.1% (29.0 mg/dL) vs. 1.8% (3.1 mg/day) (*P* = 0.005); NS changes in HDL, TG	
Cugnet-Anceau 2010	*n* = 53 adults with type 2 diabetes/8 weeks	Daily supplementation of usual diet with β-glucan–enriched soup (providing 3.5 g/day β-glucan) vs. control soup (0 g β-glucan) (RCT)	TG ↓ in the β-glucan group by 19.6 mg/dL vs. ↑ 10.6 mg/dL in the control (*P* = 0.03): NS changes in TC, LDL, HDL, apoB, A1C, and FBG; β-glucan group compared to baseline ↑ HDL by 5.4% (*P* = 0.01)	Authors' note: half of subjects were on a lipid-lowering treatment, which may have blunted effect, but results were not modified in the subgroup without lipid-lowering treatment

Table 13.1 Studies on Nutrition Therapy and Lipid Outcomes Published During and After 2007 (*continued*)

	Population/ Duration of Study	Intervention (type of study)	Major Findings	Comments
Othman 2011	n = 22 studies (1997–2010) investigating oat β-glucan and lipid profile/NA	Examines evidence for cholesterol-lowering effects of oat β-glucan (review article)	When at least 3 g/ day oat β-glucan are consumed, TC and LDL may decrease 5–10%	Includes studies with subjects with type 2 diabetes
Other Eating Patterns and Lipids				
Jönsson 2009	n = 13 adults with type 2 diabetes/6 months (3 months on each diet)	Diabetes diet (higher in fiber, whole grains; lower in SFA) vs. Paleolithic diet (lean meat, fish, fruit, vegetables, eggs, nuts, no dairy); CVD risk factors (RCT)	Paleolithic diet vs. diabetes diet ↑ HDL and ↓ TG (P = 0.03 for both) and ↓ A1C (P = 0.02)	Paleolithic diet lower in kilocalories; subjects lost weight compared to baseline; P = 0.005
Cadario 2011	n = 96 children and adolescents with type 1 diabetes/6 months	Changes in lipid profile and nutritional intake after a structured dietitian training to a Med diet (prospective cohort study)	LDL, non-HDL cholesterol, and TC:HDL ratio ↓ (P < 0.0001 for all); dietary fats and cholesterol ↓ and fiber ↑ (P < 0.0001 for all)	Author conclusions: training to Med diet improves nutrient intake quality and lipid profile
Solá 2011	n = 772 adults with type 2 diabetes or three or more CHD risk factors (hypertension, smoking, dyslipidemia, obesity, family history of CVD), recruited into the PREDIMED (Prevención con Dieta Mediterránea) Study/3 months	Effect on apoB and apoA-1: intervention (Med diet supplemented with virgin olive oil or Med diet supplemented with mixed nuts: walnuts (15 g/day), hazelnuts (7.5 g/ day), and almonds (7.5 g/ day) vs. control (advice for low-fat diet) (RCT)	Med diet + virgin olive oil vs. control diet: −2.9 mg/dL for apoB; 3.3 mg/dL for apoA-1; −0.03 mg/ dL for apoB/apoA-1 ratio	Apolipoproteins assessed in a randomly selected subpopulation with similar characteristics to entire group
Azadbakht 2011	n = 33 adults with type 2 diabetes/8 weeks	DASH diet vs. control diet (50–60% CHO, 15–20% protein, <30% total fat, <5% kcal from simple sugars) (RCT)	DASH diet ↓ LDL (−17.2 mg/dL, P = 0.02), ↑ HDL (4.3 mg/dL, P = 0.001), ↓ A1C (−1.7%, P = 0.04), FBG (−29.4 mg/dL, P = 0.04)	

	Population/ Duration of Study	Intervention (type of study)	Major Findings	Comments
Liese 2011	*n* = 2,130 youth with type 1 diabetes (1,810) or type 2 diabetes (320) participating in the SEARCH for Diabetes in Youth Study/NA	Association of DASH diet with CVD risk factors, including blood lipid levels, lipoproteins, and glycemic control; diet assessed by SEARCH FFQ and scored for adherence to DASH dietary pattern; overall score range: 0–80 (cross-sectional study)	In youth with type 1 diabetes, as DASH adherence increased, NS ↓ in TC, LDL, and apoB and significant ↓ in A1C (0.2%) and LDL:HDL ratio; NS DASH adherence with TC, LDL, HDL, and TG; in youth with type 2 diabetes, as DASH adherence increased, NS ↓ TC, TG, apoB, and HDL; significant association of DASH score and LDL particle density	Authors note association of DASH score with TC and LDL was inconsistent

Other Food Sources/Components and Lipids

	Population/ Duration of Study	Intervention (type of study)	Major Findings	Comments
Pan 2007 (flax)	*n* = 68 adults with type 2 diabetes/12 weeks	Three flaxseed-derived lignin capsules (0.6 g/capsule) per day providing 360 mg/day isolated flaxseed lignan total vs. placebo (crossover RCT)	NS differences in blood lipid profile, fasting insulin, FBG, insulin resistance; A1C ↓ after supplement (–0.10 vs. 0.09%, *P* = 0.001)	
Vuksan 2007 (chia)	*n* = 20 adults with type 2 diabetes/12 weeks	Supplementation of diet with 37 g/day Salba chia seeds vs. wheat bran control; all subjects counseled to follow the Canadian Diabetes Association's nutrition recommendations (crossover RCT)	NS differences in TC, LDL, HDL, TG, fasting insulin, or FBG levels	
Baker 2008 (cinnamon)	*n* = 5 RCTs (282 subjects total; adults with type 2 diabetes or adolescents with type 1 diabetes)/NA	Effect of cinnamon on glucose control and lipid parameters; all studies used *cinnamomum cassia*, doses ranged from 1 to 6 g/day (meta-analysis)	NS changes in lipid parameters, A1C, or FBG	

Table 13.1 Studies on Nutrition Therapy and Lipid Outcomes Published During and After 2007 (*continued*)

	Population/ Duration of Study	Intervention (type of study)	Major Findings	Comments
Sobenin 2008 (garlic)	*n* = 60 adults with type 2 diabetes and taking sulfo-nylurea deriva-tives/4 weeks	Group 1: Allicor garlic powder (300 mg, twice daily) or placebo (oral diabetes medications dis-continued) vs. Group 2: Allicor garlic powder (300 mg, twice daily) or placebo (oral diabetes medications con-tinued); patients on "standard diet" for diabetes (RCT)	Compared to base-line: TG ↓ in both groups receiving Alli-cor (monotherapy: 262 vs. 168 mg/dL; combined: 268 vs. 199 mg/dL, *P* < 0.05 for both); NS changes in TC, HDL, and LDL	6 out of 10 subjects from placebo group without medications withdrew because of increases in blood glu-cose
GI/GL				
Jenkins 2008a	*n* = 155 adults with type 2 diabe-tes/6 months	Low-GI diet (10–20% ↓ in usual GI) vs. high–cereal fiber diet; fiber constant; both groups advised to avoid muffins, pan-cakes, donuts, bagels, cookies, cakes, popcorn, fries, and chips and to have three servings of fruit and five servings of vegetables (RCT)	Low-GI diet ↑ HDL (1.7 mg/dL, *P* = 0.005); high–cereal fiber diet ↓ HDL (–0.2 mg/dL, *P* = 0.005) and ↓ A1C (–0.2%, *P* < 0.001); LDL:HDL ratio ↓ with low-GI diet (–0.12) vs. high–cereal fiber diet (–0.01, *P* = 0.047)	Actual fiber higher in low-GI group at week 24: 18.7 g/1,000 kcal vs. 15.7 g/1,000 kcal in high–cereal fiber group (*P* < 0.001)
Livesey 2008	*n* = 45 studies published before January 2005 (*n* = 972), included subjects with impaired glucose tolerance, type 1 and type 2 diabe-tes/NA	Low-GI diet effects on glyce-mic response and health outcomes using meta-anal-ysis and meta-regression models (system-atic review and meta-analysis)	Statistically signifi-cant effects lowering fasting TG were evi-dent for lower GL (dependent on GI) and higher fat intake (independent of GI)	10% drop in fasting TG requires drop of GL by 30–100 glu-cose equiva-lents/day

	Population/ Duration of Study	Intervention (type of study)	Major Findings	Comments
Westman 2008	n = 84 obese adults with type 2 diabetes/6 months	Low-GI, reduced kcal (55% CHO) vs. low-CHO (goal <20 g/day; actual 49 g/day), ketogenic (randomized parallel trial)	Low CHO, ketogenic diet ↑ HDL cholesterol 5.6 mg/dL ($P <$ 0.05) and ↓ A1C 1.5% (P = 0.03); no change in HDL cholesterol with low-GI diet	Definition of low-GI not specified; only 49 participants completed study
Studies Using Other Approaches for Lipid-Lowering Effects				
Look AHEAD Research Group 2010	n = 5,145 adults with type 2 diabetes, all Look AHEAD Trial participants/4 years	4-year effects of ILI vs. DSE (control) (prospective cohort study)	ILI vs. DSE: HDL cholesterol (3.7 vs. 2.0 mg/dL, $P <$ 0.001); TG (−25.6 vs. −19.8 mg/dL, $P <$ 0.001); DSE vs. ILI: LDL cholesterol (−11.3 vs. −12.8 mg/dL, P = 0.009)	ILI vs. DSE: weight loss (−6.2 vs. −0.9%, $P <$ 0.001); author conclusions: ILI → sustained weight loss, improvements in glycemic control, fitness, and CVD risk factors
Bruckert 2011	n = 35 studies/NA	Summarizing approaches to ↓ LDL cholesterol: step 1 and 2 diets, plant stanols/sterols, fiber, nuts, soy protein/isoflavones, Portfolio diet, Med diet, omega-3 fatty acids (review article)	Significant and additive effect on ↓ LDL cholesterol: step 1 diet (−10%), fiber (−5 to 10%), plant stanols/sterols (−10%), nuts (−8%), and soy protein (−3 to 10%)	Includes studies with subjects with diabetes

CHD, coronary heart disease; CHO, carbohydrate; DASH, dietary approaches to stop hypertension; FA, fatty acid; FBG, fasting blood glucose; FFQ, food frequency questionnaire; HC, high-carbohydrate; HF, high-fiber; HPHchol, high-protein, high-cholesterol; HPLchol, high-protein, low-cholesterol; ILI, intensive lifestyle intervention; mO-3FA, marine omega-3 fatty acids; Med diet, Mediterranean-style eating pattern; NS, nonsignificant; TG, triglyceride.

Weight loss has been shown to improve glycemic control and reduce insulin resistance as well as improve lipoproteins (decrease triglycerides and raise HDL cholesterol) (Look AHEAD [Action for Health in Diabetes] 2010; Belalcazar 2010).

Using cardioprotective nutrition interventions that include reduction in SFAs, TFAs, and dietary cholesterol and interventions to improve blood pressure can lead to a reduction in cardiovascular risk and improved cardiovascular outcomes (Vergès 2009). Because data showing the specific effects of fatty acids and cholesterol intakes on lipids and lipoproteins in patients with diabetes are limited but growing in the past few years, it is recommended that the nutrition goals for individuals with diabetes be the same as for people with preexisting CVD (ADA 2008).

The recommendations for a cardioprotective eating pattern are based on the best available scientific evidence to attain goals. The cardioprotective eating pattern should provide 25–35% of calories from fat with <7% of calories from SFAs and TFAs and be based on the individual's needs. Because TFAs raise TC and LDL cholesterol and may decrease HDL cholesterol, TFA consumption should be as low as possible. Cholesterol intake should be <200 mg/day. The majority of total fat intake should be derived from unsaturated fat sources. Robust evidence indicates that a cardioprotective diet reduces LDL cholesterol by 9–16% in both normo- and hyperlipidemic individuals (Acad Nutr Diet 2010).

The *Dietary Guidelines for Americans, 2010,* nutrition recommendations that are relevant to lipid management and diabetes include the following: reducing sodium intake to 1,500 mg/day and consuming <10% of calories from SFAs by replacing them with MUFAs and PUFAs (USDA USDHHS 2010).

Carbohydrate Versus Fat Restrictions

The recommendations for nutrition interventions for diabetes have varied over the past several decades, with shifting emphasis on carbohydrate versus fat restriction. Several studies have suggested that replacing saturated fats with carbohydrate may have a deleterious effect on both diabetes control and dyslipidemia (Siri-Tarino 2010). As a consequence, several researchers have proposed alternative eating patterns in which the level of total dietary fat intake is maintained by replacing SFAs with MUFAs. The USDA Nutrition Evidence Library reports moderate evidence indicating that replacing SFAs with MUFAs, rather than carbohydrate, may be beneficial for people with type 2 diabetes (USDA NEL 2010) and results in improved biomarkers of glucose tolerance and diabetes control. After 4 weeks of consuming a high-carbohydrate, high-fiber diet (52% carbohydrate, 28 g fiber/1,000 kcal), subjects with type 2 diabetes had significant decreases in TC, LDL cholesterol, and HDL cholesterol (De Natale 2009). In a meta-analysis of 19 short-term studies in subjects with type 2 diabetes, low-fat, high-carbohydrate diets significantly increased fasting insulin (+8%) and triglycerides (+13%) and lowered HDL cholesterol (–6%) (Kodama 2009), whereas low-carbohydrate diets raised HDL cholesterol (Haimoto 2009).

Protein Intake

The role of protein in diabetes nutrition therapy is discussed in Chapter 2. Recent publications include a study comparing a standard diet and high-protein diet with and without resistance training in adults with type 2 diabetes. All groups had reductions in triglycerides, TC, and HDL cholesterol (Wycherley 2010). In a study on adults with type 2 diabetes or impaired glucose tolerance receiving high-protein, high-cholesterol versus high-protein, low-cholesterol hypocaloric diets, HDL cholesterol increased on the high-protein, high-cholesterol diet. All subjects lost weight and reduced triglycerides, TC, A1C, fasting blood glucose, and fasting insulin. There was no change in LDL cholesterol (Pearce 2011).

Saturated Fatty Acids and Insulin Resistance

Strong evidence indicates that intake of dietary SFAs is positively associated with intermediate and end point health outcomes for two distinct pathways: *1)* increased TC, LDL cholesterol, and risk of CVD and *2)* increased markers of insulin resistance and increased risk of type 2 diabetes. A systematic review of 15 trials (9 trials in subjects without diabetes and 6 trials in subjects with diabetes) analyzed the effect of specific dietary fatty acids on insulin sensitivity (Galgani 2008). Three studies reported a differential effect on insulin sensitivity, showing decreased insulin sensitivity in healthy subjects and subjects with type 2 diabetes after SFA diets versus MUFA or PUFA diets.

Trans Fatty Acids and Lipids

TFAs raise TC and LDL cholesterol. Unlike SFAs, TFAs do not increase and may decrease HDL cholesterol. TFAs increase the TC/HDL cholesterol ratio in a dose-dependent manner (Acad Nutr Diet 2010). Although the studies are not in subjects with diabetes, replacing carbohydrates with TFAs significantly increases TC and LDL cholesterol (Mensink 2003; Judd 2002). Diet quality scores that included intake of TFAs were inversely associated with the risk for type 2 diabetes (de Koning 2011).

It is recommended to keep TFA consumption as low as possible by limiting foods that contain synthetic and natural sources of *trans* fats, such as partially hydrogenated oils, and by limiting other solid fats. There is insufficient evidence to suggest ruminant TFA and industrial TFA be considered differentially in their metabolic effect. Total TFA intake should be considered the target for change. However, it is best to avoid industrial TFAs, while leaving small amounts of ruminant TFAs in the diet (USDA NEL 2010).

Dietary Cholesterol

The current recommendation is to consume <200 mg/day dietary cholesterol for people with or at high risk for CVD and type 2 diabetes. Increased dietary cholesterol intake is associated with CVD risk (Acad Nutr Diet 2010). No studies have been published since 2008.

Monounsaturated Fatty Acids

Much interest has been paid to the effects of MUFAs on health because of the low rates of CVD and atherosclerotic CVD in the Mediterranean area, where diets are high in fat, but the fatty acids are mainly from olive oil. Strong evidence indicates that dietary MUFAs are associated with improved blood lipids related to both CVD and type 2 diabetes, when MUFA replaces dietary SFA. The evidence shows that when 5% of SFA is replaced with MUFA, it decreases intermediate markers and the risk of CVD and type 2 diabetes in healthy adults and improves insulin responsiveness in insulin-resistant individuals and individuals with type 2 diabetes (USDA NEL 2010). In a small study with 30 nonobese adults with well-controlled type 1 diabetes, there were no significant differences in lipids when a lower-carbohydrate, higher-MUFA diet was compared to a higher-carbohydrate, lower-fat diet (Strychar 2009).

Polyunsaturated Fatty Acids

Strong and consistent evidence indicates that dietary omega-6 PUFAs are associated with improved blood lipids related to CVD, in particular when PUFAs are a replacement for dietary SFAs or TFAs. Eating patterns high in PUFAs have similar effects on plasma lipid concentrations as patterns high in MUFAs (ADA

2008). Energy replacement of SFAs with PUFAs decreases TC, LDL cholesterol, and triglycerides, as well as numerous markers of inflammation. Linoleic acid is the most potent TC and LDL cholesterol–lowering fatty acid (Mensink 1990) and has a bigger cholesterol-lowering effect than MUFAs (Howard 1995). However, subjects in these studies did not have diabetes.

Omega-3 Fatty Acids

A review of literature examining the role of omega-3 fatty acids in subjects with diabetes and/or CVD reported an association with fish and omega-3 fatty acid consumption and decreased total CVD mortality (~15–19%), decreased platelet aggregation, improved lipid profiles (including decreased triglyceride levels), decreased blood pressure levels, and decreased inflammation (McEwen 2010).

A Cochrane database systematic review of trials in subjects with type 2 diabetes concluded that omega-3 PUFA supplementation lowered triglycerides (~40 mg/dL) and VLDL cholesterol (~3 mg/dL) and raised LDL cholesterol (~4 mg/dL), although results were nonsignificant in subgroups and had no statistically significant effect on glycemic control or fasting insulin (Hartweg 2008). A second systematic review and meta-analysis by Hartweg and colleagues included seven new trials in subjects with type 2 diabetes from 2007 and 2008 and concluded the results supported the triglyceride-lowering effect of omega-3 PUFAs, with no significant impact on A1C (Hartweg 2009). A trial in postmenopausal women with type 2 diabetes consuming supplemental fish oil capsules (3 g fish oil/day with 1.08 g eicosapentaenoic acid [EPA], 0.72 g docosahexaenoic acid [DHA]) had a 12% reduction in triglycerides (Kabir 2007). No effect was seen on TC, LDL cholesterol, or HDL cholesterol.

The effects of fish oil supplements on lipoprotein subclasses were measured by nuclear magnetic resonance in subjects with type 2 diabetes (Mostad 2008). Compared with corn oil, fish oil tended to increase HDL size and small LDL concentration, with no effect on oxidized LDL cholesterol. Insulin sensitivity (glucose utilization) decreased in the fish oil group compared with the corn oil group; however, the decrease did not correlate with the effects on lipoprotein subclasses.

Two reviews including studies with patients with type 2 diabetes examined the effect of marine sources of omega-3 fatty acids and concluded that 2–4 g/day (EPA/DHA combined) will lower triglyceride levels by 25–30% without adversely affecting glycemic control (Rudkowska 2010; Saravanan 2010).

To meet current recommendations and possibly lower CVD risk, patients should use plant sources of omega-3 fatty acids (α-linolenic acid, an essential fatty acid for humans) from flax and chia seeds as well as walnuts, soy, and canola oil, with an intake of 0.6–1.2% of total calories (DRI: 1.6 g/day for men, 1.1 g/day for women). No evidence is available on the effectiveness of lipid lowering with plant sources of omega-3 fatty acids. Food sources of omega-3 fatty acids are listed in Table 13.2.

Nuts and Serum Lipids

Moderate evidence indicates that consumption of unsalted peanuts and tree nuts, specifically walnuts, almonds, and pistachios, in the context of a nutritionally adequate diet and when total calorie intake is held constant, has a favorable impact on CVD risk factors, particularly serum lipid levels (Acad Nutr Diet 2010). In a recent review on almonds, the authors reported that almonds have been found to have a consistent LDL cholesterol–lowering effect in healthy individuals and in individuals with high cholesterol and diabetes, in both controlled and free-living settings (Berryman 2011). A study of Chinese adults with type 2 diabetes and mild hyperlipidemia examined the effect of a National Cholesterol Education Program (NCEP) step II diet (control) or the same diet plus almonds (60 g/day). The diet including almonds significantly decreased TC, LDL cholesterol, ratio of LDL cholesterol to HDL cholesterol, plasma apolipoprotein (apo)-B, and ratio of apoB to apoA-1 (Li 2011).

Table 13.2 Sources of Omega-3 Fatty Acids

Food	α-Linolenic acid (g)	EPA (g)	DHA (g)
Seafood, 3 oz cooked			
Flounder and sole	0.02	0.14	0.11
Halibut, Atlantic and Pacific	0.01	0.07	0.13
Herring, Atlantic	0.11	0.77	0.94
Herring, Atlantic, pickled	0	0.72	0.46
Herring, Pacific	0.06	1.06	0.75
King mackerel	n/a	0.15	0.19
Salmon, Atlantic, farmed	0.10	0.59	1.24
Salmon, Pacific, Sockeye	0.07	0.23	0.45
Trout, mixed species	0.17	0.22	0.58
Tuna, white, canned in water, drained	0.06	0.20	0.54
Tuna, white, canned in oil, drained	0.17	0.06	0.15
Oyster, Eastern, farmed	0.05	0.20	0.18
Sardine, Atlantic, canned in oil, drained	0.42	0.40	0.43
Sardine, Pacific, canned in tomato sauce	0.20	0.45	0.74
Scallop, bay and sea	0.01	0.06	0.09
Tilapia	0.04	0.01	0.11
Flax seed, 14 g (~2 Tbsp)	3.37	0	0
Chia seed, 14 g (~2 Tbsp)	2.49	0	0
Walnuts, 1 oz (14 halves)	2.57	0	0
Canola oil, 1 tsp	0.41	0	0
Purslane, ½ cup, raw*	0.01*	0	0
Purslane, ½ cup, cooked*	0.03*	0	0
Kale, ½ cup, cooked	0.07	0	0
Spinach, ½ cup, cooked	0.08	0	0

Adapted from the U.S. Department of Agriculture, Agricultural Research Service, 2010. USDA National Nutrient Database for Standard Reference, Release 24. Nutrient Data Laboratory Home Page, www.ars.usda.gov/nutrientdata/sr
*Nutrition Data System for Research, software version 2011, developed by the Nutrition Coordinating Center (NCC), University of Minnesota, Minneapolis, MN.

Replacement of carbohydrate with 75 g nuts produced significant decreases in TC and LDL cholesterol and showed promise in improving glycemic measures in subjects with type 2 diabetes (Jenkins 2011). In another trial, adults with type 2 diabetes followed an ad libitum diet (control) and a diet supplemented with 56 g unroasted, shelled walnuts (isocalorically substituted) per day (Ma 2010). When compared to baseline, the walnut diet decreased TC and LDL cholesterol and increased fasting plasma glucose. Two recent reviews (Kendall 2010; Jenkins 2008b) highlight the benefit of nut consumption in people with type 2 diabetes, including improvement of blood lipid profile.

Stanols/Sterols and Dyslipidemia in Diabetes

The NCEP Adult Treatment Panel III guidelines include adding foods fortified with plant stanols/sterols (2 g/day) as options to enhance LDL cholesterol lowering. A meta-analysis examined the effect on lipid parameters of plant sterols or stanols in patients with type 2 diabetes (Baker 2009). Stanol/sterol doses ranged from 1.6 to 3 g/day and were found to significantly reduce total and LDL cholesterol. HDL cholesterol showed a trend towards improvement but was not significant, and no beneficial effect was seen on triglyceride levels. Two randomized controlled trials (RCTs) investigated the effect on lipid parameters of daily consumption of 2–3 g plant stanol/sterol esters in subjects with type 1 diabetes (Hallikainen 2011; Hallikainen 2008). Both statin-treated (Hallikainen 2011) and non–statin-treated participants (Hallikainen 2008) experienced significantly reduced TC and LDL cholesterol. In both studies, no significant effects were seen on HDL cholesterol or triglycerides.

Soluble Fiber and CVD Risk Factors

A recent review examined the evidence pertaining to the cholesterol-lowering effect of oat β-glucan published between 1997 and 2010 (Othman 2011). Studies included subjects with and without diabetes. Intervention doses of β-glucan ranged from 2.8 to 10.3 g/day. Overall, research from the past 13 years demonstrates a daily consumption of 3 g oat β-glucan is associated with an average 5% reduction in TC and a 7% reduction in LDL cholesterol.

Subjects with type 2 diabetes consumed a soup enriched with 3.5 g β-glucan per day or a placebo soup in addition to the subjects' regular diet (Cugnet-Anceau 2010). At the end of 2 months, the group consuming the β-glucan soup had a significant lowering of triglycerides compared to the control group, whose levels actually increased. No significant between-group differences were seen in TC, LDL cholesterol, HDL cholesterol, A1C, or fasting blood glucose levels. In the β-glucan group, HDL cholesterol increased significantly from baseline. Another study on adults with type 2 diabetes and LDL cholesterol >130 mg/dL receiving a bread enriched with β-glucan (3 g/day) showed significant reductions in both LDL cholesterol and TC compared to the control group (Liatis 2009).

Food sources of total and soluble fiber are listed in Table 13.3.

Soy Protein and Lipids

Soy protein intake may have small effects on TC and LDL cholesterol in adults with normal or elevated blood lipids, although results from systematic reviews are inconsistent (USDA NEL 2010). In a crossover study to determine the effect of 40 g soy protein isolate consumption on serum lipids in adults with diet-controlled type 2 diabetes, LDL cholesterol was significantly reduced, but there was no effect on TC, HDL, non-HDL cholesterol, triglycerides, apoB, or apoA-1 (Pipe 2009).

Other Eating Patterns and Lipids

A Paleolithic dietary pattern characterized by increased consumption of whole grains, vegetables, fruits, nuts, olive oil, legumes, and fish, moderate in alcohol and low in red and processed meats, refined carbohydrates, and full-fat dairy, has been shown to lower triglyceride levels in patients with diabetes (Jönsson 2009).

A large trial assessed the effects of a traditional Mediterranean-style eating pattern on primary coronary heart disease prevention in patients with type 2 diabetes or with three or more other coronary heart disease risk factors. A low-fat diet or Mediterranean diet plus olive oil or Mediterranean diet plus nuts were compared. Individuals who improved their diet toward a Mediterranean diet pattern rich in olive oil reduced their apoB/apoA-1 ratio and apoA-1 concentrations. Changes in the Framingham score were significant between the Mediterranean diet plus olive oil group versus the low-fat group (Solá 2011).

Weight Loss and Lipids

Lifestyle-based weight-loss interventions are also recommended to improve glycemic control and CVD risk factors such as dyslipidemia. The Look AHEAD

Table 13.3 Sources of Total and Soluble Fiber

Food	Soluble Fiber (g)	Total Fiber (g)	Food	Soluble Fiber (g)	Total Fiber (g)
Cereal Grains, ½ cup cooked			Legumes, ½ cup cooked		
Barley	0.9	4.3	Black beans	0.6	9.0
Oatmeal	1.0	2.1	Kidney beans	1.3	5.7
Oat bran	1.1	2.9	Lima beans	0.9	4.4
Seeds (14 g)			Lentils	0.4	5.8
Chia (~2 Tbsp)	0.7	5.3	Black-eyed peas	0.7	5.6
Flax (~2 Tbsp)	1.2	3.9	Vegetables, ½ cup cooked		
Psyllium (~3 1/3 Tbsp)	9.9	11.0	Bok choy	0.1	0.9
Fruit, 1 medium			Broccoli	0.3	2.6
Apple	1.3	4.4	Brussels sprouts	0.3	2.0
Banana	1.0	3.1	Carrots	0.5	2.3
Blackberries (½ cup)	0.3	3.8	Kale	1.1	1.3
Pear	1.6	5.6	Okra	0.6	2.0
Prunes (¼ cup)	1.7	3.1	Spinach	0.3	2.2

Adapted from Nutrition Data System for Research, software version 2011, developed by the Nutrition Coordinating Center (NCC), University of Minnesota, Minneapolis, MN.

study is examining the long-term impact of an intensive lifestyle intervention, compared with usual care (diabetes support and education [DSE]), on cardiovascular morbidity and mortality in overweight or obese individuals with type 2 diabetes. Averaged over 4 years, participants in the intensive lifestyle intervention experienced significantly greater improvements in weight, fitness, glycemic control, blood pressure, HDL cholesterol, and triglycerides than individuals in the DSE group. The DSE group experienced greater overall reductions in LDL cholesterol, but after adjusting for medication use, changes in LDL cholesterol did not differ between the intensive lifestyle intervention and DSE groups (Look AHEAD 2010).

Alcohol and Lipids

The effect of alcohol on lipids is discussed in Chapter 4.

Other Food Sources/Components and Lipids

Supplementation with chia seeds or flaxseed-derived lignan capsules had no effect on the lipid profiles of adults with type 2 diabetes (Vuksan 2007; Pan 2007). No other studies examining flaxseed consumption in people with diabetes were found as of the writing of this text. A meta-analysis of five RCTs showed no effect of cinnamon on the lipid profiles of subjects with type 1 or type 2 diabetes (Baker 2008).

Preliminary evidence from studies before 2008 suggests fenugreek seeds may lower triglycerides and raise HDL cholesterol in subjects with type 2 diabetes (Gupta 2001) and decrease TC in subjects with type 2 diabetes also diagnosed with coronary artery disease (Bordia 1997). In a double-blind, placebo-controlled study, 25 subjects newly diagnosed with type 2 diabetes received 1 g/day fenugreek seed extract or placebo capsules along with usual care (Gupta 2001). After 2 months, serum triglycerides decreased and HDL cholesterol increased ($P < 0.05$ for both) in the fenugreek group compared to the control group.

Fenugreek, 2.5 g twice daily (5 g/day total), or placebo was administered to 60 subjects with type 2 diabetes also diagnosed with coronary artery disease (Bordia 1997). After 3 months, TC and triglycerides decreased significantly from baseline levels in the fenugreek group (240.2 ± 10.5 vs. 225.0 ± 10.2 mg/dL, $P < 0.01$, and 160.5 ± 12.2 vs. 135.3 ± 10.3 mg/dL, $P < 0.01$, respectively). However, the authors did not report any significant between-group changes. In another arm of this study, 5 g/day fenugreek was administered to healthy subjects and produced no significant effect on any outcome measure.

Supplementation with garlic powder in people with type 2 diabetes has demonstrated a significant lowering of triglycerides (Sobenin 2008). Research in healthy subjects produced contradictory evidence about the effects of garlic on cholesterol and triglyceride levels (Khoo 2009; Reinhart 2009).

Glycemic Index/Glycemic Load and Lipids

Both the Acad Nutr Diet Evidence Analysis Library and USDA DGAC state that because of limited evidence, no conclusion can be drawn regarding the relationship between glycemic index (GI) or glycemic load (GL) and CVD (Acad Nutr Diet 2008; USDA NEL 2010). A systematic review and meta-analysis of 45 studies including subjects with type 1 and type 2 diabetes or impaired glucose tolerance showed low GL (a decrease in available carbohydrate intake) reduced fasting triglycerides compared to low-GI diets (Livesey 2008). In patients with type 2 diabetes following either a low-GI or high–cereal fiber diet, the low-GI diet increased HDL cholesterol and lowered the LDL cholesterol–to–HDL cholesterol ratio, whereas the high–cereal fiber diet decreased HDL cholesterol and A1C (Jenkins 2008a). In a study in obese patients with type 2 diabetes, a low-GI, moderate-carbohydrate diet (55% carbohydrate), compared to a lower-carbohydrate (goal <20 g/day; actual intake 49 g/day), ketogenic diet, showed no effect on HDL cholesterol. However, the low-carbohydrate, ketogenic diet significantly increased HDL cholesterol and lowered A1C (Westman 2008). See Chapter 2 for further discussion of GI and GL in diabetes nutrition therapy.

NUTRITION RECOMMENDATIONS FOR DISORDERS OF LIPID METABOLISM IN DIABETES

There is no one diet for diabetes or ADA diet. The recommended eating pattern can only be defined as a nutrition prescription based on assessment and treatment goals and outcomes. Nutrition therapy for people with diabetes should be individualized, with consideration given to usual eating habits and other lifestyle factors. Monitoring metabolic parameters including blood glucose levels, A1C, lipids, blood pressure, body weight, and renal function, if appropriate, as well as quality of life, is crucial to ensure successful outcomes.

Scientific evidence strongly supports the effectiveness of nutrition therapy as a means to manage dyslipidemia and reduce risk factors associated with CVD. In addition to the well-documented role of SFAs and TFAs on LDL cholesterol and CVD, the nutrition prescription incorporates the use of foods containing specific key nutrients, with proven benefits for achieving optimal lipid management and CVD outcomes.

Medical nutrition therapy provided by a registered dietitian to patients with an abnormal lipid profile has been shown to reduce patients' daily dietary fat (5–8%), saturated fat (2–4%), and energy intake (232–710 kcal/day), resulting in a reduction in serum TC ($\downarrow$7–21%), LDL cholesterol ($\downarrow$7–22%), and triglycerides ($\downarrow$11–31%) (Acad Nutr Diet 2010).

The eating pattern based on the individual's needs should provide a total fat intake of 25–35% of calories, with <7% of calories from SFAs and TFAs. Because TFAs raise TC and LDL cholesterol and may decrease HDL cholesterol, TFA consumption should be as low as possible. Cholesterol consumption should be <200 mg/day. The majority of total fat intake should be derived from unsaturated fat sources. For individuals at their appropriate body weight, without elevated LDL cholesterol or triglyceride levels, and with normal HDL cholesterol levels, saturated fat calories should be replaced by unsaturated fat. This eating pattern can lower LDL cholesterol up to 16% and decrease risk of CVD and CVD events (Acad Nutr Diet 2010). A recommended energy intake can be developed with consideration of whether the goal is weight maintenance or weight loss.

Because of their beneficial fatty acid profile, as well as other nutritional components, nuts may be isocalorically incorporated into the eating pattern to achieve lipid lowering. Calorie adjustments may be required because of the high caloric contribution of nuts. Food sources of omega-3 fatty acids and/or MUFAs, and a reduction of refined carbohydrate, may also be effective in reducing serum triglycerides without an adverse impact on HDL cholesterol (Acad Nutr Diet 2010).

For individuals with elevated triglycerides (≥150 mg/dL), a calorie-controlled eating pattern that avoids extremes in carbohydrate and fat intake and includes physical activity should be recommended. Non–nutrient-dense calorie sources including alcohol and added sugars should be limited as much as possible. Weight loss of 7–10% of body weight should be encouraged, if indicated. These lifestyle changes have been shown to lower triglyceride levels. In addition to lifestyle modification, supplemental EPA and DHA (2–4 g/day) may be used under medical supervision. These high doses of supplemental EPA and DHA have been shown to lower triglycerides in patients with elevated levels (>200 mg/dL) (Acad Nutr Diet 2010).

Eating patterns should incorporate fiber-rich foods that contribute at least 25–30 g fiber per day, with special emphasis on soluble fiber sources (7–13 g). Foods rich in soluble fiber include fruits, vegetables, and whole grains, especially high-fiber cereals, oatmeal, and legumes (particularly beans). Eating patterns high in total and soluble fiber can further reduce TC by 2–3% and LDL cholesterol up to 7%.

Foods enriched with plant sterol and stanol ester may be incorporated into the diet, over two or three times per day, for a total consumption of 2–3 g plant sterol/stanol esters per day. These doses further lower TC by 4–11% and LDL cholesterol by 7–15%. Doses beyond 3 g have not been shown to provide additional benefit. Plant stanols and plant sterols are also effective in people taking statin drugs. To prevent weight gain, isocaloric substitutions of nuts and plant stanol/sterol– and fiber-containing foods must be made with other foods.

BIBLIOGRAPHY

Adiels M, Olofsson SO, Taskinen MR, Borén J: Overproduction of very low-density lipoproteins is the hallmark of the dyslipidemia in the metabolic syndrome. *Arterioscler Throm Vasc Biol* 28:1225–1236, 2008

Academy of Nutrition and Dietetics: Disorders of lipid metabolism evidence-based nutrition practice guideline, 2010. Available from http://www.adaevidencelibrary.com/topic.cfm?cat=4527. Accessed November 2011

Academy of Nutrition and Dietetics: Type 1 and type 2 diabetes evidence-based nutrition practice guidelines for adults, 2008. Available from http://www.adaevidencelibrary.com/topic.cfm?=3252. Accessed November 2011

American Diabetes Association: Standards of medical care in diabetes: 2012. *Diabetes Care* 35 (Suppl. 1):S11–S63, 2012

American Diabetes Association: 2011 National Diabetes Fact Sheet (released Jan. 26, 2011). Available from http://www.diabetes.org/diabetes-basics/diabetes-statistics. Accessed November 2011

American Diabetes Association, Bantle JP, Wylie-Rosett J, Albright AL, Apovian CM, Clark NG, Franz MJ, Hoogwerf BJ, Lichtenstein AH, Mayer-Davis E,

Mooradian AD, Wheeler ML: Nutrition recommendations and interventions for diabetes (Position Statement). *Diabetes Care* 31 (Suppl. 1):S61–S78, 2008

Azadbakht L, Fard NRP, Karimi M, Baghaei MH, Surkan PJ, Rahimi M, Esmail-lzadeh A, Willett WC: Effects of the Dietary Approaches to Stop Hypertension (DASH) eating plan on cardiovascular risks among type 2 diabetic patients. *Diabetes Care* 34:55–57, 2011

Baker WL, Baker EL, Coleman CI: The effect of plant sterols or stanols on lipid parameters in patients with type 2 diabetes: a meta-analysis. *Diabetes Res Clin Pract* 84:E33–E37, 2009

Baker WL, Gutierrez-Williams G, White CM, Kluger J, Coleman CI: Effect of cinnamon on glucose control and lipid parameters. *Diabetes Care* 31:41–43, 2008

Belalcazar LM, Reboussin DM, Haffner SM, Reeves RS, Schwenke DC, Hoogeveen RC, Pi-Sunyer FX, Ballantyne CM: Marine omega-3 fatty acid intake: associations with cardiometabolic risk and response to weight loss intervention in the Look AHEAD (Action for Health in Diabetes) study. *Diabetes Care* 33:197–199, 2010

Berryman CE, Preston AG, Karmally W, Deckelbaum RJ, Kris-Etherton PM: Effects of almond consumption on the reduction of LDL-cholesterol: a discussion of potential mechanisms and future research directions. *Nutr Rev* 69:171–185, 2011

Bordia A, Verma SK, Srivastava KC: Effect of ginger (Zingiber officinale Rosc.) and fenugreek (Trigonella foenumgraecum L.) on blood lipids, blood sugar and platelet aggregation in patients with coronary artery disease. *Prostaglandins Leukot Essent Fatty Acids* 56:379–384, 1997

Bruckert E, Rosenbaum D: Lowering LDL-cholesterol through diet: potential role in the statin era. *Curr Opin Lipidol* 22:43–48, 2011

Buse JB, Ginsberg HN, Bakris GL, Clark NG, Costa F, Eckel R, Fonseca V, Gerstein HC, Grundy S, Nesto RW, Pignone MP, Plutzky J, Porte D, Redberg R, Stitzel KF, Stone NJ: Primary prevention of cardiovascular diseases in people with diabetes mellitus: a scientific statement from the American Heart Association and the American Diabetes Association. *Circulation* 115:114–126, 2007

Cadario F, Prodam F, Pasqualicchio S, Bellone S, Bonsignori I, Demarchi I, Monzani A, Bona G: Lipid profile and nutritional intake in children and adolescents with type 1 diabetes improve after a structured dietician training to a Mediterranean-style diet. *J Endocrinol Invest* 27 May 2011 [Epub ahead of print]

Ciccarone E, Di Castelnuovo A, Salcuni M, Siani M, Giacco A, Donati MB, De Gaetano G, Capani F, Iacoviello L, Gendiabe Investigators: A high-score Mediterranean dietary pattern is associated with a reduced risk of peripheral arterial disease in Italian patients with type 2 diabetes. *J Thromb Haemost* 1:1744–1752, 2003

Cugnet-Anceau C, Nazare JA, Biorklund M, Le Coquil E, Sassolas A, Sothier M, Holm J, Landin-Olsson M, Onning G, Laville M, Moulin P: A controlled study of consumption of beta-glucan-enriched soups for 2 months by type 2 diabetic free-living subjects. *Br J Nutr* 103:422–428, 2010

de Koning L, Chiuve SE, Fung TT, Willett WC, Rimm EB, Hu FB: Diet-quality scores and the risk of type 2 diabetes in men. *Diabetes Care* 34:1150–1156, 2011

De Natale C, Annuzzi G, Bozzetto L, Mazzarella R, Costabile G, Ciano O, Riccardi G, Rivellese AA: Effects of a plant-based high-carbohydrate/high-fiber diet versus high-monounsaturated fat/low-carbohydrate diet on postprandial lipids in type 2 diabetic patients. *Diabetes Care* 32:2168–2173, 2009

Diakoumopoulou E, Tentolouris N, Kirlaki E, Perrea D, Kitsou E, Psallas M, Doulgerakis D, Katsilambros N: Plasma homocysteine levels in patients with type 2 diabetes in a Mediterranean population: relation with nutritional and other factors. *Nutr Metab Cardiovasc Dis* 15:109–117, 2005

Ervin RB: Prevalence of metabolic syndrome among adults 20 years of age and over, by sex, age, race and ethnicity, and body mass index: United States, 2003–2006. *Natl Health Stat Report* 5:1–7, 2009

Franz MJ, Powers MA, Leontos C, Holzmeister LA, Kulkarni K, Monk A, Wedel N, Gradwell E: The evidence for medical nutrition therapy for type 1 and type 2 diabetes in adults. *J Am Diet Assoc* 110:1852–1889, 2010

Galgani JE, Uauy RD, Aguirre CA, Diaz EO: Effect of the dietary fat quality on insulin sensitivity. *Br J Nutr* 100:471–479, 2008

Grant RW, Cagliero E, Murphy-Sheehy P, Singer DE, Nathan DM, Meigs JB: Comparison of hyperglycemia, hypertension, and hypercholesterolemia management in patients with type 2 diabetes. *Am J Med* 112:603–609, 2002

Gupta A, Gupta R, Lal B: Effect of Trigonella foenum-graecum (fenugreek) seeds on glycaemic control and insulin resistance in type 2 diabetes mellitus: a double blind placebo controlled study. *J Assoc Physicians India* 49:1057–1061, 2001

Haimoto H, Sasakabe T, Wakai K, Umegaki H: Effects of a low-carbohydrate diet on glycemic control in outpatients with severe type 2 diabetes. *Nutr Metab (Lond)* 6:21, 2009

Hallikainen M, Kurl S, Laakso M, Miettinen TA, Gylling H: Plant stanol esters lower LDL cholesterol level in statin-treated subjects with type 1 diabetes by interfering with the absorption and synthesis of cholesterol. *Atherosclerosis* 217:473–478, 2011

Hallikainen M, Lyyra-Laitinen T, Laitinen T, Moilanen L, Miettinen TA, Gylling H: Effects of plant stanol esters on serum cholesterol concentrations, relative markers of cholesterol metabolism and endothelial function in type 1 diabetes. *Atherosclerosis* 199:432–439, 2008

Hartweg J, Farmer AJ, Holman RR, Neil A: Potential impact of omega-3 treatment on cardiovascular disease in type 2 diabetes. *Curr Opin Lipidol* 20:30–38, 2009

Hartweg J, Perera R, Montori V, Dinneen S, Neil HA, Farmer A: Omega-3 polyunsaturated fatty acids (PUFA) for type 2 diabetes mellitus. *Cochrane Database Syst Rev* CD003205, 2008

Howard BV, Hannah JS, Heiser CC, Jablonski KA, Paidi MC, Alarif L, Robbins DC, Howard WJ: Polyunsaturated fatty acids result in greater cholesterol lowering and less triacylglycerol elevation than do monounsaturated fatty acids in a dose-response comparison in a multiracial study group. *Am J Clin Nutr* 62:392–402, 1995

Jenkins DJ, Kendall CW, Banach MS, Srichaikul K, Vidgen E, Mitchell S, Parker T, Nishi S, Bashyam B, de Souza R, Ireland C, Josse RG: Nuts as a replacement for carbohydrates in the diabetic diet. *Diabetes Care* 34:1706–1711, 2011

Jenkins DJ, Hu FB, Tapsell LC, Josse AR, Kendall CW: Possible benefit of nuts in type 2 diabetes. *J Nutr* 138:1752S–1756S, 2008b

Jenkins DJ, Kendall CW, McKeown-Eyssen G, Josse RG, Silverberg J, Booth GL, Vidgen E, Josse AR, Nguyen TH, Corrigan S, Banach MS, Ares S, Mitchell S, Emam A, Augustin LSA, Parker TL, Leiter LA: Effect of a low–glycemic index or a high–cereal fiber diet on type 2 diabetes: a randomized trial. *JAMA* 300:2742–2753, 2008a

Jönsson T, Granfeldt Y, Ahrén B, Branell UC, Pålsson G, Hansson A, Söderström M, Lindeberg S: Beneficial effects of a Paleolithic diet on cardiovascular risk factors in type 2 diabetes: a randomized cross-over pilot study. *Cardiovasc Diabetol* 8:35, 2009

Judd JT, Baer DJ, Clevidence BA, Kris-Etherton P, Muesing RA, Iwane M: Dietary cis and trans monounsaturated and saturated FA and plasma lipids and lipoproteins in men. *Lipids* 37:123–131, 2002

Kabir M, Skurnik G, Naour N, Pechtner V, Meugnier E, Rome S, Quignard-Boulangé A, Vidal H, Slama G, Clément K, Guerre-Millo M, Rizkalla SW: Treatment for 2 months with n-3 polyunsaturated fatty acids reduces adiposity and some atherogenic factors but does not improve insulin sensitivity in women with type 2 diabetes: a randomized controlled study. *Am J Clin Nutr* 86:1670–1679, 2007

Kendall CW, Josse AR, Esfahani A, Jenkins DJ: Nuts, metabolic syndrome and diabetes. *Br J Nutr* 104:465–473, 2010

Khoo YS, Aziz Z: Garlic supplementation and serum cholesterol: a meta-analysis. *J Clin Pharm Ther* 34:133–145, 2009

Kodama S, Saito K, Tanaka S, Maki M, Yachi Y, Sato M, Sugawara A, Totsuka K, Shimano H, Ohashi Y, Yamada N, Sone H: Influence of fat and carbohydrate proportions on the metabolic profile in patients with type 2 diabetes: a meta-analysis. *Diabetes Care* 32:959–965, 2009

Li SC, Liu YH, Liu JF, Chang WH, Chen CM, Chen CY: Almond consumption improved glycemic control and lipid profiles in patients with type 2 diabetes mellitus. *Metabolism* 60:474–479, 2011

Liatis S, Tsapogas P, Chala E, Dimosthenopoulos C, Kyriakopoulos K, Kapantais E, Katsilambros N: The consumption of bread enriched with betaglucan reduces LDL-cholesterol and improves insulin resistance in patients with type 2 diabetes. *Diabetes Metab* 35:115–120, 2009

Liese AD, Bortsov A, Günther AL, Dabelea D, Reynolds K, Standiford DA, Liu L, Williams DE, Mayer-Davis EJ, D'Agostino RB Jr, Bell R, Marcovina S: Association of DASH diet with cardiovascular risk factors in youth with diabetes mellitus: the SEARCH for Diabetes in Youth study. *Circulation* 123:1410–1417, 2011

Livesey G, Taylor R, Hulshof T, Howlett J: Glycemic response and health: a systematic review and meta-analysis: relations between dietary glycemic properties and health outcomes. *Am J Clin Nutr* 87 (Suppl.):258S–268S, 2008

Look AHEAD Research Group, Wing RR: Long-term effects of a lifestyle intervention on weight and cardiovascular risk factors in individuals with type 2 diabetes mellitus: four-year results of the Look AHEAD trial. *Arch Intern Med* 170:1566–1575, 2010

Ma Y, Njike VY, Millet J, Dutta S, Doughty K, Treu JA, Katz DL: Effects of walnut consumption on endothelial function in type 2 diabetic subjects: a randomized controlled crossover trial. *Diabetes Care* 33:227–232, 2010

Massing MW, Foley KA, Sueta CA, Chowdhury M, Biggs DP, Alexander CM, Simpson RJ Jr: Trends in lipid management among patients with coronary artery disease: has diabetes received the attention it deserves? *Diabetes Care* 26:991–997, 2003

McEwen B, Morel-Kopp MC, Tofler G, Ward C: Effect of omega-3 fish oil on cardiovascular risk in diabetes. *Diabetes Educ* 36:565–584, 2010

Mensink RP, Katan MB: Effect of dietary trans fatty acids on high-density and low-density lipoprotein cholesterol levels in healthy subjects. *N Engl J Med* 323:439–445, 1990

Mensink RP, Zock PL, Kester AD, Katan MB: Effects of dietary fatty acids and carbohydrates on the ratio of serum total to HDL cholesterol and on serum lipids and apolipoproteins: a meta-analysis of 60 controlled trials. *Am J Clin Nutr* 77:1146–1155, 2003

Mostad IL, Bjerve KS, Lydersen S, Grill V: Effects of marine n-3 fatty acid supplementation on lipoprotein subclasses measured by nuclear magnetic resonance in subjects with type II diabetes. *Eur J Clin Nutr* 62:419–429, 2008

Othman RA, Moghadasian MH, Jones PJ: Cholesterol-lowering effects of oat β-glucan. *Nutr Rev* 69:299–309, 2011

Packard CJ: Triacylglycerol-rich lipoproteins and the generation of small, dense low-density lipoprotein. *Biochem Soc Trans* 31:1066–1069, 2003

Pan A, Sun J, Chen Y, Ye X, Li H, Yu Z, Wang Y, Gu W, Zhang X, Chen X, Demark-Wahnefried W, Liu Y, Lin X: Effects of a flaxseed-derived lignan supplement in type 2 diabetic patients: a randomized, double-blind, cross-over trial. *PLoS One* 2:e1148, 2007

Pearce KL, Clifton PM, Noakes M: Egg consumption as part of an energy-restricted high-protein diet improves blood lipid and blood glucose profiles in individuals with type 2 diabetes. *Br J Nutr* 105:584–592, 2011

Pipe EA, Gobert CP, Capes SE, Darlington GA, Lampe JW, Duncan AM: Soy protein reduces serum LDL cholesterol and the LDL cholesterol:HDL cholesterol and apolipoprotein B:apolipoprotein A-1 ratios in adults with type 2 diabetes. *J Nutr* 139:1700–1706, 2009

Pyörälä K, Lehto S, De Bacquer D, De Sutter J, Sans S, Keil U, Wood D, De Backer G, EUROASPIRE I Group, EUROASPIRE II Group: Risk factor management in diabetic and non-diabetic patients with coronary heart disease: findings from the EUROASPIRE I AND II surveys. *Diabetologia* 47:1257–1265, 2004

Reinhart KM, Talati R, White CM, Coleman CI: The impact of garlic on lipid parameters: a systematic review and meta-analysis. *Nutr Res Rev* 22:39–48, 2009

Rudkowska I: Fish oils for cardiovascular disease: impact on diabetes. *Maturitas* 67:25–28, 2010

Saravanan P, Davidson NC, Schmidt EB, Calder PC: Cardiovascular effects of marine omega-3 fatty acids. *Lancet* 376:540–550, 2010

Siri-Tarino PW, Sun Q, Hu FB, Krauss RM: Saturated fat, carbohydrate, and cardiovascular disease. *Am J Clin Nutr* 91:502–509, 2010

Snell-Bergeon JK, Chartier-Logan C, Maahs DM, Ogden LG, Hokanson JE, Kinney GL, Eckel RH, Ehrlich J, Rewers M: Adults with type 1 diabetes eat a high-fat atherogenic diet that is associated with coronary artery calcium. *Diabetologia* 52:801–809, 2009

Sobenin IA, Nedosugova LV, Filatova LV, Balabolkin MI, Gorchakova TV, Orekhov AN: Metabolic effects of time-released garlic powder tablets in type 2 diabetes mellitus: the results of double-blinded placebo-controlled study. *Acta Diabetol* 45:1–6, 2008

Solá R, Fitó M, Estruch R, Salas-Salvadó J, Corella D, de La Torre R, Muñoz MA, Del Carmen López-Sabater M, Martínez-González MA, Arós F, Ruiz-Gutierrez V, Fiol M, Casals E, Wärnberg J, Buil-Cosiales P, Ros E, Konstantinidou V, Lapetra J, Serra-Majem L, Covas MI: Effect of a traditional Mediterranean diet on apolipoproteins B, A-I, and their ratio: a randomized, controlled trial. *Atherosclerosis* 218:174–180, 2011

Strychar I, Cohn JS, Renier G, Rivard M, Aris-Jilwan N, Beauregard H, Meltzer S, Bélanger A, Dumas R, Ishac A, Radwan F, Yale JF: Effects of a diet higher in carbohydrate/lower in fat versus lower in carbohydrate/higher in monounsaturated fat on postmeal triglyceride concentrations and other cardiovascular risk factors in type 1 diabetes. *Diabetes Care* 32:1597–1599, 2009

Taskinen MR: Type 2 diabetes as a lipid disorder. *Curr Mol Med* 5:297–308, 2005

U.S. Department of Agriculture, Center for Nutrition Policy and Promotion, Nutrition Evidence Library (USDA NEL): Evidence from the Report of the Dietary Guidelines Advisory Committee on the Dietary Guidelines for Americans, 2010. Available at http://www.nutritionevidencelibrary.gov. Accessed November 2011

U.S. Department of Agriculture and U.S. Department of Health and Human Services (USDA USDHHS): *Dietary Guidelines for Americans, 2010.* 7th ed. Washington, DC, U.S. Government Printing Office, December 2010. Available at www.dietaryguidelines.gov. Accessed November 2011

Vergès B: Lipid disorders in type 1 diabetes. *Diabetes Metab* 35:353–360, 2009

Vuksan V, Whitham D, Sievenpiper JL, Jenkins AL, Rogovik AL, Bazinet RP, Vidgen E, Hanna A: Supplementation of conventional therapy with the novel grain salba (salvia hispanica L.) improves major and emerging cardiovascular risk factors in type 2 diabetes: results of a randomized controlled trial. *Diabetes Care* 30:2804–2810, 2007

Westman EC, Yancy WS Jr, Mavropoulos JC, Marquart M, McDuffie JR: The effect of a low-carbohydrate, ketogenic diet versus a low-glycemic index diet on glycemic control in type 2 diabetes mellitus. *Nutr Metab (Lond)* 5:36, 2008

Wycherley TP, Noakes M, Clifton PM, Cleanthous X, Keogh JB, Brinkworth GD: A high-protein diet with resistance exercise training improves weight loss and body composition in overweight and obese patients with type 2 diabetes. *Diabetes Care* 33:969–976, 2010

Wahida Karmally, DrPH, RD, CDE, CLS, is an Associate Research Scientist and Director of Nutrition at the Irving Institute for Clinical and Translational Research, Columbia University, New York, NY. Jacqueline Santora Zimmerman, MS, RD, is a Research Nutritionist at the Irving Institute for Clinical and Translational Research, Columbia University, New York, NY.

Chapter 14

Nutrition Therapy for Diabetes and Hypertension

Karin Aebersold, MPH; Natania Wright Ostrovsky, PhD; and Judith Wylie-Rosett, EdD, RD

Highlights
Nutrition Therapy for
Diabetes and Hypertension

■ Randomized controlled trials have demonstrated that lowering blood pressure to <140 mmHg systolic and <80 mmHg diastolic can reduce cardiovascular heart disease events and stroke in individuals with diabetes.

■ Although there are no well-controlled studies of nutrition therapy and exercise among people with diabetes and hypertension, the American Diabetes Association (ADA) recommends adopting the DASH (Dietary Approaches to Stop Hypertension) eating pattern to lower blood pressure.

■ Although there are no well-controlled studies of sodium effects on blood pressure among people with diabetes and hypertension, the ADA recommends reducing sodium intake to <1,500 mg/day in persons with diabetes and hypertension.

Nutrition Therapy for Diabetes and Hypertension

Hypertension is a risk factor for developing diabetes, and in people who have diabetes, hypertension is a risk factor for developing complications. The American Diabetes Association (ADA) defines hypertension as blood pressure levels >140/90 mmHg among the general population and the population at risk for developing diabetes and suggests a lower diagnostic cut point of >130/80 mmHg among people with diabetes (ADA 2012). From 1999 to 2008, there has been a dramatic increase in the rates of awareness, treatment, and control of hypertension (Yoon 2010). In the general population, this improvement in control of hypertension was associated with a decrease in age-adjusted mortality rate of nearly 60% for stroke and 53% for coronary heart disease (Chobanian 2003).

Diabetes and hypertension both increase in prevalence by age. Among people aged ≥65 years, 26.9% have diabetes (ADA 2012) and nearly 70% have hypertension (Gillespie 2011), compared to 11.3 and 30.9%, respectively, for people aged ≥20 years. Isolated systolic hypertension is the most common type of hypertension among the older population (Franklin 2006). Isolated systolic hypertension arises more commonly from preexisting normal blood pressure or high-normal blood pressure than from preexisting diastolic hypertension. Additionally, prevalence rates for hypertension vary by race, with non-Hispanic African Americans most affected at 38.6% (Gillespie 2011).

Hypertension is a serious concern for people with diabetes; it is estimated that 67% have blood pressure ≥140/90 mmHg or use prescription drugs for hypertension (ADA 2012). The overall prevalence of hypertension in people with diabetes (57.3%) is substantially higher than in people without diabetes (28.6%) (Keenan 2011). In type 2 diabetes, essential hypertension often precedes the development of diabetes as a concomitant condition associated with the metabolic syndrome. Hypertension can also develop as the result of diabetic nephropathy. Irrespective of the etiology of hypertension in diabetes, it is considered a major factor in the development of the cardiovascular complications of diabetes. Elevated blood pressure increases risk of macrovascular complications associated with diabetes, such as heart attack, stroke, renal failure, and peripheral vascular disease (Chobanian 2003). As such, individuals with diabetes are given a higher risk status than individuals without diabetes with similar blood pressure levels.

This chapter reviews the evidence that reducing blood pressure in people with diabetes decreases mortality and reviews strategies to reduce blood pressure levels in people with diabetes through nutrition therapy interventions that assist in achieving ADA treatment goals. Evidence regarding specific medication options is beyond the scope of this chapter. Excellent resources on pharmacological therapy are available (Chobanian 2003; ADA 2012).

OVERVIEW OF TREATMENT GOALS

The ADA has established the treatment goal for systolic blood pressure of <130 mmHg and goal for diastolic blood pressure of <80 mmHg for patients with diabetes, although the systolic blood pressure target may be higher or lower based on patient characteristics and response to therapy (ADA 2012). Table 14.1 provides an overview of treatment goals and therapy strategies.

Treatment strategies couple nutrition therapy and physical activity with pharmacological agents. The ADA recommends patients with a systolic blood pressure of 130–139 mmHg or a diastolic blood pressure of 80–89 mmHg receive 3 months of nutrition therapy. If targets are not met, a pharmacological component should be added. For patients with more severe hypertension (systolic blood pressure ≥140 mmHg or diastolic blood pressure ≥90 mmHg), pharmacological therapy should be initiated in addition to the nutrition therapy. Pharmacological therapy for patients with diabetes and hypertension should include either an angiotensin-converting enzyme inhibitor or an angiotensin receptor blocker.

Decreases in Mortality in People with Diabetes as a Result of Reducing Blood Pressure

Lowering blood pressure is a major strategy for reducing morbidity and mortality related to hypertension (ADA 2012). A 2002 meta-analysis of 61 prospective, observational, general population studies found that each 20-mmHg increase in systolic blood pressure above 115/75 mmHg was associated with more than a twofold increase in stroke mortality and death from coronary heart disease as well as other vascular causes of death at ages 40–69 years (Gillespie 2011).

Studies conducted in people with diabetes have reported similar findings. In the U.K. Prospective Diabetes Study (UKPDS) in individuals with type 2 diabetes, lowering blood pressure to a mean of 144/82 mmHg significantly reduced the incidence of stroke, diabetes-elevated death, heart failure, microvascular complications, and visual loss (UKPDS 1998). A 10-year follow-up study of patients in the UKPDS reported that the benefits of previously improved blood pressure control were not sustained when between-group differences in blood pressure were lost. Therefore, it appears that good blood pressure control must be continued if the

Table 14.1 ADA Blood Pressure Treatment Goals

Blood Pressure Level	Therapy
<130/80 mmHg	Nutrition therapy* (optional)
130–139 mmHg systolic blood pressure or 80–89 mmHg diastolic blood pressure	1) 3-month nutrition therapy 2) If no change, add treatment with pharmacological agents
≥140 mmHg systolic blood pressure or ≥90 mmHg diastolic blood pressure	Treatment with pharmacological agents and nutrition therapy

*Nutrition therapy includes the DASH eating pattern, reduced sodium intake, weight loss, increased physical activity, and moderation of alcohol intake. From ADA 2012.

benefits are to be maintained (Holman 2008). Results from the randomized controlled trial (RCT) Appropriate Blood Pressure Control in Diabetes (ABCD) indicated that all-cause mortality in the hypertensive cohort was lower in the intensive blood pressure group (blood pressure decreased from 156/98 mmHg at baseline to 132/78 mmHg after treatment) than the moderate blood pressure group (154/98 mmHg at baseline to 138/89 mmHg) (Schrier 2007).

NUTRITION THERAPY FOR DIABETES AND HYPERTENSION

A literature search was conducted using PubMed MEDLINE to identify research related to diabetes, hypertension, and nutrition therapy after the publication of the chapter on diabetes and hypertension in the 1999 book *American Diabetes Association Guide to Medical Nutrition Therapy for Diabetes* (Wylie-Rosett 1999). Search criteria included diabetes, nutrition therapy, diet, and hypertension, restricted to humans, adults, and clinical trials. The initial search identified 62 articles, of which all were excluded because title or abstracts did not indicate that the study addressed the effects of nutrition therapy in human subjects with diabetes and hypertension. Additional literature searches were conducted using the same restriction, with blood glucose, diabetes, hypertension, and nutrition therapy as search terms. Of the 41 articles identified, none were trials focusing on the effects of nutrition therapy in human subjects with diabetes and hypertension. We used publications from multicenter studies that specifically looked at a blood pressure or hypertension question among a population of study subjects with diabetes to whom nutrition therapy was provided and with results that reported blood pressure changes related to nutrition therapy. We identified 98 articles, 18 articles were retrieved for more detailed evaluation, and 5 articles are included in the evidence table (Table 14.2). However, none of the articles retrieved included a comprehensive approach to nutrition therapy, so we did an additional search of known trials that were conducted with study subjects who had high blood pressure, in which nutrition therapy was provided and blood pressure was likely to have been reported as an outcome. These studies, although not conducted specifically in subjects with diabetes, provide insight into nutrition therapy for hypertension and diabetes.

Research conducted for management of hypertension using nutrition therapy interventions primarily includes the Dietary Approaches to Stop Hypertension (DASH) eating pattern, weight reduction, and sodium restriction. Additionally, physical activity and behavior modifications are important components of weight-loss programs and should be included in weight maintenance strategies (Franz 2007). In addition to the DASH eating pattern, the OmniHeart study investigated the use of two other eating patterns—a higher-protein diet (48% carbohydrate, 25% protein, and 27% fat) and a higher–unsaturated fat diet (48% carbohydrate, 15% protein, and 27% fat, primarily unsaturated fats) for treatment of individuals with hypertension (Swain 2008). All three eating patterns reduced blood pressure, total, and LDL cholesterol and estimated coronary heart disease risk.

DASH Eating Pattern

The DASH trial was a multicenter, randomized controlled diet trial that provided food to participants to study the effects of eating patterns rather than single

Table 14.2 Nutrition Therapy Evidence for Diabetes and Hypertension

	Population/ Duration of Study	Intervention (type of study)	Major Findings	Comments
Imanishi 2001	$n = 32$ patients with type 2 diabetes (11 normo-, 12 micro-, 9 macroalbuminuria/1 week on each diet	Usual sodium diet (4,600 mg) vs. low-sodium diet (1,840 mg); urinary excretion of sodium and albumin, SBP measured daily (crossover trial)	Increased sodium sensitivity of blood pressure in patients with albuminuria but normal creatinine levels; sodium sensitivity of blood pressure appears before hypertension	Sodium restriction is important in early nephropathy, even when patient is normotensive
Houlihan 2002	$n = 20$ with type 2 diabetes/two 4-week phases	Losartan, 50 mg/day, vs. placebo; in last 2 weeks of each phase, low- (~2,000 mg) or regular-sodium diets (RCT)	Losartan plus low-sodium vs. regular-sodium diet: SBP ↓ 9.7 and DBP ↓ 5.5 mmHg; ACR ↓ 8.5% (both $P = 0.002$); in placebo, no change in BP or ACR between diets	Low-sodium diet potentiates antihypertensive and antiproteinuric effects of losartan, similar to addition of second antihypertensive agent
Wing 2011	$n = 5,145$ adults with type 2 diabetes (45–76 years in age) and with a BMI ≥25 kg/m²/4 years	ILI (10% weight loss and 175 min of physical activity/week) vs. DSE (three group sessions per year) (multi-centered RCT)	Weight loss (4 years): 4.7% (ILI) vs. 1.1% (DSE) ($P < 0.001$); in both groups, a 2–5% weight loss increased odds of improvements in SBP (odds ratio 1.24), glucose (1.75); 5–10% weight loss improved all risk factors	
Ekinci 2011	$n = 638$ patients with type 2 diabetes/9.9 years	Relationship between dietary salt intake and mortality in patients with type 2 diabetes; baseline sodium excretion estimated from 24-h urine collections (prospective cohort study)	For every 2,300 mg rise in 24hU$_{Na}$, all-cause mortality was 28% lower ($P = 0.02$); 24hU$_{Na}$ also associated with cardiovascular mortality ($P = 0.03$)	Lower 24-h urinary sodium excretion paradoxically associated with increased all-cause and cardiovascular mortality
Thomas 2011	$n = 2,807$ adults with type 1 diabetes without ESRD/10 years	Predictors of all-cause mortality and ESRD determined; baseline sodium excretion estimated from 24-h urine collections (prospective cohort study)	217 (7.7%) deaths, patients with highest and lowest sodium excretion had reduced survival; 126 (4.5%) developed ESRD, patients with lowest sodium excretion had the highest incidence of ESRD	Sodium was independently associated with all-cause mortality and ESRD; suggests caution with universal salt restriction

24hU$_{Na}$, 24-h urinary collections of sodium excretion; ACR, albumin-to-creatinine ratio; DBP, diastolic blood pressure; DSE, diabetes support and education; ESRD, end-stage renal disease; ILI, intensive lifestyle intervention.

nutrients. Participants were randomized to an eating pattern: *1*) combination diet—a diet rich in fiber, whole grains, fruits, vegetables, and low-fat dairy products that was also low in fat—or *2*) a DASH control diet—based on the typical American diet. Calorie level was designed to maintain body weight (Appel 1997). The 8-week results demonstrated a blood pressure–lowering effect of the dietary pattern that was high in fruits and vegetables, low in total and saturated fat and cholesterol, and high in whole grains, as well as being moderately low in sodium (3,000 mg). This landmark study reduced systolic blood pressure by 5.5 mmHg and diastolic blood pressure by 3.0 mmHg more than a control diet, and an even greater reduction (11.4 mmHg/5.5 mmHg) was seen among people with hypertension. The DASH diet lowered blood pressure regardless of age, sex, or BMI and was particularly effective among the African-American participants (Svetkey 1999). The DASH eating plan, when implemented along with exercise and weight loss, also improved insulin sensitivity (Hinderliter 2011).

Table 14.3 compares the DASH eating pattern suggested intake and the usual U.S intake between 2002 and 2004. The table highlights particularly noteworthy disparities between suggested intake of fruit, vegetables, fats and oils, and sweets and added sugar and average consumption.

Weight Reduction

Data from RCTs indicate that a comprehensive approach to lifestyle modification can be effective in lowering blood pressure to prevent the development of overt hypertension and in treating hypertension. A 4.5-kg (10-lb) weight loss can

Table 14.3 Estimated Food Intake for DASH Dietary Pattern Versus Usual U.S. Intake

	DASH Dietary Pattern	NHANES 2002–2004 Daily Mean U.S. Intake
	Servings per day	
Grains* (1 oz or ½ cup)	6–8	6.4
Vegetables (1 cup raw, ½ cup cooked)	4–5	1.6
Fruits (1 medium fruit, ½ cup fresh, ¼ cup dried)	4–5	1.0
Fat-free or low-fat milk and milk products† (1 cup milk, 1½ oz cheese)	2–3	1.5
Lean meats, poultry, fish† (1 oz cooked)	≤6	4.6
Nuts, seeds, and legumes (1½ oz nuts, ½ oz seeds, ½ cup cooked legumes)	4–5 per week	0.5
Fats and oils (1 tsp)	2–3	12.2
Sweets and added sugar (1 Tbsp)	≤5 per week	5.3/day

From the U.S. Department of Agriculture and U.S. Department of Health and Human Services 2010. Serving sizes are comparable to exchanges.
*DASH recommendations are most grain servings should be whole grains; usual U.S. intake of whole grains is 0.6/day.
†Usual U.S. intake servings may not be restricted to fat-free milk, low-fat milk, or lean meats.

be effective in controlling stage 1 hypertension (Chobanian 2003). The ENCORE (Exercise and Nutrition interventions for CardiOvascular hEalth) study, which asked participants to adopt the DASH eating pattern and provided an additional weight management component, demonstrated a decrease in weight and blood pressure (Blumenthal 2010).

The Look AHEAD (Action for Health in Diabetes) study randomly assigned 5,145 participants with type 2 diabetes to either an intensive lifestyle intervention (ILI) or a usual care group called diabetes support and education (DSE). ILI participants received weekly comprehensive nutrition education and physical activity counseling, compared with three educational sessions for DSE participants. After the first year, ILI participants found a weight loss of 8.6% was associated with improved diabetes control. Four-year results indicated a 4.7% overall weight reduction, compared to baseline in the ILI group, compared to a 1.1% weight loss in the DSE group (Wadden 2011; Wing 2011). ILI also demonstrated a decrease of systolic blood pressure by 6.8 mmHg and diastolic blood pressure by 3.0 mmHg compared to baseline (Delahanty 2008).

Sodium Restriction

To lower blood pressure, it is recommended to reduce dietary sodium to ≤2,000 mg/day for patients with diabetes and symptomatic congestive heart failure and ≤2,300 mg/day in normotensive people with diabetes, and <1,500 mg/day for those with diabetes and hypertension, while following an eating pattern high in fruits, vegetables, and low-fat dairy products (ADA 2008). The *Dietary Guidelines for Americans, 2010*, recommends that daily sodium intake be reduced to <2,300 mg and that people who are ≥51 years of age and individuals of any age who are African American or have hypertension, diabetes, or chronic kidney disease further reduce their daily sodium intake to 1,500 mg (U.S. Department of Agriculture and U.S. Department of Health and Human Services 2010).

Maintaining sodium intake to 2,400 mg/day has an approximate systolic blood pressure (SBP) reduction range of 2–8 mmHg among a general population (Chobanian 2003). The efficacy of sodium reduction below 2,300 mg/day on blood pressure was demonstrated with the DASH-sodium diet study (Sacks 2001). The DASH eating pattern lowered blood pressure levels at high (3,500 mg/day), medium (2,300 mg/day), and low (1,150 mg/day) sodium intakes; however, a greater difference was observed with the low sodium level than high sodium level. Blood pressure reductions were seen among both hypertensive and non-hypertensive participants, although the effects were greater among hypertensive participants.

Hypertension in almost all people with diabetes is sodium sensitive compared to individuals without diabetes (Tuck 1990). People with diabetes also differ from the nondiabetic population by having an increase in total body sodium, an increase in renal tubular sodium reabsorption, and an impaired ability to excrete a sodium load (Weir 1998). This result suggests that restriction of dietary sodium intake may play a greater role in the management of hypertension in people with diabetes than in people without diabetes. In a study in patients with type 2 diabetes with albuminuria but normal serum creatinine levels, sodium sensitivity of blood pressure appeared before hypertension. Sodium restriction (~1,800 mg/day) without medication decreased blood pressure from high-normal (~140 mmHg) to lower (~125 mmHg) values and decreased urinary excretion of albumin, making restriction of sodium intake an effective treatment (Imanishi 2001). In another study in patients with type 2 diabetes, a low-sodium diet had equivalent effects on blood pressure reduction as the effect of adding a second antihypertensive agent and led to an approximate doubling of the antihypertensive effect of losartan (Houlihan 2002).

However, in patients with type 2 diabetes, lower 24-h urinary sodium excretion (suggesting a lower sodium intake) was associated with increased all-cause and cardiovascular mortality (Ekinci 2011). Similarly, in adults with type 1 diabetes, lower sodium excretion was associated with all-cause mortality and end-stage renal disease (Thomas 2011). Although associations do not demonstrate causality, these findings caused the authors to recommend caution before applying salt restriction universally.

Concurrent Medication Prescription

The Action to Control Cardiovascular Risk in Diabetes (ACCORD), a study of patients with type 2 diabetes, demonstrated the effectiveness of lowering blood pressure in interventions that combined nutrition therapy with medication. The intensive interventions aimed to reduce cardiovascular disease (CVD) risk in type 2 diabetes in individuals whose risk for CVD was elevated because of having hypertension or dyslipidemia. The study was conducted as an open-label trial in which investigators could use various combinations of medications in addition to lifestyle intervention for participants in the intensive treatment arms. In the blood pressure trial, participants in the intensive therapy arm were treated with an average of 3.4 medications, whereas participants in the standard-therapy arm were treated with an average of 2.1 medications (Gerstein 2011). At baseline, the mean systolic and diastolic blood pressures of the participants at baseline were 139 and 76 mmHg, respectively, for both groups. After the first year of therapy, the average systolic blood pressure was 119 mmHg in the intensive-therapy group and 133 mmHg in the standard-therapy group, resulting in an average between-group difference of 14 mmHg. The corresponding mean diastolic blood pressures were 64 and 70 mmHg, for an average difference of 6 mmHg (Cushman 2010). However, there was no significant difference in primary end point—a composite of fatal and nonfatal CVD events—between the groups, suggesting that a systolic blood pressure around or below 140 mmHg is a reasonable goal for people with diabetes. Combining nutrition therapy with medications is effective therapy for achieving this goal.

SUMMARY

The scientific evidence strongly supports controlling hypertension to prevent complications of diabetes. In the UKPDS, lowering blood pressure to a mean of 144/82 mmHg greatly reduced complications associated with diabetes. Results of the ABCD trial found that all-cause mortality was lower in the intensive blood pressure control group of the hypertension cohort. The DASH trial showed that eating patterns that are high in fruits, vegetables, whole grains, and low-fat dairy products and low in total and saturated fat and cholesterol had a blood pressure–lowering effect. Finally, controlling sodium intake to 2,400 mg/day has an approximate SBP reduction range of 2–8 mmHg. Extrapolating from more general studies, reduced energy intake, hopefully leading to weight reduction, appears to be the treatment of choice for hypertension in diabetes. Sodium restriction appears to be effective in lowering blood pressure in sodium-sensitive individuals. However, concern has been expressed about too severe a sodium restriction in people with diabetes.

BIBLIOGRAPHY

American Diabetes Association: Nutrition recommendations and interventions for diabetes (Position Statement). *Diabetes Care* 31 (Suppl. 1):S61–S78, 2008

American Diabetes Association: Standards of medical care in diabetes: 2012. *Diabetes Care* 35 (Suppl. 1):S11–S63, 2012

Appel LJ, Moore TJ, Obarzanek E, Vollmer VM, Svetkey LP, Sacks FM, Bray GA, Vogt TM, Cutler JA, Windhauser MM, Lin PH, Karanja N: A clinical trial of the effects of dietary patterns on blood pressure: DASH Collaborative Research Group. *N Engl J Med* 336:1117–1124, 1997

Blumenthal JA, Babyak MA, Hinderliter A, Watkins LL, Craighead L, Lin PH, Caccia C, Johnson J, Waugh R, Sherwood A: Effects of the DASH diet alone and in combination with exercise and weight loss on blood pressure and cardiovascular biomarkers in men and women with high blood pressure: the ENCORE Study. *Arch Intern Med* 170:126–135, 2010

Chobanian AV, Bakris GL, Black HR, Cushman WC, Green LA, Izzo JL Jr, Jones W, Materson BJ, Oparil S, Wright JT Jr, Roccella EJ: The Seventh Report of the Joint National Committee on Prevention, Detection, Evaluation, and Treatment of High Blood Pressure: the JNC 7 report. *JAMA* 289:2560–2572, 2003

Cushman WC, Evans GW, Byington RB, Goff DC Jr, Grimm RH Jr, Cutler JA, Simons-Morton DG, Basile JN, Corson MA, Probstfield JL, Katz L, Peterson KA, Friedewald WT, Buse JB, Bigger JT, Gerstein HC, Ismail-Beigi F: Effects of intensive blood-pressure control in type 2 diabetes mellitus: the ACCORD Study Group. *N Engl J Med* 362:1575–1585, 2010

Delahanty LM, Nathan DM: Implications of the Diabetes Prevention Program and Look AHEAD clinical trials for lifestyle interventions. *J Am Diet Assoc* 108 (Suppl. 1):S66–S72, 2008

Ekinci EI, Clarke S, Thomas MC, Moran JL, Cheong K, MacIsaac RJ, Jerums G: Dietary salt intake and mortality in patients with type 2 diabetes. *Diabetes Care* 34:703–709, 2011

Franklin SS, Barboza MG, Pio JR, Wong ND: Blood pressure categories, hypertensive subtypes, and the metabolic syndrome. *J Hypertens* 24:2009–2016, 2006

Franz M, VanWormer JJ, Crain AL, Boucher JL, Histon T, Caplan W, Bowman JD, Pronk NP: Weight loss outcomes: a systematic review and meta-analysis of weight loss clinical trials with a minimum 1-year follow-up. *J Am Diet Assoc* 107:1755–1767, 2007

Gerstein HC, Miller ME, Genuth S, Ismail-Beigi F, Buse JB, Goff DC Jr, Probstfield JL, Cushman WC, Ginsberg HN, Bigger JT, Grimm RH Jr, Byington RP, Rosenberg YD, Friedewald WT: Long-term effects of intensive glucose lowering on cardiovascular outcomes. *N Engl J Med* 364:818–828, 2011

Gillespie C, Kuklina EV, Briss PA, Blair NA, Hong Y: Vital signs: prevalence, treatment, and control of hypertension: United States, 1999–2002 and 2005–2008. *MMWR Morb Mortal Wkly Rep* 60:103–108, 2011

Hinderliter AL, Babyak MA, Sherwood A, Blumenthal JA: The DASH diet and insulin sensitivity. *Curr Hypertens Rep* 13:67–73, 2011

Holman RR, Paul SK, Bethel A, Neil HAW, Matthews DR: Long-term follow-up after tight control of blood pressure in type 2 diabetes. *N Engl J Med* 359:1565–1576, 2008

Houlihan CA, Allen TJ, Baxter AL, Panangiotopoulos S, Casley DJ, Cooper ME, Jerums G: A low-sodium diet potentiates the effects of losartan in type 2 diabetes. *Diabetes Care* 25:663–671, 2002

Imanishi M, Yoshioka K, Okumura M, Konishi Y, Okada N, Morikawa T, Sato T, Tanaka S, Fujii S: Sodium sensitivity related to albuminuria appearing before hypertension in type 2 diabetic patients. *Diabetes Care* 24:111–116, 2001

Keenan NL, Rosendorf KA: Prevalence of hypertension and controlled hypertension: United States, 2005–2008. *MMWR Surveill Summ* 60 (Suppl.):94–97, 2011

Sacks FM, Svetkey LP, Vollmer WM, Appel LJ, Bray GA, Harsha D, Obarzanek E, Conlin PR, Miller ER 3rd, Simons-Morton DG, Karanja N, Lin PH: Effects on blood pressure of reduced dietary sodium and the Dietary Approaches to Stop Hypertension (DASH) diet: Dash-Sodium Collaborative Research Group. *N Engl J Med* 344:3–10, 2001

Schrier RW, Estacio RO, Mehler PS, Hiatt WR: Appropriate blood pressure control in hypertensive and normotensive type 2 diabetes mellitus: a summary of the ABCD trial. *Nat Clin Pract Nephrol* 3:428–438, 2007

Svetkey LP, Simons-Morton D, Vollmer WM, Appel LJ, Conlin PR, Ryan DH, Ard J, Kennedy BM: Effects of dietary patterns on blood pressure: subgroup analysis of the Dietary Approaches to Stop Hypertension (DASH) randomized clinical trial. *Arch Intern Med* 159:285–293, 1999

Swain JF, McCarron PB, Hamilton EF, Sacks FM, Appel LJ: Characteristics of the diet patterns tested in the optimal macronutrient intake trial to prevent heart disease (OmniHeart): options for a heart-healthy diet. *J Am Diet Assoc* 108:257–265, 2008

Thomas MC, Moran J, Forsblom C, Harjutsalo V, Thorn L, Ahola A, Waden J, Tolonen N, Saraheimo M, Gordin D, Groop P-H, for the FinnDiane Study Group: The association between dietary sodium intake, ESRD, and all-cause mortality in patients with type 1 diabetes. *Diabetes Care* 34:861–866, 2011

Tuck M, Corry D, Trujillo A: Salt-sensitive blood pressure and exaggerated vascular reactivity in the hypertension of diabetes mellitus. *Am J Med* 88:210–216, 1990

U.K. Prospective Diabetes Study Group: Tight blood pressure control and risk of macrovascular and microvascular complications in type 2 diabetes: UKPDS 38. *BMJ* 317:703, 1998

U.S. Department of Agriculture and U.S. Department of Health and Human Services: *Dietary Guidelines for Americans, 2010*. 7th ed. Washington, DC, U.S. Government Printing Office, 2010

Wadden TA, Neiberg RH, Wing RR, Clark JM, Delahanty LM, Hill JO, Krakoff J, Otto A, Ryan DH, Vitolins MZ: Four-year weight losses in the Look AHEAD study: factors associated with long-term success. *Obesity (Silver Spring)* 19:1987–1998, 2011

Weir MR: Impact of salt intake on blood pressure and proteinuria in diabetes: importance of the renin-angiotensin system. *Miner Electrolyte Metab* 24:438–445, 1998

Wing RR, Lang W, Wadden TA, Safford M, Knowler WC, Bertoni AG, Hill JO, Brancati JL, Peters A, Wagenknecht L: Benefits of modest weight loss in improving cardiovascular risk factors in overweight and obese individuals with type 2 diabetes. *Diabetes Care* 34:1481–1486, 2011

Wylie-Rosett J: Hypertension and medical nutrition therapy. In *American Diabetes Association Guide to Medical Nutrition Therapy for Diabetes*. Franz MJ, Bantle JP, Eds. Alexandria, VA, American Diabetes Association, 1999, p. 295–311

Yoon S, Ostchega SY, Louis T: Recent trends in the prevalence of high blood pressure and its treatment and control, 1999–2008. *NCHS Data Brief* 48:1–8, 2010

Karin Aebersold, MPH, is a Research Program Manager at Albert Einstein College of Medicine, New York, NY. Natania Wright Ostrovsky, PhD, is an instructor in the Department of Epidemiology and Population Health at Albert Einstein College of Medicine, New York, NY. Judith Wylie-Rosett, EdD, RD, is a Professor of Epidemiology and Population Health and Division Head of Health Promotion and Nutrition Research at Albert Einstein College of Medicine, New York, NY.

Chapter 15

Nutrition Therapy for Diabetic Kidney Disease

Madelyn L. Wheeler, MS, RD, CDE, FADA

Highlights

Review of Existing Diabetes Nutrition Recommendations and Guidelines for Diabetes and CKD

Translation of Evidence into Nutrition Interventions

Summary

Highlights
Nutrition Therapy for
Diabetic Kidney Disease

■ Earlier stages of diabetic kidney disease (DKD) are essentially a component of diabetes treatment, and later stages are a component of chronic kidney disease (CKD) treatment. Strict control of blood glucose and hypertension is necessary in all stages of DKD.

■ Although there is not a linear relationship between glomerular filtration rate (GFR) and albuminuria, in general, microalbuminuria is found in CKD stages 1 and 2, whereas macroalbuminuria is commonly found in CKD stages 3 and 4.

■ Protein has been the macronutrient most studied in DKD. Lower-protein diets (achieved average 0.9 g/kg/day) versus usual-protein diets (average 1.2 g/kg/day):
  • Do not significantly improve the rate of decline of GFR.
  • May possibly improve the albumin excretion rate in individuals with macroalbuminuria but not in individuals with microalbuminuria.

■ Malnutrition, as defined by reduced serum albumin, may be an issue for protein intakes below 0.7 g/kg/day; however, it appears to remain stable at intakes ≥0.8 g/kg/day.

■ Adherence to prescribed lower-protein diets is poor. Protein intake, on average, was 0.9 g/kg/day when 0.7 g/kg/day was prescribed.

■ Blood pressure control is a major treatment for DKD. Reducing salt (and therefore sodium) in individuals with microalbuminuria can reduce blood pressure and should be considered a nutrition therapy objective.

■ Other macronutrients (carbohydrate, fat), micronutrients (potassium, phosphorus, calcium), or lifestyle interventions (physical activity, obesity intervention, prevention of weight loss) lack evidence-based DKD studies and may be areas for future research.

Nutrition Therapy for Diabetic Kidney Disease

One of the major microvascular complications of diabetes (both type 1 and type 2) is kidney disease. Diabetic kidney disease (DKD) is the leading cause of kidney failure (44% of all new cases) among adults in the U.S. (Centers for Disease Control and Prevention [CDC] 2011). DKD is also known as "diabetes in chronic kidney disease," "incipient nephropathy" (microalbuminuria), and "diabetic nephropathy" (macroalbuminuria) (National Kidney Foundation Kidney Disease Outcomes Quality Initiative [KDOQI] 2007).

Glomerular filtration rate (GFR) is a measure of the filtering capacity of the kidneys, with a low or decreasing GFR being a good index of chronic kidney disease (CKD). CKD is therefore defined as either kidney damage or GFR <60 mL/min/1.73 m² body surface area for ≥3 months. CKD is divided into five stages (Table 15.1) ranging from normal GFR to significantly reduced GFR, indicative of end-stage renal disease (KDOQI 2002).

Persistently increased protein (especially albumin) excretion is usually a marker of kidney damage and is a surrogate end point for clinical outcomes in DKD in both type 1 and type 2 diabetes. Albuminuria is defined as follows (KDOQI 2007; American Diabetes Association [ADA] 2012):

- Microalbuminuria, a modest elevation of albumin thought to be associated with stable kidney function, but a greater risk of macroalbuminuria and kidney failure
- Macroalbuminuria, a higher elevation of albumin associated with progressive decline in GFR, an increase in systemic blood pressure, and a high risk of kidney failure

Relationships between glomerular structural lesions and the presence or absence of microalbuminuria in diabetes are not straightforward (see Table 15.1), particularly because a substantial proportion of patients with type 1 and type 2 diabetes and microalbuminuria can spontaneously revert to normoalbuminuria (KDOQI 2007).

Interventions that have proven to be effective in slowing the progression of DKD include strict glucose control and strict blood pressure control (KDOQI 2002; ADA 2012). In general, every percentage drop in A1C can reduce the risk of microvascular complications such as kidney disease by 40% (CDC 2011). Detecting and treating early kidney disease by lowering blood pressure can reduce the decline in kidney function by 30–70% (CDC 2011). Lifestyle interventions such as protein restriction have also been proposed to slow or prevent the progression of DKD.

Table 15.1 CKD Stage Markers and Possible Relationship with Albuminuria

Stage	Description	GFR (ml/min/1.73 m² body surface area)	Albuminuria
1	Kidney damage* with normal or increased GFR	≥90	Normal- or microalbuminuria
2	Kidney damage* with mildly decreased GFR	60–89	Microalbuminuria or possibly macroalbuminuria
3	Moderately decreased GFR	30–59	Macroalbuminuria
4	Severely decreased GFR	15–29	Macroalbuminuria
5	Kidney failure	<15 or dialysis	

Stage markers are from KDOQI 2002. Relationships between glomerular structural lesions and the presence of microalbuminuria in DKD are not straightforward. Normal GFR is ~90–125 mL/min/1.73 m² body surface area. Albuminuria is defined as the normal mean value for urine albumin excretion in adults of ~10 mg/24 h. Microalbuminuria is present when the AER is 30–300 mg/24 h (20–200 µg/min) or the albumin-to-creatinine ratio is 30–300 mg/g; macroalbuminuria is defined as an albumin-to-creatinine ratio of ≥300 mg/g creatinine.

*As defined by structural or functional abnormalities of the kidney (with or without decreased GFR) as manifested by either pathological abnormalities or markers of kidney damage (proteinuria, hematuria, pyuria, or abnormal imaging studies).

Adapted from KDOQI 2002.

Because protein is excreted during kidney disease, reducing dietary protein "to reduce kidney load" has been a practice for patients with and without diabetes, with an extreme being the 1960s era Giovannetti-Maggiore diet for severe chronic uremia (6–9 g protein/day). However, what are lower-protein diets, and can they reduce or slow the rate of decline in kidney function in DKD? There are also questions concerning the ability of patients to comply with lower-protein diets. And finally, at what lower level of protein will malnutrition occur?

While protein has been the main focus for nutrition studies of diabetes and CKD, other macronutrients (carbohydrate and fat) and micronutrients (sodium, potassium, and phosphorus) are or may be factors in DKD. Also, physical activity and obesity should be considered.

REVIEW OF EXISTING DIABETES NUTRITION RECOMMENDATIONS AND GUIDELINES FOR DIABETES AND CKD

The Evidence Analysis Library (EAL) of the Academy of Nutrition and Dietetics (formerly the American Dietetic Association) (Acad Nutr Diet) contains systematic reviews pertaining to DKD. Both the diabetes (Acad Nutr Diet 2008) and CKD (Acad Nutr Diet 2010) sections of the EAL contain reviews for DKD and protein, as does the ADA in its systematic review of diabetes and macronutrients (Wheeler 2012) The CKD EAL also provides some information about DKD and energy, sodium, and physical activity (Acad Nutr Diet 2010).

Protein

The diabetes section of the Acad Nutr Diet EAL (diabetes EAL) conducted a systematic review to answer the question, "What is the evidence to support protein restriction (with or without amino acid or ketoacid supplementation) for the effective treatment of patients with diabetic nephropathy?" (Acad Nutr Diet 2008). Inclusion dates were 2001 to July 2006, with two earlier studies (from 1994 and 1999). The sample size of each study group was ≥10 individuals, and the dropout rate was <20%. In addition, an update search was done (from July 2006 to July 2009). The original review, an update, and evidence tables are published in the article "The Evidence for Medical Nutrition Therapy for Type 1 and Type 2 Diabetes in Adults" (Franz 2010). A further search was done to cover the period of July 2009 to May 2011, but no newer studies meeting the sample size and dropout rate criteria were found.

Amount of protein. (Evidence summaries for protein research are provided in Table 8 from the article by Franz, 2010.) Three parallel-type randomized controlled trials (RCTs) examined the effects of lower versus usual protein intake on renal function markers in patients with diabetes and microalbuminuria (Pijls 2002; Dussol 2005; Velázquez 2008), and seven parallel-type RCTs examined the effects of lower versus usual protein intake on renal function markers in patients with diabetes and macroalbuminuria (Raal 1994; Hansen 1999; Meloni 2002; Hansen 2002; Meloni 2004; Dussol 2005; Velázquez 2008). Studies included individuals with type 1 and type 2 diabetes. Duration of follow-up ranged from 4 weeks to 4 years, and sample sizes were small (range 11–63 participants in the intervention groups). All studies had completion rates of >80%. Only two studies blinded physicians to diet treatment (Pijls 2002; Velázquez 2008). In most of the studies, there were confounding factors, such as weight not controlled (Pijls 2002), significant weight loss in the lower protein group versus control (Meloni 2002; Meloni 2004), and poor (Raal 1994) or moderate (Hansen 1999; Hansen 2002; Dussol 2005; Velázquez 2008) blood glucose control. Two meta-analyses also addressed the topic of protein restriction and DKD (Robertson 2007; Pan 2008).

Of the studies involving subjects with microalbuminuria (Pijls 2002; Dussol 2005; Velázquez 2008) or normoalbuminuria (Pijls 2002), only one achieved a lower protein intake (0.82 g/kg/day vs. usual protein intake [1.2 g/kg/day]) (Velázquez 2008). The other two studies found that subjects on the lower-protein diet consumed more protein per day than the group randomized to "usual protein" (Pijls 2002; Dussol 2005). All three studies found no significant change between groups or from beginning to end in either group for GFR or albumin excretion rate (AER).

In the studies of subjects with macroalbuminuria (Raal 1994; Hansen 1999; Hansen 2002; Meloni 2002; Meloni 2004; Dussol 2005; Velázquez 2008), one study achieved a significant difference between the lower-protein group of 0.68 versus 1.39 g/kg/day for the usual protein group (Meloni 2002). In one study, the lower-protein group was actually higher in protein (1.1 g/kg/day) than the usual protein group (Dussol 2005). In the other studies, the lower-protein groups achieved a range from 0.8 to 0.87 g/kg/day, and the usual protein groups achieved a range from 1.03 to 2.0 g/kg/day (Raal 1994; Hansen 1999; Hansen 2002; Meloni 2004; Velázquez 2008). All seven studies found no significant change between groups in GFR. Whereas five studies found no significant change in AER between groups, two did find significantly reduced AERs—the lower-protein group and the usual-protein group (Hansen 1999; Meloni 2002).

The two meta-analyses included subjects with diabetes who had either micro- or macroalbuminuria, with a range for the lower-protein diet of 0.6–1.1 g/kg/day versus the usual-protein diet of 1–2 g/kg/day (Robertson 2007) and an average of 0.91 versus 1.27 g/kg/day (Pan 2008), respectively. Neither meta-analysis found a significant difference between groups for GFR. Pan found no significant difference between groups for AER (Pan 2008), and Robertson (Robertson 2007) did not report AER as an outcome.

Five studies provided information about serum albumin levels. All but one of these studies found no significant difference in serum albumin between lower- and usual-protein groups (achieved protein intakes ranged from 0.8 to 1.1 in the lower-protein group and 1.0 to 1.2 in the usual-protein group). The one study where intervention subjects were able to stay on the prescribed lower-protein diet (0.68 g/kg/day) found significantly reduced serum albumin levels (a marker of malnutrition) after the ninth month in the lower-protein group versus the usual-protein group (Meloni 2002). In addition, the Pan meta-analysis, in a subgroup analysis, found that the lower-protein diets resulted in significantly lower serum albumin concentrations (Pan 2008).

From the above information, the following can be derived:

- The terms "low protein," "lower protein," "high protein," "higher protein," "usual protein," "free protein," etc., do not have widely accepted definitions. In this chapter, the terms "lower-protein" (average 0.9 g/kg/day, range 0.7–1.1) and "usual-protein" (average 1.2 g/kg/day, range 1.0–1.4) are used to reflect the average and range of protein achieved in either group. In general, these terms agree with the meta-analyses' average (0.9 vs. 1.3 g/kg/day) (Pan 2008) or range (0.6–1.1 vs. 1–2 g/kg/day) (Robertson 2007).
- Adherence to lower-protein diets is poor. When lower-protein diets (average 0.7 g/kg/day, range 0.6–0.8) were prescribed, subjects consumed an average of 0.9 g/kg/day.
- Lower-protein diets (0.7–1.1 g/kg/day) versus usual-protein diets (1.0–1.4 g/kg/day):
  - Do not significantly improve GFR.
  - May improve AER in individuals with macroalbuminuria (two studies out of seven) but not in individuals with microalbuminuria; however, it is not known if improvement in AER will improve the rate of decline in GFR.
- Hypoalbuminemia, a marker of malnutrition, may be associated with a decrease in protein intake to about or below 0.7 g/kg/day.

The ADA's systematic review of macronutrients (Wheeler 2012) and the CKD EAL (Acad Nutr Diet 2010) reviews came to basically the same conclusions.

Type of protein. (Evidence summaries for type of protein research are provided in Table 7 from the article by Franz, 2010.) The diabetes EAL (Acad Nutr Diet 2008; Franz 2010) found only one study meeting criteria that addressed *type* of protein (Azadbakht 2008). This study of 41 individuals with type 2 diabetes and macroalbuminuria, lasting for 4 years, found that (when replacing some animal protein with textured soy) there were no significant differences between groups for GFR or proteinuria. However, as expected, CVD risk measures (total cholesterol, LDL cholesterol, and triglycerides) were reduced significantly in the soy group versus the control group. These results essentially agree with previously published studies in the area (Wheeler 1999).

Other Nutrition-Related Topics

Carbohydrate, fat, and energy. The CKD EAL (Acad Nutr Diet 2010) found no studies examining the effects of carbohydrate/fat modification on CKD progression among adult non-dialyzed patients with DKD. Although some studies cited in the diabetes EAL (Acad Nutr Diet 2008; Franz 2010) attempted isocaloric diets (e.g., replacing protein mainly with carbohydrate), several studies did not ask subjects with macroalbuminuria to replace the reduced protein, resulting in significantly lower calories in the lower-protein group (Hansen 1999; Meloni 2002; Meloni 2004). The study that maintained protein at ~0.7 g/kg/day with lowered energy also found a significant decrease in serum albumin from 9 months to the end of the study (Meloni 2002).

Salt and sodium. A recently published meta-analysis (Suckling 2010) identified 13 studies involving individuals with diabetes and normo- or microalbuminuria and with lower-salt (0.6–8 g/day [233–3,100 mg sodium/day]) versus higher-salt (9.8–18.9 g/day [3,800–7,325 mg sodium/day]) diets. This analysis found that reducing salt by an average of 8.5 g/day (3,300 mg sodium/day) lowers blood pressure on average 7/3 mmHg, with no significant change in GFR. Because of diversity of data, no AER information was provided. One of the studies included in this meta-analysis was also included in the CKD EAL (Acad Nutr Diet 2010) question addressing sodium (Imanishi 2001). Imanishi and colleagues found that blood pressure decreased significantly when subjects with diabetes and albuminuria consumed ~1,800 mg/day sodium (Imanishi 2001).

Reducing salt (and thus sodium) levels could reduce blood pressure substantially in individuals with diabetes and microalbuminuria, depending on initial salt consumption and salt sensitivity of individuals. There is no research concerning salt reduction and individuals with diabetes and macroalbuminuria.

Physical activity. Individuals with DKD are generally inactive and may benefit from increased physical activity; however, this issue has not been addressed in the literature, except for one small pilot study (11 subjects) (Leehey 2009). Aerobic exercise plus optimal medical management was compared to medical management alone in individuals with type 2 diabetes, obesity, and stage 2–4 CKD. Exercise over 24 weeks produced slight, insignificant decreases in resting systolic blood pressure and 24-h proteinuria, but did not alter GFR or other measured parameters.

Table 15.2 Studies Reporting the Effectiveness of Salt/Sodium Restriction in DKD

	Population/ Duration of Study	Intervention (type of study)	Major Findings	Comments
Imanishi 2001	$n = 32$ adults with type 2 diabetes (11 normo, 12 micro, 9 macro)/1 week	Sodium restriction (80 mmol/day [1,812 mg]) vs. usual sodium (200 mmol/day [4,530 mg]) (RCT crossover)	Urinary sodium excretion: slope of pressure-natriuresis curve higher in albuminuric patients than normo ($P < 0.001$) AER: ↓ in micro and normo with sodium restricted vs. usual sodium (36.6 vs. 48.6 mg/day, $P < 0.02$) BP higher in macro vs. normo at start of study ($P < 0.025$) BP ↓ in albuminuric patients during sodium restriction ($P < 0.02$)	
Suckling 2010	$n = 13$ studies with 254 adults with types 1 and type 2 diabetes and normo or micro/5 day to 12 weeks	Lower-salt diet (0.6–8 g salt/day) vs. higher-salt diet (9.8–18.9 g salt/day) (Cochrane meta-analysis, 1966 to January 2010)	↓ in salt to 8.5 g/day lowers BP 7/3 mmHg; equally effective in both types of diabetes Small ↓ creatinine clearance (6 mL/min) No change in GFR	Only six studies reported urinary albumin/protein excretion and authors unable to do a pooled analysis because of diversity of data reported

BP, blood pressure; macro, macroalbuminuric; micro, microalbuminuric; normo, normoalbuminuric.

Although there is no evidence that physical activity per se produces a change in renal function, regular aerobic and anaerobic exercises have a number of benefits, such as improving cardiovascular function and preventing muscle breakdown or wasting, and should be explored with patients who have DKD.

Potassium, phosphorus, and calcium. As kidney function declines, the ability to eliminate excess potassium, phosphorus, and calcium from the blood is reduced. In the later stages of CKD, and based on laboratory serum values and medications taken, foods containing high levels of these nutrients may need to be restricted. The CKD EAL found no studies examining the effects of potassium, phosphorus, and calcium modification on CKD progression among adult non-dialyzed patients with DKD (Acad Nutr Diet 2010).

TRANSLATION OF EVIDENCE INTO NUTRITION INTERVENTIONS

In individuals with diabetes and microalbuminuria, protein restriction is not warranted. Reducing protein levels to <1 g/kg/day in individuals with diabetes and macroalbuminuria may improve albuminuria somewhat but does not appear to have significant effects on GFR. In individuals with diabetes and macroalbuminuria, serum albumin and energy intake must be monitored and changes in protein and energy intake made to correct deficits and to prevent potential risk of malnutrition. Salt (sodium) reduction, particularly in individuals with diabetes and microalbuminuria, can reduce blood pressure significantly. Because there is no evidence base for restrictions or increases of micronutrients (potassium, phosphorus, and calcium) in DKD, individual prescriptions should be based on laboratory values and prescribed medications as well as the CKD EAL nondiabetic evidence base.

SUMMARY

DKD is a microvascular complication of diabetes and is usually expressed as microalbuminuria or macroalbuminuria. Recent research has focused on the effect of lower-protein diets and risk reduction for the development of end-stage renal disease. The most recent evidence-based guidelines indicate that protein need not be restricted in individuals with diabetes and microalbuminuria. Lowering protein intake to <1 g/kg/day in individuals with macroalbuminuria may improve albuminuria somewhat; however, this decrease does not appear to reduce the rate of decline of kidney function (GFR) and may be a cause of malnutrition. Strictly controlling blood glucose levels and blood pressure is a proven intervention in DKD.

BIBLIOGRAPHY

Academy of Nutrition and Dietetics: Chronic kidney disease evidence-based nutrition practice guidelines. American Dietetic Association Evidence Analysis Library, 2010. Available from http://www.adaevidencelibrary.com/topic.cfm?cat=3927. Accessed 4 June 2011

Academy of Nutrition and Dietetics: Type 1 and 2 evidence-based nutrition practice guidelines for adults. American Dietetic Association Evidence Analysis Library, 2008. Available from http://www.adaevidencelibrary.com/topic.cfm?cat=3251. Accessed 4 June 2011

American Diabetes Association: Standards of medical care in diabetes—2012 (Position Statement). *Diabetes Care* 35 (Suppl. 1):S11–S63, 2012

Azadbakht L, Atabak S, Esmailizadeh A: Soy protein intake, cardiorenal indices, and C-reactive protein in type 2 diabetes with nephropathy. *Diabetes Care* 31:648–654, 2008

Centers for Disease Control and Prevention: National diabetes fact sheet: national estimates and general information on diabetes and prediabetes in the United States, 2011. Atlanta, GA, U.S. Department of Health and Human Services, Centers for Disease Control and Prevention, 2011. Available from http://apps. nccd.cdc.gov/DDTSTRS/FactSheet.aspx. Accessed 1 June 2011

Dussol B, Iovanna C, Raccah D, Darmon P, Morange S, Vague P, Vialettes B, Oliver C, Loundoun A, Berland Y: A randomized trial of low-protein diet in type 1 and type 2 diabetes mellitus patients with incipient and overt nephropathy. *J Ren Nutr* 15:398–406, 2005

Franz MJ, Powers MA, Leontos C, Holzmeister LA, Kulkarni K, Monk A, Wedel N, Gradwell E: The evidence for medical nutrition therapy for type 1 and type 2 diabetes in adults. *J Am Diet Assoc* 110:1852–1889, 2010

Hansen HP, Christensen PK, Tauber-Lassen E, Klausen A, Jensen BR, Parving H-H: Low-protein diet and kidney function in insulin-dependent diabetic patients with diabetic nephropathy. *Kidney Int* 55:621–628, 1999

Hansen HP, Tauber-Lassen E, Jensen BR, Parving H-H: Effect of dietary protein restriction on prognosis in patients with diabetic nephropathy. *Kidney Int* 62:220–228, 2002

Imanishi M, Yoshioka K, Okumura M, Konishi Y, Okada N, Morikawa T, Sato T, Tanaka S, Fujii S: Sodium sensitivity related to albuminuria appearing before hypertension in type 2 diabetic patients. *Diabetes Care* 24:111–116, 2001

National Kidney Foundation Kidney Disease Outcomes Quality Initiative (KDOQI): Clinical practice guidelines for chronic kidney disease: evaluation, classification, and stratification. 2002. Available from http://www.kidney.org/ professionals/kdoqi/guidelines_commentaries.cfm#guidelines. Accessed 4 June 2011

National Kidney Foundation Kidney Disease Outcomes Quality Initiative (KDOQI): Clinical practice guidelines and clinical practice recommendations for diabetes and chronic kidney disease. *Am J Kidney Dis* 49 (Suppl. 2):S1–S180, 2007

Leehey DJ, Moinuddin I, Bast JP, Qureshi S, Jelinek CS, Cooper C, Edwards LC, Smith BM, Collins EG: Aerobic exercise in obese diabetic patients with chronic kidney disease: a randomized and controlled pilot study. *Cardiovasc Diabetol* 8:62–70, 2009

Meloni C, Morosetti M, Suraci C, Pennafina MG, Tozzo C, Taccone-Gallucci M, Casciani CU: Severe dietary protein restriction in overt diabetic nephropathy: benefits or risks? *J Ren Nutr* 12:96–101, 2002

Meloni C, Tatangelo P, Cipriani S, Rossi V, Curaci C, Tozzo C, Rossini B, Cecilia A, DiFranco D, Straccialano E, Casciani CU: Adequate protein dietary restriction in diabetic and nondiabetic patients with chronic renal failure. *J Ren Nutr* 14:208–213, 2004

Pan Y, Guo LL, Min Jin H: Low-protein diet for diabetic nephropathy: a meta-analysis of randomized controlled trials. *Am J Clin Nutr* 88:660–666, 2008

Pijls LTJ, de Vries H, van Eijk JThM, Donker AJM: Protein restriction, glomerular filtration rate and albuminuria in patients with type 2 diabetes mellitus: a randomized trial. *Eur J Clin Nutr* 56:1200–1207, 2002

Raal FJ, Kalk WJ, Lawson M, Esser JD, Buys R, Fourie L, Panz VR: Effect of moderate dietary protein restriction on the progression of overt diabetic nephropathy: a 6-mo prospective study. *Am J Clin Nutr* 60:579–585, 1994

Robertson LM, Waugh N, Robertson A: Protein restriction for diabetic renal disease. *Cochrane Database Syst Rev* CD002181, 2007

Suckling RJ, He FJ, MacGregor GA: Altered dietary salt intake for preventing and treating diabetic kidney disease. *Cochrane Database Syst Rev* CD006763, 2010.

Velázquez López L, Sil Acosta MJ, Goycochea Robles MV, Torres Tamayo M, Castañeda Limones R: Effect of protein restriction diet on renal function and metabolic control in patients with type 2 diabetes: a randomized clinical trial. *Nutr Hosp* 23:141–147, 2008

Wheeler ML, Dunbar SA, Jaacks LM, Karmally W, Mayer-Davis EJ, Wylie-Rosett J, Yancy WS Jr: Macronutrients, food groups, and eating patterns in the management of diabetes: a systematic review of the literature, 2010. *Diabetes Care* 35:434–445, 2012

Wheeler ML: Nephropathy and medical nutrition therapy. In *American Diabetes Association Guide to Medical Nutrition Therapy for Diabetes*. Franz MJ, Bantle JP, Eds. Alexandria VA, American Diabetes Association, 1999, p. 312–329

Madelyn L. Wheeler, MS, RD, CDE, FADA, is Co-Owner, Nutritional Computing Concepts, Zionsville, IN.

Chapter 16

Nutrition Therapy for Diabetes and Celiac Disease

Carol Brunzell, RD, CDE

Highlights
Nutrition Therapy for
Diabetes and Celiac Disease

- People with diabetes and celiac disease must follow a strict gluten-free diet (GFD) for life.

- The GFD is complex, and ongoing nutrition therapy education and support is necessary for best clinical outcomes.

- Adherence to a GFD will normalize growth, nutrient deficiencies, and bone density in people with type 1 diabetes and celiac disease.

Nutrition Therapy for Diabetes and Celiac Disease

Celiac disease (CD) is an autoimmune disorder that occurs more frequently in individuals with preexisting type 1 diabetes. Approximately 1–16% of people with type 1 diabetes have CD, compared with 0.3–1% in the general population (Holmes 2002; Rewers 2004). There is limited evidence for combined nutrition therapy for CD and diabetes available in the literature; however, there is ample evidence for nutrition therapy for CD and diabetes respectively. Registered dietitians (RDs) and other health care providers who work in diabetes care must be well versed on the intricacies of the gluten-free diet (GFD) and CD in relation to its influence on nutritional status and metabolic control.

The American Diabetes Association (ADA) recommends that children with type 1 diabetes be screened for CD by measuring tissue transglutaminase or anti-endomysial antibodies, with documentation of normal serum IgA levels, soon after the diagnosis of diabetes. Testing should be repeated in children with growth failure, failure to gain weight, weight loss, or gastroenterological symptoms or with frequent unexplained hypoglycemia or deterioration of glycemic control. Children with biopsy-confirmed CD should be placed on a GFD and consult with an RD experienced in managing both diabetes and CD (ADA 2012).

The National Institutes of Health (NIH) statement on CD also recommends that populations at higher risk for CD, which includes individuals with type 1 diabetes (especially with unexplained hypoglycemia), be tested for CD. Recommendations for the management of CD include consultation with a skilled RD, education about the disease, lifelong adherence to a GFD, identification and treatment of nutritional deficiencies, access to an advocacy group, and continuous long-term follow-up by a multidisciplinary team (NIH 2005).

This chapter begins with a brief overview of CD symptoms from undiagnosed or untreated CD, followed by a summary of the research available on nutrition therapy for diabetes complicated by CD. Nutrition therapy recommendations for people with diabetes and CD are similar to the recommendations for all people with CD; therefore, the Academy of Nutrition and Dietetics (formerly the American Dietetic Association) (Acad Nutr Diet) Evidence Analysis Library (EAL) (http://www.adaevidencelibrary.com) recommendations for CD and the GFD are reviewed.

CELIAC DISEASE: SYMPTOMS AND TREATMENT

Celiac disease is a multisystem immunological disorder occurring in genetically susceptible individuals characterized by an abnormal T-cell response against specific prolamins: gliadin in wheat, secalin in rye, and hordein in barley, collectively referred to as gluten (Vader 2003). Ingestion of gluten results in small-bowel mucosal injury. CD is systemic and not restricted to the gastrointestinal tract, and clinical presentation can be highly variable (Green 2005b; Murray 2003). People with CD may or may not have symptoms. The only treatment for CD is a lifelong strict GFD (Fasano 2001).

The skin manifestation of CD, present in 15–25% of people with CD, is dermatitis herpetiformis, an intensely pruritic, blistering rash primarily affecting the knees, elbows, buttocks, scalp, and back in a symmetrical pattern. Diagnosis is made by biopsying the skin next to the lesions. Dapsone is a medication prescribed for relieving the irritation to the skin. Sulfapyridine or sulfamethoxypyridazine may also be used, but these drugs are not as effective as dapsone (Nicolas 2003). People with dermatitis herpetiformis are less likely to have gastrointestinal manifestations of CD, but they do exhibit positive serology as well as damage to the small-bowel mucosa; therefore, the treatment for dermatitis herpetiformis is a lifelong GFD (Oxentenko 2003; Rodrigo 2006).

There are four main categories of CD (NIH 2005):

1. **Classical celiac disease** is dominated by symptoms and sequelae of gastrointestinal malabsorption. The diagnosis is established by serological testing, biopsy evidence of villous atrophy, and improvement of symptoms on a GFD.

2. **Celiac disease with atypical symptoms** is characterized by few or no gastrointestinal symptoms, and extra-intestinal manifestations predominate (e.g., iron deficiency anemia, osteopenia, osteoporosis, and vitamin deficiencies). Recognition of atypical features of CD is responsible for much of the increased prevalence and now may be the most common presentation. As with classical CD, the diagnosis is established by serological testing, biopsy evidence of villous atrophy, and improvement of symptoms on a GFD.

3. **Silent celiac disease** refers to individuals who are asymptomatic but have a positive serological test and villous atrophy on biopsy. These individuals usually are detected via screening of high-risk individuals, or villous atrophy occasionally may be detected by endoscopy and biopsy conducted for another reason.

4. **Latent celiac disease** is defined by a positive serology but no villous atrophy on biopsy. These individuals are asymptomatic, but later may develop symptoms and/or histological changes.

Damage to the intestinal epithelium can cause an array of symptoms and complications. Some symptoms of undiagnosed or untreated CD include diarrhea, weight loss or poor weight gain, growth failure, abdominal pain, bloating and distention, fatigue, constipation, vomiting, malnutrition due to malabsorption of macro- and micronutrients, osteopenia, osteoporosis, and unexplained hypoglycemia or erratic blood glucose levels. Other presentations are delayed puberty, infertility, recurrent fetal loss, recurrent aphthous stomatitis, elevated transaminases, and dental enamel hypoplasia. In addition, a variety of neuropsychiatric conditions such as depression, anxiety, peripheral neuropathy, ataxia, epilepsy with or without cerebral calcifications, and migraine headaches have been reported in people with CD (Green 2005a; Fasano 2005a). There is an increased risk of intestinal lymphoma, adenocarcinoma of the small intestine, and carcinoma elsewhere in the gastrointestinal tract, however, these are very rare complications (Green 2001; Card 2004).

The GFD should never be recommended unless diagnosis is firmly established after a complete diagnostic evaluation, including positive serology and intestinal biopsy, which is considered the gold standard for diagnosis of CD. Eating a GFD before biopsy can lead to false test results; therefore, these tests must occur while the individual is consuming gluten to ensure an accurate diagnosis (Green 2005b). The absence of detectable symptoms with intentional or inadvertent gluten ingestion does not mean ongoing intestinal injury does not occur. Once gluten is removed from the diet, the intestinal damage heals completely (Fasano 2005b). However, complete histological resolution may take up to 2 years (Grefte 1988).

If gastrointestinal symptoms, such as bloating, gas, constipation, and diarrhea, persist after ruling out gluten exposure, there may be other potential causes, such as leaky gut; lactose, fructose, and carbohydrate intolerances; bacterial overgrowth; refractory sprue; related cancers; and other gastrointestinal diseases and conditions that require evaluation.

NUTRITION THERAPY FOR CELIAC DISEASE AND DIABETES

A literature search was conducted using PubMed MEDLINE, and additional articles were identified from reference lists. Search criteria included gluten-free diet, celiac disease and diabetes, and English language articles since 1999. The PubMed MEDLINE search resulted in 141 articles. Of these, 126 were excluded because titles or abstracts did not meet inclusion criteria. An additional six articles were identified from reference lists. A total of 22 articles met inclusion criteria and are summarized in Table 16.1.

Pediatric patients with type 1 diabetes and CD were found to have at diagnosis of CD lower weight standard deviation scores (SDSs) (Artz 2008), lower height and weight SDSs (Kaspers 2004; Hansen 2006), lower BMI SDSs (Amin 2002; Kaspers 2004; Simmons 2007; Artz 2008), lower A1C levels (Kaspers 2004), and no difference in daily insulin doses (Amin 2002; Kaspers 2004). No differences were observed for height (Valetta 2007; Artz 2008) and height and weight at CD diagnosis (Sun 2009). No differences in A1C values were observed in pediatric subjects at CD diagnosis (Valetta 2007; Poulain 2007; Simmons 2007) and 2 years before CD diagnosis (Simmons 2007). One pediatric study reported lower hemoglobin (Hb) at diagnosis of CD compared to controls (Valleta 2007). However, adults with type 1 diabetes were found to have worse A1C levels at CD diagnosis than matched control subjects (Leeds 2011).

Gluten-Free Diet and Effects on Nutritional Status

The implementation of a GFD in pediatric patients with type 1 diabetes and its effects on nutritional status are mixed. Height (SDS) was reported to increase in people who were compliant with a GFD in one study (Sanchez-Albisua 2005) and in children <14 years old (Hansen 2006). Other studies reported no significant improvements or differences (Westman 1999; Saukkonen 2002; Saadah 2004;

Table 16.1 Studies on Nutritional Status and Metabolic Outcomes from Nutrition Therapy for Type 1 Diabetes and CD (Gluten-Free Diet)

	Population/ Duration of Study	Intervention (type of study)	Major Findings	Comments
Westman 1999	n = 20 youth with type 1 diabetes and CD (on GFD) and 40 youth with type 1 diabetes and no CD/not applicable	Compared 3-day food records and 7-day food frequency questionnaire for associations to A1C, ht SDS, wt SDS, BMI SDS, energy, and macro- and micronutrient intake (cross-sectional study)	No differences in A1C; ht, wt, or BMI SDS; energy or nutrient intake; CD patients had a higher saturated fat intake	Only 30% of CD patients compliant with GFD; IgA results available in 12 patients only, none elevated
Kaukinen 1999	n = 28 adults with type 1 diabetes and CD/3 years before and 5 years after starting a GFD n = 22 adults with type 1 diabetes and CD and 22 diabetes control subjects/1 year	Analyzed influence of GFD on metabolic control, insulin doses, BMI, and hypoglycemic episodes (retrospective and prospective cohort study)	GFD had no effect on metabolic control (P = 0.02), insulin doses, BMI, or hypoglycemic episodes in retrospective or prospective surveys	Small sample size; GFD compliance low in both surveys, patients with better compliance had no differences in metabolic control
Mohn 2001	n = 18 youth with type 1 diabetes and CD (on GFD) and 26 with type 1 diabetes without CD/36 months	Compared frequency of hypoglycemia, A1C, total insulin doses before (18 months) and after (18 months) diagnosis of CD and GFD (retrospective cohort study)	More hypoglycemic episodes 6 months before and 6 months after CD (P = 0.01); total insulin doses same at 18 months as before CD, ↓ in patients with CD, reached nadir at diagnosis (P = 0.05), and ↑ slowly after GFD; no difference in A1C (~8%)	Small sample size; GFD compliance assessed by AGA/EMA, which became negative during first 6 months in all subjects
Sauk-konen 2002	n = 18 youth with type 1 diabetes and CD/2 years	Analyzed ht SDS, weight-for-height, and changes in A1C before (1 year) and after (1 year) diagnosis of CD (retrospective cohort study)	No changes in ht SDS before or after CD diagnosis (P = 0.47); mean weight-for-height: no change before CD diagnosis (P = 0.87), ↑ after diagnosis (P = 0.02); no change in A1C before or after CD diagnosis (P = 0.12)	Small sample size; GFD compliance was established by questionnaire only

	Population/ Duration of Study	Intervention (type of study)	Major Findings	Comments
Amin 2002	$n = 11$ youth with type 1 diabetes and CD and 22 with type 1 diabetes and no CD/4 years	Measure ht, wt, and BMI SDS and glycemic control before CD diagnosis and after initiation of a GFD (cohort study)	Between diabetes and CD diagnosis, mean BMI SDS lower in CD patients ($P = 0.015$) as was A1C (9.3%) ($P = 0.002$); no difference in daily insulin dose ($P = 0.54$); after GFD, BMI SDS reversed over 1 year ($P = 0.11$); no difference in BMI SDS; A1C lower on GFD vs. before GFD ($P = 0.02$); insulin doses ↑ in both groups before the GFD ($P < 0.001$) but no difference in daily insulin dose between groups ($P = 0.33$)	Small sample size; GFD compliance good in 6 patients verified by re-biopsy, remaining patients maintained negative AGA/EMA antibody status throughout study period
Kaspers 2004	$n = 127$ youth with type 1 diabetes and CD and 18,470 type 1 diabetes controls/9 years	Reviewed ht, wt, BMI, A1C, insulin doses, severe hypoglycemia episodes, and thyroid autoimmunity (observational retrospective study)	Patients with CD and diabetes: impaired ht SDS ($P < 0.05$) and BMI SDS ($P < 0.05$), lower wt, and lower A1C ($P < 0.0011$); insulin doses and rates of severe hypoglycemia the same between groups	GFD adherence was not available in the database
Saadah 2004	$n = 21$ youth with type 1 diabetes and CD (on GFD) and 42 diabetes control subjects/2 years	Measured wt, ht, and BMI Z scores, A1C, and insulin doses before (1 year) and after (1 year) GFD initiation (retrospective cohort study)	After 1 year GFD, mean wt-for-age Z score ↑ ($P = 0.049$); mean ht ↑ but was NS ($P = 0.14$); mean BMI-for-age Z score ↑ ($P = 0.015$); control group no changes in wt, ht, or BMI	GFD compliance assessed by questionnaire only; 80% reported good adherence to GFD
Franzese 2004	$n = 33$ youth with type 1 diabetes and CD (18 had asymptomatic CD)/2–15 years	Studied asymptomatic CD in type 1 diabetes and relationship to wt/ht ratio and growth velocity (observational case control study)	After 2–15 years, 18 asymptomatic patients remained asymptomatic and showed normal wt/ht ratio and satisfactory growth velocity	GFD adherence was found in only 7 patients; methods to assess adherence not available
Sanchez-Albisua 2005	$n = 9$ youth with type 1 diabetes and CD/mean of 43 months (range 12–84)	Assessed changes in ht SDS and wt-for-ht SDS, A1C, and iron status (retrospective cohort study)	Ht SDS ↑ for GFD-adherent patients ($P = 0.03$); wt-for-ht changes NS ($P = 0.28$); trend toward improvement in A1C ($P = 0.05$); iron deficiency anemia in four patients, normalized in three patients who followed the GFD	Small sample size; GFD adherence assessed by questionnaire and negative antibody tests

Table 16.1 Studies on Nutritional Status and Metabolic Outcomes from Nutrition Therapy for Type 1 Diabetes and CD (Gluten-Free Diet) (*continued*)

	Population/ Duration of Study	Intervention (type of study)	Major Findings	Comments
Rami 2005	n = 98 youth with type 1 diabetes and CD on GFD (74 patients had silent CD) and 195 type 1 diabetes control subjects/3.3 years	A1C, severe hypoglycemia, DKA, insulin dosage, BMI SDS, ht SDS, and wt gain between CD/diabetes compared to diabetes control subjects (retrospective case control study)	A1C similar ($P = 0.35$); no difference in severe hypoglycemia, DKA, and insulin doses ($P = 0.45$); BMI SDS and ht SDS no difference at diagnosis, wt gain ↓ after diagnosis in boys with CD ($P < 0.05$); girls with CD had lower BMI but NS ($P = 0.067$)	GFD compliance was variable and was measured by EMA titers
Hansen 2006	n = 33 youth with type 1 diabetes and CD (on GFD) and 236 diabetes control subjects/CD patients 2 years, control subject parameters at diagnosis of CD	Examined growth, ht, and wt SDS for CD/diabetes and only diabetes at diagnosis of CD; iron deficiency anemia, wt and ht SDS, and A1C after 2 years on GFD (retrospective cohort study)	At baseline, CD patients had lower ht SDS ($P < 0.001$) and wt SDS ($P = 0.002$) vs. diabetes controls; 2-year data on GFD showed ↑ in wt SDS ($P = 0.006$) and in patients <14 years an ↑ in ht SDS ($p=0.036$); ht SDS in patients >14 years NS ($P = 0.073$); ↑ in Hb ($P = 0.002$) and ferritin ($P = 0.020$); A1C unchanged ($P = 0.311$)	GFD was followed by 31 patients (2 without symptoms refused the GFD); GFD compliance was determined by IgA EMA and tTGA and showed variable compliance
Simmons 2007	n = 71 youth with type 1 diabetes and CD (on GFD) and 63 youth with diabetes/ baseline CD diagnosis/ baseline and prior 2 years	Examined growth, body composition, BMD, and metabolic control compared between CD/ diabetes patients using IgA tTG+ and diabetes without CD (case control study)	Wt Z scores ($P = 0.024$), BMI scores ($P = 0.005$), and midarm circumference ($P = 0.031$) lower in IgA tTG + group vs. controls; A1C same in groups at baseline and 2 years before CD ($P = 0.245$); no differences in severe hypoglycemia or BMD ($P = 0.412$); in 35 biopsy-proven CD patients, BMI score lower than controls ($P = 0.05$)	20% of CD subjects had been following a GFD for ≥6 months at baseline; however, the mean IgA tTG index similar to remainder of IgA tTG group ($P = 0.768$); only 49.3% of patients had biopsy-confirmed CD

	Population/ Duration of Study	Intervention (type of study)	Major Findings	Comments
Poulain 2007	n = 15 youth with biopsy-confirmed CD (on GFD) out of 950 children with type 1 diabetes/3 years (2 months to 16.2 years)	Examined wt SDS, ht SDS, BMI percentile, A1C, and insulin doses at baseline and at study end (retrospective cohort study)	A1C: poor control of diabetes at baseline, no change after GFD, increases in insulin doses (P = 0.05) and body weight (P = 0.04) after GFD; ht and BMI did not increase	Small sample size; GFD diet compliance evaluated by RD by food records; 75% assessed as good compliance with GFD
Valetta 2007	n = 27 youth with type 1 diabetes and CD (on GFD) and 43 type 1 diabetes and no CD/diagnosis of CD, 24 and 48 months	Examined effects of early screening and diagnosis of CD and effects of GFD on wt, ht, BMI Z score, Hb, A1C, and daily insulin doses (longitudinal case controlled study)	At diagnosis of CD, ht, BMI Z scores, A1C, and daily insulin doses were similar, but Hb was lower in CD patients (P < 0.05); at 24 and 48 months, no differences in ht, BMI, A1C, and insulin dose; all patients had negative serology after 12–18 months on GFD	GFD adherence assessed by RD and tested by EMA and/or TGA; study showed positive benefits of early screening and diagnosis of CD
Artz 2008	n = 30 youth with asymptomatic and positive TGA CD and type 1 diabetes (on GFD) and 34 type 1 diabetes negative TGA patients/12–48 months	Examined baseline wt, ht, BMI Z scores, and lumbar spine BMD and BMAD Z scores at baseline and after GFD initiation (observational study)	Seropositive patients had reductions in BMD (P = 0.05); wt, BMI, and BMAD were marginally lower, but ht was comparable to controls at baseline; patients with severe villous atrophy on biopsy had ↓ wt, ht, BMD, and BMAD and ↑ in parathyroid hormone (all P < 0.05); GFD for at least 1 year ↑ BMD and BMAD	GFD adherence confirmed by normalization of or marked reductions in TGA titers
Valerio 2008	n = 52 youth with type 1 diabetes and CD (on GFD) and 50 patients with type 1 diabetes and no CD/for CD/diabetes patients 6.7 years; for patients without CE 5.0 years	Examined BMD in relation to level of adherence to GFD and glycemic control (observational cross-sectional study)	No difference in quality of bone between groups; osteopenia higher in patients not compliant with the GFD; negative correlation in BMD and A1C in patients with type 1 diabetes and patients with CD who strictly adhered to the GFD	GFD adherence measured by questionnaire from RD and IgA-tTG and/or EMA and stratified into groups based on adherence

Table 16.1 Studies on Nutritional Status and Metabolic Outcomes from Nutrition Therapy for Type 1 Diabetes and CD (Gluten-Free Diet) (*continued*)

	Population/ Duration of Study	Intervention (type of study)	Major Findings	Comments
Sun 2009	*n* = 49 youth with biopsy-proven silent CD and type 1 diabetes and 49 type 1 diabetes without CD/before CD diagnosis, at diagnosis, and after 1 and 2 years on a GFD	Examined growth, ht, wt, BMI SDS, and A1C (case-control study)	No difference in growth between groups; A1C was lower before diagnosis (*P* = 0.02), at diagnosis (*P* = 0.01), and ↑ after diagnosis and 1 year on GFD; A1C same as diabetes patients without CD (*P* = 0.9)	GFD adherence assessed by IgA EMA and AGA and tTG; patients with poor compliance excluded from study
Narula 2009	*n* = 22 youth with diabetes, positive celiac serology +/- biopsy confirmed CD (on GFD) and 50 patients with diabetes and negative CD serology/1-year follow-up	Examined gastrointestinal symptoms, growth, and insulin requirements in patients with type 1 diabetes with and without CD (retrospective case review)	At diagnosis, 76.4% of CD/diabetes patients had ≥1 gastrointestinal symptom vs. 6% of diabetes patients (*P* < 0.0005); GFD-compliant patients after 1 year: improvements in BMI SDS (*P* = 0.02); wt SDS (*P* = 0.0.08), NS ↑ insulin requirement; change in wt SDS (*P* = 0.008) and BMI SDS (*P* = 0.01) found between groups	GFD adherence determined by positive TTG and EMA serology at 1 year and/or the child admitting to noncompliance; 57% were compliant with GFD and were included in results
Goh 2010	*n* = 29 youth with asymptomatic CD and diabetes and 58 diabetes without CD/2 years	Examined ht *Z* score, wt *Z* score, change in BMI *Z* score, and A1C between groups before (1 year) and after (1 year) after diagnosis of CD (observational study)	No changes in ht *Z* scores, BMI *Z* scores, or A1C noted during the study period	GFD adherence confirmed by EMA and tTG titers; compliance was good in 92% of CD patients

	Population/ Duration of Study	Intervention (type of study)	Major Findings	Comments
Abid 2011	*n* = 22 youth with type 1 diabetes and CD (on GFD)/2 years	Examined ht, wt, and BMI SDS; Hb; A1C; insulin doses; and severe hypoglycemia episodes before (1 year) and after (1 year) diagnosis of CD and on GFR (retrospective longitudinal study)	Severe hypoglycemia episodes before and after GFD, NS ($P <$ 0.07); ht (P = 0.75), wt (P = 0.63), and BMI SDS (P = 0.37), NS; Hb unchanged; A1C NS small increase (P = 0.17); insulin doses ↑ at 12 months after GFD ($P <$ 0.0005)	Small sample size; GFD adherence measured by EMA and tTG; 4 patients IgA deficient, 16 patients showed serological improvement, 2 patients lacked complete data; compliance to GFD uncertain
Frohlich-Reiterer 2011	*n* = 411 youth with type 1 diabetes and biopsy-confirmed CD (*n* = 183) and 17,661 patients with type 1 diabetes and no CD/5-yr follow up	Examined ht, wt, and BMI SDS; A1C; insulin dosages; severe hypoglycemic events; DKA; dyslipidemia; retinopathy; and microalbuminuria in the most recent treatment year and 5-year follow-up of 9,805 patients (183 with CD) (observational prospective cohort study)	Ht and wt SDS lower in CD patients ($P <$ 0.001), NS difference in BMI SDS, acute or chronic complications, or metabolic control in the most recent treatment year; 5-year follow-up lower wt and ht SDS ($P <$ 0.005); no difference in BMI SDS and A1C at 5 years	GFD adherence was measured by tTGA and EMA; CD antibody positivity ↑ from 18% at 3 years to 27% at 5 years showing worse compliance with GFD over time
Leeds 2011	*n* = 1,000 patients with type 1 diabetes aged >16 years/1 year	Patients assessed for CD, A1C, lipids, quality of life, retinopathy, and nephropathy stage, degree of neuropathy before and after 1 year on GFD (case-control study)	33 patients had CD (3.3%) and at diagnosis had worse A1C (P = 0.05) and higher prevalence of retinopathy and nephropathy; treatment with GFD was safe and did not affect quality of life	

AGA, anti-gliadin antibodies; BMAD, bone mineral apparent density; DKA, diabetic ketoacidosis; EMA, anti-endomysial antibodies; ht, height; NS, nonsignificant; TGA or tGA or tTGA or tTG+, anti-tissue transglutaminase antibodies; wt, weight.

Franzese 2004; Rami 2005; Hansen 2006; Poulain 2007; Sun 2009; Goh 2010; Abid 2011), and two studies showed significantly lower height and weight after 9 years (Kaspers 2004) and 5 years on a GFD (Frohlich-Reiterer 2011). Improvements in weight (Saadah 2004; Hansen 2006; Poulain 2007; Narula 2009) and BMI (Amin 2002; Saadah 2004; Narula 2009) have also been reported, but this is not true for adults (Kaukinen 1999) and in all pediatric subjects (Westman 1999; Kaspers 2004; Rami 2005; Sanchez-Albisua 2005; Poulain 2007; Valletta 2007; Sun 2009; Goh 2010; Abid 2011; Frohlich-Reiterer 2011). One study observed a significant increase in weight-for-height in patients who were not previously underweight, suggesting introduction of a GFD may be associated with excess weight gain (Saukkonen 2002). Two studies in adults looked at mean serum fasting total cholesterol levels, which were lower at study entry in CD/diabetes subjects than in control subjects (Kaukinen 1999; Leeds 2011), and one pediatric study did not find any differences in dyslipidemia compared to control subjects (Frohlich-Reiterer 2011). A higher intake of saturated fat compared to controls was reported in one pediatric study (Westman 1999). Iron deficiency anemia normalized in pediatric subjects who followed the GFD were noted in one study (Sanchez-Albisua 2005), and increases in Hb and ferritin were noted in another (Hansen 2006). Mean Hb was normal 12 months before and 12 months after a GFD in one study (Abid 2011).

Gluten-Free Diet and Effects on Glycemic Control

An increase in A1C levels after following a GFD was reported in one pediatric study (Sun 2009), whereas others showed improvement in A1C (Amin 2002; Sanchez-Albisua 2005). Two adult studies showed improvement in A1C 1 year after diagnosis (Depczynski 2008; Leeds 2011), and another study showed a consistently lower A1C throughout the study period of 9 years (Kaspers 2004). The remaining adult and pediatric studies reported no change in A1C (Westman 1999; Kaukinen 1999; Mohn 2000; Saukkonen 2002; Saadah 2004; Rami 2005; Hansen 2006; Valetta 2007; Goh 2010; Abid 2011; Frohlich-Reiterer 2011). A decrease in the number of hypoglycemic episodes was noted in some pediatric studies (Sanchez-Albisua 2005; Hansen 2006) but not in other adult (Kaukinen 1999) or pediatric studies (Mohn 2000; Kaspers 2004; Rami 2005; Abid 2011; Frohlich-Reiterer 2011). Two pediatric studies showed no difference in diabetic ketoacidosis episodes when compared to control subjects (Rami 2005; Frohlich-Reiterer 2011).

Gluten-Free Diet and Effects on Insulin Requirements

Total insulin requirements decreased before diagnosis of CD in pediatric subjects (Mohn 2000), increased after introduction of a GFD (Mohn 2000; Poulain 2007; Narula 2009; Abid 2011), were similar to control subjects with type 1 diabetes without CD (Amin 2002; Kaspers 2004; Valetta 2007), and remained unchanged in adults (Kaukinen 1999).

Bone Health

Osteoporosis and osteopenia are the most common complications of undiagnosed or untreated CD. A few studies have examined bone mineral density (BMD) levels in adolescents and children with CD and type 1 diabetes. Results have differed, with some studies reporting lower BMD in patients with CD and type 1 diabetes (Diniz-Santos 2008; Artz 2008) and another finding no difference (Simmons 2007). One pediatric study stratified BMD results according to adherence with the GFD, showing individuals who adhere strictly have the same BMD as type 1 diabetes control subjects, but poor compliance with the GFD resulted in lower BMD (Valerio 2008). One study in adults identified lower BMD in type 1 diabetes and undiagnosed CD (Lunt 2001). Pediatric patients who followed a GFD had improvement in BMD and bone mineral apparent density Z scores (Artz 2008).

Conclusions Regarding Nutrition Therapy

The variable findings among studies, small numbers of patients studied, lack of consistent distinction between symptomatic and asymptomatic patients and degree of small bowel mucosa injury, variable time periods preceding CD diagnosis, variable study time periods after CD diagnosis, and variable methods to determine GFD compliance make interpretation of the real impact of strict adherence to a GFD in pediatric and adult patients with type 1 diabetes difficult. Therefore, the nutrition therapy recommendations for people with CD and type 1 diabetes should emphasize strict adherence to the GFD, maintenance of a well-balanced healthy eating pattern to ensure adequate nutrient intake and appropriate growth in children and adolescents, and optimal metabolic control of diabetes using insulin to cover carbohydrates consumed.

THE GLUTEN-FREE DIET

People with CD who carefully follow a well-balanced, healthy GFD have the same nutrition requirements as other individuals once the intestinal mucosa is healed. However, careful nutrition assessments must be conducted to ensure adequate intake of nutrients, since some deficiencies have been noted while on the GFD for many years (Thompson 2005; Hallert 2002). The complexities of the GFD can be extremely challenging, since ongoing monitoring of ingredients in foods and food processing are intricate parts of nutrition interventions.

The Acad Nutr Diet EAL published their findings after a review of the evidence related to the following questions: *1*) what is the evidence to support the nutritional adequacy of a gluten-free eating pattern in people newly diagnosed with CD; *2*) what is the long-term effectiveness of following a gluten-free eating pattern on bone density, hematological variables related to iron deficiency anemia, villous atrophy, and gastrointestinal symptoms; *3*) can oats be incorporated into the eating pattern; and *4*) what is the long-term effectiveness of following a gluten-free eating pattern on pregnancy outcomes and on neurological symptoms? A summary of the conclusion statements follows (Acad Nutr Diet 2009).

For newly diagnosed children and adults with CD, studies report that adherence to a gluten-free eating pattern results in significant improvements in nutritional laboratory values, such as serum Hb, iron, zinc, and calcium, as a result of intestinal healing and improved absorption. However, adherence to the gluten-free eating pattern may result in a diet that is high in fat and low in carbohydrates and fiber, as well as low in iron, folate, niacin, vitamin B_{12}, calcium, phosphorus, and zinc, and a small number of studies in adults show a trend toward weight gain after diagnosis (Acad Nutr Diet 2009).

It is concerning that clinical trials and cross-sectional studies have reported reduced bone mineral content and BMD in untreated children, adolescents, and adults with CD; both of these parameters improve significantly with compliance to a gluten-free eating pattern for at least 1 year. Adherence to nutrition therapy initiated during childhood or adolescence allows normal bone mineralization. However, studies in untreated adults have shown that a gluten-free eating pattern improves but may not normalize BMD; successful treatment depends on the age at diagnosis, since patients who do not receive treatment in childhood and adolescence may never reach peak bone mass. Further studies are needed regarding the effects of calcium and vitamin D supplementation on bone mineral content and BMD, as well as hormone replacement therapy for postmenopausal women.

Studies report that for most children and adults with CD, adherence to a gluten-free eating pattern results in significant improvements in hematological parameters including serum Hb, iron, ferritin, mean corpuscular volume, mean corpuscular Hb, and red cell distribution width. Recovery of anemia (normalization of Hb concentrations) generally occurs within 6 months, whereas recovery from iron deficiency (normalization of ferritin concentrations) may take longer than 1 year. Iron supplementation in the form of a multivitamin with iron or additional therapeutic doses of iron may be necessary to achieve normal values of these hematological variables within these time periods.

It is reported that individuals who adhere to a gluten-free eating pattern have substantial improvement in villous atrophy; however, mucosal abnormalities may persist in some individuals. Normalization of abnormalities may occur within 1 year, but generally takes longer, depending on the severity of villous atrophy, level of dietary adherence, and age at diagnosis. One study indicated that recovery in children may progress faster and more completely than in adults. Several studies report that improvement in villous atrophy does not depend on the type of gluten-free eating pattern (wheat starch–based [specially processed to remove gluten] or naturally gluten-free); however, villous atrophy is significantly associated with adherence to a gluten-free eating pattern. Further research is needed to determine the factors involved in the persistence of mucosal abnormalities in people adhering to a GFD.

With regard to the long-term effect on gastrointestinal symptoms when following a gluten-free eating pattern, several studies reported that people with CD (treated and untreated) are more likely to experience gastrointestinal symptoms such as diarrhea, constipation, abdominal pain and bloating, nausea or vomiting, reduced gut motility, and delayed gastric emptying than healthy control subjects. However, adherence to a GFD has been shown to reduce the prevalence of these symptoms.

Oats

Questions are often asked about the inclusion of oats in an eating pattern for CD. It is reported that incorporating oats uncontaminated with wheat, barley, or rye into a gluten-free eating pattern for people with CD, at intake levels of ~50 g dry oats per day, is generally safe and improves compliance (Acad Nutr Diet 2009). However, many studies report that the introduction of oats may result in gastrointestinal symptoms such as diarrhea and abdominal discomfort. Additional adverse effects that have been reported include dermatitis herpetiformis, villous atrophy, and an increased density of intra-epithelial lymphocytes, indicating that some people with CD may be unable to tolerate oats. Further research is needed in this area.

Pregnancy and Women's Health

Several cohort and case-control studies have reported that women with undiagnosed or untreated CD have an increased risk of spontaneous abortion and miscarriage, low-birth-weight and small-for-gestational-age newborns, stillbirth, perinatal disease and mortality, low Apgar scores, delayed menarche and early menopause, premature delivery, intrauterine growth retardation, breech presentation, and cesarean delivery, whereas compliance with a gluten-free dietary pattern results in risks similar to those of healthy control subjects (Acad Nutr Diet 2009). Despite the increased risks of complications, the overall number of pregnancies does not appear to be influenced by CD. Evidence is limited in the areas of fertility, breast-feeding duration, threatened abortion, secondary amenorrhea, and labor induction. Further research is needed in these areas.

Neurological Symptoms

Several studies reported that people with CD are more likely to experience neurological symptoms such as depression, cerebellar ataxia, headaches and migraines, and neuropathy than healthy control subjects. Early diagnosis and adherence to a gluten-free eating pattern may reduce the prevalence of symptoms related to cerebellar ataxia, headaches, and migraines. Six studies report that adherence to a GFD has not been shown to have an effect on depressive symptoms; one study suggests that this may relate more to family history of depression. Evidence is less conclusive and/or limited regarding the effect of a gluten-free eating pattern on epilepsy, anxiety, regional cerebral perfusion, hypotonia, learning disorders, and disruptive behavior disorders; additional research needs to be conducted in these areas.

Implementing the Gluten-Free Diet

It is also known that a GFD can be more expensive than a normal eating pattern and requires extensive, repeated counseling and instruction by an RD. People with CD must become scrupulous label-readers every time they purchase food and must be knowledgeable regarding food processing, preparation, and handling practices to avoid cross contamination with gluten-containing grains. As little as 10 mg gluten (1/50th a slice of bread) can cause significant mucosal inflammation in some individuals; therefore, the study authors recommended the ingestion of contaminating gluten should be kept to <50 mg/day in the treatment of CD (Catassi 2007). A recent study found contamination in gluten-free grains, seeds, and flours; therefore, food manufacturers are being urged to test gluten-free products for gluten contamination using validated testing methods (Thompson 2010). The U.S. Food and Drug Administration's (FDA) final ruling on the definition of gluten-free under the Food Allergen Labeling and Consumer Protection Act proposed in 2004 (FALCPA 2004) has yet to be determined as of spring 2011 (Federal Register Proposed Rule 2007). FDA is proposing gluten-free products would contain <20 parts per million gluten, using validated testing methods. Unfortunately, this testing would be voluntary. Gluten-free certification programs exist to assist consumers with selection of gluten-free foods. Gluten can also be found in pre-

Table 16.2 Resources for Gluten-Free Food Determination and Certification Programs

Celiac Sprue Association GF Product Listing	http://www.csaceliacs.info/product_listing.jsp
Zeer	http://www.zeer.com
Gluten Free Watchdog	http://www.glutenfreewatchdog.org
Gluten-Free Certification Organization	http://www.gfco.org
National Foundation for Celiac Awareness	http://www.celiaccentral.org
Quality Assurance International	http://www.qai-inc.com/resources/gluten_free_process.asp
Canadian Celiac Association	http://www.celiac.ca/certification.php
Celiac Sprue Recognition Seal Program	http://www.csaceliacs.info/csa_recognition_seal_program_requirements.jsp

scription and over-the-counter medications, vitamins, minerals and supplements, and non-food items such as play dough. Table 16.2 lists resources for GF food determination and CD patients.

SUMMARY

The Academy of Nutrition and Dietetics, after conducting a literature review, published the following guidelines for CD and nutrition therapy (Acad Nutr Diet 2009):

- After a thorough assessment, individuals with CD and family members should be provided with and educated on a gluten-free eating pattern. Individuals are advised to consume whole or enriched gluten-free grains and products and to avoid gluten-containing grains (Table 16.3).
- If usual food intake shows nutritional inadequacies that cannot be alleviated through improved eating habits, a daily gluten-free age- and sex-specific multivitamin and mineral supplement may be needed. Gluten-free foods may be low in iron, folate, niacin, vitamin B12, calcium, phosphorus, and zinc.
- Individuals who enjoy and can tolerate gluten-free oats can gradually include them in their gluten-free eating pattern. Incorporating oats uncontaminated with wheat, barley, or rye at intake levels of ~50 g dry oats per day is generally reported to be safe and improves adherence to a gluten-free eating pattern.
- Education about the disease, about label reading, and on food cross-contamination within manufacturing plants, restaurants, and home kitchens is essential.

Table 16.3 Listing of Gluten-Free Grains, Starches, and Flours and Unsafe Gluten-Containing Grains

Gluten-Free Grains, Starches, and Flours (partial listing)	Unsafe Gluten-Containing Grains, Starches, and Flours (partial listing)
Amaranth	Barley
Arrowroot	Bran
Buckwheat, kasha	Bulgur
Beans, peas, legumes	Cereal binding
Corn, cornmeal, corn gluten, corn malt, cornstarch, corn bran	Communion wafers
Flaxseed	Couscous
Job's tears	Cracked wheat
Kudzo	Dinkle
Manioc	Durum
Millet	Einkorn
Montina® (Indian Rice Grass)	Emmer
Nut, tree nut, peanut, and seed flours (almond, hazelnut, pecan, sesame, sunflower, etc.)	Farina
	Farro
	Fu
Oats, oat bran, oat gum (use uncontaminated sources)	Graham flour
	Kamut
Popcorn	Malt (malt extract, malt flavoring, malt syrup, malt beverages, malted milk, malt vinegar)
Potato, sweet potato, yam, potato flour, potato starch	
	Matzo
Quinoa	Mir
Rice: brown, white, wild, rice bran, rice flour	Rye
	Seitan
Soy	Semolina
Sago	Spelt
Sorghum, milo	Triticale
Tapioca (also called cassava or manioc)	Wheat (wheat bran, berry, germ, gluten, grass, nut)
Teff	
	Any unidentifiable flour product

Adapted from the Celiac Sprue Association (http://www.csaceliacs.org). Accessed October 2011.

BIBLIOGRAPHY

Abid N, McGlone O, Cardwell C, McCallion W, Carson D: Clinical and metabolic effects of gluten free diet in children with type 1 diabetes and celiac disease. *Pediatr Diabetes* 12:322–325, 2011

Academy of Nutrition and Dietetics: Celiac disease evidence analysis project, 2009. Available from http://www.adaevidencelibrary.com/topic.cfm?cat=3055

American Diabetes Association: Standards of medical care in diabetes: 2012. *Diabetes Care* 35 (Suppl. 1):S11–S63, 2012

Amin R, Murphy N, Edge J, Ahmed M, Acerini C, Dunger D: A longitudinal study of the effects of a gluten-free diet on glycemic control and weight gain in subjects with type 1 diabetes and celiac disease. *Diabetes Care* 25:1117–1122, 2002

Artz E, Warren-Ulanch J, Becker D, Greenspan S, Freemark M: Seropositivity to celiac antigens in asymptomatic children with type 1 diabetes mellitus: association with weight, height, and bone mineralization. *Pediatr Diabetes* 9:277–284, 2008

Card TR, West J, Holmes GK: Risk of malignancy in diagnosed celiac disease: a 24-year prospective, population-based, cohort study. *Aliment Pharmacol Ther* 20:769–775, 2004

Catassi C, Fabian E, Iacono G, D'Agate C, Francavilla R, Biagi F, Volta U, Accomando S, Picarelli A, De Vitis I, Pianelli G, Gesuita R, Carle F, Mandolesi A, Bearzi I, Fasano A: A prospective, double-blind, placebo-controlled trial to establish a safe gluten threshold for patients with celiac disease. *Am J Clin Nutr* 85:160–166, 2007

Depczynski B: Coeliac disease and its relation to glycaemic control in adults with type 1 diabetes mellitus. *Diabetes Res Clin Pract* 79:10, 2008

Diniz-Santos DR, Brandão F, Adan L, Moreira A, Vicente EJ, Silva LR: Bone mineralization in young patients with type 1 diabetes mellitus and screening-identified evidence of celiac disease. *Dig Dis Sci* 53:1240–1245, 2008

Fasano A: Clinical presentation of celiac disease in the pediatric population. *Gastroenterology* 128 (Suppl. 1):S68–S73, 2005a

Fasano A, Catassi C: Current approaches to diagnosis and treatment of celiac disease: an evolving spectrum. *Gastroenterology* 120:636–651, 2001

Fasano A, Shea-Donohue T: Mechanisms of disease: the role of intestinal barrier function in the pathogenesis of gastrointestinal autoimmune diseases. *Nat Clin Pract Gastroenterol Hepatol* 2:416–422, 2005b

Federal Register Proposed Rule, 72 FR 2795, January 23, 2007: Food Labeling; Gluten-Free Labeling of Foods, 2007. Available from http://www.fda.gov/Food/LabelingNutrition/FoodAllergensLabeling/GuidanceComplianceRegulatoryInformation/ucm077926.htm

Food Allergen Labeling and Consumer Protection Act (FALCPA) of 2004 (Public Law 108-282, Title II, 2004). Available from http://www.fda.gov/Food/LabelingNutrition/FoodAllergensLabeling/GuidanceComplianceRegulatoryInformation/ucm106187.htm

Franzese A, Spagnuolo MI, Valerio G: Diabetic children with asymptomatic celiac disease: is it necessary to stress gluten-free diet? (Letter) *Clin Nutr* 23:281–282, 2004

Frohlich-Reiterer E, Kaspers S, Hofer S, Schober E, Kordonouri O, Bechtold-Dalla Pozza S, Reinhard W, Holl RW: Anthropometry, metabolic control, and follow-up in children and adolescents with type 1 diabetes mellitus and biopsy-proven celiac disease. *J Pediatr* 158:589–593, 2011

Goh VL, Estrada DE, Lerer T, Balarezo F, Sylvester FA: Effect of gluten-free diet on growth and glycemic control in children with type 1 diabetes and asymptomatic celiac disease. *J Pediatr Endocrinol Metab* 23:1169–1173, 2010

Green PH: The many faces of celiac disease: clinical presentation of celiac disease in the adult population. *Gastroenterology* 128:S74–S78, 2005a

Green PH, Rostami K; Marsh MN: Diagnosis of coeliac disease. *Best Pract Res Clin Gastroenterol* 19:389–400, 2005b

Green PH, Stavropoulos SN, Panagi SG, Goldstein SL, McMahon DJ, Absan H, Neugut AI: Characteristics of adult celiac disease in the USA: results of a national survey. *Am J Gastroenterol* 96:126–131, 2001

Grefte JM, Bouman JG, Grond J, Jansen W, Kleibeuker JH: Slow and incomplete histological and functional recovery in adult gluten sensitive enteropathy. *J Clin Pathol* 41:886–891, 1988

Hallert C, Grant C, Grehn S, Granno C, Hulten S, Midhagen G, Strom M, Svensson H, Valdimarsson T: Evidence of poor vitamin status in coeliac patients on a gluten free diet for 10 years. *Aliment Pharmacol Ther* 15:1333–1339, 2002

Hansen D, Brock-Jacobsen B, Lund E, Bjørn C, Hansen LP, Nielsen C, Fenger C, Fenger C, Lillevang ST, Husby S: Clinical benefit of a gluten-free diet in type 1 diabetic children with screening-detected celiac disease: a population-based screening study with 2 years' follow-up. *Diabetes Care* 29:2452–2456, 2006

Holmes GK: Screening for coeliac disease in type 1 diabetes. *Arch Dis Child* 87:495–498, 2002

Kaspers S, Kordonouri O, Schober E, Grabert M, Hauffa BP, Holl RW; German Working Group for Pediatric Diabetology: Anthropometry, metabolic control, and thyroid autoimmunity in type 1 diabetes with celiac disease: a multicenter survey. *J Pediatr* 145:790–795, 2004

Kaukinen K, Salmi J, Lahtela J, Siljamaki-Ojansuu U, Koivisto AM, Oksa H, Collin P: No effect of gluten-free diet on the metabolic control of type 1 diabetes in patients with diabetes and celiac disease (Letter). *Diabetes Care* 22:1747–1748, 1999

Leeds JS, Hopper AD, Hadjivassilioou M, Tesfaye S, Sanders DS: High prevalence of microvascular complications in adults with type 1 diabetes and newly diagnosed celiac disease. *Diabetes Care* 34:2158–2163, 2011

Lunt H, Florkowski CM, Bramwell Cook H, Whitehead MR: Bone mineral density, type 1 diabetes, and celiac disease (Letter). *Diabetes Care* 24:791–792, 2001

Mohn A, Cerruto M, Iafusco D, Prisco F, Tumini S, Stoppoloni O, Chiarelli F: Celiac disease in children and adolescents with type 1 diabetes: importance of hypoglycemia. *J Pediatr Gastroenterol Nutr* 32:37–40, 2001

American Diabetes Association Guide to Nutrition Therapy for Diabetes

Murray JA, Van Dyke C, Plevak MF, Dierkhising RA, Zinsmeister AR, Melton L: Trends in the identification and clinical features of celiac disease in a North American community, 1950–2001. *Clin Gastroenterol Hepatol* 1:9–27, 2003

Narula P, Porter L, Langton J, Rao V, Davies P, Cummins C, Kirk J, Barrett T, Protheroe S: Gastrointestinal symptoms in children with type 1 diabetes screened for celiac disease. *Pediatrics* 124:489–495, 2009

National Institutes of Health: NIH Consensus Development Conference on Celiac Disease, June 28–30, 2004. *Gastroenterology* 128 (Suppl. 1):S1–S9, 2005

Nicolas MEO, Krause PK, Gibson LE, Murray JA: Dermatitis herpetiformis. *Int J Dermatol* 42:588–600, 2003

Oxentenko AS, Murray JA: Celiac disease and dermatitis herpatiformis: the spectrum of gluten-sensitive enteropathy. *Int J Dermatol* 42:585–587, 2003

Poulain C, Johanet C, Delcroix C, Levy-Marchal C, Tubiana-Rufi N: Prevalence and clinical features of celiac disease in 950 children with type 1 diabetes in France. *Diabetes Metab* 33:453–458, 2007

Rami B, Sumnik Z, Schober E, Waldhör T, Battelino T, Bratanic N, Kürti K, Lebl J, Limbert C, Madacsy L, Odink RJ, Paskova M, Soltesz G: Screening detected celiac disease in children with type 1 diabetes mellitus: effect on the clinical course (a case control study). *J Pediatr Gastroenterol Nutr* 41:317–321, 2005

Rewers M, Liu E, Simmons J, Redondo MJ, Hoffenberg EJ: Celiac disease associated with type 1 diabetes mellitus. *Endocrinol Metab Clin North Am* 33:197–214, 2004

Rodrigo L: Celiac disease. *World J Gastroenterol* 12:6585–6593, 2006

Saadah OI, Zacharin M, O'Callaghan A, Oliver MR, Catto-Smith AG: Effect of gluten-free diet and adherence on growth and diabetic control in diabetics with coeliac disease. *Arch Dis Child* 89:871–876, 2004

Sanchez-Albisua I, Wolf J, Neu A, Geiger H, Wäscher I, Stern M: Coeliac disease in children with type 1 diabetes mellitus: the effect of the gluten-free diet. *Diabet Med* 22:1079–1082, 2005

Saukkonen T, Vaisanen S, Akerblom HK, Savilahti E, the Childhood Diabetes in Finland Study Group: Coeliac disease in children and adolescents with type 1 diabetes: a study of growth, glycaemic control, and experiences of families. *Acta Paediatr* 91:297–302, 2002

Simmons JH, Klingensmith GJ, McFann K, Rewers M, Taylor J, Emery LM, Taki I, Vanyi S, Liu E, Hoffenberg EJ: Impact of celiac autoimmunity on children with type 1 diabetes. *J Pediatr* 150:461–466, 2007

Sun S, Puttha R, Ghezaiel S, Skae M, Cooper C, Amin R: The effect of biopsy-positive silent coeliac disease and treatment with a gluten-free diet on growth and glycaemic control in children with type 1 diabetes. *Diabet Med* 26:1250–1254, 2009

Thompson T, Dennis M, Higgins LA, Lee AR, Sharrett MK: Gluten-free diet survey: are Americans with celiac disease consuming recommended amounts of fibre, iron, calcium and grain foods? *J Hum Nutr Diet* 18:163–169, 2005

Thompson T, Lee A, Grace T: Gluten contamination of grains, seeds, and flours in the United States: a pilot study. *J Am Diet Assoc* 110:937–940, 2010

Vader LW, Stepniak DT, Bunnik EM, Kooy YM, de Haan W, Drijfhout JW, Van Veelen PA, Konig F: Characterization of cereal toxicity for celiac disease patients based on protein homology in grains. *Gastroenterology* 125:1105–1113, 2003

Valerio G, Spandaro R, Iafusco D, Lombardi F, del Puente A, Esposito A, De Terlizzi F, Prisco F, Troncone R, Franzese A: The influence of gluten free diet on quantitative ultrasound of proximal phalanxes in children and adolescents with type 1 diabetes mellitus and celiac disease. *Bone* 43:322–326, 2008

Valletta E, Ulmi D, Mabboni I, Tomasselli F, Pinelli L: Early diagnosis and treatment of celiac disease in type 1 diabetes: a longitudinal, case-control study. *Pediatr Med Chir* 29:99–104, 2007

Westman E, Ambler GF, Royle M, Peat J, Chan A: Children with coeliac disease and insulin dependent diabetes-growth, diabetes control and dietary intake. *J Pediatr Endocrinol Metab* 12:433–422, 1999

Carol Brunzell, RD, CDE, is a Diabetes Educator at the Diabetes Care Centers, University of Minnesota Medical Center, Fairview, Minneapolis, MN.

Chapter 17
Nutrition Therapy for Cystic Fibrosis–Related Diabetes

Carol Brunzell, RD, CDE

Highlights
Nutrition Therapy for Cystic Fibrosis–Related Diabetes

■ Cystic fibrosis–related diabetes (CFRD) occurs with increasing frequency, since people with cystic fibrosis (CF) are living longer.

■ There are critical differences in nutrition therapy for CFRD compared to type 1 and type 2 diabetes that must be understood to ensure survival in these individuals. A higher energy intake is essential as well as routine vitamin and mineral supplementation; restricting fats, protein, and sodium is not recommended.

Nutrition Therapy for Cystic Fibrosis–Related Diabetes

About 1 in 3,500 children in the U.S. is born with cystic fibrosis (CF) each year. CF affects all racial and ethnic groups and is more common among Caucasians. An estimated 30,000 people in the U.S. have CF. In the 1950s, the life expectancy was <5 years. In 2009, it was 35.9 years; however, many people live well into their sixth and seventh decades (Cystic Fibrosis Foundation [CFF] 2009). Cystic fibrosis–related diabetes (CFRD) has become the most common comorbidity in people with CF as the population ages and is associated with worse survival. It occurs in ~20% of adolescents and 40–50% of adults (Moran 2009a). The etiology for diabetes in CF is not related to either type 1 or type 2 diabetes; however, there are some shared similarities (Moran 1998). Nutrition therapy for CFRD drastically differs from type 1 and 2 diabetes (Moran 2010). These critical nutrition therapy differences are essential to understand for individuals with CFRD to have the best clinical outcomes.

This chapter begins with the Cystic Fibrosis Foundation care guidelines and goals (CFF 2009). A selected summary of the evidence-based nutrition recommendations for adults and children with CF will be reviewed (Stallings 2008). Differences in nutrition therapy and selected medical management for CFRD versus type 1 and type 2 diabetes, pregnancy with CFRD and gestational diabetes mellitus (GDM), treatment for hypoglycemia, and prediabetes are summarized (Moran 2010). A literature search was also conducted using PubMed MEDLINE for articles related to CFRD nutrition therapy. Search criteria included nutrition and cystic fibrosis–related diabetes, and additional articles were identified from reference lists. The initial search of potentially relevant articles identified 61 articles, of which 60 were excluded because titles or abstracts did not meet inclusion criteria. Three articles were identified from reference lists. Two articles met inclusion criteria and are included in Table 17.1.

NUTRITION THERAPY FOR CYSTIC FIBROSIS

Nutrition therapy is the cornerstone of treatment for people with CF, and optimization of growth and nutritional status is essential for survival. Nutrition therapy goals for CF include normal growth and nutrition for children, teens, and adults with CF and aggressively screening and managing people with CF for complications of the disease, particularly CFRD (CFF 2009; CFF 2011a). The following recommendations are for nutrition and growth status, which includes weight, stature, and weight-for-stature (CFF 2011b). For children older than 2 years of age and adults, energy intakes greater than the standard for the general population

Table 17.1 Studies on Nutrition Therapy for CFRD

	Population/ Duration of Study	Intervention (type of study)	Major Findings	Comments
White 2009	n = 96 adults, 48 with CFRD, 48 with CF/8 years (6 years before until 2 years after diagnosis)	Nutrition monitoring every 2 months at outpatient clinic appointments; high-calorie oral supplements used and overnight enteral tube feedings initiated with nutritional decline (case-control study)	Intensive nutritional intervention prevented clinical decline in the prediabetic period but is influenced by age of onset; in younger patients with CFRD, actively growing, BMI was 5–11% lower than control subjects, with some improvement after insulin therapy; children continuing to grow through the prediabetic years, had level of nutritional decline absent in older adults	44% of CFRD patients vs. 19% of control subjects required enteral tube feedings at the time of diagnosis, starting 2 years before diagnosis
Moran 2009b	n = 81 patients (61 with CFRD but without fasting hyperglycemia and 20 with severe IGT)/2 years	One year of therapy with premeal insulin aspart, repaglinide, or oral placebo compared in patients with CF and abnormal glucose tolerance before (1 year) and after (1 year) treatment (randomized controlled trial)	One year before therapy, BMI ↓ in all groups; after 1 year of insulin therapy, patients gained more weight (P = 0.02) than repaglinide-treated patients who had an initial BMI gain (P = 0.01) but lost weight after 6 months, and at 12 months, there was no difference in rate of BMI change compared to the year before (P = 0.33); no change in rate of BMI decline was seen in patients with IGT on insulin or repaglinide	Insulin is superior to oral agents in improving weight and nutritional status in patients with CFRD

IGT, impaired glucose tolerance.

are recommended to support weight maintenance in adults and weight gain at an age-appropriate rate in children.

Improved weight status was found at intakes ranging from 110 to 200% of energy needs for the non-CF population of similar age, sex, and size. To achieve energy intakes of 110–200% of requirements for the non-CF population, the following is recommended for patients with CF:

- For children aged 1–12 years with growth deficits, intensive treatment with behavioral intervention in conjunction with nutrition counseling is recommended to promote weight gain.
- For children with growth deficits and adults with weight deficits, use of nutritional supplements (oral and enteral) in addition to usual food intake is recommended to improve the rate of weight gain.
- For children aged ≥13 years with growth deficits and for adults with weight deficits, there is insufficient evidence to make a recommendation regarding intensive treatment with behavioral intervention in conjunction with nutrition counseling to promote weight gain.

There is good evidence from population-based studies that normal ranges of weight-for-age, height-for-age, and weight-for-height percentiles are associated with better pulmonary function, as indicated by the percent predicted forced expiratory volume in 1 second (FEV1) and survival for adults and children. Therefore, the following recommendations have been made (Stallings 2008):

- For children, maintenance of normal ranges of weight- and stature-for-age are recommended, since normal growth status is associated with better FEV1 and survival.
- For adults, maintenance of normal weight-for-height is recommended, since it is associated with better FEV1 and survival.
- For children and adults with nutritional deficits, there is insufficient evidence to make a recommendation concerning the relationship between improved rate of weight gain after nutrition interventions and improved FEV1. The patient registry shows a strong link between a higher BMI percentile and better lung function in children. One important measure of lung function in CF is FEV1, or over 1 second FEV1 percent predicted. The connection between a higher BMI and better lung function is also seen in adults with CF.
- For adults aged ≥20 years, weight-for-stature assessment should use the BMI method, and women should maintain a BMI of ≥22 kg/m^2 and men a BMI of ≥23 kg/m^2.

Nutrition Therapy Interventions for CFRD

Achieving nutrition therapy goals requires management of gastrointestinal symptoms, pulmonary symptoms, and nutrient and energy intake. Malnutrition in CF results from a combination of factors: *1)* inadequate energy and micronutrient intake complicated by malabsorption due to pancreatic exocrine deficiency requiring pancreatic enzyme replacement therapy, *2)* increased resting metabolic rate due to decreased pulmonary function and increased work of breathing, *3)* insulin deficiency with catabolism of lean body mass and adipose stores from fibrosis of β-cells and reduced β-cell mass, and *4*) recurrent sinopulmonary infections and chronic inflammation (Gaskin 2004; Orenstein 2002; Moran 1991; Tofé 2005).

Body weight and lean body mass are directly related to pulmonary function in CF. Insulin is a potent anabolic hormone necessary for maintaining body weight and lean body mass. Insulin deficiency and hyperglycemia lead to protein and lipid catabolism in CF with loss of lean body mass and adipose stores, even in the face of relatively normal blood glucose levels. Deterioration of nutritional status was shown to occur 4 years before diagnosis of CFRD, negatively affecting lung function and increasing morbidity and mortality (Milla 2000). Most individuals die from inflammatory lung disease (Milla 2000; Rosenecker 2001). When compared to repaglinide, insulin therapy was demonstrated to safely reverse chronic weight loss and improve BMI in people with CFRD without fasting hyperglycemia. Insulin is superior to oral agents in breaking the cycle of protein catabolism, weight loss, and pulmonary function decline because of its anabolic effects (Moran 2009b).

Aggressive nutritional interventions with oral nutritional supplements and overnight enteral tube feedings have been demonstrated to prevent the nutritional decline before the diagnosis of CFRD in adults, but is influenced by age of onset. Younger people who continued to grow throughout the prediabetic years had a lower BMI 2 years before CFRD diagnosis than people without CFRD and showed a level of nutritional decline not found in older adults (White 2009).

Abnormal glucose tolerance and diabetes are present in the majority of individuals with CF due to insulin insufficiency and, to a lesser extent, to insulin resistance. Recognition of glycemic abnormalities through aggressive screening has led to improvements in nutritional status, pulmonary function, and mortality rates (Moran 2009b).

There are many critical differences in nutrition therapy recommendations for CFRD that must be understood to ensure survival in these individuals, specifically with regard to calories, fat, protein, sodium, supplemental vitamins and minerals, and nutrition therapy for GDM and prediabetes. Adequate calorie intake to maintain the recommended BMI for children and adults is critical for health and survival. The additional diagnosis of CFRD does not change the CF nutrition recommendations. Normalization of blood glucose is essential to optimize nutrient metabolism and to improve BMI and lean body mass (Moran 2009b). Calories should almost never be restricted. The high-calorie eating pattern does not replace the need for a healthy, nutrient-dense food and nutrient intake, but people with CF will still need routine vitamin and mineral supplementation because of malabsorption. Pancreatic exocrine deficiency is present in 85–90% of all people with CF, and these patients require pancreatic enzyme replacement therapy with all meals and snacks. Adequate dosing of pancreatic enzyme replacement therapy facilitates absorption of macronutrients and micronutrients, minimizes symptoms of malabsorption, promotes adequate weight gain and growth, and optimizes nutritional status (Borowitz 1995). A high-sodium diet is necessary for all people with CF because of an increased risk for hyponatremia from excess salt loss through sweating, especially in hot weather, during extensive exercise and outdoor sports, or during a fever.

Appetite can be highly variable from day to day in people with CF, who frequently require oral high-calorie supplements and/or enteral tube feedings to meet caloric requirements (Borowitz 2002; Yankaskas 2004; White 2009). For these reasons, meal plans are not practical. Using carbohydrate counting and insulin-to-carbohydrate ratios in conjunction with the CF eating pattern to guide insulin therapy can help to optimize glycemic control (Moran 2010).

Whereas some individuals with CF are now living into their sixth and seventh decades, there have not been any deaths reported from atherosclerotic cardiovascular disease. Cholesterol levels are generally low despite a diet high in saturated fatty acids. Low cholesterol levels have been attributed to fat malabsorption, but there may also be some intrinsic connection to the basic CF gene defect, since lipids are low even in well-nourished patients (Figueroa 2002). However, dyslipidemia does occur in individuals with CF, but no differences in lipid profiles were seen between people with diabetes and people without. As survival in the CF population increases, the prevalence of dyslipidemia may increase, resulting in clinically important complications; however, current recommendations for a high-fat diet have not changed (Rhodes 2010).

Microvascular complications do occur in CFRD and are related to the duration and metabolic control of diabetes. Restrictions for protein and sodium are not recommended if microvascular complications occur. Low-protein diets increase the risk of malnutrition. Low-sodium diets for people with CF can lead to hyponatremia, seizures, and death due to increased losses of sodium in sweat, especially in hot weather, with fever, or during extensive exercise in outdoor sports (Borowitz 2002; Yankaskas 2004). Table 17.2 lists the percentage of patients with CFRD of >10 years' duration with microvascular complications compared to patients with type 1 and type 2 diabetes (Schwarzenberg 2007).

Table 17.2 Microvascular Complications in Patients with CFRD >10 Years' Duration Compared to Microvascular Complications in Patients with Type 1 and Type 2 Diabetes

Complication	CFRD (%)	Type 1 and Type 2 Diabetes (%)
Retinopathy	15	60
Nephropathy	16	20–30
Neuropathy	55	50
Gastropathy	50*	50
Macrovascular	0	60

*Higher rates of gastroparesis are observed in patients with CF without diabetes; therefore, it is difficult to determine etiology. Adapted from Schwarzenberg 2007.

CLINICAL CARE GUIDELINES FOR CYSTIC FIBROSIS–RELATED DIABETES

The following are recommendations for CFRD and nutrition therapy for CFRD developed by a committee of experts from the CFF, the American Diabetes Association (ADA), and the Pediatric Endocrine Society:

- Nutritional management is recommended for patients with CFRD. Patients with CFRD diagnosed with hypertension or microvascular complications should receive treatment as recommended by the ADA for all people with diabetes, except that there is no restriction of sodium and, in general, no protein restriction.
- An annual lipid profile is recommended for patients with CFRD and pancreatic exocrine sufficiency or if any of the following risk factors are present: obesity, family history of coronary artery disease, or immunosuppressive therapy after transplantation.
- Oral diabetes agents are not as effective as insulin in improving nutrition and metabolic outcomes in CFRD and are not recommended outside the context of clinical research trials.
- Women with CF who are planning a pregnancy or confirmed pregnant should be screened for preexisting CFRD with a 2-h 75-g fasting oral glucose tolerance test (OGTT) if they have not had a normal CFRD screen in the last 6 months.
- Screening for GDM is recommended at both 12–16 and 24–28 weeks' gestation in pregnant women with CF not known to have CFRD, using a 2-h 75-g OGTT with blood glucose measures at 0, 1, and 2 h. Screening for CFRD using a 2-h 75-g fasting OGTT is recommended 6–12 weeks after the end of the pregnancy in women with GDM.
- The A1C test used for standard screening for type 1 and type 2 diabetes is not sufficiently sensitive for diagnosis of CFRD. This is the case because of increased red blood cell turnover due to chronic inflammation, resulting in a spuriously low A1C; therefore, the A1C test should not be used for screening. The OGTT is the screening test of choice for CFRD (Moran 2010).
- Table 17.3 lists nutrition therapy recommendations for CFRD and compares them to nutrition therapy recommendations for type 1 and type 2 diabetes.

NUTRITION THERAPY FOR PREGNANCY WITH CYSTIC FIBROSIS–RELATED DIABETES AND GDM IN CYSTIC FIBROSIS

Pregnancy in women with CF is now quite commonplace and is generally considered safe, with good fetal and maternal outcomes in women with mild-to-moderate disease (CFF 2009). Preconception counseling and normalization of blood glucose are necessary in women with preexisting CFRD, as with type 1 and type 2 diabetes. Women with CF are also at higher risk for GDM because of underlying insulin deficiency and therefore should be screened more aggressively

Table 17.3 Nutrition Recommendations for CFRD Compared to Nutrition Recommendations for Type 1 and Type 2 Diabetes

Nutrient	CFRD	Type 1 and Type 2 Diabetes
Calories	1.2–1.5 times dietary reference intake (DRI) for age; individualized based on weight gain and growth	As needed for growth, maintenance, or weight reduction
Carbohydrate	Individualized; carbohydrates should be monitored to achieve glycemic control; artificial sweeteners should be used sparingly because of lower calorie content	Individualized; monitor carbohydrates to achieve glycemic control; choose from fruits, vegetables, whole grains and fiber-containing foods, legumes, and low-fat milk; sugar alcohols and nonnutritive sweeteners are safe within FDA-established consumption guidelines
Fat	No restriction on type of fat; high fat necessary for weight maintenance; aim for 35–40% total calories	Limit saturated fat to <7% of total calories, minimize intake of *trans* fat, and limit dietary cholesterol to <200 mg/day; consume two or more servings per week of fish high in n-3 polyunsaturated fatty acids
Protein	Approximately 1.5–2.0 times the DRI for age; no reduction for nephropathy	15–20% of total calories; reduction to <1.0 g/kg with nephropathy
Sodium	Liberal, high-salt diet, especially in warm conditions and/or when exercising	<2,300 mg/day for blood pressure control
Vitamins, minerals	Routine supplementation with CF-specific multivitamins or a multivitamin and additional fat-soluble vitamins A, D, E, and K	No supplementation necessary unless deficiency noted
Alcohol	Consult with physician due to the higher prevalence of liver disease in CF and possible use of hepatotoxic drugs	If consumed, limit to a moderate amount; 1 drink/day for women, ≤2 drinks/day for men
Special Circumstances:		
GDM Prediabetes	No calorie or carbohydrate restriction; adequate kilocalories for weight gain; no weight loss, spread carbohydrate throughout day, consume nutrient-dense beverages	Restricted calories/carbohydrate for weight and blood glucose control; weight loss of 5–10% recommended, low-fat eating pattern

FDA, U.S. Food and Drug Administration. Adapted from Moran 2010.

(Moran 2010). All pregnant women with CF and diabetes require increased energy intake and require close monitoring of weight gain and nutritional status for best outcomes. Prepregnancy weight will determine the weight gain goals during pregnancy. Standard prenatal weight gain charts can be used to determine goals. Additional calorie needs will vary based on prepregnancy weight, degree of malabsorption, pulmonary status, and presence of infections. The use of oral supplements may be necessary to promote adequate weight gain. Because of the risk of suboptimal weight gain, current practice does not encourage the restriction of calories or carbohydrate during pregnancy. However, empty calories should be replaced with nutrient-dense foods. In pregnant women with CFRD or CF with GDM requiring insulin therapy, insulin should be matched to carbohydrate intake to optimize blood glucose control without restricting carbohydrate intake (Moran 2010).

HYPOGLYCEMIA IN CFRD

Hypoglycemia risk is not different from that of individuals with type 1 or type 2 diabetes requiring insulin. Absorption of fat-free carbohydrates is not compromised, since patients with CF are able to secrete amylase in their saliva (Borowitz 1995). Therefore, low blood glucose should be treated with fat-free carbohydrate sources that do not require pancreatic enzyme replacement.

PREDIABETES IN CYSTIC FIBROSIS

Because prediabetes in CF is due to underlying insulin deficiency, it is not preventable in people with CF, unlike in the general population; therefore, nutrition therapy guidelines for prediabetes in the general population are not applicable for people with CF. Weight loss is almost never recommended for people with CF. Exercise in people with CF is beneficial for overall health; however, since people with CF in their baseline state of health are insulin sensitive, exercise will not help to slow the progression towards CFRD because of the progressive insulin deficiency. Most people with CF, including people with severe pulmonary disease, are capable of engaging in strength and aerobic exercise and are advised to do moderate aerobic exercise for at least 150 min/week. Spreading carbohydrates throughout the day and replacing empty-calorie carbohydrates with nutrient-dense carbohydrates are recommended. Maintenance of a healthy weight and nutritional status must be monitored closely (Moran 2010). A few studies have looked at using once-daily low-dose basal insulin for this population; however, larger randomized controlled trials are needed to verify efficacy and safety (Rolon 2001; Bizzarri 2006; Mozzillo 2009; Frohnert 2010; Sterescu 2010; Hameed 2011).

SUMMARY

CFRD is a unique clinical entity with very different approaches to clinical management and nutrition therapy. It is important to be aware of these important differences to optimize care for people living with CFRD. An education manual is available from the CFF to assist health care providers when educating individuals with CFRD (Brunzell 2011).)

BIBLIOGRAPHY

Bizzarri C, Lucidi V, Ciampalini P, Bella S, Russo B, Cappa M: Clinical effects of early treatment with insulin glargine in patients with cystic fibrosis and impaired glucose tolerance. *Endocrinol Invest* 29:RC1–RC4, 2006

Brunzell C, Hardin D Moran A, Schindler T: *Managing Cystic Fibrosis Related Diabetes (CFRD): An Instruction Guide for Patients and Families.* 5th ed. Bethesda, MD, Cystic Fibrosis Foundation, 2011. Available from http://www.cff.org/UploadedFiles/LivingWithCF/StayingHealthy/Diet/Diabetes/CFRD-Manual-5th-edition.pdf

Borowitz D, Baker RD, Stallings V: Consensus report on nutrition for pediatric patients with cystic fibrosis. *J Pediatr Gastroenterol Nutr* 35:246–259, 2002

Borowitz D, Grand R, Durie P, Beker L, Dodge J, Fink R, Fitzsimmons S, Freiman J, Kalnins D, Kimura R, Kirschner B, Lloyd-Still J, Lowenfels A, Maguiness K, Roberts I, Schwarzenberg S, Smyth R, Stevens J, Stone R, Thompson B, Vanvelzen D, West K, Zerin J: Use of pancreatic enzyme supplements for patients with cystic fibrosis in the context of fibrosing colonopathy. *J Pediatr* 127:681–684, 1995

Cystic Fibrosis Care Guidelines, Nutrition/GI, 2011b. Available from http://www.cff.org/treatments/CFCareGuidelines/Nutrition/#Nutrition_in_Children_and_Adults. Accessed 14 July 2011

Cystic Fibrosis Foundation Patient Registry 2009 Annual Data Report. Bethesda, MD, Cystic Fibrosis Foundation, 2011a. Available from http://www.cff.org/UploadedFiles/research/ClinicalResearch/Patient-Registry-Report-2009.pdf

Figueroa V, Milla C, Parks E, Schwarzenberg SJ, Moran A: Abnormal lipid levels in cystic fibrosis. *Am J Clin Nutr* 75:1005–1011, 2002

Frohnert BI, Ode KL, Moran A, Nathan BM, Laguna T, Holme B, Thomas W: Impaired fasting glucose in cystic fibrosis. *Diabetes Care* 33:2660–2664, 2010

Gaskin KJ: Exocrine pancreatic function. In *Pediatric Gastrointestinal Disease.* Walker WA, Goulet O, Kleinman RE, Sherman PM, Schneider BL, Sanderson IR, Eds. Hamilton, ON, Canada, Decker, 2004, p. 1607–1623

Hameed S, Morton JR, Field PI, Belessis Y, Yoong T, Katz T, Woodhead HJ, Walker JL, Neville KA, Campbell TA, Jaffé A, Verge CF: Once daily insulin detemir in cystic fibrosis with insulin deficiency. *Arch Dis Child* 14 April 2011. http://adc.bmj.com/content/early/2011/04/14/adc.2010.204636.full?sid=9745ff40-d72a-4167-ab23-cb20e9ec8d41 [Epub ahead of print]

Milla C, Warwick J, Moran A: Trends in pulmonary function in patients with cystic fibrosis correlate with the degree of glucose intolerance at baseline. *Am J Respir Crit Care Med* 162:891–895, 2000

Moran A, Brunzell C, Cohen R, Katz M, Marshall B, Onady G, Robinson K, Sabodosa K, Stecenko A, Slovis B, the CFRD Guidelines Committee: Clinical care guidelines for cystic fibrosis–related diabetes: a position statement of the American Diabetes Association and a clinical practice guideline of the Cystic Fibrosis Foundation, endorsed by the Pediatric Endocrine Society. *Diabetes Care* 33:2697–2708, 2010

Moran A, Diem P, Klein D, Levitt M, Robertson R: Pancreatic endocrine function in cystic fibrosis. *J Pediatr* 118:715–723, 1991

Moran A, Doherty L, Wang X, Thomas W: Abnormal glucose metabolism in cystic fibrosis. *J Pediatr* 133:10–16, 1998

Moran A, Dunitz J, Nathan B, Saeed A, Holmes B, Thomas W: Cystic fibrosis-related diabetes: current trends in prevalence, incidence, and mortality. *Diabetes Care* 32:1626–1631, 2009a

Moran A, Pekow P, Grover P, Zorn M, Slovis B, Pilewski J, Tullis E, Liou T, Allen H, the CFRDT Study Group: Insulin therapy to improve BMI in cystic fibrosis related diabetes without fasting hyperglycemia: results of the CFRDT trial. *Diabetes Care* 32:1783–1788, 2009b

Mozzillo E, Franzese A, Valerio G, Sepe A, De Simone I, Mazzarella G, Ferri P, Raia V: One-year glargine treatment can improve the course of lung disease in children and adolescents with cystic fibrosis and early glucose derangements. *Pediatr Diabetes* 10:162–167, 2009

Orenstein DM: Cystic fibrosis. In *Rudolph's Pediatrics*. Rudolph CD, Rudolph AM, Hostetter MK, Lister G, Siegel NJ, Eds. New York, McGraw-Hill, 2002, p. 1969–1980

Rhodes B, Nash EF, Tullis E, Pencharz PB, Brotherwood M, Dupuis A, Stephenson A: Prevalence of dyslipidemia in adults with cystic fibrosis. *J Cyst Fibrosis* 9:24–28, 2010

Rolon MA, Benali K, Munck A, Navarro J, Clement A, Tubiana-Rufi N, Czernichow P, Polak M: Cystic fibrosis-related diabetes mellitus: clinical impact of prediabetes and effects of insulin therapy. *Acta Paediatr* 90:860–867, 2001

Rosenecker J, Hofler R, Steinkamp G, Eichler I, Smaczny C, Ballmann M, Posselt H, Bargon J, von der Hardt H: Diabetes mellitus in patients with cystic fibrosis: the impact of diabetes mellitus on pulmonary function and clinical outcome. *Eur J Med Res* 6:345–350, 2001

Schwarzenberg SJ, Thomas W, Olsen T, Grover T, Walk D, Milla C, Moran A: Microvascular complications in cystic fibrosis-related diabetes. *Diabetes Care* 30:1056–1061, 2007

Stallings VA, Stark LJ, Robinson KA, Feranchak AP, Quinton H: Clinical Practice Guidelines on Growth and Nutrition Subcommittee; Ad Hoc Working

Group: Evidence-based practice recommendations for nutrition-related management of children and adults with cystic fibrosis and pancreatic insufficiency: results of a systematic review. *J Am Diet Assoc* 108:832–839, 2008

Sterescu AE, Rhodes B, Jackson R, Dupuis A, Hanna A, Wilson DC, Tullis E, Pencharz PB: Natural history of glucose intolerance in patients with cystic fibrosis: ten-year prospective observation program. *J Pediatr* 156:613–617, 2010

Tofé S, Moreno JC, Máz L, Alonso M, Escobar H, Barrio R: Insulin secretion abnormalities and clinical deterioration related to impaired glucose tolerance in cystic fibrosis. *Eur J Endocrinol* 152:241–247, 2005

White H, Pollard K, Etherington C, Clifton I, Morton AM, Owen D, Conway SP, Peckham DG: Nutritional decline in cystic fibrosis related diabetes: the effect of intensive nutritional intervention. *J Cyst Fibros* 8:179–185, 2009

Yankaskas JR, Marshall BC, Sufian B, Simon RH, Rodman D: Cystic fibrosis adult care: consensus conference report. *Chest* 125 (Suppl. 1):1S–39S, 2004

Carol Brunzell, RD, CDE, is Diabetes Educator at the Diabetes Care Centers, University of Minnesota Medical Center, Fairview, Minneapolis, MN.

Chapter 18

Nutrition Therapy for Diabetic Gastropathy

Meghann Moore, MPH, RD, CDE

Highlights

Diagnosing Gastroparesis

Pathophysiology

Symptoms of Gastroparesis

Treating Gastroparesis

Review of Existing Nutrition Recommendations and
Translation of Evidence into Nutrition Interventions

Pharmacology and Alternative Therapies

Surgery

Summary

Highlights
Nutrition Therapy for Diabetic Gastropathy

■ Correcting hyperglycemia and maintaining good glycemic control is advised, since acute hyperglycemia delays gastric emptying.

■ There is limited research supporting the efficacy of nutrition therapy in gastroparesis treatment. However, the current eating pattern recommendations for low-fiber, small, frequent meals, with a greater proportion of liquid calories to meet nutrition needs, are reasonable.

■ Recent research demonstrates that high-protein meals and large-particle meals delay gastric emptying and should be avoided.

Nutrition Therapy for Diabetic Gastropathy

Gastroparesis is considered the most significant and challenging manifestation of diabetic gastropathy, or gastroenteropathy, which more generally refers to all gastrointestinal (GI) complications of diabetes (Ordog 2009). Other GI complications include dysphagia, heartburn, abdominal pain or discomfort, early satiety, nausea, vomiting, postprandial fullness and bloating, constipation, diarrhea, and fecal incontinence. Many of these symptoms also accompany gastroparesis. Gastroparesis (Greek for "a weakness of movement") is a neuromuscular disorder of the stomach involving both motor and sensory dysfunction and is characterized by delayed gastric emptying, particularly of solid foods, in the absence of mechanical obstruction.

Gastroparesis is increasingly recognized and, although the population-wide prevalence is not well defined, is estimated to affect 4% of the U.S. population, or up to 12 million individuals in the U.S., based on the current population (Hasler 2008). Diabetes is the second leading cause of gastroparesis, with 24–29% of cases attributed to this disease (Parkman 2010), and between 30 and 50% of people with diabetes may be affected by it (Abrahamsson 2007). Gastroparesis is primarily associated with type 1 diabetes, affecting 25–55% of patients, but has also been exhibited in 30% of patients with type 2 diabetes (Hasler 2008).

The mean age of onset of gastroparesis is 34 years, and this disease usually develops after diabetes has been present for >10 years and patients have evidence for autonomic dysfunction. Women are approximately four times more likely than men to be affected by gastroparesis (Parkman 2010). One hypothesis for this significant gender disparity is due to the apparent slower gastric emptying in women than in men, in particular during the luteal phase of the female menstrual cycle (Parkman 2009).

Complications of gastroparesis include esophagitis, Mallory-Weiss tear from chronic nausea/vomiting, malnutrition, volume depletion with acute renal failure (secondarily), electrolyte disturbances, and bezoar formation (Waseem 2009). The long-term prognosis of gastroparesis has not been well studied. A study of 20 patients with diabetic gastroparesis found no change in gastric emptying rates at 12 years of follow-up (Masaoka 2009). In addition, patients with diabetic gastroparesis have an increased mortality rate, but this is usually related to other organ dysfunction, such as cardiovascular or renal disease (Kong 1999).

DIAGNOSING GASTROPARESIS

The gold standard method used to diagnose gastroparesis is scintigraphy with a radionuclide solid meal gastric emptying measurement. This method involves the patient ingesting a meal labeled with a radioisotope and use of a camera and mathematics to determine gastric emptying time and meal retention up to 4 h postprandially (Masaoka 2009). Gastric retention >60% at 2 h and >10% at 4 h is diagnostic of the disorder, with greater retention at 4 h associated with increased gastroparesis severity. Although no current standard exists for the radionuclide food, a low-fat Egg Beater meal was established by an international collaborative study as the meal of choice; other foods such as chicken, liver, eggs, oatmeal, or pancakes are also used as test meals. Variables of meal content such as food density, indigestible residue, fat content, calories, and volume all alter gastric emptying time and should be taken into account in performing gastric emptying tests. Wireless motility capsule and gastric emptying breath testing are alternative and noninvasive diagnostic methods for gastroparesis that allow for standardization among centers. Ultrasound is also a diagnostic option, but its utility is limited, since it is not suitable for solid meals, and liquid emptying rate is often preserved until advanced progression of gastroparesis. Magnetic resonance imaging and single-photon emission computed tomography are diagnostic tools primarily used in research settings.

PATHOPHYSIOLOGY

Normal Digestive Physiology

Understanding the pathophysiology of gastroparesis begins with an understanding of normal digestive physiology. During and after ingestion of a meal where there is normal gastric motor function, the proximal stomach (fundus) relaxes, providing a reservoir for the meal with an accompanying increase in gastric volume, without a rise in pressure. This process also allows passage of food to the duodenum at a rate that matches the duodenal absorptive capacity. In diabetes, independent of any autonomic neuropathy, there can be impaired meal-induced relaxation of the fundus, increased pyloric motor activity, fewer antral contractions in the distal part of the stomach, and impaired antroduodenal coordination (Parkman 2010). Glucagon-like peptide-1, an antihyperglycemia gut hormone normally secreted in response to nutrients in the small intestine, exerts its glucoregulatory effect by slowing gastric emptying; this result may further exacerbate impaired gastric motor function in gastroparesis (Baggio 2007).

Gastroparesis Pathophysiology

Autonomic neuropathy, with vagal parasympathetic dysfunction, is a likely contributor to the pathogenesis of gastroparesis, especially among patients with longstanding diabetes (Parkman 2010). Autonomic neuropathy affects between 20 and 40% of patients with diabetes. Other contributors to the pathogenesis of gastroparesis include hyperglycemia and loss of expression of neuronal nitric oxide synthesis (nNOS), the enzyme responsible for the synthesis of neuronal nitric oxide, which has emerged as a key molecule important in the pathogenesis of this disorder (Parkman 2009).

Hyperglycemia and electrolyte imbalances are associated with delayed gastric emptying in people with diabetes. Delayed gastric emptying can lead to worsening blood glucose control by altering the pharmacokinetics of oral hypoglycemic agents and preprandial insulin, disrupting glucose absorption, and affecting postprandial insulin levels. These occurrences result in wide swings of glycemia and unexpected episodes of postprandial hypoglycemia (Parkman 2010). Blood glucose levels between 288 and 360 mg/dL have been associated with a median change delay in gastric emptying of 17 min for solids and 6 min for liquids (Fraser 1990). However, glycemia levels >250 mg/dL were shown to cause near-absent gastric emptying, and glucose levels of 140–175 mg/dL may correlate with delayed gastric emptying in people with diabetes compared to euglycemic patients (Barnett 1988). Once glucose levels are corrected, GI symptoms typically resolve.

SYMPTOMS OF GASTROPARESIS

Gastroparesis symptoms may be present in up to as many as 86% of patients with diabetes (Ordog 2009); however, these high rates may be associated with patients in academic centers compared to the general community, where the symptom prevalence may be much lower, at 5–27%. The prevalence and incidence of the most common and debilitating of these symptoms include nausea, vomiting, and dyspepsia. Other symptoms often attributed to gastroparesis include postprandial fullness (early satiety), upper abdominal pain, abdominal distension and bloating, anorexia and weight loss, weight gain, and constipation. More than 80% of patients with gastroparesis may experience nausea, pain, and vomiting.

Gastric stasis and delayed gastric emptying have also been associated with diabetic gastroparesis (Abell 2006). However, some patients with delayed gastric emptying may have little to no GI symptoms. Delayed gastric emptying can lead to prolonged gastric retention of food, which may result in reflux and cause or exacerbate existing symptoms of gastroesophageal reflux disease (GERD) (Parkman 2009).

An increased frequency of hypoglycemic events in people with insulin-treated diabetes has been associated with abnormal gastric emptying. This result is due to a mismatch of the prandial insulin action with the impaired digestion of the meal. Psychological distress is linked to the GI symptoms of nausea and early satiety in people with diabetes. Gastroparesis is further associated with impaired quality of life and increased levels of anxiety, depression, and somatization (a chronic condition characterized by physical symptoms affecting multiple parts of the body without any associated physical cause) (Abell 2006).

The gastroparesis cardinal symptom index was developed as a patient-based symptom instrument for assessing gastroparesis severity, and a clinical grading scale was also proposed to classify gastroparesis severity (Table 18.1) (Abell 2006). Use of these symptom and severity assessment tools for patient classification may offer benefits to improving patient care.

Table 18.1 Proposed Classification of Gastroparesis Severity with Corresponding Treatment Recommendations: Confirmation of Gastroparesis Must Occur First

Grade	Symptoms	Nutrition Therapy	Treatment	Hospital-izations
1: mild gastroparesis	Easily controlled	Able to maintain weight and nutrition with regular eating patterns or minor nutrition interventions	Eating pattern modifications, avoid medications that delay gastric emptying, low doses of antiemetic or prokinetic medications as needed (prn), optimize glycemia	None
2: compensated gastroparesis	Moderate, with partial control with pharmacological agents	Able to maintain weight with eating pattern and lifestyle adjustments	Combination of antiemetic and prokinetic medications given at regularly scheduled intervals to relieve chronic symptoms, continuation of nutrition modifications and pain control prn	Rare
3: gastroparesis with gastric failure	Refractory despite medical therapy	Inability to maintain weight via oral route	Hospitalization for intravenous hydration, insulin administration and intravenous administration of antiemetic and prokinetic agents, enteral or parenteral nutrition support prn, consideration of GES and gastrectomy or other surgeries	Frequent emergency room visits or admissions

Adapted from Abell 2006.

TREATING GASTROPARESIS

Despite the fact that gastroparesis has been recognized and treated as a distinct disorder for decades, fully validated and adequate treatment options are lacking. Effective management of gastroparesis may be enhanced by involvement of a team of collaborative providers, including a primary care provider, gastroenterologist, endocrinologist, registered dietitian, psychologist, interventional radiologist, and surgeon, with the latter two health care professionals indicated more so in severe cases (Abell 2006).

Treatment goals include reducing symptoms; correcting fluid, electrolyte, and nutritional deficiencies and glycemic imbalances; and correcting the precipitating cause(s) with appropriate drug therapy. Patient education and explanation of the condition should be included in the treatment plan. Treatment is aimed at controlling, not curing, the disorder. Modification of the eating pattern is the primary treatment strategy, especially among patients with mild symptoms. If nutrition therapy does not control symptoms, low doses of prokinetic and antiemetic medications can be prescribed as well as pain control medicine. Endoscopic or surgical options may be warranted to manage severe symptoms.

The chronic symptoms of gastroparesis can have significant impacts on patients' quality of life, and many patients may benefit from professional counseling to cope with this disability. Psychosocial support, education, and rehabilitation are important, and relaxation techniques, cognitive restructuring, and distraction can offer a sense of control to the patient. Treatment recommendations based on symptom severity and proposed grading scale are summarized in Table 18.1.

Acute hyperglycemia slows gastric emptying, even in patients where the autonomic nervous system is intact; therefore, a focus on glycemic control should occur with initial treatment of diabetic gastroparesis (Parkman 2010). Correcting hyperglycemia may facilitate and augment the benefits of other treatments and is advised. Despite what is known about the impact of hyperglycemia on gastric emptying, the first study using scintigraphy to assess the relationship between A1C and delayed gastric emptying in people with diabetes did not demonstrate a significant association between A1C level and delayed gastric emptying (Reddy 2010). It is possible that day-to-day management of glycemic control with prevention of wide glucose variations is more relative to gastric emptying time than A1C, since normal A1C values may exist in a patient with marked fluctuations in glucose levels.

REVIEW OF EXISTING NUTRITION RECOMMENDATIONS AND TRANSLATION OF EVIDENCE INTO NUTRITION INTERVENTIONS

There is limited research on nutrition therapy interventions in patients with diabetic gastroparesis, and as a result, evidence supporting the efficacy of many nutrition recommendations is not available. To update this chapter from that published in 1999, a literature search was conducted using PubMed MEDLINE for research published on or after January 1, 1999, on nutrition therapy in diabetic gastroparesis. Search criteria included: gastric emptying, gastroparesis, and diabetes mellitus, with the search limited to human subjects and English language articles. Such a broad search on the subject was intentional in order to collect comprehensive data on gastroparesis not limited to nutrition therapy. The literature search identified 1005 articles. Twenty-four were retrieved for more detailed evaluation and three additional articles were identified from reference lists. Of these, four met the following study inclusion criteria for nutrition interventions in diabetic gastroparesis: randomized controlled trials, clinical controlled studies, large nonrandomized observational studies, cohort studies, or case-controlled studies. Table 18.2 summarizes available data.

Nutrition recommendations are based on the knowledge of the pathophysiology of gastroparesis and professional clinical judgment rather than on study outcomes. Nutrition and eating pattern modifications will likely provide the greatest benefit for people with mild gastroparesis but should be recommended to all patients with gastroparesis regardless of degree of severity.

Table 18.2 Nutrition Interventions in People with Diabetes Involving Gastric Emptying and Gastroparesis

	Population/ Duration of Study	Intervention (type of study)	Major Findings	Comments
Hlebowicz 2007	*n* = 10 patients with type 1 diabetes and diabetes gastroparesis/ one meal	GER measured after rice pudding and water with and without apple cider vinegar (clinical trial)	Lower GER with vinegar meal vs. non-vinegar meal (*P* < 0.05)	Vinegar may ↑ gastric emptying in people with diabetes and gastroparesis
Olausson 2008	*n* = 7 patients with type 1 diabetes and gastroparesis and 7 matched controls/2 meals	Two solid meals, identical composition but different particle size (clinical trial)	Gastric emptying was faster with the small-particle meal than the large-particle meal	Small-particle diet may aid in glycemic control compared to large-particle diet
Ma 2009	*n* = 8 patients with diet-controlled type 2 diabetes and gastroparesis/ 3 meals	Beef soup 30 min before potato meal with 20 g glucose; 55 g whey added to soup, potato meal, or neither (clinical trial)	Gastric emptying slowest with whey in soup, slower with whey in meal than no whey	High-protein meals may worsen delayed gastric emptying in gastroparesis
Reddy 2010	*n* = 250 patients with diabetes and GES and A1C tested within a 3-month period over 5 years/not applicable	GES liquid egg-white meal with white bread, jam, and water = 255 kcal (2% fat meal); delayed gastric emptying = half-life >90 min (retrospective cross-sectional)	No correlation observed between gastric emptying time, A1C, and age	A1C is not as important as daily glycemic control in gastric emptying

GER, gastric emptying rate; GES, gastric electrical stimulation.

A patient food and nutrition history should be collected to identify any food intolerances, and a physical examination should be performed, including assessment of dentition to assess potential impairments in mastication. Patients with gastroparesis may self-impose food restrictions, putting them at risk for developing nutrient deficiencies (Hsu 1995). As such, laboratory assessments and ongoing monitoring of magnesium, glucose and A1C, iron and ferritin, vitamin B12, and 25-hydroxy vitamin D (25-OHD) are recommended, and supplementation is recommended if deficiency is determined. Chewable or liquid versions may be better tolerated than tablets (Parrish 2007). Conventional nutritional laboratory assessments of serum albumin and pre-albumin levels are affected by a variety of factors in gastroparesis and may not be reliable measures of nutritional status. Identifying the severity of gastroparesis in a patient first is advised, since patients with more severe malnutrition due to the disorder will require more aggressive nutrition interventions initially, compared to a patient with mild gastroparesis and symptoms. The patient with mild gastroparesis may only need eating pattern adjustments.

The amount of carbohydrate ingested is usually the primary determinant of postprandial response. There is not a specific recommendation for carbohydrate intake (American Diabetes Association 2008). Incorporating general nutrition recommendations for diabetes into a patient's meal plan is likely to be appropriate. A daily multivitamin/mineral supplement can be taken if food and nutrition intake is inadequate. A small study in patients with type 2 diabetes demonstrated delayed gastric emptying when a relatively large amount of whey protein (55 g) was consumed before or with a carbohydrate meal, possibly indicating that protein consumption greater than the current general recommendations may exacerbate gastroparesis (Ma 2009).

A low-fiber eating plan is recommended because of the presumption that fibrous meals increase risk for bezoar formation (an indigestible concretion of food residue retained within the stomach) in patients with gastroparesis. Bezoars decrease ability for clearing indigestible fiber from the stomach and may produce a palpable epigastric mass, gastric ulceration, small intestinal obstruction, or gastric perforation and must be eliminated by endoscopic disruption and lavage, enzymatic digestion, and exclusion of high-residue foods (Hasler 2008). Fiber-dense foods should also be avoided in patients who have difficulty with small bowel bacterial overgrowth because of fermentation in the upper gut, which can cause gas, cramping, and bloating.

Small, nutritionally balanced meals eaten throughout the day may lessen the possibility of impaired nutritional status and help the patient reach nutrient needs. Large-volume meals are associated with longer emptying times, which can aggravate existing early satiety. Large meals can also decrease the lower esophageal sphincter pressure, which may cause gastric reflux, providing further aggravation (Parrish 2007).

A study in patients with diabetes and gastroparesis demonstrated that gastric emptying was faster when a small-particle mixed-meal (meat, pasta, carrots, and oil) was consumed compared to a large-particle meal of identical composition (Olausson 2008). Therefore, a small-particle diet may improve glycemic control more than a large-particle diet. Meal particle size <2 mm is advised.

Table 18.3 lists nutrition therapy recommendations by health care professionals with clinical experience in treating gastroparesis. In addition, patients may benefit from avoiding vinegar, since meals including apple cider vinegar have been associated with lower gastric emptying rates than control meals (Hlebowicz 2007).

Nutrition Support

Nutrition support—oral, enteral, or parenteral—should be considered when a patient with gastroparesis falls below the goal or target weight (Parrish 2007). When gastroparesis is associated with weight loss and the patient requires nutritional support to maintain body weight, the gastroparesis is considered to be severe. A 5% loss of usual body weight over 3 months or 10% loss over 6 months is indicative of severe malnutrition. Other nutritional risk parameters include weight <80% of ideal weight, BMI <20 kg/m^2, or a loss of 5 lb or 2.5% of baseline

Table 18.3 Nutrition Therapy Interventions for Treating Gastroparesis

- Restrict meal volumes.
- Use consistent carbohydrates in meals: suggested 30–45 g carbohydrate per meal.
- Increase meal frequency: six small meals/snacks per day.
- Use small-particle meals (<2 mm).
- Eat slowly (e.g., 30 min per meal) and chew foods well.
- Solid foods may be better tolerated earlier in the day, with liquid meals the rest of the day.
- High-fat foods may delay stomach emptying; however, fat-containing liquids are better tolerated and can be used to increase calories.
- Avoid excess dietary fiber.
- Avoid eating on-the-go.
- Avoid late-evening snacks.
- Avoid caffeine, alcohol, tobacco, and stress.
- Avoid gum chewing.
- Avoid peppermint and chocolate.
- Remain upright while eating and drinking.
- Sit or walk for 1–2 h after meals.
- Elevate head of bed 6–8 inches when sleeping.
- Use supplementary nutrition (liquid formula).
- Gain support from a specialized registered dietitian.

Adapted from Abrahamsson 2007; Parrish 2007; and Abell 2006.

weight in 1 month. When assessing changes in weight, consideration of hydration status is important. Chronic hemodialysis patients are an often-overlooked population at high risk for gastroparesis, since their chronic fluid issues may mask significant weight changes truly indicative of malnutrition and gastroparesis. If a patient with diabetes has declining weight and complains of early satiety, notably in the morning after an overnight fast, assessment for gastroparesis is prudent (Parrish 2007).

Enteral Nutrition

In certain situations, initiation of enteral feedings may be warranted to maintain hydration, nutrition, and glycemic control. These situations include drug refractory cases and patients who experience significant unintentional weight loss of 5–10% over 3–6 months; have been unable to achieve the weight goal identified by the health care team via the oral route; are unresponsive to nutrition and eating pattern modifications; exhibit essential mineral deficiencies or electrolyte disturbances; require gastric decompression; have repeated hospitalizations for hydration or nutrition medication delivery; need nasogastric intubation to relieve symptoms; or experience nausea and vomiting resulting in poor quality of life (Parkman 2010). There are several options for enteral feeding routes, and superiority of one enteral access modality over another has not been shown; however, nasogastric and gastrostomy tubes may worsen gastroparesis and increase risk of pulmonary aspiration. Subjective reports of symptoms among patients with diabetic gastroparesis and a jejunostomy feeding tube indicate improvement, although the evidence is not substantial. Enteral feeding is usually initiated 24 h after jejunostomy tube placement and may be given overnight so that oral intake can continue, as tolerated during the day (Abell 2006). Jejunostomy is associated with complications, and hospitalization or surgery is required in more than half of the cases (Masaoka 2009). In patients suspected as having dysmotility in the small intestine, a 48-h nasojejunal feeding trial to determine if enteral feedings are tolerated may be prudent before endoscopic or surgical placement. For some patients, a venting gastrostomy was successful in reducing hospitalizations by a factor of 5 during the year after placement (Parkman 2010).

Upon initiation of enteral feeding, it is advised to restrict nutrition to "nothing per oral" (NPO) status for the first 48 h, so that enteral intolerance and oral intolerance are not confused if complications develop. The enteral formula should be a standard polymeric, nonfiber variety, since fiber may cause or increase gas, bloating, and cramping. Low-osmolarity formulas with a caloric density of 1.0–1.5 kcal/mL are recommended (Abell 2006). Some enteral products contain fructooligosaccharides, which may need to be avoided because of patient intolerance. If diarrhea occurs, medications and liquids should be assessed for sugar alcohols, since these may cause osmotic diarrhea. Reducing the infusion rate while increasing the formula concentration to maintain caloric intake or diluting the enteral feeding may also resolve diarrhea if the diarrhea is caused by the hyperosmolar nutrient fluid (Parkman 2010).

As previously mentioned, maintenance of glucose control is important to maximize use of nutrients and avoid further aggravation of gastroparesis symptoms due to hyperglycemia (Parkman 2010). An additional benefit of enteral nutrition therapy is provision of ready access for medication delivery, which can be followed by low-volume water flushes (Parrish 2007). Initially, enteral feedings should be delivered continuously 24 h/day; over time, if appropriate, they can be given at night to free up daytime hours for oral intake and offer some daily living normalcy. In these cases, insulin may be needed to correct for the additional calories and to prevent overnight hyperglycemia (Abell 2006).

Parenteral Nutrition

Parenteral nutrition is another nutrition therapy option. However, this treatment should be reserved for patients who have failed an enteral feeding trial with several formulas or who have a dysmotility that extends throughout the small and large intestines, because parenteral nutrition is associated with septicemia, thrombo-embolism, intravenous access problems, and liver disease (Masaoka 2009; Waseem 2009). However, short-term parenteral nutrition can improve acute fluid and nutrient deficiencies and effect weight gain in severely malnourished patients and may further help optimize glycemic control (Hasler 2008).

In such cases, regular insulin may need to be added to each liter of parenteral nutrition according to the patient's insulin requirements and individual institutional protocols (Abell 2006).

PHARMACOLOGY AND ALTERNATIVE THERAPIES

Providers should assess a patient's current medication regimen, and the reduction or withdrawal of medications that may further decrease gastric emptying is warranted. Specific examples of such drugs include incretin mimetics, such as exenatide and liraglutide. Alternative therapies for such medications may include dipeptidyl peptidase-4 inhibitors, which do not delay gastric emptying or reduce food intake (Parkman 2010). Bulk-forming agents used in the treatment of constipation and narcotics are associated with delayed gastric emptying and should be decreased or avoided if possible (Parrish 2007).

Postprandial hypoglycemia or hyperglycemia may develop depending on the timing of nutrient delivery and peak medication absorption. Effective measures in the optimization of glycemic control include frequent blood glucose monitoring to determine postprandial blood glucose levels. A once- or twice-daily basal dose of a long-acting insulin analog (glargine or determir) with a rapid-acting analog (lispro, aspart, or glulisine) is an insulin regimen strategy that may help to optimize glycemic control while reducing risk of hypoglycemia (Abell 2006). Some patients may benefit from taking bolus insulin doses of rapid-acting (aspart, lispro, or glulisine) insulin up to 30 min after eating meals, once certain the meal will not be vomited. Delayed insulin dosing may help to prevent postprandial hypoglycemia by better correlating insulin with gastric emptying and blood glucose response (Olausson 2008). Insulin pump therapy is a viable option for some patients, since it offers consistent basal insulin infusion in addition to control over mealtime boluses, with the ability to alter doses and dose delivery as needed. Short-acting insulin (regular) and premixed insulin may be a poor choice with delayed or unpredictable gastric emptying. Patients with type 2 diabetes taking oral hypoglycemia agents may experience dramatic swings in blood glucose control due to the mismatch between nutrient and medication absorption. For these patients, the addition of basal insulin therapy to oral therapy should be considered, since it is associated with better glycemic control and limited hypoglycemic episodes (Abell 2006).

Common pharmacological treatment of gastroparesis includes prokinetic agents such as domperidone, metoclopramide, and erythromycin. These medications generally will improve gastric emptying rates, but no consistent effects on gastroparesis symptoms or glycemic control have been demonstrated (Masaoka 2009). The U.S. Food and Drug Administration (FDA) withdrew approval of domperidone; however, outside of the U.S., it is still available. In February 2009, manufacturers of metoclopramide were required to include a black box warning on the drug because of the risks associated with long-term or high-dose use, such as somnolence and reduction in mental acuity (Parkman 2010). Gastroparesis may affect drug administration and absorption, and acute hyperglycemia can weaken the efficacy of prokinetic drugs because of the associated delay in gastric emptying (Parkman 2009, Masaoka 2009).

Limited research exists regarding the use of antiemetic agents in gastroparesis; however, they may be beneficial in cases where prokinetic drug therapy is ineffective or produces unacceptable toxicity. Antiemetic agents include the commonly prescribed phenothiazines (prochlorperazine and thiethylperazine); transdermal scopolamine is also occasionally used to treat nausea and vomiting in gastroparesis

(Abell 2006). Antidepressant medications may help with gastroparesis-associated symptoms such as vomiting and neuropathic pain (Hasler 2008; Waseem 2009). Ginger has antiemetic properties in some settings, but its benefit in gastroparesis has not been sufficiently explored (Hasler 2008). Injection of botulinum toxin into the pyloric sphincter for treatment of spasm and to improve gastric emptying and associated symptoms of delayed gastric emptying is another drug treatment option; however, results of two controlled studies failed to show any benefits of this treatment over saline injection (Masaoka 2009).

Acupuncture and biofeedback may be helpful in the treatment of visceral pain with few side effects (Parkman 2010). Acupressure and acustimulation have been shown to reduce nausea in other treatment settings and may have benefits with diabetic gastroparesis. Biofeedback and hypnosis are associated with psychological symptom benefits, such as anxiety, depression, and somatization, which are commonly experienced by people with gastroparesis (Hasler 2008).

SURGERY

In cases of difficult and severe gastroparesis in which a patient has chronic diabetic gastroparesis with relentless nausea and vomiting not responsive to nutrition and medication therapy, implantation of a gastric stimulation device subcutaneously in the abdominal wall is an option (Abell 2006). This gastric electrical stimulation (GES) device (Enterra, Medtronic) received FDA approval as a humanitarian device exemption in March 2000. Symptomatic improvement (reduced vomiting and improved quality of life) with this device has been reported, although the mechanism underlying this improvement has not been established, and the long-term efficacy of this treatment remains unclear. Some researchers suggest that, given the high cost of this device and the lack of conclusive data, generalized use of it is not to be recommended and treatment with it should be limited to research settings (Masaoka 2009). Alternative approaches and refinements to current GES therapy are currently being explored (Parkman 2010).

In the most advanced cases of gastroparesis, near-total gastrectomy has been performed to bypass a non-emptying stomach and decrease symptoms, although its success has been limited. Drainage procedures such as pyloromyotomy or pyloroplasty are other surgical options for treatment of gastroparesis that can be considered (Abell 2006). Pancreatic transplantation has resulted in halted progression or partly reversed peripheral polyneuropathy; however, limited data exist regarding the correction of diabetic gastroparesis status after pancreas transplant or after pancreas-kidney transplant in patients with type 1 diabetes (Abell 2006; Waseem 2009). New experimental treatments are also available and include possible future use of stem cell transplantation of enteric nerves and interstitial cell of Cajal (ICC) networks—cells in the GI tract that affect smooth muscle contraction (Parkman 2010).

SUMMARY

Gastroparesis is arguably the most complicated and challenging manifestation of diabetic gastropathy, associated with chronic and in some cases debilitating GI symptoms. Nutrition therapy is certainly at the foundation of treatment strategies, despite the lack of research supporting its efficacy, and is reasonable and prudent to use given an understanding of the physiology of delayed gastric emptying that defines gastroparesis. Future research is warranted to determine the best nutrition therapy practices and eating pattern recommendations for people who suffer with gastroparesis.

BIBLIOGRAPHY

Abell TL, Bernstein RK, Cutts T, Farrugia G, Forster J, Hasler WL, McCallum RW, Olden KW, Parkman HP, Parrish CR, Pascricha PJ, Prather CM, Soffer EE, Twillman R, Vinik AI: Treatment of gastroparesis: a multidisciplinary clinical review. *Neurogastroenterol Motil* 18:263–283, 2006

Abrahamsson H: Treatment options for patients with severe gastroparesis. *Gut* 56:877–883, 2007

American Diabetes Association: Nutrition recommendations and interventions for diabetes: a position statement of the American Diabetes Association. *Diabetes Care* 31 (Suppl. 1):S61–S78, 2008

Baggio LL, Drucker DJ: Biology of incretins: GLP-1 and GIP. *Gastroenterology* 132:2131–2157, 2007

Barnett JL, Owyang C: Serum glucose concentration as a modulator of interdigestive gastric motility. *Gastroenterology* 94:739–744, 1988

Fraser R, Horowitz M, Maddox A, Harding P, Chatterton B, Dent J: Hyperglycaemia slows gastric emptying in type 1 (insulin-dependent) diabetes mellitus. *Diabetologia* 33:675–680, 1990

Hasler WL: Gastroparesis: current concepts and considerations. *Medscape J Med* 10:16, 2008

Hlebowicz J, Darwiche G, Bjorgell L, Almer LO: Effect of apple cider vinegar on delayed gastric emptying in patients with type 1 diabetes mellitus: a pilot study. *BMC Gastroenterol* 7:46, 2007

Hsu JJ, Lee ST, Glena RC, Hach J, Nelson DK, Kim CH: Gastroparesis syndrome: nutritional sequelae and the impact of dietary manipulation on symptoms. *Gastroenterology* 108:A17, 1995

Kong MF, Horowitz M, Jones KL, Wishart JM, Harding PE: Natural history of diabetic gastroparesis. *Diabetes Care* 22:503–507, 1999

Ma J, Stevens JE, Cukier K, Maddox AF, Wishart JM, Jones KL, Clifton PM, Horowitz M, Rayner CK: Effects of a protein preload on gastric emptying, glycemia, and gut hormones after a carbohydrate meal in diet-controlled type 2 diabetes. *Diabetes Care* 32:1600–1602, 2009

Masaoka T, Tack J: Gastroparesis: current concepts and management. *Gut and Liver* 3:166–173, 2009

Olausson EA, Alpsten M, Larsson A, Mattsson H, Andersson H, Attvall S: Small particle size of a solid meal increases gastric emptying and late postprandial glycaemic response in diabetic subjects with gastroparesis. *Diabetes Res Clin Pract* 80:231–237, 2008

Ordog T, Hayashi Y, Gibbons SJ: Cellular pathogenesis of diabetic gastroenteropathy. *Minerva Gastroeneterol Dietol* 55:315–343, 2009

Parkman HP: Pathophysiologic relationship between gastroparesis and GERD. *Gastroenterol Hepatol* 5 (Suppl. 18):4–8, 2009

Parkman HP, Camilleri M, Farrugia G, McCallum RW, Bharucha AE, Mayer EA, Tack JF, Spiller R, Horowitz M, Vinik AI, Galligan JJ, Pasricha J, Kuo B, Szarka LA, Marciani L, Jones K, Parrish CR, Sandroni P, Abell T, Ordog T, Hasler W, Koch KL, Sanders K, Norton NJ, Hamilton F: Gastroparesis and functional dyspepsia: excerpts from the AGA/ANMS meeting. *Neurogastroenterol Motil* 22:113–133, 2010

Parrish CR, Pastors JG: Nutritional management of gastroparesis in people with diabetes. *Diabetes Spectrum* 20:231–234, 2007

Reddy S, Ramsubeik K, Vega KJ, Federico J, Palacio C: Do HbA1c levels correlate with delayed gastric emptying in diabetic patients? *J Neurogastroenterol Motil* 16:414–417, 2010

Waseem S, Moshiree B, Draganov PV: Gastroparesis: current diagnostic challenges and management considerations. *World J Gastroenterol* 15:25–37, 2009

Meghann Moore, MPH, RD, CDE, is Program Coordinator of the Diabetes Self-Management Education Program and Dietitian/Nutrition Management Consultant at The Polyclinic, Seattle, WA.

Chapter 19
Nutrition Therapy for Bariatric Surgery and Diabetes

Margaret Furtado, MS, RD, and Alison B. Evert, MS, RD, CDE

Highlights

Pathophysiology of Obesity

Types of Bariatric Procedures

Medical Indications for Bariatric Surgery

Bariatric Surgery Procedures and Diabetes-Related Outcomes

Nutrition Therapy and Related Interventions for Bariatric Surgery

Conclusion

Highlights
Nutrition Therapy for
Bariatric Surgery and Diabetes

■ Patients challenged by impaired glucose tolerance may benefit from bariatric surgery, since most studies report 99–100% prevention of progression to diabetes, whereas individuals with diabetes before surgery have remission rates ranging from 55 to 95%.

■ A meta-analysis of 136 weight-loss surgery studies, including 22,094 individuals, revealed an overall type 2 diabetes remission rate of 84% after Roux-en-Y gastric bypass (RYGBP), whereas, after adjustable gastric banding, the diabetes remission rate was 48%.

■ Parameters for bariatric surgery are a BMI of 40 kg/m² or higher without comorbidities or 35 kg/m² or higher with significant comorbidities. Small trials have shown glycemic benefit of bariatric surgery in patients with type 2 diabetes and a BMI 30–35 kg/m²; however, there is currently insufficient evidence to generally recommend surgery in patients with type 2 diabetes and a BMI <35 kg/m² outside of research protocols.

■ After bariatric surgery, nutrition therapy progresses from a clear liquid diet to full liquids to pureed foods to a mechanically altered soft eating pattern. An important concern is adequate protein intake.

Nutrition Therapy for Bariatric Surgery and Diabetes

O besity has reached epidemic proportions, with estimates that >65% of the U.S. population is either overweight or obese (Hill 2003). Using National Health and Nutrition Examination Survey (NHANES) data collected between 1999 to 2004, the prevalence of overweight among children and adolescents and obesity among men increased significantly with no change in women (Ogden 2006). In addition, there has been a worrisome increase in the prevalence of extreme or severe obesity (McTigue 2006). From 1986 to 2000 in adults the prevalence of obesity (BMI $\geq$30 kg/m^2) doubled, morbid obesity (BMI $\geq$40 kg/m^2) quadrupled, and super obesity (BMI $\geq$50 kg/m^2) increased fivefold in the United States (Sturm 2003). The prevalence of obesity among children, suggests there is no end in sight for this epidemic (McTigue 2006).

Medical weight loss via lifestyle intervention programs, including nutrition therapy, behavior modification, physical activity regimens, and pharmacotherapy, have not been extensively studied to determine effectiveness in the treatment of morbid obesity (Buchwald 2005; Tsai 2005). A 2004 consensus statement prepared by a panel of experts in obesity and bariatric surgery concluded that long-term weight loss in this population is difficult to achieve with diet, exercise, and pharmacotherapy (Buchwald 2005). Among people with overweight and/or obesity, studies have found only 20% are able to sustain weight loss long term (Wing 2005). Other research reveals that severe obesity is a refractory condition that is particularly difficult to ameliorate long term via conventional treatments, including various diet regimens, modification in lifestyle, and the use of pharmaceutical agents (Ostman 2004). Most patients who present for bariatric surgery have already failed multiple attempts to achieve a sustained weight loss by using non-surgical treatment options (Buchwald 2005). Therefore, surgical treatment for obesity, which has been found not only to attenuate obesity but also major risk factors for type 2 diabetes, appears to be an effective means of treating both comorbidities (Sjöström 2004). Presently, bariatric surgery has been deemed the sole treatment alternative capable of producing sustained and significant weight loss, as well as improvements in health status and quality of life (Buchwald 2004).

This chapter begins with a brief review of the pathophysiology of obesity and how bariatric surgery procedures can affect outcome measures such as inflammation, insulin resistance, and glycemia. The next sections provide a brief description of the different types of bariatric surgery procedures, a review of the medical implications for bariatric surgery, and research findings on the remission rates of diabetes after bariatric surgery. The chapter concludes with a summary of nutrition therapy and other interventions for patients with diabetes as they prepare for bariatric surgery and after.

PATHOPHYSIOLOGY OF OBESITY

Evidence suggests that adipose tissue and abnormal lipid metabolism play pivotal roles in the pathophysiology of obesity, although the cellular and molecular mechanisms have not been elucidated (Samuel 2010). Furthermore, there is speculation that a chronic state of low-grade inflammation, perhaps perpetuated by proinflammatory cytokines and peptides produced by adipose tissue, may be involved in the relationship between obesity and cardiovascular disease and insulin resistance (Tretjakovs 2009; Vázquez 2005). Gastric bypass procedures have been linked to decreases in insulin resistance, levels of inflammatory mediators, and functional markers of coronary atherosclerosis (Habib 2009; Batsis 2008; Kashyap 2010).

In light of the possible role of plasma ceramide as a mediator of inflammation, insulin resistance, and weight loss, changes in ceramide levels after gastric bypass surgery may serve as an indicator of improvement in insulin resistance and lipid-induced inflammation. The effects of a bariatric procedure on weight loss, insulin sensitivity, plasma ceramides, cardiovascular risk factors, and proinflammatory markers before and 3 and 6 months after surgery have been examined (Huang 2011). Six months after the operation, improvement in insulin sensitivity correlated with the change in total ceramide levels and with plasma tumor necrosis factor. The researchers concluded that there is a potential role for ceramide levels as mediators of a proinflammatory state, as well as improved insulin sensitivity after gastric bypass procedures.

Patients challenged by impaired glucose tolerance may benefit from bariatric surgery, since most studies report 99–100% prevention of progression to diabetes. In patients with diabetes before surgery, diabetes remission rates range from 55 to 95% (ADA 2012). Remission rates may vary, depending on the type of bariatric procedure (e.g., gastric banding vs. gastric bypass) and how long the individual has had diabetes. Individuals with the shortest duration and mildest form of type 2 diabetes are reported to have higher rates of diabetes remission (Schauer 2003). However, all of the bariatric procedures generally result in improved weight loss and glycemic control when compared to lifestyle modification. Some procedures offer superior weight loss and diabetes remission rates and will be summarized later in this chapter. It is believed that these results are due to the bypassing of the foregut, leading to elevation of the enteroglucagon level and increased weight loss (Greenway 2002).

As the obesity epidemic worsens, there is enhanced interest in weight-loss surgery, since it is at present the most effective therapy to combat the disease of severe obesity. In addition, there is significant interest in the decrease of mortality and morbidity linked with bariatric surgery. Since 2005, over 200,000 bariatric surgery procedures are performed annually in the U.S., with an estimated half a million completed worldwide each year (Buchwald 2005).

TYPES OF BARIATRIC PROCEDURES

Roux-en Y Gastric Bypass (RYGBP)

Figure 19.1 illustrates the 4 common bariatric surgery procedures. The RYGBP technique was developed by Mason and Ito in 1967 using a surgical stapler to create a gastric pouch holding only ~30 cc (Mason 1967). The upper pouch is entirely divided from the gastric remnant and anastomosed to the jejunum via a narrow gastrojejunal anastomosis. An entero-entero anastomosis between the excluded biliopancreatic limb and the alimentary limb is made, typically performed 100–150 cm distal to the gastrojejunostomy. However, in some patients with severe obesity and/or with BMI levels >50 kg/m², the anastomosis may be up to 250 cm to allow for greater weight loss (Keidar 2011).

Laparoscopic Adjustable Banding (LAGB)

LAGB is a purely restrictive procedure involving implanting silicon band-like tubing along the upper portion of the stomach to encircle it, forming a pouch-like area of stomach above the band and the larger part of the stomach below it. LAGB constricts the cardia of the stomach and is secured in place to help decrease the risk of retrograde slippage of the stomach through the band. Adjustments can be made to the band by injecting or withdrawing saline solution from the hollow core of the band via a subcutaneous port that is connected to the tubing and subsequent ring that encircles the top part of the stomach (Keidar 2011).

Vertical Sleeve Gastrectomy (VSG)

VSG, commonly referred to as a "sleeve," creates a 100- to 150-mL stomach via the creation of a partial gastrectomy of the greater curvature side of the stomach, whereas the last 6–8 cm of antrum stays intact. Therefore, with the sleeve, the pylorus is kept intact, which aids in preventing gastric emptying issues (Keidar 2011). A two-staged approach in high-risk patients seeking laparoscopic biliopancreatic diversion with duodenal switch (BPD-DS) is a higher-risk, malabsorptive surgery that will be discussed in the next section (Gagner 2005). The VSG is performed first and the BPD-DS several months later as a second procedure among high-risk patients and/or patients with very high BMIs (e.g., >60 kg/m²). This procedure was found to lower the surgical morbidity and mortality versus the one-stage approach. Surprisingly, individuals often exhibit significant weight loss after the VSG/first stage, and the VSG is now gaining ground as an independent bariatric procedure, with some insurance carriers reimbursing for it as a stand-alone procedure.

Biliopancreatic Diversion (BPD)

The BPD procedure consists of a distal, horizontal gastrectomy that allows for a functional upper stomach of 200–500 mL (variable with patient's needs) and leaving the fundus intact (Scopinaro 2005). The gastric remnant is then anastomosed to the distal 250 cm of small intestine (the alimentary limb). The small bowel that is excluded, including the duodenum, jejunum, and a section of the proximal ileum, carries bile and pancreatic secretions (bilipancreatic limb) and is connected to the alimentary channel 50 cm proximal to the ileocecal valve. Therefore, the only section of the small bowel where digestive secretions and nutrients mix is the 50-cm "common limb." The alimentary limb (~200–250 cm in length) allows absorption of some protein and simple carbohydrates, whereas fat and starches are absorbed in the short common limb (Keidar 2011).

Biliopancreatic Diversion with Duodenal Switch (BPD-DS)

The BPD-DS involves the "sleeve" cited above, leaving a 150- to 200-mL gastric reservoir. The duodenum is closed 2 cm distal to the pylorus, and a duodeno-ileal anastomosis is created (DS) (Hess 2005; Marceau 1998). The gastric fundus is virtually completely removed, whereas the antrum, pylorus, and a very small segment of duodenum are left intact, along with the vagus nerve. With the BPD-DS procedure, the entero-entero anastomosis is created more proximally on the alimentary limb, allowing for a longer common channel of 100 cm versus the original BPD procedure (Keidar 2011).

MEDICAL INDICATIONS FOR BARIATRIC SURGERY

To be considered a candidate for bariatric surgery, an individual should meet the following criteria: BMI of at least 40 kg/m^2 if no significant comorbidities exist or a BMI of at least 35 kg/m^2 if at least one significant comorbidity exists, such as cardiovascular disease, type 2 diabetes, obstructive sleep apnea, and hypertension (Yermilov 2009). Recently, surgeons were granted permission to insert the LAP-

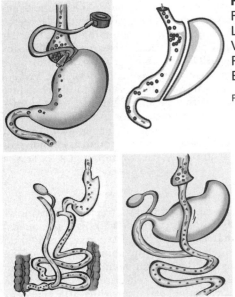

Figure 19.1

Four common bariatric surgeries: LABG (upper left panel), VSG (upper right panel), RYGBP (lower right panel), and BPD-DS (lower left panel).

Reproduced with permission from Keidar 2011.

BAND® System (trademarked by Allergan, Inc.) of adjustable gastric banding in patients with lower BMI levels of 30–35 kg/m², but this procedure is not currently covered by insurance.

Type 2 Diabetes and Indications for Surgery

For patients with type 2 diabetes, the International Diabetes Federation (IDF) outlined eligibility and prioritization criteria (IDF 2011). In all cases, patients should have failed to lose and sustain significant weight loss through nonsurgical weight management programs and have type 2 diabetes that has not responded to lifestyle intervention strategies (with or without metformin) and an A1C <7%. A team that specializes in diabetes should determine conditional eligibility or prioritization. Contraindications for surgery include alcohol and drug abuse, uncontrolled psychiatric illness, and lack of understanding of the risks/benefits, expected surgical outcomes, and alternative and lifestyle changes required with these types of procedures. Table 19.1 summarizes the IDF's eligibility and prioritization for bariatric surgery.

The American Diabetes Association (ADA) also made recommendations for people with type 2 diabetes and bariatric surgery (ADA 2012). Adults may be considered for bariatric surgery with a BMI >35 kg/m² and type 2 diabetes, especially if the diabetes or associated comorbidities are difficult to control with lifestyle and pharmacological therapy, may be considered for bariatric surgery. The ADA notes that although small trials have shown glycemic benefits of bariatric surgery in patients with type 2 diabetes and BMI levels of 30–35 kg/m², there is currently insufficient evidence to generally recommend surgery in patients with BMIs <35 kg/m² outside of a research protocol.

Table 19.1 Eligibility and Prioritization for Bariatric Surgery Based on Failed Nonsurgical Weight Loss Therapy, BMI*, and Disease Control

BMI Range	Eligible for Surgery	Prioritized for Surgery
<30	No	No
30–35	Yes, conditional†	No
35–40	Yes	Yes, conditional†
>40	Yes	Yes

* BMI should be lowered by 2.5 BMI points for Asians.

†For individuals with A1C levels >7.5%, despite being fully optimized on conventional therapies, especially if weight is increasing, or other weight-responsive comorbidities not achieving targets (such as lipids, blood pressure, and obstructive sleep apnea), bariatric surgery may be considered conditionally.

Adapted from IDF 2011.

BARIATRIC SURGERY PROCEDURES AND DIABETES-RELATED OUTCOMES

Bariatric surgery may offer a novel end point: major improvement and even complete remission of diabetes for some individuals. The RYGBP, BPD, and/or BPD-DS procedures offer superior weight loss and diabetes remission rates than less invasive, non-diversionary procedures such as the LAGB (IDF 2011). There is no evidence to support the use of subcutaneous lipectomy (liposuction) as a treatment for type 2 diabetes in obese patients (Klein 2004).

A retrospective analysis reported the results in 330 of 608 (50.6%) morbidly obese patients who had either type 2 diabetes or impaired glucose tolerance who had undergone gastric bypass surgery (Pories 1995). In addition to significant, long-lasting weight loss (37% of total body weight 1 year post-operation and 30% total weight loss 14 years after surgery), these patients achieved an outstanding result with regard to remission of type 2 diabetes. In 121 of 146 (82.9%) patients with type 2 diabetes, and in 150 of 152 patients (98.7%) with impaired glucose tolerance, normal glucose, A1C, and insulin levels were maintained. Of note, blood glucose levels returned to normal levels within a few days after the RYGBP procedure (thus before significant weight loss).

Additional research reported similar results. In a meta-analysis of 136 weight-loss surgery studies that included 22,094 subjects undergoing a variety of bariatric surgery procedures, diabetes was completely resolved in 76.8% of the patients and resolved or improved in 86% (Buchwald 2004).

The Swedish Obesity Study (which was a prospective, contemporaneously matched, multicenter bariatric surgery trial) compared surgery to medical treatment of obesity after 2 years among 4,047 patients, and 1,703 patients at 10 years (Sjöström 2004). Two years after bariatric surgery, no patients had developed type 2 diabetes, whereas 5% of the medical treatment group had; at 10 years, the risk of developing type 2 diabetes was three times higher for the medically treated group, whereas recovery from type 2 diabetes was three times more common among the bariatric surgery group. A small number of RYGBP patients did not experience complete remission of diabetes. These individuals were characterized as having had type 2 diabetes for a longer duration, suggesting they may have had insufficient residual β-cell mass to allow for euglycemia after surgery (Sjöström 2004). A later analysis of the Swedish Obesity Study data revealed that patients undergoing bariatric surgery also had a decrease in mortality rates (Sjöström 2007).

A meta-analysis and systematic review conducted in 2009 revealed that in 78.1% of the cases of type 2 diabetes, complete resolution was obtained (blood glucose levels normal without diabetes-related medications) (Buchwald 2009). When including individuals who cited improvement in their glycemic control, the percentage increased to 86.6%. Resolution of diabetes occurred simultaneously, with an average weight loss of 38.5 kg, which represented 55.9% of excess body-weight loss.

Despite the traditionally set parameters for bariatric surgery of a BMI of ≥40 kg/m² without comorbidities, or ≥35 kg/m² with significant comorbidities, recent trials among individuals with BMI levels <35 kg/m² reported complete remission of type 2 diabetes at the same or higher percentage of cases than seen among patients with severe obesity status after RYGBP (Cohen 2006; Lee 2008). There is evidence that this surgery may induce anti-diabetes help beyond that seen with weight loss alone (Cummings 2009). Cummings discovered that the insulin sensitivity index, which was calculated via intravenous glucose tolerance testing and minimal modeling, increased by four- to fivefold. This increase was linked to the enhancement of the insulin-sensitizing hormone adiponectin, particularly the high-molecular-weight form, which increases in response to the amount of decrease in fat mass and predicts the extent of improvement in insulin sensitivity estimated by the homeostatic model assessment. The amount of lipid found in muscle drops after RYGBP, as it does in the liver. This fall in hepatic and muscle lipid levels may also help increase insulin sensitivity, since accumulation of lipid in these two tissues is thought to be a key factor in elevated blood glucose levels (Cummings 2009).

The effect of the BPD procedure on remission of diabetes has also been evaluated, and it is hypothesized that positive changes occur in genes that control fatty acid and glucose metabolism in muscle. Insulin sensitivity improved by 6 months after BPD and remained improved, with no additional improvements from 2 to 10 years after the operation (Cummings 2009). As promising as these reports are, a critical caveat lies in the fact that these observations were post-surgery, anywhere from many months to several years post-operation, at the point where significant weight loss had already been witnessed (Cummings 2009).

Unfortunately, postoperative type 2 diabetes remission rates do not appear as dramatic with the LAGB, since improvement in blood glucose levels from this procedure generally appear only after significant weight loss (Cummings 2008; Dixon 2008). A systematic review and meta-analysis of post-LAGB procedures reveal a diabetes remission rate of 48% of cases, whereas remission rate was 84% in RYGBP cases (Buchwald 2004). In addition, the time point of type 2 diabetes remission after LAGB is much longer than with RYGBP and may be significantly linked to the pace and extent of weight loss. Studies among individuals with mild type 2 diabetes at baseline have shown that, while there was 73% remission at 2 years after LAGB, none of the patients had achieved remission of type 2 diabetes at 6 months postoperatively, suggesting a significant role of weight loss as etiology of remission among band patients (Cummings 2008; Dixon 2008).

NUTRITION THERAPY AND RELATED INTERVENTIONS FOR BARIATRIC SURGERY

A literature search was conducted using PubMed MEDLINE to determine the evidence-based recommendations and guidelines for diabetes nutrition therapy interventions before and after bariatric surgery. Search criteria included the following: nutrition, diet, lifestyle intervention, diabetes, type 2 diabetes, bariatric surgery and bypass surgery, and English language since 1999. No articles related to nutrition therapy interventions in subjects with type 2 diabetes, before or after bariatric surgery, were found. In general, nutrition therapy recommendations are based on studies done in subjects without diabetes and professionals' clinical experiences and judgments rather than diabetes-specific study outcomes.

Preoperative Bariatric Surgery Interventions

Guidelines were developed by a joint effort of the American Association of Clinical Endocrinologists, the Obesity Society, and the American Society for Metabolic and Bariatric Surgery (ASMBS) to help inform health care providers working with patients with diabetes and obesity both before and after bariatric surgery (Mechanick 2008). It is recommended that all patients requiring insulin before bariatric surgery have their blood glucose concentrations monitored regularly and insulin administered to control significant hyperglycemia.

Preoperative nutrition assessment. The ASMBS also independently published general pre- and postoperative nutrition guidelines for RYGBP, LAGB, and BPD with and without duodenal switch (BPD-DS) procedures (Aills 2008). The preoperative nutrition assessment includes anthropometrics, including an accurate height and weight, BMI, and excess body weight; weight history, including previous and recent weight-loss attempts, if required by the program (and/or the patient's insurance carrier); and a medical history with current comorbidities, prescription medications, and all over-the-counter supplements, including vitamins/minerals and herbal or other supplements. It also includes a history of food intake on weekdays and weekends as well as a review of food logs, if available; dining-out habits; and assessment of potential disordered eating patterns, including binge eating disorder. If binge eating disorder is suspected, referral to a behavioral provider and/or registered dietitian specializing in eating disorders may be helpful. In addition, the patient should be asked about his or her ability to purchase vitamin/mineral and/or protein supplements prescribed after surgery to reduce risk of nutritional deficiencies. There may be at least short-term assistance for financially needy patients, such as from the Obesity Action Coalition (OAC), which allows clinicians affiliated with a bariatric surgery program to request 3 months of free vitamin/mineral supplements.

A common misconception is that the patient with severe obesity is well nourished, but that is certainly not the case for many preoperative patients, particularly when it comes to micronutrients. Some preoperative patients may have a significant dieting history or an eating pattern that does not include regular consumption of fruits, vegetables, and whole grains. These individuals may be at increased risk of osteopenia, sarcopenia, and/or other nutrition-related deficiencies. It is imperative that the clinician working with preoperative bariatric patients screen for the adequacy of the current diet, as well as perceived risk for vitamin/mineral deficiencies. A daily vitamin/mineral supplement may be advised preoperatively to help ensure adequate micronutrient intake (Aills 2008).

Vitamin/Mineral Deficiencies

It is important to monitor vitamin and mineral deficiencies both preoperatively and postoperatively (Aills 2008; IDF 2011). Preoperatively, patients with severe obesity may be at risk for deficiencies of several of the B-complex vitamins, vital for adequate metabolism of carbohydrates as well as neural functioning, which affect appetite (Flancbaum 2006; Boylan 1988). Additionally, as many as 50% of preoperative patients may be iron deficient (Flancbaum 2006), as well as have deficiencies related to zinc, selenium, and vitamins A, E, and C (Buffington 1993; Boylan 1988; Reitman 2002). Nutritional concerns and risk for bariatric surgery procedures are summarized in Table 19.2.

Vitamin D. Research has indicated that 60–80% of severely obese patients may be deficient in vitamin D (Buffington 1993; Ybarra 2005; Flancbaum 2006; Carlin 2006). Vitamin D deficiency may decrease the absorption of dietary calcium and increase calcitriol, possibly resulting in metabolic adaptations favoring adipose tissue deposition, potentially further exacerbating weight gain (El-Kadre 2004; Schrager 2005). It is also known that the risk of vitamin D deficiency is generally increased after bariatric surgery. Additionally, the higher the patient's BMI, the greater the risk of deficiency (Aills 2008).

Thiamin. Patients who present for bariatric surgery already low in thiamin may be at significantly higher risk for developing beriberi (Aills 2008). Preoperative thiamin deficiency has been documented to be as high as 29% overall and may vary among specific ethnicities, with 6.7% of whites, nearly 31% of African Americans, and 47% of Hispanics with preoperative deficits in one study (Flancbaum 2006). These results suggest the importance of preoperative thiamin testing.

Vitamin B12. Many medications taken by preoperative bariatric patients may affect vitamin B12 absorption and/or stores. For example, it is reported that among patients taking metformin, 10–30% had issues with reduced vitamin B12 absorption (Bauman 2000). Additionally, the high rate of bariatric patients who suffer from gastroesophageal reflux disease and need to take proton pump inhibitors may exacerbate the risk for vitamin B12 deficiency (Aills 2008). In a group of preoperative gastric bypass patients, vitamin B12 levels were evaluated, and 13% exhibited vitamin B12 deficiency (Madan 2006). Another researcher reported preoperative vitamin B12 levels among both gastric bypass and BPD patients to be in the low-normal range for both groups (Skroubis 2006). These results suggest it would be prudent to check preoperative vitamin B12 levels among prospective bariatric surgery patients.

Folic acid. It was estimated that between 23 and 33% of women aged 15–44 years of age in the general population do not meet the recommended dietary intake of 400 mg/day folic acid (Bentley 2006). Possible contributors include the popularity of low-carbohydrate/high-protein diets, which diminish the likelihood of adequate servings of good folate food sources, such as fortified grain products and fresh fruits and vegetables. Among preoperative gastric bypass patients, folate deficiency as high as 56% has been documented. Therefore, folic acid levels need to be assessed preoperatively (Boylan 1988).

Iron. It is estimated that women of childbearing age represent >80% of the population of bariatric surgery patients in the U.S., and among menstruating women, iron deficiency and related anemia may be risk factors independent of surgery (Aills 2008). The use of oral contraceptives may decrease menstrual blood losses as much as 60%, but still necessitate iron supplementation (Wood 2006). Perhaps surprisingly, obese men and surgical candidates younger than 25 years of age may also be at risk for iron deficiency preoperatively. Among 379 consecutive bariatric cases studied, 44% of preoperative patients were found to be iron deficient, with male patients more likely to be anemic than female patients (41% males vs. 19% females) (Flancbaum 2006). However, the female patients had a higher

Table 19.2 Nutritional Concerns/Risks for Bariatric Surgery Procedures

Nutrient	RYGBP	BPD	BPD-DS	VSG	LAGB
Thiamin	+	+	+	++	+
Vitamin B12	+++	++	++	++	+
Folic acid	++	++	++	++	++
Iron	+++	+++	++	++	+
Vitamin D	++	+++	+++	+	+

+Recommended daily intake (allowance) or standard multivitamin preparation likely to be sufficient.

++Significant risk of deficiency or increased requirements.

+++High risk of deficiency. Additional supplementation is necessary to prevent deficiency. Careful monitoring recommended. Patient may need to supplement in levels in excess of daily requirements.

Adapted from IDF 2011.

incidence of abnormal ferritin levels. Overall, iron deficiency (as measured by serum iron levels) and anemia were more prevalent in patients younger than 25 years of age when compared to patients >60 years of age (79 vs. 42%, respectively). These reports highlight the importance of preoperative screening for iron deficiency and anemia.

Postoperative Bariatric Surgery Diabetes Recommendations

Recommendations have been made for postoperative bariatric surgery (Aills 2008; Mechanick 2008). In the immediate postoperative period (within 4 days of surgery), in patients with type 2 diabetes, periodic fasting blood glucose levels should be measured. In patients hospitalized in the non–intensive care unit, fasting blood glucose levels should be maintained between 80 and 110 mg/dL. This step may require the use of a long-acting insulin, such as insulin glargine or detemir. It is also recommended that maximal postprandial glucose values be below 180 mg/dL. Achieving these values may require a rapid-acing insulin analog before meals and at bedtime. In the intensive care unit, it is recommended that all blood glucose values be maintained ideally within the range of 80–110 mg/dL by using an intravenous insulin infusion (Mechanick 2008).

In the late postoperative period (>4 days after surgery), routine metabolic and nutritional monitoring is recommended. It is noted that patients who have undergone RYGBP, BPD, or BPD-DS who have postprandial hypoglycemic symptoms that have not responded to nutritional manipulation should be evaluated for the possibility of endogenous hyperinsulinemic hypoglycemia associated with nesidioblastosis. Hyperinsulinemic hypoglycemia is theorized to be potentially related to changes in glucagon-like peptide (GLP)-1 and other gut hormones (Meneghini 2007). Gut hormones secreted by the L-cells of the small intestine, GLP-1, and gastric inhibitory polypeptide (GIP) are impaired with type 2 diabetes. Metabolic surgery, including gastric bypass and BPD with duodenal switch procedures, may restore this function. Both RYGBP and BPD-DS allow for consistent GLP-1 production during fasting, as well as postprandially, resulting in L-cell stimulation via early arrival of nutrients to the distal ileum (Patriti 2004). The production of GLP-1 may affect glucose metabolism by inhibiting the production of glucagon, stimulating insulin secretion, delaying gastric emptying, and stimulating glycogenogenesis (Patriti 2004).

Patients also should be encouraged to increase their physical activity (aerobic and strength training) to a minimum of 30 min/day as well as increase physical activity throughout the day as soon as tolerated. They are also encouraged to participate in ongoing support groups after discharge from the hospital.

Post-surgery nutrition recommendations. Clinical guidelines have been developed for nutrition care after surgical weight-loss procedures and detection and management of complications such as vitamin and mineral deficiencies, osteoporosis, and hypoglycemia from insulin hypersecretion (Aills 2008). Although not specifically geared toward patients with diabetes, the overall guidelines also pertain to patients with type 2 diabetes. The goals of nutrition care after surgery are *1*) to provide adequate energy and nutrients to support preservation of lean body mass during extreme weight loss and support tissue healing and *2*) to encourage beverages and foods that maximize weight loss and promote weight maintenance while minimizing the reflux, dumping syndrome, and early satiety.

A multiphase post-surgery eating pattern is often recommended to achieve these goals and includes a progression in food choices and texture. Clear liquid diets are often prescribed initially in the first day or two. The diet is then typically advanced to full liquids and then to a pureed diet. A mechanically altered soft diet is usually the next step, and after 5–8 weeks, the diet is finally advanced to a regular surgical weight-loss diet. Patients should be advised to eat slowly, generally no more than 1 oz every 10 min, and they should stop eating if they feel full. Patients should also be advised to not consume beverages and food at the same time. Most patients quickly learn to control portion sizes, since overeating can result in vomiting. It is also important to teach patients to thoroughly chew their food and to practice mindful eating and avoiding distractions when eating.

Clinical practice recommendations for protein intake after a non-complicated surgery are similar to those for medically supervised modified protein fasts (70 g/day on very-low-calorie diets) (Mahan 2000). Many bariatric centers recommend a protein intake of 60–80 g/day or 1.0–1.5 g/kg ideal body weight; research studies are currently lacking to confirm exact requirements. After BPD-DS procedures, the amount of protein should be increased by 30% to accommodate for malabsorption (~90 g/day) (Slater 2004). Incorporating liquid supplements into the patient's daily oral intake during the early postoperative period provides an important source of protein as well as calories that help prevent the loss of lean body mass. Experts in clinical practice have noted that adding 100 g/day carbohydrate decreases nitrogen loss by 40% in modified protein fasts (Scopinaro 1998).

General post-bariatric surgery eating phases and recommendations are summarized in Table 19.3. Table 19.4 lists foods and beverages to delay reintroduction or avoid post-bariatric surgery.

Table 19.3 General Post-Bariatric Surgery Eating Phases: Advancement of Food and Beverages in the Non-Complicated Patient

Diet Phase	Duration	Foods Commonly Included	Additional Comments
Clear liquid	1–2 days	Broth, herbal/decaffeinated tea, sugar-free popsicles, sugar-free gelatin, artificially sweetened beverages, and protein supplements	Post-operation day 1 patients undergo a gastrogaffin swallow test for leaks; once tested, begin sips of clear liquids; serve foods at body temperature; these types of fluids provide electrolytes and a limited amount of energy to encourage resolution of gut activity and leave a minimal amount of gastrointestinal residue; this diet is nutritionally inadequate
Full liquid	10–14 days	Milk and milk alternatives, artificially sweetened yogurt, strained creamed soups, cream cereals, vegetable juices, and sugar-free puddings; also included are protein supplements (2 oz or ¼ cup protein supplement every hour while awake)	Patients should consume a minimum of 48–64 oz of total fluids per day; 24–32 oz of any combination of full liquids; this phase of the eating pattern has slightly more texture and increased gastric residue; liquid texture is thought to further allow healing; the eating pattern provides caloric restriction with energy and protein equivalent to very-low-calorie diets
Pureed	10–14+ Days	Emphasis on protein-rich foods such as pureed meat, flaked fish, scrambled eggs and egg substitute, soft cheeses, pureed fruit and vegetables, and hot cereal	Protein food choices are encouraged for 3–6 small meals per day; patients may only be able to tolerate a couple of tablespoons at each meal/snack; total liquids 48–64+ oz per day; patients are encouraged not to drink fluids with meals and to wait ~30 min after each meal before resuming fluids; foods are blended or liquefied with sufficient fluid to create a food texture that ranges from a milkshake to mashed potato consistency
Mechanically soft	≥14 days	Foods in this phase include chopped tender or ground cuts of meat and meat alternatives, soft fresh or canned fruit, soft cooked or canned vegetables, and grains as tolerated	This phase provides foods that are texture-modified to require minimal chewing by pureeing, mashing, grinding, chopping, or flaking; food texture should easily pass through adjustable band or gastrojejunostomy into the jejunum
Weight loss regular	5–8 weeks post-surgery	Vitamin and mineral supplement daily; healthy, balanced eating pattern consisting of adequate protein, fruits, vegetables, and whole grains; calorie needs based on height, weight, age	Patients should be counseled about setting realistic weight-loss goals; few patients will achieve a normal weight (BMI <25 kg/m²); long-term maintenance will depend on a patient's ability to commit to regular physical activity and a healthy eating pattern

Adapted from Aills 2008.

Table 19.4 Post-Bariatric Surgery: Food and Beverages to Delay Reintroduction or Avoid

Food or Beverage	Recommendation
Alcohol	Avoid/delay in moderation
Caffeine	Avoid/delay in moderation
Carbonated beverages	Avoid/delay
Fruit juice	Avoid
Fatty foods, high saturated fat/fried food	Avoid
Nuts, popcorn, other fibrous foods	Delay
Soft "doughy" bread, pasta, rice	Avoid/delay
Sugar, sugar-containing foods, concentrated sweets	Avoid
Tough, dry, red meat	Avoid/delay

Adapted from Aills 2008.

CONCLUSION

Although there has been groundbreaking research in the field of bariatric surgery, the complex, underlying mechanisms responsible for remission of type 2 diabetes have yet to be fully elucidated. Well-designed controlled trials need to be conducted that compare the long-term benefits, cost-effectiveness, and risks of bariatric surgery in individuals with type 2 diabetes with optimal medical and lifestyle therapy (ADA 2012). In addition, future research may aid in the development of new medications that may mimic the significant anti-diabetes effects of bariatric surgery without the need for surgery itself. It appears evident that bariatric surgery is changing the paradigm in which diabetes is managed in the present day and may be a significant tool in helping to prevent and/or attenuate the devastating disease of diabetes, as well as obesity. Even if complete remission of diabetes does not occur, bariatric surgery can offer major benefits in glucose control, in addition to weight loss (Pournaras 2012). The long-term benefit of improved gllycemic control may be the reduction of diabetes complications. Despite the numerous studies conducted on individuals with bariatric surgery pre- and postoperatively, at this time, diabetes nutrition therapy interventions are based on the knowledge of the professional and clinical judgment rather than study outcomes.

BIBLIOGRAPHY

Aills L, Blankenship J, Buffington C, Furtado M, Parrott J: ASMBS Allied Health Nutritional Guidelines for the Surgical Weight Loss Patient. *Surg Obes Relat Dis* 4:S73–S108, 2008

American Diabetes Association: Standards of medical care in diabetes: 2012. *Diabetes Care* 35 (Suppl. 1):S11–S63, 2012

Batsis JA, Romero-Corral A, Coliazo-Clavell ML, Sarr MG, Somers VK, Lopez-Jimenez F: Effect of bariatric surgery on the metabolic syndrome: a population-based, long-term controlled study. *Mayo Clin Proc* 83:897–907, 2008

Bauman WA, Shaw S, Jayatilleke K, Spungen AM, Herbert V: Increased intake of calcium reverses the B-12 malabsorption induced by metformin. *Diabetes Care* 23:1227–1231, 2000

Bentley TGK, Willett W, Weinstein MC, Kuntz KM: Population-level changes in folate intake by age, gender, race/ethnicity after folic acid fortification. *Am J Pub Health* 96:2040–2047, 2006

Boylan LM, Sugerman JH, Driskell JA: Vitamin E, vitamin B-6, vitamin B-12, and folate status of gastric bypass surgery patients. *J Am Diet Assoc* 88:579–585, 1988

Buchwald H: Health implications of bariatric surgery. *J Am Coll Surg* 200:593–604, 2005

Buchwald H, Avidor Y, Braunwald E, Jensen MD, Pories WJ, Fahrbach K, Schoelles K: Bariatric surgery: a systematic review and meta-analysis. *JAMA* 292:1724–1737, 2004

Buchwald H, Estok R, Fahrbach K, Banel D, Jensen MD, Pories WJ, Bantle JP, Sledge I: Weight and type 2 diabetes after bariatric surgery: systematic review and meta-analysis. *Am J Med* 122:248–256, 2009

Buffington CK, Walker B, Cowan GS, Scruggs D: Vitamin D deficiency in the morbidly obese. *Obes Surg* 3:421–424, 1993

Carlin AM, Rao DS, Meslemani AM, Genaw JA, Parikh NJ, Levy S, Bhan A, Talpos GB: Prevalence of vitamin D depletion among morbidly obese patients seeking bypass surgery. *Surg Obes Related Dis* 2:98–103, 2006

Cohen R, Pinheiro JS, Correa JL, Schiavon CA: Laparoscopic Roux-en-Y gastric bypass for BMI < 35 kg/m²: a tailored approach. *Surg Obes Relat Dis* 2:401–404, 2006

Cummings DE: Endocrine mechanisms mediating remission of diabetes after gastric bypass surgery. *Int J Obes* 33:533–540, 2009

Cummings DE, Flum DR: Gastrointestinal surgery as a treatment for diabetes. *JAMA* 299:341–343, 2008

Dixon JB, O'Brien PE, Playfair J, Chapman L, Schachter LM, Skinner S, Proietto J, Bailey M, Anderson M: Adjustable gastric banding and conventional therapy for type 2 diabetes: a randomized controlled trial. *JAMA* 299:316–323, 2008

El-Kadre LJ, Savassi Roca PR, de Almeida Tinoco AC, Tinoco RC: Calcium metabolism in pre- and post-menopausal morbidly obese women at baseline and after laparoscopic Roux-en-Y gastric bypass. *Obes Surg* 14:1062–1066, 2004

Flancbaum L, Belsley S, Drake V, Colarusso T, Tayler E: Preoperative nutritional status of patients undergoing Roux-en-Y gastric bypass for morbid obesity. *J Gastrointest Surg* 10:1033–1037, 2006

Gagner M, Inabnet WB, Pomp A: Laparoscopic gastrectomy with second stage biliopancreatic diversion and duodenal switch in the super-obese. In *Laparoscopic Bariatric Surgery*. Inabnet WB, DeMaria EJ, Ikramuddin S, Eds. Philadelphia, Lippincott Williams & Wilkins, p. 143–149, 2005

Greenway SE, Greenway FL 3rd, Klein S: Effects of obesity surgery on non-insulin-dependent diabetes mellitus. *Arch Surg* 137:1109–1117, 2002

Habib R, Scrocco JD, Terek M, Vanek V, Mikolich JR: Effects of bariatric surgery on inflammatory, functional and structural markers of coronary atherosclerosis. *Am J Cardiol* 104:1251–1255, 2009

Hess DS, Hess DW, Oakley RS: The biliopancreatic diversion with duodenal switch: results beyond 10 years. *Obes Surg* 15:408–416, 2005

Hill JO, Wyatt HR, Reed GW, Peters JC: Obesity and the environment: where do we go from here? *Science* 299:853–855, 2003

Huang H, Kasumov T, Gatmaitan P, Heneghan H, Kashyap S, Schauer P, Brethauer S, Kirwan J: Gastric bypass surgery reduces plasma ceramide subspecies and improves insulin sensitivity in severely obese patients. *Obesity* 19:2235–2240, 2011

International Diabetes Federation: Bariatric surgical and procedural interventions in the treatment of obese patients with type 2 diabetes: a position statement from the International Diabetes Federation Taskforce on Epidemiology and Prevention. Available at http://www.idf.org/position-statements. Accessed on 6 November 2011

Kashyap SR, Daud S, Kelly KR, Gastaldelli A, Win H, Brethauer S, Kirwan JP, Schauer PR: Acute effects of gastric bypass versus gastric restrictive surgery on beta-cell function and insulinotropic hormones in severely obese patients with type 2 diabetes. *Int J Obes (Lond)* 34:462–471, 2010

Keidar A: Bariatric surgery for type 2 diabetes reversal: the risks. *Diabetes Care* 34 (Suppl. 2):S362–S366, 2011

Klein S, Fontana L, Young VL, Coggan AR, Kilo C, Patterson BW, Mohammed SB: Absence of an effect of liposuction on insulin action and risk factors for coronary heart disease. *N Engl J Med* 350:2549–2557, 2004

Lee WJ, Wang W, Lee YC, Huang MT, Ser KH, Chen JC: Effect of laparoscopic mini-gastric bypass for type 2 diabetes mellitus: comparison of BMI >35 and < 35kg/m². *J Gastrointest Surg* 12:945–952, 2008

Madan AK, Orth WS, Tichansky DS, Ternovits CA: Vitamin and trace mineral levels after laparoscopic gastric bypass. *Obes Surg* 16:603–606, 2006

Mahan LK, Escott-Stump S (Eds). *Medical Nutrition Therapy for Anemia: Krause's Food, Nutrition, and Diet Therapy.* 10th ed. Philadelphia, WB Saunders, p. 469, 2000

Marceau P, Hould FS, Simard, S, Lebel S, Bourque RA, Potvin M, Biron S: Bilio-pancreatic diversion with duodenal switch. *World J Surg* 22:947–954, 1998

Mason EE, Ito C: Gastric bypass in obesity. *Obes Res* 4:316–319, 1967

McTigue K, Lason JC, Valoski A, Burke G, Kotchen J, Lewis CE, Stefanick ML, Van Horn L, Kuller L: Mortality and cardiac and vascular outcomes in extremely obese women. *JAMA* 296:79–86, 2006

Mechanick JI, Kushner RF, Sugerman HJ, Gonzalez-Campoy JM, Collazo-Clavell ML, Guven S, Spitz AF, Apovian CM, Livington EH, Brolin R, Sarwer DB, Anderson WA, Dixon J: American Association of Clinical Endocrinologists, The Obesity Society, and American Society for Metabolic & Bariatric Surgery medical guidelines for clinical practice for the perioperative nutritional, meta-bolic, and nonsurgical support of the bariatric surgery patient. *Endocr Pract* 14 (Suppl. 1):1–83, 2008

Ogden CL, Carrol MD, Curtin LR, McDowell MA, Tabak CJ, Flegal KM: Preva-lence of overweight and obesity in the United States, 1999–2004. *JAMA* 295:1549–1555, 2006

Ostman J, Britton M, Jonsson E (Eds.): *Treating and Preventing Obesity: An Evi-dence-Based Review.* Weinheim, Germany, Wiley, 2004

Patriti A, Facchiano E, Sanna A, Gulla N, Donini A: The enteroinsular axis and the recovery from type 2 diabetes after bariatric surgery. *Obes Surg* 14:840–848, 2004

Pories WJ, Swanson MS, MacDonald KG, Long SB, Morris PG, Brown BM, Barakat HA, deRamon RA, Israel G, Dolezal JM, Dohm L: Who would have thought it? An operation proves to be the most effective therapy for adult-onset diabetes mellitus. *Ann Surg* 222:339–350, 1995

Reitman A, Friedrich I, Ben-Amotz A, Levy Y: Low plasma antioxidants and nor-mal plasma B vitamins and homocysteine in patients with severe obesity. *Isr Med Assoc J* 4:590–593, 2002

Pournaras DJ, Aasheim ET, Sovik TT, Andrews R, Mahon D, Welbourn R, Olbers T, le Roux CW: Effect of the definition of type II diabetes remission in the evaluation of bariatric surgery for metabolic changes. *Br J Surg* 99:100–103, 2012

Samuel VT, Petersen KF, Shulman GI: Lipid-induced insulin resistance: unravel-ing the mechanism. *Lancet* 375:2267–2277, 2010

Schauer PR, Burguera B, Ikramuddin S, Cottam D, Gourash W, Hamad G, Eid GM, Mattar S, Ramanathan R, Barinas-Mitchel E, Rao HR, Kuller L, Kelley D: Effect of laparoscopic Roux-en Y gastric bypass on type 2 diabetes mellitus. *Ann Surg* 238:467–484, 2003

Schrager S: Dietary calcium intake and obesity. *J Am Board Fam Pract* 18:205–210, 2005

Scopinaro N, Adami GF, Marinari GM, Gianetta E, Traverso E, Friedman D, Camerini G, Baschieri G, Simonelli S: Biliopancreatic diversion. *World J Surg* 22:936–924, 1998

Scopinaro N, Marinari GM, Camerini G, Papadia F, 2004 ABS Consensus Conference: Biliopancreatic diversion for obesity: state of the art. *Surg Obes* 1:317–328, 2005

Sjöström L, Lindroos AK, Peltonen M, Torgerson J, Bouchard C, Carlsson B, Dahlgren S, Larsson B, Narbro K, Sjöström CD, Sullivan M, Wedel H, for Swedish Obese Subjects Study Scientific Group: Lifestyle, diabetes and cardiovascular risk factors 10 years after bariatric surgery. *N Engl J Med* 351:2683–2693, 2004

Sjöström L, Narbro K, Sjöström CD, Karason K, Larsson B, Wedel H, Lystig T, Sullivan M, Bouchard C, Bengtsson C, Dahlgren S, Gummesson A, Jacobson P, Karlsson J, Lindroos AK, Lonroth H, Näslund I, Olbers T, Stenlöf K, Torgerson J, Ågren G, Carlsson MS, for the Swedish Obese Subjects Study Scientific Group: Effects of bariatric surgery on mortality in Swedish obese subjects. *N Engl J Med* 357:741–752, 2007

Skroubis G, Anesidis S, Kehagias L, Mead N, Vagenas K, Kalfarentzos F: Roux-en-Y gastric bypass versus a variant of BPD in a non-superobese population: prospective comparison of the efficacy and the incidence of metabolic deficiencies. *Obes Surg* 16:488–495, 2006

Slater GH, Ren CJ, Seigel N, Williams T, Barr D, Wolf B, Dolan K, Fielding GA: Serum fat-soluble vitamin deficiency and abnormal calcium metabolism after malabsorptive bariatric surgery. *J Gastrointest Surg* 8:48–55, 2004

Sturm R: Increases in clinically severe obesity in the United States, 1986–2000. *Arch Intern Med* 163:2146–2148, 2003

Tretjakovs P, Jurka A, Bormane I, Mackevics V, Mikelsone I, Balode L, Reihmane D, Stukena I, Bahs G, Aviars JI, Pirage V: Relation of inflammatory chemokines to insulin resistance and hypoadiponectinemia in coronary artery disease patients. *Eur J Intern Med* 20:712–717, 2009

Tsai AG, Wadden TA: Systematic review: an evaluation of major commercial weight loss programs in the United States. *Ann Intern Med* 142:56–66, 2005

Vázquez LA, Pazos F, Berrazueta JR, Fernández-Escalante C, García-Unzueta MT, Freijanes J, Amado JA: Effects of changes in body weight and insulin resistance on inflammation and endothelial function in morbid obesity after bariatric surgery. *J Clin Endocrinol Metab* 90:316–322, 2005

Wing RR, Phelan S: Long-term weight loss maintenance. *Am J Clin Nutr* 82 (Suppl. 1):222S–225S, 2005

Wood RJ, Ronnenberg AG: Iron. In *Modern Nutrition in Health and Disease.* Shils ME, Shike M, Ross AC, Cabellero B, Cousins RJ, Eds. 10th ed. Philadelphia, Lippincott Williams & Wilkins, 2006

Ybarra J, Sanchez-Hernandez J, Gich I, De Levia A, Ruis X, Rodriguez-Espinosa J, Perez A: Unchanged hypovitaminosis D and secondary hyperparathyroidism in morbid obesity after bariatric surgery. *Obes Surg* 15:330–335, 2005

Yermilov I, McGory, M, Shekelle PW, Ko CY, Maggard MA: Appropriateness criteria for bariatric surgery: beyond the NIH guidelines. *Obesity (Silver Spring)* 17:1521–1527, 2009

Margaret Furtado, MS, RD, is a Clinical Dietitian Specialist at Johns Hopkins Bayview Medical Center and The Johns Hopkins Center for Bariatric Surgery in Baltimore, MD. Alison B. Evert, MS, RD, CDE, is a Diabetes Nutrition Educator and the Coordinator of Diabetes Education Programs at the University of Washington Medical Center, Diabetes Care Center in Seattle, WA.

Chapter 20

Integrating Nutrition Therapy, Blood Glucose Monitoring, and Continuous Glucose Monitoring

Margaret A. Powers, PhD, RD, CDE, and Mary M. Austin, MA, RD, CDE, FAADE

Highlights

Translation of Evidence into Nutrition Recommendations

Current Perspectives

New Evidence for SMBG and CGM

Summary

Highlights
Integrating Nutrition Therapy, Blood Glucose Monitoring, and Continuous Glucose Monitoring

■ Glucose monitoring is a valuable tool for assessing the glycemic response to food, activity, and medications when data are used for decision-making.

■ A monitoring schedule should be individualized and based on eating patterns, medications, activity schedule, current glucose control, cost, convenience, and the patient's willingness to monitor.

■ Glucose monitoring can be used to reduce glycemic variability and increase stability in glucose levels, thus reducing the oxidative stress that leads to complications.

■ Continuous glucose monitoring (CGM) data are a better indicator of overall glycemic management than A1C.

Integrating Nutrition Therapy, Blood Glucose Monitoring, and Continuous Glucose Monitoring

Glucose monitoring has been widely available for over three decades. Currently, there are almost 75 blood glucose meters available in the U.S., and they perform a variety of functions. Some offer glucose testing with a memory of 100–450 test results, whereas others have a memory capacity of over 3,000 results. Some are quite sophisticated and have markers for when meals are eaten, medications are taken, and when an activity occurs. In addition, some meters have alarms to check blood glucose, graphs to show results for different times of the day, and options to download data to smartphones. These glucose meters measure blood (plasma) glucose, whereas continuous glucose sensors measure interstitial glucose. An annual review of the meters and continuous glucose monitoring (CGM) systems is available in the Consumer Product Guide, published each January in *Diabetes Forecast* and available online (American Diabetes Association [ADA] 2012a).

In the 1990s, a great amount of effort was directed at obtaining reimbursement for blood glucose monitoring (BGM) supplies as self-monitored glucose data were seen as a tool to improve glucose control. However, in the 2000s, questions were raised about the value of BGM in reducing A1C levels, especially in people with type 2 diabetes. The research showed that if the data were not used for management decision-making, they were not valuable. Thus, it is important to know how to best use the data, so that the information can have a positive effect on diabetes outcomes. Factors that affect the frequency and timing of self-monitoring of blood glucose (SMBG) include the following: type of diabetes, individual's willingness to monitor, level of diabetes control, medication regimen, lifestyle and daily schedule with regard to activity, food intake and work, physical ability to check blood glucose, ability to problem-solve and take action, financial limitations, and comorbid conditions (Austin 2010).

This chapter will summarize the nutrition-related glucose monitoring recommendations from the ADA 2008 position statement on nutrition recommendations (ADA 2008) and the Academy of Nutrition and Dietetics (Acad Nutr Diet) evidence-based nutrition practice guidelines for adults with type 1 and type 2 diabetes published in the Acad Nutr Diet Evidence Analysis Library (EAL) (Acad Nutr Diet 2008; Franz 2010). The chapter also includes research related to the use of glucose monitoring for diabetes management.

TRANSLATION OF EVIDENCE INTO NUTRITION RECOMMENDATIONS

ADA Nutrition Recommendations and Interventions for Diabetes

The ADA nutrition recommendations and interventions for diabetes position statement highlights the use of BGM in type 1 diabetes, in type 2 diabetes, and during acute illness (ADA 2008). The recommendations state the following:

- For people with type 1 diabetes who take multiple injections of insulin a day, including mealtime insulin, glucose monitoring is valuable in deciding how to best match insulin to carbohydrate intake to achieve glucose goals.
- For people with type 2 diabetes, glucose monitoring can be used to determine whether adjustments in foods and meals will be sufficient to achieve blood glucose goals or if medication(s) needs to be combined with nutrition therapy.
- During acute illness, testing plasma glucose and ketones, drinking adequate amounts of fluids, and ingesting carbohydrate are all important to avoid hyper- and hypoglycemia.

Acad Nutr Diet EAL Recommendations

In 2008, the Acad Nutr Diet EAL published their findings related to BGM (Acad Nutr Diet 2008; Franz 2010). Three questions related to glucose monitoring were asked: *1*) what is the relationship between SMBG and metabolic outcomes in people with type 1 diabetes; *2*) what is the relationship between SMBG and metabolic outcomes in people with type 2 diabetes; and *3*) what is the relationship between CGM and metabolic outcomes in people with type 1 and type 2 diabetes?

A total of 34 studies were reviewed to address these questions, and three recommendations were made. The recommendations are as follows:

1. **BGM.** For individuals on nutrition therapy alone or nutrition therapy in combination with glucose-lowering medications, SMBG is recommended. Frequency and timing depends on diabetes management goals and therapies (e.g., nutrition therapy, diabetes medications, and physical activity). Evidence showed that when SMBG is incorporated into diabetes education programs and the information from SMBG is used to make changes in diabetes management, SMBG is associated with improved glycemic control.

2. **Frequency of BGM.** For people with type 1 or type 2 diabetes on insulin therapy, at least three to eight blood glucose tests per day are recommended to determine the efficacy of the insulin dose(s) and guide adjustments in insulin dose(s), food intake, and physical activity. Some insulin regimens require more testing to establish the best integrated therapy (insulin, food, and activity). Once established, some insulin regimens will require less frequent SMBG. Intervention studies that include self-management training and adjustment of insulin doses based on SMBG report improvements in glycemic control.

3. **Possible need for CGM or more frequent SMBG.** People experiencing unexplained elevations in A1C or unexplained hypoglycemia and hyperglycemia may benefit from use of CGM or more frequent SMBG. It is essential that people with diabetes receive education on how to calibrate CGM and how to interpret CGM results. Studies have proven the accuracy of CGM, and most show that using the trend/pattern data from CGM can result in less glucose variability and improved glucose control.

CURRENT PERSPECTIVES

Since the 2000s, several dozen consensus statements, reviews, and commentaries on SMBG and CGM have been published by professional associations, health care organizations, and renowned diabetes clinicians (Cameron 2010; Hirsch 2008; Klonoff 2008; St. John 2010; Towfigh 2008). The primary focus was exploring the value of glucose monitoring on diabetes outcomes, specifically the A1C value. A long-held tenet of diabetes care has been that the A1C value is correlated with development of complications (Diabetes Control and Complications Trial [DCCT] 1993). Lately, however, the focus has changed to the role of glucose stability and variability and their effect in the development of diabetes complications. BGM, either from SMBG or CGM, provides data on these factors, whereas an A1C level does not. Glucose monitoring from either SMBG or CGM is more useful in providing real-time feedback that can be used to guide therapy sooner and improve outcomes rather than using monthly or quarterly A1C test results (Polonsky 2011).

The ADA established four goals for nutrition therapy (ADA 2008). Glucose monitoring is an essential component of each goal, since it provides feedback data on the impact of food that is eaten and allows individuals to learn how to make the best food choices for themselves. There is evidence that glucose monitoring is valuable in attaining all four goals. The following highlights the value of glucose monitoring in achieving each goal.

The first goal is *achieve and maintain desirable blood glucose, lipid and lipoprotein profile, and blood pressure*. This goal highlights the influence of nutritional intake in controlling blood glucose levels. Even when medication therapy is needed as an adjunct to nutrition therapy, it is important to evaluate the synchronization of the therapies to achieve a glycemic balance (Powers 2010). Glucose monitoring provides the data to make decisions about the best blend of food, medication, and activity. Without this glucose feedback, it would be impossible to know if a particular combination of food, medication, and activity is optimizing the daily diurnal glucose pattern.

The second goal is *prevent, or at least slow, the rate of developing chronic complications of diabetes by modifying nutrient intake and lifestyle*. Variations in daily glucose levels have been shown to contribute to the complications of diabetes (Ceriello 2004). Thus, it is important to assess and correct variations, so individuals can maintain a stable glucose pattern within the normal range, or as close to normal as is safely possible. Glucose monitoring provides feedback on daily variations (diurnal patterns). Previously, the A1C value was viewed as the hallmark of diabetes control (DCCT 1993) and the reference value for indicating risk of diabetes complications. Although A1C value indicates the average blood glucose value over the previous 2–3 months, it does not indicate key factors in glucose control, including stability and variability of blood glucose levels throughout a day (Monnier 2003; Mazze 2008). These factors have been shown to increase oxidative stress and thus can promote the development of the chronic complications of diabetes (Ceriello 2004).

The third and fourth goals relate to meeting individual nutritional needs and pleasure of eating: *address individual nutrition needs, taking into account personal and cultural preferences and willingness to change, and maintain the pleasure of eating by limiting food choices when indicated by scientific evidence.* Glucose monitoring helps achieve these goals by providing data about individual food and various combinations of foods and their glycemic response. This information allows individuals to make informed decisions about their food choices, so they can attain these goals as well as goals one and two.

NEW EVIDENCE FOR SMBG AND CGM

Since the publication of the 2008 ADA nutrition recommendations and the findings of the Acad Nutr Diet EAL, there have been additional studies published related to the value of SMBG and CGM in diabetes management.

A literature search was conducted using PubMed MEDLINE, and additional articles were identified from reference lists. Search criteria included the following: monitoring, glycemic control, and English language articles published after 2008. The PubMed MEDLINE search produced 50 articles, and an additional eight articles were identified from reference lists. Of these, 24 were excluded because titles or abstracts did not meet inclusion criteria, or they were previously reviewed by the EAL. Of note, a 2006 article (Siebolds 2006) was found that met our criteria, but was not included previously in the Acad Nutr Diet EAL and is included in this review. A total of 34 articles were considered for further review. Of the 34 articles, 9 met inclusion criteria and were retrieved for more detailed evaluation. These nine studies are summarized in Tables 20.1 and 20.2. Studies that appear in the tables in "The Evidence for Medical Nutrition Therapy for Type 1 and Type 2 Diabetes in Adults" (Franz 2010) and in the Acad Nutr Diet EAL (http://www.adaevidencelibrary.com) are not included.

SMBG Evidence

Table 20.1 summarizes three studies that looked at the relationship between SMBG and metabolic outcomes. All of the studies focused on using the data obtained from SMBG to guide decision-making by both the patient and health care provider. When the data were used as part of structured counseling, an improvement in A1C was achieved.

The Siebolds study is unique in that it looked at the impact of structured counseling on patient decision-making. This study was not included in the EAL review but was considered and included in Table 20.1 because it examined the actions taken by the patient as a result of counseling on SMBG results. It concluded that SMBG coupled with structured counseling provided patients a tool for more self-directed action and improved outlook (Siebolds 2006). This approach is analogous to what a registered dietitian might do when combining SMBG and nutrition therapy.

The meta-analysis by Poolsup reinforced previous findings that SMBG in non–insulin-using type 2 diabetes patients positively affects A1C, especially within the first 6 months of use, when the data are used for decision-making (Poolsup 2009).

A clinic-based intervention study, examining use of SMBG versus A1C results in making therapy recommendations, showed not only a significant improvement in A1C using SMBG results, but also an unexpected decrease in body weight (Durán 2010). Additionally, there was a significant increase in the consumption of vegetables, nuts, high-fat fish, high-fiber cereals, legumes, low-fat milk, and juices in the SMBG group compared to the A1C group.

A 12-month study sought to eliminate many of the study design issues of previous SMBG trials. A reduction of 1.2% in A1C was seen in patients who were enrolled in the structured testing group, and a 0.9% reduction in A1C was seen in the active control group (Polonsky 2011). A unique finding of this study was that therapy changes by the provider were implemented sooner in the structured testing group, thus increasing the likelihood of improving glycemic control sooner.

Continuous Glucose Monitoring Evidence

Table 20.2 summarizes six studies that have recently studied the relationship between CGM and diabetes therapy. Two studies specifically addressed the impact of food on glucose values. The other four studies focused on the use of CGM with insulin pump therapy. One of the studies was conducted in people with type 2 diabetes, whereas the other five studies were on patients with type 1 diabetes wearing an insulin pump.

In one of the food studies, four different meals and bolus-type pump settings on meals with various glycemic index values were compared. Ten people without diabetes served as controls. High–glycemic index meals resulted in higher postprandial glucose values regardless of the type of bolus insulin dose provided (O'Connell 2008). Another food study was done in people with type 2 diabetes who were on metformin (Powers 2010). The objective of the study was to define the 4-h glycemic response to two meals that differed only in the amount of carbohydrate; protein and fat content were similar, whereas carbohydrate was either 45 or 90 g. Although doubling the carbohydrate did not double any glycemic parameters, there were statistical differences in peak glucose, change from baseline glucose to peak, time to return to preprandial glucose, 4-h glucose area under the curve, and 4-h mean glucose. This study highlights the value of CGM in evaluating the glycemic response of food and the value of using fixed meals to study the glycemic response to food. The difference in time to peak glucose did not achieve significance between 45- and 90-g lunch meals (83.9 ± 18.5 vs. 103.2 ± 30.5 min; $P = 0.101$); yet it is important to note that, for both lunches, the peak averaged substantially earlier than the commonly recommended SMBG test 2 h postprandially.

Ten people with type 1 diabetes on insulin pumps for 4 weeks with CGM and 4 weeks without CGM were followed (Rigla 2008). Glucose values were more stable during the CGM phase, and A1C decreased more after the intervention phase of CGM, yet no changes were observed during the control phase. The Real Trend Study switched 115 children and adults from multiple daily insulin injections to an insulin pump with or without CGM. All had A1C levels of ≥8% (Rac-cah 2009). A1C levels improved in both groups, with no significant difference between the two. However, when the analysis included individuals in the CGM group who wore the CGM device ≥70% of the time, there was a significant differ-ence. This result indicates the value of using glucose data for decision-making and may indicate a timeframe for its impact. Both studies found that when CGM was used, more bolus insulin doses were given. Neither study identified the protocol for nutrition therapy. The studies did not determine whether insulin-to-carbohy-drate ratios were used or, if used, how they were determined or whether patients were taught to use insulin correction factors. Despite the knowledge and skills required to accurately implement carbohydrate counting and insulin-to-carbohy-drate ratios, there was no assessment of whether the study participants accurately implemented these therapies.

The STAR 3 study stated that all study participants received training in carbo-hydrate counting and insulin correction doses (Bergenstal 2010). The key findings of this study were similar to the Raccah study; the more individuals used the CGM device, the lower their A1C level. This study also provided data on who wore the device the most and who achieved the greatest decrease in A1C, since it included 329 adults and 156 children. The Chase study was an ancillary study to the Juvenile Diabetes Research Foundation (JDRF) trial previously included in the EAL (JDRF 2008). The results showed that, in 80 patients aged 8–17 years, individuals who used the CGM device ≥6 days had greater improvements in A1C than individuals who did not. However, only 44% used the device at this frequency at the end of the first 6 months and only 18% at the end of 12 months (Chase 2010).

SUMMARY

National and international organizations have published statements based on scientific evidence regarding glucose monitoring (American Association of Clini-cal Endocrinologists 2007; ADA 2012b; IDF 2009) and have consistently raised questions regarding its value in clinical care, how often it should be performed, and whether it is a wise investment that should be reimbursed. Yet, as demon-strated with the literature review, glucose monitoring is a critical component of diabetes care for two distinct reasons. First, glucose monitoring provides data on glucose response to a specific combination of food, medication, and activity, so that decisions regarding these three therapies can be better synchronized to improve overall glycemic control. Second, glucose monitoring provides data on glucose stability and variations, unlike A1C values, so that therapies can be adjusted sooner to improve these aspects, thus decreasing the risk of diabetes complications. However, as the research shows, the glucose data need to be used for decision-making; otherwise, the value in reducing A1C and complications is questionable. For the most part, studies examining the benefits of monitoring center around when, if, or how the data are used to modify or intensify medication therapy in achieving improved A1C levels. Few studies have examined how moni-toring data are used to make decisions regarding nutritional intake.

Kerr suggested that the lack of structure in the use of SMBG for type 2 diabetes patients raises the question of its value (Kerr 2011). The data need to be obtained in a structured approach; there is no value unless the glucose monitoring data captured

Table 20.1 Studies Evaluating the Relationship Between SMBG and Outcomes

	Population/ Duration of Study	Intervention (type of study)	Major Findings	Comments
Siebolds 2006	n = 223 adults with type 2 diabetes controlled with either diet or diet + oral medication/6 months	SMBG group (BGM device, BGM eating diary, counseling, algorithm used in weeks 0, 4, 12, and 20) vs. control group (no SMBG, nonstandardized counseling)/RCT	SMBG group: A1C ↓ 1.0% vs. ↓ 0.54% in control group (P = 0.0086)	SMBG coupled with structured counseling provided patients a tool for self-directed action and improved outlook
Poolsup 2009	n = 9 studies with 2,419 non–insulin-treated adults with type 2 diabetes/studies' duration ≥6 months	SMBG vs. non-SMBG RCT/meta-analysis	SMBG vs. non-SMBG: in all patients, difference in mean A1C –0.24% (P < 0.00001); in patients with A1C >8%, difference in mean A1C –0.27% (P < 0.0001); in patients with A1C >10%, mean difference in mean A1C –1.23% (P = 0.03); A1C ↓ in trials lasting 6 months but not at ≥12 months	Follow-up study to Poolsup 2008 systematic review
Duràn 2010	n = 161 newly diagnosed patients with type 2 diabetes/1 year	SMBG-based intervention (n = 99) vs. A1C-based control group (n = 62) (prospective randomized clinical trial)	SMBG vs. control: A1C <6%, 39 vs. 5% (P < 0.001); A1C between 6 and 6.4%, 37 vs. 30% (P < 0.01); lifestyle score >12, 38.4 vs. 9.7% (P > 0.001); ↓ in BMI for SMBG group, 29.6 → 27.9 kg/m² (P < 0.001)	SMBG-based education and medication recommendations empower patients to achieve nutrition and physical activity goals; nutrition score was evaluated with significant differences in dietary factors between groups
Polonsky 2011	Total n = 483 adults with type 2 diabetes, non–insulin-treated with A1C >7.5% (n = 227 in ACG; n = 256 in STG) in 34 primary care practices in the U.S./12 months	ACG (enhanced usual care including quarterly clinic visits focused on diabetes, free meters and strips, and office point-of-care A1C) vs. STG (enhanced usual care plus seven-point SMBG profile on 3 consecutive days) (cluster-randomized multicenter trial)	Mean reduction in A1C of –1.2% for STG vs. –0.9% for ACG (P < 0.004); STG vs. ACG: A1C ↓ 1.2 vs. 0.9% (P < 0.004); 179 (75%) STG vs. 61 (28%) ACG patients received treatment changes at 1-month visit (P < 0.0001)	Study aimed to eliminate some of the study design controversies of previous SMBG effectiveness studies

ACG, active control group; RCT, randomized controlled trial; STG, structured testing group.

Table 20.2 Studies Evaluating the Relationship Between CGM and Metabolic Outcomes

	Population/ Duration of Study	Intervention (type of study)	Major Findings	Comments
O'Connell 2008	n = 20 people with type 1 diabetes ages 8–18 years on insulin pumps and 10 control subjects without diabetes/ four meals	Compared four different meal and bolus-type pump settings on meals with varying glycemic index value (crossover study)	Dual-wave (50:50% over 2 h) before low-GI meals decreased PPG AUC up to 47% (P = 0.004) and lowered risk of hypoglycemia for same premeal glucose (P = 0.005) vs. standard bolus	High-GI meals resulted in higher PPG regardless of bolus type
Rigla 2008	n = 10 peple with type 1 diabetes on insulin pumps/14 weeks	CGM (4 weeks, 6 weeks wash-out) vs. control (4 weeks no CGM); DIABTel telemedicine system and CGM for 3 days/week during intervention (randomized crossover study)	A1C ↓ after CGM phase (8.1 vs. 7.3%, P = 0.007); no change during control phase; bolus dose ↑ per day (5.23 vs. 4.4., P < 0.05)	The Glycemic Risk Index (GRI) was used to quantify glucose variability.
Raccah 2009	n = 115 children and adults with type 1 diabetes on MDI switched to insulin pump, the Real Trend Study, A1C ≥8%/6 months	Pump therapy with or without CGM (with CGM required to wear pump 70% of time) (RCT)	A1C ↓ in both groups (CGM −0.81%, P < 0.001; without CGM −0.57%, P < 0.001); nonsignificant between groups; when adjusted for only those protocol compliant, significant difference between groups	CGM: more bolus and total insulin doses delivered; 20% made changes in eating habits and/or lifestyle (only 10% without CGM); 93% used CGM to adjust insulin doses and 60% used CGM to modify response to glycemic excursions
Bergenstal 2010	n = 443 people with type 1 diabetes (329 adults and 156 children), A1C 7.4–9.5%/1 year	Pump therapy with CGM vs. MDI and no CGM (RCT)	A1C: CGM pump group, 8.3% → 7.5%; MDI no CGM, 8.3% → 8.1% (P < 0.001); increased use of CGM resulted in lower A1C	All patients trained in intensive diabetes management including carbohydrate counting and insulin correction doses

	Population/ Duration of Study	Intervention (type of study)	Major Findings	Comments
Chase 2010	n = 80 patients aged 8–17 years with type 1 diabetes, A1C $\geq$7%, randomized to CGM as part of a larger study/6 months randomized and 6-month follow-up	Patients were randomized to SMBG alone or with 1 of 3 CGM systems (insulin-to-carbohydrate ratios used to dose and adjust mealtime insulin) (cohort study on patients using CGM)	17 who used CGM $\geq$6 days/week in month 12 had greater improvement in A1C than 63 who used CGM <6 days/week (mean change –0.8% vs. +0.1%, P < 0.0001); also reported greater satisfaction and low incidence of severe hypoglycemia	In first 6 months only, 44% used CGM for $\geq$6 days/week; this fell to 18% at 12 months; daily use was lower for ages 13–17 years than for 8–12 years
Powers 2010	n = 14 people with type 2 diabetes on metformin only/four meals followed for 4 h	45-g vs. 90-g carbohydrate meal 4-h glycemic response (crossover study)	Double the carbohydrate content did not double the glycemic response (210.6 vs. 190.6 mg/dL peak glucose, P = 0.028); change from baseline glucose to peak (80.7 vs. 60.6 mg/dL, P = 0.043); time to return to preprandial glucose (201 vs. 163 min, P = 0.021); 4-h glucose AUC (787.1 vs. 718.2 mg-4 h/dL, P = 0.036); 4-h mean glucose (164.3 vs. 147.9 mg/dL, P = 0.026)	CGM provides a description of the glycemic response to food/meals; data can be used to improve PPG by synchronization of food intake, diabetes medication, and/or physical activity

AUC, area under the curve; MDI, multiple daily insulin injections; PPG, postprandial glucose; RCT, randomized controlled trial.

is used in decision-making. Suggesting timing and frequency of monitoring to coincide with mealtimes, designated postprandial glucose peaks, activity, and medication are integral to nutrition therapy for diabetes. Health care providers can provide the structure necessary to maximize the value of glucose monitoring.

In practice, registered dietitians and health care providers currently use glucose values as feedback for nutrition therapy in the synchronization of food, activity, and medication. Used in this manner, monitoring serves as a behavior modification tool and is used to determine and reinforce nutrition therapy recommendations. Yet, we need more research that provides guidance on food combinations and timing of glucose tests to increase the ease of implementing nutrition therapy. The decision-making regarding food intake based on glucose monitoring results needs to be better researched, so it can be better described and understood.

BIBLIOGRAPHY

Academy of Nutrition and Dietetics: Type 1 and type 2 diabetes evidence-based nutrition practice guidelines for adults, 2008. Available from http://www.adaevidencelibrary.com/topic.cfm?cat=3252. Accessed June 2011

American Association of Clinical Endocrinologists: American Association of Clinical Endocrinologists medical guidelines for clinical practice for the management of diabetes mellitus. *Endocr Pract* 13 (Suppl. 1):1–68, 2007

American Diabetes Association: Consumer Product Guide. *Diabetes Forecast.* January, 2012a. Available from http://forecast.diabetes.org/magazine/features/2012-consumer-guide. Accessed February 2012

American Diabetes Association: Nutrition recommendations and interventions for diabetes (Position Statement). *Diabetes Care* 31 (Suppl. 1):S61–S78, 2008

American Diabetes Association: Standards of medical care in diabetes: 2012. *Diabetes Care* 35 (Suppl. 1):S11–S63, 2012b

Austin MM, Powers MA: Monitoring. In *The Art and Science of Diabetes Self-Management Education Desk Reference.* 2nd ed. Mensing C, Ed. Chicago, American Association of Diabetes Educators, 2010, p. 167–193

Bergenstal RM, Tamborlane WW, Ahmann A, Buse JB, Dailey G, Davis SN, Joyce C, People T, Perkins BA, Welsh JB, Willi SM, Wood MA; STAR 3 Study Group: Effectiveness of sensor-augmented insulin-pump therapy in type 1 diabetes. *N Engl J Med* 363:311–320, 2010

Cameron F, Baghurst P, Rodbard D: Assessing glycemic variation: why, when and how? *Pediatric Endocr Reviews* 7 (Suppl. 3):432–444, 2010

Ceriello A, Hanefeld M, Leiter L, Monnier L, Moses A, Owens D, Tajima N, Tuomilehto J, for the International Prandial Glucose Regulation Study Group: Postprandial glucose regulation and diabetic complications. *Arch Intern Med* 164:2090–2095, 2004

Chase P, Beck R, Dongyuan X, Tamborlane W, Coffey J, Fox L, Ives B, Keady J, Kollman C, Laffel L, Ruedy K: Continuous glucose monitoring in youth with type 1 diabetes: 12-month follow-up of the juvenile diabetes research foundation continuous glucose monitoring randomized trial. *Diabetes Technol Ther* 12:507–515, 2010

Diabetes Control and Complications Trial Research Group: The effect of intensive treatment of diabetes on the development and progression of long-term complications in insulin-dependent diabetes mellitus. *N Engl J Med* 329:683–689, 1993

Durán A, Martin P, Runkle I, Pérez N, Abad R, Fernández M, Del Valle L, Sanz MF, Calle-Pascual AL: Benefits of self-monitoring blood glucose in the management of new-onset type 2 diabetes mellitus: the St Carlos Study, a prospective randomized clinic-based interventional study with parallel groups. *J Diabetes* 2:203–211, 2010

Franz MJ, Powers MA, Leontos C, Holzmeister LA, Kulkarni K, Monk A, Wedel N, Gradwell E: The evidence for medical nutrition therapy for type 1 and type 2 diabetes in adults. *J Am Diet Assoc* 110:1852–1889, 2010

Hirsch I, Bode B, Childs B, Close K, Fisher W, Gavin J, Ginsberg B, Raine C, Verderese C: Self-monitoring of blood glucose (SMBG) in insulin-and non-insulin-using adults with diabetes: consensus recommendations for improving SMBG accuracy, utilization, and research. *Diabetes Technol Ther* 10:419–439, 2008

International Diabetes Federation: Clinical Guidelines Taskforce and SMBG International Working Group: Guideline on self-monitoring of blood glucose in non-insulin treated type 2 diabetes, 2009, p. 1–44. Available at http://www.idf.org/guidelines/self-monitoring

JDRF CGM Study Group: JDRF randomized clinical trial to assess the efficacy of real-time continuous glucose monitoring in the management of type 1 diabetes: research design and methods. *Diabetes Technol Ther* 10:310–321, 2008

Kerr D: Self-monitoring of blood glucose and type 2 diabetes: new tricks for the old dog? *J Diabetes Sci Technol* 5:209–211, 2011

Klonoff D, Bergenstal R, Blonde L, Boren SA, Church T, Gafaney J, Jovanovic L, Kendall D, Kollman C, Kovatchev B, Leippert C, Diabetesberaterin DDG, Owens D, Polonsky W, Reach G, Renard E, Riddell M, Rubin R, Schnell O, Siminiero L, Vigersky RE, Wilson D, Wollitzer A: Consensus report of the coalition of clinical research: self-monitoring of blood glucose. *J Diabetes Sci Technol* 2:1030–1053, 2008

Mazze RS, Strock E, Wesley D, Borgman S, Morgan B, Bergenstal R, Cuddihy R: Characterizing glucose exposure for individuals with normal glucose tolerance using continuous glucose monitoring and ambulatory glucose profile analysis. *Diabetes Technol Ther* 10:149–160, 2008

Monnier L, Lapinski H, Colette C: Contributions of fasting and postprandial plasma glucose increments to the overall diurnal hyperglycemia of type 2 diabetic patients. *Diabetes Care* 26:3:881–885, 2003

O'Connell M, Donath S, Gilbertson H, Cameron F: Optimizing postprandial glycemia in pediatric patients with type 1 diabetes using insulin pump therapy. *Diabetes Care* 31:1491–1495, 2008

Polonsky WH, Fisher L, Schikman CH, Hinnen DA, Parkin CG, Jelsovsky Z, Petersen B, Schweitzer M, Wagner R: Structured self-monitoring of blood glucose significantly reduces A1C levels in poorly controlled, noninsulin-treated type 2 diabetes. *Diabetes Care* 34:262–267, 2011

Poolsup N, Suksomboon N, Jiamsathit W: Systematic review of the benefits of self-monitoring of blood glucose on glycemic control in type 2 diabetes patients. *Diabetes Technol Ther* 10 (Suppl. 1):S51–S65, 2008

Poolsup N, Suksomboon N, Rattanasookchit S: Meta-analysis of the benefits of self-monitoring of blood glucose on glycemic control in type 2 diabetes patients: an update. *Diabetes Technol Ther* 11:775–784, 2009

Powers MA, Cuddihy R, Wesley D, Morgan B: Continuous glucose monitoring reveals different glycemic responses of moderate-vs-high-carbohydrate lunch meals in people with type 2 diabetes. *J Am Diet Assoc* 110:1912–1915, 2010

Raccah D, Sulmont V, Reznik Y, Guerci B, Renard E, Hanaire H, Jeandidier N, Nicolino M: Incremental value of continuous glucose monitoring when starting pump therapy in patients with poorly controlled type 1 diabetes (The RealTrend Study). *Diabetes Care* 32:2245–2250, 2009

Rigla M, Hernando E, Gomez E, Brugues E, Garcia-Saez G, Capel I, Pons B, DeLeiva A: Real-time continuous glucose monitoring together with telemedical assistance improves glycemic control and glucose stability in pump-treated patients. *Diabetes Techol Ther* 10:194–199, 2008

Siebolds M, Gaedeke O, Schwedes U; SMBG Study Group: Self-monitoring of blood glucose: psychological aspects relevant to the changes in HbA1c in type 2 diabetic patients treated with diet or diet plus oral antidiabetic medication. *Patient Educ Couns* 62:104–110, 2006

St. John A, Davis WA, Price CP, Davis TM: The value of self-monitoring of blood glucose: a review of recent evidence. *J Diabetes Complications* 24:129–141, 2010

Towfigh A, Romanova M, Weinreb J, Munjas B, Suttorp M, Zhou A, Shekelle P: Self-monitoring of blood glucose levels in patients with type 2 diabetes mellitus not taking insulin: a meta-analysis. *Am J Manag Care* 14:468–475, 2008

Margaret A. Powers, PhD, RD, CDE, is a Research Scientist, International Diabetes Center at Park Nicollet, Minneapolis, MN. Mary M. Austin, MA, RD, CDE, FAADE, is a Registered Dietitian and Diabetes Educator and Owner of The Austin Group, LLC, Shelby Township, MI.

Chapter 21

Integrating Nutrition Therapy into Insulin Pump Therapy

ALISON B. EVERT, MS, RD, CDE

Highlights
Integrating Nutrition Therapy into Insulin Pump Therapy

■ Use of continuous subcutaneous insulin infusion (CSII) is growing worldwide.

■ A method of accurately estimating the carbohydrate content of meals and snacks (carbohydrate counting) is a prerequisite for successfully determining the bolus insulin requirement for individuals using CSII.

■ The bolus calculator feature on insulin pumps has been shown to effectively reduce postprandial blood glucose levels.

■ "Active insulin" or "insulin on board" from a previous bolus should be taken into consideration when determining the subsequent bolus dose, to prevent "stacking" of correction insulin boluses.

■ Missed boluses can contribute to postprandial hyperglycemia and may result in suboptimal glycemic control.

■ Use of carbohydrate ranges versus precise carbohydrate (gram) counting for determining prandial bolus doses can result in satisfactory postprandial glycemic control.

■ A few small studies suggest that the use of a combination (dual-wave) bolus feature for prandial bolus infusion may provide better insulin coverage for high-fat, high-protein, and/or high-fiber meals and help reduce postprandial hyperglycemia.

■ Use of a novel fat-protein bolus algorithm in addition to a traditional carbohydrate bolus algorithm may result in more desirable postprandial blood glucose levels.

Integrating Nutrition Therapy into Insulin Pump Therapy

For individuals with type 1 diabetes and a growing number of people with insulin-requiring type 2 diabetes, intensive glucose control can be achieved through use of continuous subcutaneous insulin infusion (CSII) via an insulin pump. Several clinical trials have demonstrated that both youth and adults with type 1 diabetes can use CSII to achieve better glycemic control (Pickup 2008; Doyle 2004).

The use of CSII has been gaining popularity since the late 1970s. The industry estimates that there are over 300,000 people using insulin pumps in the U.S. (Schneiner 2009). Over the last several years, insulin pump manufacturers have developed new features that can enable the person with diabetes to obtain more optimal glycemic control. A meta-analysis concluded that the use of CSII compared to multiple daily injections (MDI) delivery was associated with significantly lower rates of severe hypoglycemia (Pickup 2008). Research has also been conducted to determine the impact of insulin pump therapy on quality of life. A recent meta-analysis in pediatric subjects revealed a significantly higher level of satisfaction with CSII treatment over MDI (Pańkowska 2009a). Few studies to date have been conducted in subjects with type 2 diabetes and CSII (Raskin 2003; Bode 2010).

Individuals with type 1 diabetes or insulin-requiring type 2 diabetes of Medicare age can obtain coverage for CSII if they meet specific criteria. Some individuals with profound insulin resistance may use U-500 insulin in their pumps rather than rapid-acting insulin analogs (Lane 2009). These topics will not be discussed in this chapter.

This chapter will summarize the limited nutrition-related insulin pump recommendations. In the absence of American Diabetes Association (ADA) nutrition therapy recommendations for adult insulin pump use, the nutrition recommendations from the ADA consensus statement on the use of insulin pump therapy in the pediatric age-group will be provided (ADA 2007). The bolus calculator feature that is used to determine prandial and correction of insulin doses (or boluses) is discussed, followed by a description of the small number of studies conducted regarding use of carbohydrate ranges to estimate the prandial bolus dose and how missed prandial boluses contribute to suboptimal glycemic control. The limited research is summarized on the use of bolus calculators/tools and dual-wave bolus features for prandial insulin delivery to reduce postprandial glycemic excursions when higher-fat, -protein, and/or -fiber meals are consumed. Use of these features is optional and it is important to determine if they are associated with better glycemic control (Cukierman-Yaffe 2011).

TRANSLATION OF EVIDENCE INTO NUTRITION RECOMMENDATIONS

There are few specific references regarding the integration of nutrition therapy and insulin pump therapy by the ADA. As reviewed in previous chapters, the recommended therapy for type 1 diabetes is intensive insulin therapy, using basal and bolus insulin to reproduce or mimic normal physiological insulin secretion. This step involves use of multiple-dose insulin injections (three to four injections per day of basal and prandial insulin) or insulin pump therapy and matching of prandial insulin to carbohydrate intake, premeal blood glucose levels, and anticipated activity (ADA 2012). Monitoring carbohydrate, whether by carbohydrate counting, choices, or experience-based estimation, remains a key strategy in achieving glycemic control (ADA 2008). For individuals who adjust mealtime (prandial) insulin or who are on CSII, it is optimal to adjust insulin doses to carbohydrate intake (insulin-to-carbohydrate ratios). Comprehensive nutrition education and counseling should be provided that includes instruction on interpretation of blood glucose monitoring patterns and nutrition-related medication management (Academy of Nutrition and Dietetics 2008; Franz 2010).

A consensus statement titled the "Use of Insulin Pump Therapy in the Pediatric Age-Group" was published by the ADA (ADA 2007). Although there is no section in the statement that specifically addresses nutrition therapy, recommendations can be found throughout the document. The authors state, "the child and caregivers should be educated on the following concepts: nutrition therapy including carbohydrate counting/estimation and prandial boluses are dependent on carbohydrate intake as well as circadian variation in insulin sensitivity, current blood glucose levels, and planned physical activity."

A method of accurately estimating the carbohydrate content of meals and snacks (carbohydrate counting) is a prerequisite for successfully determining the bolus insulin requirement (Waldron 2002). A discussion about the calculation and timing of prandial (bolus) insulin requirements includes the following:

1. Patients with CSII must have a method to calculate the appropriate insulin dose.
   a. Various algorithms exist that assist in calculating insulin-to-carbohydrate ratios.
   b. Receiving more than seven daily boluses has been associated with significantly lower A1C levels (Danne 2005).
   c. A dual-wave bolus may be beneficial when eating foods that are gradually absorbed, such as pizza, beans, and meals with high fat content (Chase 2002).
2. Prandial bolus should be designed to preserve the physiological variation in blood glucose, e.g., blood glucose ~30–40 mg/dL higher 2 h after a meal and returning to preprandial level by 4 h after a meal.
3. In children or fussy eaters, parents may prefer to administer the bolus after the meal to choose an insulin dose that is appropriate for the amount of food actually eaten (Rutledge 1997). However, if postprandial insulin doses are frequently forgotten, administration of bolus after the meal should not be encouraged (Burdick 2004).

4. The amount of insulin per gram of carbohydrate is usually the highest in the morning (breakfast).

Another section addresses calculation of the correction dose. The correction insulin dose depends on the individually prescribed insulin sensitivity or blood glucose correction factor as well as the blood glucose target. Similar to the insulin-to-carbohydrate ratio, the insulin sensitivity factor is determined by a variety of different methods or formulae. An important component of bolus insulin administration is the "insulin on board" and the bolus calculator features (Glaser 2004; Hirsch 2010). Key nutrition recommendations in this section include the following:

1. "Active insulin" or "insulin on board" from a previous bolus should be taken into consideration when determining the subsequent bolus dose to prevent "stacking" of correction insulin boluses.
   a. The duration of action of large boluses is generally longer than small doses of insulin.
   b. If the pump does not have an "insulin on board" function, a second correction dose should not be given within 2 h of the first.

The monitoring section states that nutrition therapy recommendations should be reviewed as part of regularly scheduled outpatient visits to optimize use of CSII—evaluation of insulin-to-carbohydrate ratios, correction dose, and target blood glucose levels; average number of boluses per day (to assess for missed boluses); appropriateness of the total grams of carbohydrate entered into the bolus calculator for the child's age; weight gain; average (7 days) total daily insulin dose compared to body weight; glycemic control (blood glucose values including postprandial and overnight); and basal-to-bolus ratio (ADA 2007).

CURRENT PERSPECTIVES

Key Feature of Insulin Pumps: Bolus Calculators

One of the major problems associated with CSII use is accurately determining the insulin boluses (Pickup 2002). To optimize glycemic control, bolus insulin doses must take into account multiple factors, such as target blood glucose, current blood glucose, individualized insulin-to-carbohydrate ratios and insulin sensitivity factor, determination of grams of carbohydrate consumed in a meal or snack, and active insulin. Unfortunately, many patients often neglect these factors and rely on empirical estimations (Klupa 2008). To simplify calculation of prandial bolus doses, insulin pumps now include bolus calculators that can be preprogrammed with individualized settings. The diabetes care provider works with the individual pump user to determine the bolus calculator settings. (See Chapter 5 for methods of prandial insulin dosing.)

One of the features in the bolus calculator is the "active insulin" or "insulin on board" feature. Insulin analogs are typically prescribed for use in insulin pumps. The insulin action times of the currently available rapid-acting insulin analogs are in general onset at 5–15 min, a peak between 30 and 90 min, and duration of ~4–6 h (Hirsch 2005). The main activity of the insulin analog occurs during the first 3 h after the injection, followed by a prolonged tail of decreasing effect (ADA 2007). Based on the needs of the individual patient, the diabetes care provider can set the "insulin on board" duration to a variable length. Most patients use a time somewhere between 3 and 6 h. Currently, there are no published studies on the appropriate duration for the active insulin time. Individuals seeking tight control may prefer a shorter duration of action, whereas subjects concerned about hypoglycemia may prefer a longer duration of insulin action (ADA 2007). Unfortunately, each pump manufacturer uses a slightly different calculation for active insulin. Individuals using this feature to quickly perform complex mathematical equations should be well educated on the functionality of their particular bolus calculator to reduce the risk of hypo- or hyperglycemia (Zisser 2008). In clinical practice, the bolus calculator has been the most important advancement in CSII therapy in the past decade (Hirsch 2010). Future areas of research should include investigation of the calculation of bolus insulin doses with glucose sensor–augmented insulin pumps.

To use the bolus calculator, a premeal blood glucose level (some blood glucose meters can wirelessly transmit these data to the pump) is inputted along with the amount of carbohydrate (in grams or exchanges) to be eaten. Using these two values, in addition to the "insulin on board" information, the bolus calculator in the pump calculates a recommended dose (Hirsch 2010). Manual dose calculations do not take into account the effect of the active insulin that remains from a previous bolus (insulin on board). Currently available insulin pumps cannot compute insulin doses for physical activity. Based on factors such as planned sessions of physical activity or periods of sedentary activity occurring soon after eating, the individual wearing the pump must decrease or increase the recommended dose.

Use of different bolus calculators effectively controls postprandial blood glucose levels. A 3-month randomized crossover study in 49 subjects with type 1 diabetes who counted carbohydrate grams and delivered appropriate premeal insulin doses reported that using a handheld bolus calculator was more effective in controlling postprandial blood glucose than determining a dose based on standard bolus (their current insulin dosing method) (Gross 2003). Additionally, during the standard bolus period, more correction boluses were administered to reduce postprandial hyperglycemia, and more supplemental carbohydrate was consumed to treat low blood glucose levels.

A small study ($n = 18$) was conducted to assess the metabolic control in young, active professionals with type 1 diabetes treated with CSII with or without the use of a bolus calculator (Klupa 2008). All the subjects were trained in food-counting (including carbohydrate, protein, and fat content counting and carbohydrate glycemic index [GI] estimation) and were using insulin analogs. Mean A1C and fasting blood glucose levels were not significantly different between the two groups, but mean postprandial blood glucose was significantly lower in the bolus calculator group.

A prospective crossover clinical trial was conducted in pediatric subjects with type 1 diabetes ($n = 36$, mean age 13.9 years) who used CSII and carbohydrate counting to assess the efficacy in pre- and postprandial glycemic control and the impact of treatment satisfaction of a bolus calculator incorporated into an insulin pump (Shashaj 2008). In study periods lasting 2 weeks, subjects in phase A used a bolus calculator or in phase B used their current conventional insulin-dosing method to determine premeal boluses. A questionnaire assessing treatment satisfaction with the bolus calculator was also completed. During phase A, subjects had significant reductions in blood glucose levels before and 2 h after meals and required fewer correction boluses, without modifying prandial insulin requirements and without restricting carbohydrate intake, compared to phase B. Estimation of the prandial bolus was more precise and accurate using the bolus calculator and resulted in a reduction of postprandial hyperglycemia. In addition, use of the bolus calculator was easy and associated with a high level of treatment satisfaction in these participants.

A randomized clinical trial demonstrated that subjects who used a diabetes interactive diary (a tool incorporating a bolus calculator) and subjects who were provided carbohydrate-counting education had similar reductions in A1C levels (Rossi 2010). However, participants using a diabetes interactive diary experienced greater improvements in diabetes treatment satisfaction and in some aspects of health-related quality of life.

Use of Carbohydrate Ranges to Estimate Bolus Insulin Dose

Effective integration of CSII into diabetes self-care is based on three components: 1) self-monitoring of blood glucose (SMBG), 2) determination of food (carbohydrate) intake, and 3) bolus insulin administration. A study investigated how precise carbohydrate quantification needs to be to maintain postprandial glycemic control (Smart 2009). The study found that in 31 youth, using either CSII or MDI, an individually calculated insulin dose for 60 g carbohydrate maintained postprandial blood glucose levels for meals containing between 50 and 70 g carbohydrate. They concluded that a single mealtime insulin dose would cover a range of carbohydrate amounts without deterioration in postprandial glycemic control. However, other researchers reported that youth (ages 4–12 years, 70% using CSII/30% insulin injections) or their caregivers estimated carbohydrate content of meals accurately and precisely and achieved better glycemic control (Mehra 2009).

In another study, human error factor in food (carbohydrate) counting in eight different meals of known carbohydrate value was assessed in 60 subjects, between 18 and 60 years of age (Shapira 2010). They proposed that use of a "bolus guide," based on carbohydrate range selection, might have advantages over a bolus calculator in terms of ease of use and therefore could lead to higher treatment satisfaction and adherence and ultimately improved glycemic control. Carbohydrate estimation accuracy using the bolus calculator or the bolus guide, an alternative system based on ranges of carbohydrate load, was compared using simulated outcome blood glucose (OBG). The estimated error distribution (coefficient of variation [CV]) was the basis for the computer simulation ($n = 1.6$ million observations) of insulin recommendations for the bolus calculator and bolus guide, translated in OBG ranges (≤60, 61–200, and >200 mg/dL). Thirty of the participants completed questionnaires to assess their treatment satisfaction with the bolus guide. Mean percentage error tended to get larger with increasing carbohydrate load, and the CV of the estimated carbohydrate for all meals ranged from 28 to 46%. The percentages of simulated OBG for the bolus calculator and the bolus guide in the <60 mg/dL range were 21 and 17%, respectively, and 14 and 16%, respectively, in the >200 mg/dL range. In terms of bolus guide treatment satisfaction and ease of learning, the mean and medium scores were 4.17 and 4.2, respectively (out of 5). The researchers concluded that the bolus guide recommendations based on carbohydrate range selection are similar to the bolus calculator based on carbohydrate gram estimation.

Missed Boluses: Impact on Glycemic Control

Two studies were conducted to investigate the relationship between insulin omission and metabolic control in pediatric populations with type 1 diabetes. In one study (n = 48), children and adolescents (mean age 15.3 years) using CSII therapy and glucose meters for ≥6 months with data that could be downloaded from their insulin pumps participated in a cross-sectional study (Burdick 2004). All of the participants received pump training and instruction on carbohydrate counting for estimation of prandial insulin boluses and completed a questionnaire about reasons for suboptimal glycemic control. During the study visit, subjects were questioned about their prandial bolus habits to identify possible reasons for suboptimal control, they were asked about frequency of blood glucose monitoring, and their pumps were downloaded. Their physicians estimated boluses missed from the 4 weeks preceding the study visit. The download data and participant questionnaires revealed that a major cause of suboptimal glycemic control was missed meal boluses. Participants who missed <1 bolus per week had a mean A1C of 8.0%, whereas participants who missed ≥1 bolus per week had a mean A1C of 8.8%. Significant correlations were found between number of missed mealtime boluses per week and mean blood glucose levels and A1C levels.

Another cross-sectional study investigated the management in adolescents with type 1 diabetes (n = 90, mean age 14.8 years) using CSII >6 months, including their administration of prandial bolus doses (Lindholm-Olinder 2009a). Also evaluated were relationships between metabolic control and insulin omission, BMI, daily frequency of bolus doses and SMBG, health-related quality of life, treatment satisfaction, and the burden of diabetes. All patients had received pump training and were educated about the importance of taking a bolus when they ate a meal or snack. Researchers found that 38% of subjects had missed >15% of the doses the previous day; these patients had higher A1C levels (7.8 vs. 7.0%, P = 0.001), took fewer daily boluses (3.8 vs. 5.3, P < 0.001) and did less SMBG (2.4 vs. 3.6, P = 0.003), were less satisfied with treatment (4.8 vs. 5.3, scale 0–6, P = 0.029), and perceived the medical treatment more negatively (72.1 vs. 79.7, scale 0–100, P = 0.029). It was concluded that omission of bolus insulin was common, and frequencies of daily SMBG and boluses were associated with glycemic control. The subjects who missed boluses were also less satisfied and perceived more impact with the treatment. It was suggested that diabetes care providers need to assist youth using CSII to develop creative strategies to reduce missed boluses. In youth treated with CSII, it is easy to determine if insulin omission is occurring by reviewing download data reports from the pump memory, whereas with youth using MDI, this is not possible.

EVIDENCE FOR USE OF VARIABLE BOLUS FEATURES TO DELIVER A PRANDIAL DOSE

Bolus calculators can be valuable tools to determine prandial boluses and optimize glycemic control. However, the effectiveness of the bolus calculator depends on precise determination of the individual's bolus calculator settings, including the insulin-to-carbohydrate ratios, insulin sensitivity factors, individualized blood glucose targets, and active insulin time. It is recommended that the accuracy of these insulin-dosing algorithms and settings should be evaluated *after* the basal rates have been confirmed. Unfortunately, in clinical practice, both basal and bolus settings are often not evaluated. The effectiveness of the bolus calculator also depends on the knowledge and skill level of the pump user to input the grams of carbohydrate to be consumed by "counting carbohydrates" or some other method of carbohydrate estimation. Despite all of these attempts to accurately "match" the prandial insulin dose to the carbohydrate intake, many individuals continue to experience postprandial hyperglycemia.

The mismatch between the prandial bolus dose and carbohydrate intake is often attributed to the protein, fat, and/or fiber content or the GI of the meal. The postprandial glucose excursion after these types of meals has not been well studied; therefore, it is difficult to make recommendations for optimal dosing of prandial insulin for these nutrients or food components. Previous research in patients with type 1 diabetes using basal-bolus insulin regimens reported that the prandial bolus insulin doses should be based on the carbohydrate content of the meal and that the GI, fiber, fat, and caloric content of the meals did not affect premeal insulin requirements (Rabasa-Lhoret 1999). However, the protein and fat content of the meals in the study was kept constant, and the insulin needed for their metabolism was likely from the basal insulin doses. In clinical practice, based on information from glucose meters and continuous glucose monitoring (CGM) data reports, meals with larger and varying amounts of protein and fat are often found to prolong the postprandial glucose excursion up to several hours. This result suggests that these factors may delay the absorption of glucose or that additional prandial insulin may be required to cover the additional protein and fat, which are not typically accounted for in the traditional prandial bolus calculations (Pańkowska 2010).

Pump manufacturers have developed variable bolus features for insulin pumps in an attempt to match circulating insulin levels to the rate of glucose absorption from the gut to minimize postprandial blood glucose excursions (Heinemann 2009). Depending on the composition of the meal or snack, a bolus can be administered in three different ways: *1)* infusion of the total bolus all at once (or "normal" bolus [NL]), *2)* infusion of the entire bolus in an "extended" fashion (or "square-wave" bolus [SW]) over a few minutes to several hours, or *3)* infusion of part of the bolus all at once and part of the bolus over a few minutes to several hours (or "dual-wave" bolus [DW]).

Heinemann published an excellent critical evaluation of clinical experimental studies conducted from 2002 to 2009 (Heinemann 2009). The article evaluates the effectiveness of the different types of boluses on postprandial glycemic control as well as fundamental shortcomings in study design and performance.

For this chapter, a literature search was conducted using PubMed MEDLINE to locate research on the use of dual-wave boluses to reduce postprandial blood glucose excursions. Additional articles were identified from reference lists. Search criteria included research studies using continuous sustained insulin pump infusion/CSII, insulin pump, prandial insulin, bolus, dual-wave bolus, carbohydrate counting, nutrition therapy, and English language articles published after 1999.

The PubMed search produced 11 articles, and an additional two articles and one abstract were identified from reference lists. Of these, six were excluded because titles or abstracts did not meet inclusion criteria. Eight articles met inclusion criteria and were retrieved for more detailed evaluation.

Table 21.1 summarizes the studies reporting on use of insulin pump variable bolus features to deliver prandial insulin in adults and youth with type 1 diabetes and the effects on postprandial glycemia. The eight studies in the table explore the use of DW, SW, and NL bolus administration in conjunction with meals of varying composition. Many of the studies used CGM devices in addition to blood glucose monitoring to evaluate glycemic control.

Heinemann suggests that performance of meal-related research studies requires careful attention to several factors to allow meaningful evaluation of a given intervention (type of prandial bolus infusion) (Heinemann 2009). Key limitations of the current studies are the insufficient establishment of comparable premeal blood glucose levels and insulinemia on different study days with and between patients. In addition, a majority of the studies had a small sample size; four studies investigated youth with type 1 diabetes and four were conducted in adults. Only one study evaluated C-peptide levels of the participants before enrollment (Lindholm-Olinder 2009b). Confirmation of basal rate settings before investigations occurred in only two studies (Jones 2005; O'Connell 2008). One of the studies appeared to use regular insulin (Lee 2004), and two studies did not specify type of insulin (Pańkowska 2009b; Pańkowska 2012), whereas all of the remaining studies used rapid-acting analogs.

One small study evaluated the effect of different insulin bolus delivery methods with two different GI pasta meals, low (GI 34) versus high (GI 76) on 3-h postprandial blood glucose excursions (O'Connell 2008). The researchers found the DW bolus before the low-GI meal reduced postprandial glucose area under the curve by up to 47% when compared with an NL bolus.

Three small studies used pizza meals (>36% fat) to evaluate the use of a DW bolus versus an NL bolus feature to reduce the postprandial excursion (Chase 2002; Lee 2004; Jones 2005). The study conducted by Lee revealed similar 3-h postprandial glucose values using either the NL or DW bolus; however, the use of the NL bolus for the high-fat meal resulted in significantly elevated postprandial glucose 5–14 h after the bolus insulin administration. Chase reported that postprandial glucose excursions were the lowest at 90–120 min when the DW bolus was administered 70% as an NL bolus and 30% as an SW bolus over 2 h. The pizza study by Jones showed that a DW bolus (50% NL/50% SW) administered over 8 h resulted in the best glycemic control and the lowest mean glucose.

Another study reported that after a higher-fat pasta meal (>36% fat), there were no significant differences in plasma glucose levels at any time point. However, they did find that the insulin administration by only an SW bolus may be less favorable with a less fatty meal (Lindholm-Olinder 2009b).

The effectiveness of DW bolus use after switching from multiple daily injections to CSII and glycemic control was evaluated, with the authors concluding that the DW bolus might be a tool to potentially improve glycemic control in patients with type 1 diabetes (Klupa 2011). In particular, male subjects with shorter duration of diabetes seem more willing to use DW boluses.

Table 21.1 Studies Reporting on the Use of Insulin Pump Variable Bolus Features to Deliver Prandial Insulin in Adults and Youth with Type 1 Diabetes and Effects on Postprandial Glycemia

	Population/ Duration of Study	Intervention (type of study)	Major Findings	Comments
Chase 2002	$n = 9$ youth and young adults with type 1 diabetes (A1C <9%, CSII therapy >1 year)/4 weeks	Four insulin bolus deliveries on PP BG: 1) 100% insulin as NL bolus 10 min before meal; 2) 50% insulin as NL bolus 10 min before meal + 50% insulin as NL bolus 90 min later; 3) 100% bolus as SW 10 min before meal and continuing over 2 h; 4) 70% insulin as NL bolus 10 min before meal and 30% insulin delivered over 2 h as SW; pizza meal (11% protein/53% CHO/36% fat/829 kcal); FBG before study 60–200 mg/dL; BG was measured at –60 and –30 min and at 0 time and every 30 min for 6 h (randomized crossover clinical study)	After test meal, PP BG lowest at 90 min and 120 min using DW bolus; continued delivery of insulin over 2 h (DW and SW) resulted in significantly ↓ BG after 4 h in comparison with single or double NL bolus; incidence of hypoglycemia similar for all four bolus delivery methods	Gastric emptying more rapid with ↓ BG (60–200 mg/dL) before a meal and slower when premeal BG >200 mg/dL and when meal is higher in fat; lispro insulin used in study
Lee 2004	$n = 10$ adults with type 1 diabetes (average duration of diabetes 18 years)/3 days using CSII + CGM	Three combinations of evening meals and insulin bolus on PP glycemic excursions: 1) control meal with NL bolus (two bean burritos: 14% protein/62% CHO/24% fat) 100% bolus delivered ~3 min before meal; 2) high-fat meal with NL bolus (1/3 medium pizza + extra cheese: 20% protein/26% CHO/54% fat) 100% bolus delivered ~3 min before meal; 3) high-fat meal with DW bolus (pizza: same as above) 70% insulin bolus delivered as NL bolus ~3 min before meal and 30% via SW continuing over 5 h (crossover clinical study)	Baseline CGM values similar in three combinations of meal and bolus types ($P = 0.54$) and 3 h after meal ($P = 0.64, P = 0.83, P = 1.0$) when compared to control meal/NL bolus and high-fat meal/DW bolus combinations; PP glucose elevated in hours 5–14 ($P < 0.05$) after high-fat/NL bolus combination insulin delivery	Glucose levels during study measured with CGM not with laboratory system; regular insulin may have been used in the study

Table 21.1 Studies Reporting on the Use of Insulin Pump Variable Bolus Features to Deliver Prandial Insulin in Adults and Youth with Type 1 Diabetes and Effects on Postprandial Glycemia (*continued*)

	Population/ Duration of Study	Intervention (type of study)	Major Findings	Comments
Jones 2005	n = 24 adults with type 1 diabetes (average duration diabetes 21 years)/3 consecutive days using CSII + CGM	Three insulin bolus deliveries for an evening pizza meal (2–3 slices; 1 slice: 15 g protein/30 g CHO/14 g fat) on PP glycemic excursions: 1) NL bolus; 2) 4-h DW bolus (50% delivered with NL bolus/50% delivered over 4 h with SW); 3) 8-h DW bolus (50% delivered with NL bolus/50% delivered over 8 h with SW) (crossover clinical study)	8-h DW bolus provided best glycemic control and lowest mean BG (NL bolus, 133 mg/dL; 4-h DW, 145 mg/dL; 8-h DW, 104 mg/dL); divergence between glucose profiles occurred at 4–12 h after the meal and was greatest at 8–12 h	Preprandial BG or incidence of hypoglycemia not reported; lispro insulin used in study; basal rates confirmed from evening meal to 6:00 a.m., 6 months before study
O'Connell 2008	n = 20 youth with type 1 diabetes (A1C ≤8.5%, CSII therapy >1 year); n = 10 control subjects without diabetes/4 different days using CSII + CGM	Two insulin bolus deliveries (NL bolus vs. DW bolus [50%/50% over 2 h] in combination with two different GI meals [low 34 vs. high 76] on 3-h PP BG excursions on 4 days in randomized order; meals had equal macronutrient, kilocalories, and fiber and differed only in GI (randomized crossover clinical study)	DW bolus before low-GI meals ↓ PP BG AUC by up to 47% (P = 0.004) and ↓ risk of hypoglycemia for same premeal glucose (P = 0.005) vs. NL bolus; high-GI meal resulted in significant upward PP BG with greater AUC (P = 0.45) regardless of bolus type	Fasting subjects ate standardized breakfast, test meal at lunchtime; 2 weeks before study, basal and bolus calculator rates were optimized; bolus (aspart insulin) given immediately before meal

	Population/ Duration of Study	Intervention (type of study)	Major Findings	Comments
Lindholm-Olinder 2009b	*n* = 15 youth with type 1 diabetes (females; average duration of diabetes 6.5 years; A1C <9%); *n* = 10 youth without diabetes control subjects/6 different days using CSII + CGM	Three insulin bolus deliveries on PP BG after two pasta meals eaten at lunch with different amounts of fat (16% protein/54% CHO/30% fat/512 kcal/GI 38 vs. 14% protein/50% CHO/36% fat/541 kcal/GI 39): *1)* 100% insulin delivered as NL bolus before meal; *2)* 60% insulin delivered as NL bolus before meal + 40% delivered over 60 min; *3)* 100% bolus delivered as SW bolus over 2 h; BG measured over 30 min from 90 min before meal until 3 h after meal (crossover clinical study)	No differences in time to reach BG peak or AUC between different bolus deliveries for two pasta meals; SW bolus may be less favorable with a less fatty meal, giving higher glucose increase, from start to 60 min (83 vs. 50 mg/dL for NL bolus and 34 mg/dL for DW bolus, *P* = 0.018); after higher-fat meal, there were no differences in BG at any time point	Insulin used in study: aspart, *n* = 5, lispro, *n* = 10
Pańkowska 2009b	*n* = 499 children and adolescents with type 1 diabetes (246 females/253 males; average duration of diabetes 4 years; A1C 7.4%; daily insulin requirement 0.74 units; proportion basal insulin 32%)/2 weeks	Use of DW or SW boluses on metabolic control; boluses calculated using CHO (10 g CHO = 1 unit CHO) units for NL bolus and use of fat-protein units for SW bolus (100 kcal fat and/or protein = 1 FPU) multiplied by insulin ratios (dose of insulin that covers 10 g CHO product or 100 kcal from fat/protein products); high-fat foods result in delivering SW bolus over a longer time: 1 FPU = 3 h; 2 FPU = 4 h; 3 FPU = 5 h; >3 FPU = 8 h (cross-sectional clinical study)	Number of DW/SW boluses: 16.6/14 days (range 0–95), 18.8% of patients did not use variable bolus features; lowest A1C in group using 2 or more DW/SW boluses/day (*P* = 0.001) vs. the group using 1 or fewer DW/SW boluses/day; patients with <7.5% A1C had higher DW/SW boluses, 19.55 vs. 12.42 (*P* < 0.001)	Uncontrolled evaluation of the data collected in outpatient clinic setting during routine office visits; patients were able to apply use of DW/SW boluses in the daily self-treatment process based on food counting

Table 21.1 Studies Reporting on the Use of Insulin Pump Variable Bolus Features to Deliver Prandial Insulin in Adults and Youth with Type 1 Diabetes and Effects on Postprandial Glycemia (*continued*)

Study	Population/ Duration of Study	Intervention (type of study)	Major Findings	Comments
Klupa 2011	n = 56 adults with type 1 diabetes/2 years, using CSII	Evaluated DW bolus use in adults after switching from MDI to CSII; A1C. BMI, frequency of BG monitoring measured before and 12 and 24 months after change to CSII; after CSII started, two study cohorts: frequent DW+ bolus (>20% daily bolus dose delivered as SW), n = 32; and infrequent DW− bolus (≤20% of daily bolus dose delivered as SW), n = 24 (observational study)	Frequent DW bolus use by males (59 vs. 17%, P = 0.001) and shorter duration of type 1 diabetes (3.4 vs. 11.3 years, P < 0.0001), but not patient age (25.7 vs. 27.0 years, P = 0.6); A1C improved by 0.45% in DW+ patients vs. DW− patients (P = 0.0009)	Author conclusions: DW bolus might be a tool to improve glycemic control in type 1 diabetes; males with shorter duration of diabetes more willing to use DW bolus; aspart and lispro used in study
Pańkowska 2012	n = 24 adults using CSII with type 1 diabetes/1 week	Impact of the inclusion of FPUs in the general algorithm for mealtime insulin dose calculator on 6-h PP BG. Meal = pizza dinner, 45 g CHO/400 kcal fat; Group A: used DW bolus algorithm (nCHO units ´ ICR + nFPU ´ ICR/6 h [standard deviation + SW bolus] vs. Group B (control): used algorithm (nCHO units ´ ICR); glucose, C-peptide, glucagon evaluated before and at 30, 60, 120, 240, and 360 min PP (randomized clinical trial)	Group A: glucose increment occurred at 120–360 min, with maximum at 240 min; 60 vs. −3 mg/dL in Group B (P = 0.04)	Author conclusions: mixed meal elevates PP glucose after 4–6 h; DW bolus calculated for both CHO and fat/protein is effective in controlling PP glycemia

AUC, area under the curve; BG, blood glucose; CHO, carbohydrate; CGM, continuous glucose monitoring; DW, "dual-wave" bolus: insulin bolus delivered as a combination of an instant standard "normal" bolus followed by a "square-wave" bolus infused over minutes to several hours; FBG, fasting blood glucose; ICR, insulin-to-carbohydrate ratio; nCHO units, number of calculated carbohydrate units; nFPU units, number of calculated Fat/Protein units; NL, "normal" bolus: prandial insulin infused in an instant, over several seconds to minutes depending on the amount of insulin calculated to cover carbohydrate (protein/fat) intake determined at the meal; PP, postprandial; SW, "square-wave" bolus: prandial insulin infused over minutes to several hours.

Two studies evaluated the application of a novel DW meal bolus for meals containing fat and/or protein in children and adolescents with type 1 diabetes collected from data downloaded from the participants' insulin pumps in routine visits to their outpatient clinic (Pańkowska 2009b; Pańkowska 2010). The algorithm was based on a formula in which carbohydrate as well as either fat and/or protein in the meal was covered by prandial insulin. The carbohydrate component of the meal was expressed by exchange/portions of carbohydrate, where 10 g carbohydrate was equivalent to 1 carbohydrate unit (CU), which was covered by 1 unit of rapid-acting insulin (Dose Adjustment for Normal Eating [DAFNE] Study Group 2002). The carbohydrate content of the meal was determined by dividing the total grams of carbohydrate by 10, and the CUs were administered by using an NL bolus. A new fat-protein unit (FPU) was then added to the prandial meal dosing equation; the FPU was defined as 100 kcal fat and/or protein foods being equivalent to 1 FPU, which was covered by 1 unit rapid-acting insulin. The grams of fat and/or protein to be consumed were converted to calories (1 g fat = 9 calories and 1 g protein = 4 calories). The FPU was administered using an SW bolus, which was extended based on the number of FPUs. The SW bolus was extended for 3 h for a meal containing 1 FPU, to 4 h for 2 FPUs, 5 h for 3 FPUs, and finally to 8 h when a meal included >3 FPUs (300 calories). Most of the currently available insulin pumps have a DW bolus feature that can be preprogrammed at the beginning of a meal to infuse the NL and SW boluses.

Because of the lengthy calculations required to determine the prandial bolus using this novel algorithm, Pańkowska and colleagues developed an online software program called "*Diabetics*," and this program is available in Polish and English at www.diabetics.pl. This system consists of two integrated parts: the bolus calculator and the nutrition database software (Pańkowska 2010). The *Diabetics* system was created to optimize prandial insulin dosing by calculating nutrition product data accurately and adjusting insulin dosages for all meal components. It is the first bolus dose calculator that suggests the optimal type of prandial bolus for a mixed meal (including carbohydrate, protein, and fat) as well as the necessary period of time that an extended bolus is needed to cover a particular type of food. When comparing the *Diabetics* to the standard method in calculating the prandial bolus dose, significantly lower postprandial blood glucose levels were observed after main meals in the *Diabetics* group (Blazik 2009). This group recommends that the *Diabetics* software that includes a bolus calculator should not be used in conjunction with other bolus calculators that may be integrated into the insulin pump. The group is in their final research stage on the safety of the *Diabetics* program.

A disadvantage of this novel algorithm is that the research studies to date were conducted exclusively in the patients from the Department of Pediatrics, Medical University of Warsaw, Poland. The results are based on uncontrolled evaluation of data collected in their outpatient clinic patients. In addition, the bolus calculator does not take into account the current blood glucose level, target blood glucose level, or active insulin time. And finally *Diabetics* was developed in Poland and therefore the foods included in database may not be applicable to other countries.

SUMMARY

There are few randomized controlled trials comparing pump therapy to an identical population using multiple daily injections; as a result, there are little data about how to best teach and use pump therapy to optimize glycemic control. When research is available, it has often been conducted in pediatric populations rather than adults. In addition to the 2007 ADA consensus statement on the use of insulin pump therapy in the pediatric age-group, the American Association of Diabetes Educators published an article on education for CSII pump users, and Hirsch wrote a review of "practical pearls" that could be used to improve diabetes control outcomes (Schneiner 2009; Hirsch 2010).

To date, there have only been a small number of research studies investigating the use of bolus calculators and the impact of the different types of bolus delivery functions. Hopefully in the near future, well-designed, sufficiently powered, meal-related studies will be conducted using CGM devices. The results of these types of studies will provide diabetes care providers with evidence-based guidelines and recommendations for the use of CSII and/or CGM features to reduce postprandial blood glucose excursions and to improve overall metabolic control. Until that time, results of variable bolus features that have been conducted to date should be cautiously applied in clinical practice.

BIBLIOGRAPHY

Academy of Nutrition and Dietetics: Type 1 and type 2 diabetes evidence-based nutrition practice guidelines for adults, 2008. Available from http://www.adaevidencelibrary.com/topic.cfm?cat=3252. Accessed November 2011

American Diabetes Association: Nutrition recommendations and interventions for diabetes (Position Statement). *Diabetes Care* 31 (Suppl. 1):S61–S78, 2008

American Diabetes Association: Standards of medical care in diabetes: 2012. *Diabetes Care* 35 (Suppl. 1):S11–S63, 2012

American Diabetes Association: Use of insulin pump therapy in the pediatric age group: a consensus statement. *Diabetes Care* 30:1653–1662, 2007

Blazik M, Szypowska A, Golicka D, Groele L, Pañkowska E: The "Diabetics" software in adjusting prandial insulin in patients treated with insulin pumps: the results of RCT study. *Pediatr Diabetes* 10 (Suppl. 11):71, 2009

Bode BW: Insulin pump use in type 2 diabetes. *Diabetes Technol Ther* 12 (Suppl.):S17–S21, 2010

Burdick J, Chase HP, Slover RH, Knievel K, Scrimgeour L, Maniatis AK, Klingensmith GJ: Missed insulin meal boluses and elevated hemoglobin A1C levels in children receiving insulin pump therapy. *Pediatrics* 113:e221–e224, 2004

Chase HP, Saib SZ, MacKenzie T, Hansen MM, Garg SK: Post-prandial glucose excursions following four methods of bolus insulin administration in subjects with type 1 diabetes. *Diabet Med* 19:317–321, 2002

Cukierman-Yaffe T, Konvalina N, Cohen O: Key elements for successful intensive insulin pump therapy in individuals with type 1 diabetes. *Diabetes Res Clin Pract* 92:69–73, 2011

DAFNE Study Group: Training in flexible, intensive insulin management to enable dietary freedom in people with type 1 diabetes: dose adjustment for normal eating (DAFNE) randomized controlled trial. *BMJ* 325:746–751, 2002

Danne T, Battelino T, Jarosz-Chobot P, Kordonouri O, Pańkowska E, Phillip M, the PedPump Study Group: The PedPump Study: a low percentage of basal insulin and more than five boluses are associated with better centralized HbA1c in 1041 children on CSII from 17 countries (Abstract). *Diabetes* 54 (Suppl. 1):A453, 2005

Doyle EA, Weinzimer SA, Steffen AT, Ahren JA, Vincent M, Tamborlane WV: A randomized, prospective trial comparing the efficacy of continuous subcutaneous insulin infusion with multiple daily insulin injections using glargine. *Diabetes Care* 27:1554–1558, 2004

Franz MJ, Powers MA, Leontos C, Holmeister LA, Kulkarni K, Monk A, Wedel N, Gradwell E: The evidence for medical nutrition therapy for type 1 and type 2 diabetes in adults. *J Am Diet Assoc* 110:1852–1889, 2010

Glaser NS, Iden SB, Green-Burgeson D, Bennett C, Hood-Johnson K, Styne DM, Goodlin-Jones B: Benefits of an insulin dosage calculation device for adolescents with type 1 diabetes mellitus. *J Pediatric Endocrinol Metab* 17:1641–1651, 2004

Gross TM, Kayne D, King A, Rother C, Juth S: A bolus calculator is an effective means of controlling postprandial glycemia in patients on insulin pump therapy. *Diabetes Technol Ther* 5:365–369, 2003

Heinemann L: Insulin pump therapy: What is the evidence for using different types of boluses for coverage of prandial insulin requirements? *J Diabetes Sci Technol* 3:1490–1500, 2009

Hirsch IB: Insulin analogues. *N Engl J Med* 352:174–183, 2005

Hirsch IB: Practical pearls in insulin pump therapy. *Diabetes Technol Ther* 12 (Suppl. 1):S23–S27, 2010

Jones SM, Quarry JL, Caldwell-McMillan M, Mauger DT, Gabbay RA: Optimal insulin pump dosing and postprandial glycemia following a pizza meal using the continuous glucose monitoring system. *Diabetes Technol Ther* 7:233–240, 2005

Klupa T, Benbenek-Klupa T, Malecki M, Szalecki M, Steradzki J: Clinical usefulness of a bolus calculator in maintaining normoglycaemia in active professional patients with type 1 diabetes treated with continuous subcutaneous insulin infusion. *J Int Med Res* 3:1112–1116, 2008

Klupa T, Skupien J, Cyganek K, Katra B, Sieradzki J, Malecki MT: The dual-wave bolus feature in type 1 diabetes adult users of insulin pumps. *Acta Diabetol* 48:11–14, 2011

Lane WS, Cochran EK, Jackson JA, Scism-Bacon JL, Corey IB, Hirsch IB, Skyler JS: High-dose insulin therapy: is it time for U-500 insulin? *Endocr Pract* 15:71–79, 2009

Lee SW, Cao M, Said S, Hayes M, Choi L, Rother C, de Leon R: The dual-wave bolus feature in continuous subcutaneous insulin infusion pumps controls prolonged post-prandial hyperglycemia better than standard bolus in type 1 diabetes. *Diabetes Nutr Metab* 17:211–216, 2004

Lindholm-Olinder A, Kernell A, Smide B: Missed bolus doses: devastating for metabolic control in CSII-treated adolescents with type 1 diabetes. *Pediatr Diabetes* 10:142–148, 2009a

Lindholm-Olinder A, Runefors J, Smide B Kernell A: Post-prandial glucose levels following three methods of insulin bolusing: a study in adolescent girls in comparison with girls without diabetes. *Pract Diabetes Int* 26:110–115, 2009b

Mehra R, Raman R, Bayless ML, Sivitz WI: Antecedent caloric intake and glucose excursion following a subsequent meal type 1 diabetes. *J Diabetes* 1:273–277, 2009

O'Connell MA, Gilbertson HR, Donath SM, Cameron FJ: Optimizing postprandial glycemia in pediatric patients with type 1 diabetes using insulin pump therapy: impact of glycemic index and prandial bolus type. *Diabetes Care* 31:1491–1495, 2008

Pańkowska E, Blazik M: Bolus calculator with nutrition database software, a new concept of prandial insulin programming for pump users. *J Diabetes Sci Technol* 4:571–576, 2010

Pańkowska E, Blazik M, Dziechciarz P, Szypowska A, Szajewska H: Continuous subcutaneous insulin infusion vs. multiple daily injections in children with type 1 diabetes: a systematic review and meta-analysis of randomized control trials. *Pediatr* 10:52–58, 2009a

Pańkowska E, Blazik M, Groele L: Does the fat-protein meal increase postprandial glucose levels in type 1 diabetes patients on insulin pump: the conclusion of a randomized study. *Diabetes Technol Ther* 14:16–22, 2012

Pańkowska E, Szypowska A, Lipka M, Szpotańska M, Blazik M, Groele L: Application of novel dual wave meal bolus and its impact glycated hemoglobin A1C level in children with type 1 diabetes. *Pediatr Diabetes* 10:298–303, 2009b

Pickup JC, Keen H: Continuous subcutaneous insulin infusion at 25 years: evidence base for expanding use of insulin pump therapy in type 1 diabetes. *Diabetes Care* 25:593–598, 2002

Pickup JC, Sutton AJ: Severe hypoglycaemia and glycaemic control in type 1 diabetes: meta-analysis of multiple daily injections compared with continuous subcutaneous insulin infusion. *Diabetic Med* 25:765–774, 2008

Rabasa-Lhoret R, Garon J, Langelier H, Poisson D, Chiasson J-L: Effects of meal carbohydrate content on insulin requirements in type 1 diabetic patients treated intensively with the basal-bolus (ultralente-regular) insulin regimen. *Diabetes Care* 22:667–673, 1999

Raskin P, Bode BW, Marks JB, Hirsch IB, Weinstein RL, McGill JB, Peterson GE, Mudaliar SR, Reinhardt RR: Continuous subcutaneous insulin infusion and multiple daily injection therapy are equally effective in type 2 diabetes: a randomized, parallel-group, 24-week study. *Diabetes Care* 26:2598–2603, 2003

Rossi MC, Nicolucci A, Di Bartolo P, Bruttomesso D, Girelli A, Ampudia FJ, Kerr D, Ceriello A, De la Mayor C, Pellegrini F, Horwitz D, Vespasiani G: Diabetes Interactive Diary: a new telemedicine system enabling flexible diet and insulin therapy while improving quality of life: an open-label, international, multi-center, randomized study. *Diabetes Care* 33:109–115, 2010

Rutledge KS, Chase HP, Klingensmith GJ, Walravens PA, Slover RH, Garg SK: Effectiveness of postprandial Humalog in toddlers with diabetes. *Pediatrics* 100:968–972, 1997

Schneiner G, Sobel RJ, Smith DE, Pick AJ, Kruger D, King J, Green K: Insulin pump therapy: guidelines for successful outcomes. *Diabetes Educ* 35 (Suppl. 2):S29–S49, 2009

Shapira G, Yodfat O, HaCohen A, Feigin P, Rubin R: Bolus guide: a novel insulin bolus dosing decision support based on selection of carbohydrate ranges. *J Diabetes Sci Technol* 4:893–902, 2010

Shashaj B, Busetto E, Sulli N: Benefits of a bolus calculator in pre- and postprandial glycaemic control and meal flexibility of paediatric patients using continuous subcutaneous insulin infusion (CSII). *Diabet Med* 25:1036–1042, 2008

Smart CE, Ross K, Edge JA, Collins CE, Colyvas K, King BR: Children and adolescents on intensive insulin therapy maintain postprandial glycaemic control without precise carbohydrate counting. *Diabet Med* 26:279–285, 2009

Waldron S, Hanas R, Palmvig B: How do you educate young people to balance carbohydrate intake with adjustments of insulin? *Horm Res* 57 (Suppl. 1):62–65, 2002

Zisser H, Robinson L, Bevier W, Dassau E, Ellingsen C, Doyle FJ, Jovanovic L: Bolus calculator: a review of four "smart" insulin pumps. *Diab Technol Ther* 10:441–444, 2008

Alison B. Evert, MS, RD, CDE, is a Diabetes Nutrition Educator and the Coordinator of Diabetes Education Programs at the University of Washington Medical Center, Diabetes Care Center, Seattle, WA.

Chapter 22
Effective Nutrition Education and Counseling

JACKIE BOUCHER, MS, RD, CDE

Highlights

Diabetes Nutrition Education and Counseling Interventions

Implications for Health Care Providers

Summary

Highlights
Effective Nutrition
Education and Counseling

■ Approximately 50% of people with diabetes report attending some type of diabetes self-management class, and only ~26% of people with diabetes reported seeing a diabetes educator in the previous year. Only ~9% of patients have at least one nutrition visit with a registered dietitian.

■ The National Standards for Diabetes Self-Management Education defines effective interventions for improving clinical outcomes and quality of life and recommends diabetes education curriculum that includes nutrition therapy. Programs should be culturally and demographically appropriate.

■ Nutrition education is defined as instruction or training intended to lead to acquired nutrition-related skills and can be provided in individual or group settings.

■ Nutrition counseling is a supportive process designed to help people with chronic diseases such as diabetes set priorities, establish goals, and create individualized action plans that acknowledge and foster responsibility and self-care. Nutrition counseling strategies are based on evidence-based methods or plans of action designed to help individuals achieve behavior change for a particular goal.

■ Clinicians are encouraged to use combinations of behavior change theories and strategies to plan effective nutrition counseling interventions. Goal-setting, problem-solving, and social support are effective nutrition counseling strategies.

■ Research has shown that when clinicians spend as little as 3 min talking about a new behavior, patients will consider and even adopt a behavior change. The 5As (Assess, Advise, Agree, Assist, Arrange) is one framework that can be used for brief counseling.

■ Technology and peer support are emerging as nutrition counseling tools.

Effective Nutrition Education and Counseling

The National Standards for Diabetes Self-Management Education (DSME) defines "quality diabetes self-management education" and provides guidelines for delivering evidence-based education (Funnell 2011). DSME is an essential component of care for people with diabetes and is necessary to improve the health and quality of life of all individuals with diabetes. DSME is a collaborative process through which individuals with diabetes gain the knowledge and skills needed to modify behavior and successfully self-manage diabetes and its related conditions. Nutrition education is considered to be one of the educational components of DSME (Funnell 2011).

Despite the recommendation that all patients receive diabetes education, national data indicate that only 54.3% of people with diabetes report attending some type of diabetes self-management class (Diabetes Prevention and Control Programs 2011). According to the 2007 Roper U.S. Diabetes Patient Market Study, out of 16,660,000 diagnosed diabetes patients in the U.S., only 26%, or 4,249,000 patients, reported that they had seen a diabetes educator in the previous 12 months. Visits with a registered dietitian (RD) for nutrition therapy are even less frequent; in one study of 18,404 diabetes patients, only 9.1% had at least one nutrition visit within a 9-year period (Robbins 2008). Whereas national data suggest more patients are achieving glycemic control (A1C <7%), the National Health and Nutrition Examination Survey (NHANES) data show that 45% of patients with diabetes still have not achieved the glycemic target of <7% (Hoerger 2008; Resnick 2006), which may be due to lack of education and/or inappropriate medical care.

Meta-analyses evaluating the effect of an educational and behavioral intervention on glycemic control for adults with type 2 diabetes observed average decreases in A1C of 0.43% and 0.76% (Gary 2003; Norris 2002). Norris and colleagues noted that contact time with the diabetes educator was the best predictor of improvements in glycemic control. Educational visits, especially nutritionist visits, are also associated with fewer hospitalizations and reductions in total hospital charges (Robbins 2008). What is less known is which specific behavioral components and/or education are necessary to support lifestyle and self-care behaviors for individuals with diabetes (Weinger 2011). However, research does suggest that when health care providers spend as little as 3 min with a patient talking about a new behavior, some patients will consider and even adopt a change (Miller 2000; Fiore 2000).

The purpose of this chapter is to review the evidence supporting nutrition education and nutrition counseling, key components of DSME. Nutrition education is defined as instruction or training intended to lead to acquired nutrition-related skills and can be provided in individual or group settings (Acad Nutr Diet 2011). Nutrition counseling is a supportive process to set priorities, establish goals, and create individualized action plans that acknowledge and foster responsibility and self-care (Curry 1998). "Nutrition counseling strategies are evidence-based methods or plans of action designed to achieve behavior change toward a particular client goal" (Acad Nutr Diet 2011). Nutrition education is necessary to teach an individual with diabetes an individualized meal plan or a diabetes program curriculum, where the focus is on information. Nutrition counseling requires a contextual understanding of the patient's individual situation, which can help support and promote health behavior change (Maurer 2005). The nutrition counseling strategies are tools to help the client achieve the collaborative goals set in the counseling process.

DIABETES NUTRITION EDUCATION AND COUNSELING INTERVENTIONS

Nutrition education and counseling are critical components of the diabetes education interventions recommended by the "National Standards for Diabetes Self-Management Education" (Funnell 2011), and healthy eating is a common behavior-change goal for individuals with diabetes. In a survey of 954 individuals with diabetes, 74% identified healthy eating as their most common goal (Zgibor 2007). From the group, 527 subjects identified goals that were mutually identified with their diabetes educator, and 94% reported setting a goal related to healthy eating.

Before setting goals with clients, the nutrition education and counseling process should begin with a thorough nutrition assessment. Ideally, the individual assessment and education plan are developed collaboratively between the individual with diabetes and the diabetes educator or health care professional. The assessment can include, but is not limited to, information about the individual's medical and family history, life stage, and cultural background; current diabetes knowledge and self-management skills and behaviors; readiness and willingness to change; health literacy level; physical abilities and limitations; social support system; and financial situation (Funnell 2011).

Once a thorough assessment is completed, the diabetes educator's or health care professional's role is to facilitate behavior change. Various behavior-change theories and strategies can be used as frameworks to help practitioners use information obtained in the nutrition assessment to select counseling strategies to achieve a specific counseling objective and to tailor nutrition interventions to help the client achieve specific health and quality-of-life outcomes (Spahn 2010). Table 22.1 outlines key theories, models, and counseling strategies used in nutrition education and counseling interventions.

To evaluate evidence related to specific behavior-change theories and strategies and their impact on the nutrition education and counseling process, articles were identified both from PubMed MEDLINE and the Academy of Nutrition and Dietetics (Acad Nutr Diet) Evidence Analysis Library (EAL). Studies included randomized controlled trials, systematic reviews, case-controlled trials, cross-sectional studies, and surveys. A systematic review conducted by the Acad

Table 22.1 Brief Definitions for Behavior-Change Theories and Strategies

Behavior-Change Theory/Model	Definition
Adult Learning Theory	Encompasses both concepts of experience and behavior change. Adults need to know why they need to learn something, have a desire to learn and discover (i.e., be self-directive), want to experience change or develop/practice new skills, and like problem-oriented learning (apply and learn).
Cognitive Behavioral Theory	Focuses on producing cognitive change (i.e., change how we act [behavior], think [cognition], and feel [emotion]). Both cognitive and behavior-change strategies are used to effect change.
Health Belief Model	Health-behavior change is a function of the individual's perceptions regarding his or her vulnerability to illness and the possible effectiveness of treatment. The following constructs determine a person's ability to change: perceived susceptibility to an illness, perceived severity of an illness, perceived barriers to change, perceived benefits of change, and costs of change (e.g., money, effort, or pain).
Self-Determination Theory	Asserts that people are motivated to act on the basis of internal/intrinsic motivation or external motivation.
Social Cognitive Theory (also called Social Learning Theory)	Emphasizes the interaction between people and their environment (e.g., social interactions, experiences, and outside media influences).
Transtheoretical Model (also called Stages of Change Model)	Proposes that at any specific time, people change health behaviors by moving through a series of stages on the basis of their "readiness to change." There are five stages: pre-contemplation, contemplation, preparation, action, and maintenance.

Behavior-Change Strategy	Definition
Cognitive Restructuring	Used to help individuals increase their awareness of destructive or distorted thoughts and beliefs about themselves. Teaches them to change their internal dialogue.
Goal-Setting	Collaborative activity between a client and a clinician in which a client determines from a number of potential courses of action what he or she is willing to do to make health behavior changes.
Motivational Interviewing	Elicits behavior change by helping clients explore and resolve ambivalence to making health behavior changes.
Problem-Solving	Process in which clients identify barriers to achieving goals, brainstorm solutions to overcoming barriers and evaluating which will work for them. Clients will try solutions and reevaluate how they work to revise strategies as needed to find something that works.
Self-Monitoring	Increases awareness of client's habit. Examples of what to self-monitor include client keeping a record of thoughts, emotions, nutrition behaviors, physical activity level, and/or health measurements (e.g., blood glucose).

Adapted from Knowles 1996; Kushner 2009; and Spahn 2010.

Nutr Diet for the EAL was used to evaluate evidence between 1986 and 2007 (Spahn 2010). A separate search for evidence from 2008 to 2011 was conducted using PubMed MEDLINE. From this search, 79 abstracts were reviewed and 8 articles were selected to be included in Table 22.2. Six additional articles were identified and included by searching reference lists in articles reviewed during the search process.

The systematic review focused on literature related to specific behavior-change theories and strategies used in nutrition counseling (Spahn 2010). Strong evidence exists to support the use of a combination of behavioral theory and cognitive behavioral theory in facilitating changes in nutrition behaviors to address diabetes risk factors. This evidence was particularly strong in patients with type 2 diabetes receiving intensive intermediate-duration (6–12 months) and long-term (>12 months' duration) interventions. Other behavioral theories with strong evidence included motivational interviewing (especially when combined with cognitive behavioral theory). In terms of behavioral strategies, self-monitoring had the strongest evidence for effectiveness and is a common tool used in the nutrition education and counseling process. Whereas goal-setting, problem-solving, and social support are effective strategies, additional research is needed to test these strategies in diverse populations. Limited research was available to assess the application of the transtheoretical (stages of change) model or the social cognitive theory to change nutrition behaviors.

For the remaining studies in Table 22.2, which were published between 2008 and 2011, study purposes included the evaluation of specific behavioral theories or strategies but also broader purposes in terms of looking at the nutrition assessment or education process. Outcomes of these studies included health outcomes (e.g., glycemic control, lipid and blood pressure levels), diabetes knowledge, self-care behaviors, and nutrient intakes. Interventions evaluated the effectiveness of structured groups (Davies 2008; Samuel-Hodge 2009; Liebbrandt 2010; Naik 2011; Weinger 2011), the impact of peer education/counseling (Perez-Escamilla 2008; Samuel-Hodge 2009), use of computerized dietary assessments (Probst 2008), adaptation of culturally relevant nutrition education materials (Kattelmann 2009), client preferences for nutrition education methods (Mian 2009), non-didactic/empowerment approaches (Liebbrandt 2010), impact of food insecurity (Homenko 2010), group versus individual counseling (Huang 2010; Vadstrup 2011), and the effect of dietary advice (Al-Sinani 2010).

Nutrition assessment is the first step in the education and counseling process. Computerized nutrition assessments may be a more helpful tool than interviewer-administered assessments (Probst 2008). During the nutrition assessment process, it is important to assess and address the issue of food insecurity. When it is addressed in the counseling process, clients are more able to follow nutrition advice (Homenko 2010). Addressing cultural influences is also important. Although the one culturally relevant study did not achieve significant health outcomes (Kattelmann 2009), which may have been due to the limited length of the intervention, participants did have high satisfaction with the intervention. Culturally relevant educational materials and resources are desired by South Asian patients with diabetes (Mian 2009) and need to be studied further in other populations.

Table 22.2 Studies Related to Nutrition Counseling for Diabetes Published After March 2008*

	Population/ Duration of Study	Intervention (type of study)	Major Findings	Comments
Davies 2008	n = 162 practices (77 control, 85 intervention), patients with type 2 diabetes referred within 4 weeks of diagnosis (n = 824 patients, 487 control, 437 intervention)/1 year	Evaluated effectiveness of structured group education (6-h program delivered over 1 or 2 days) vs. standard care (cluster RCT)	A1C: nonsignificant at 1 year; odds of not smoking at 1 year: 3.56 higher in the intervention group (P = 0.033); weight loss greater in the intervention group at 1 year (−2.98 vs. −1.86 kg, P = 0.027)	Structured education for newly diagnosed type 2 diabetes patients can result in sustainable lifestyle changes after diagnosis
Perez-Escamilla 2008	n = 9 diabetes experimental or quasi-experimental studies/not applicable	Impact of peer education/counseling in DSME programs on nutrition and health outcomes among Latinos (systematic review)	Peer-delivered nutrition education resulted in improved glycemic control, lipid profile, and blood pressure and improvement in diabetes knowledge and self-care behaviors	Author conclusions: there is a need for randomized trials testing the impact of peer nutrition education interventions
Probst 2008	n = 31 adults with type 2 diabetes/8 weeks	Four dietary assessments: *1)* three computerized, *2)* three interviewer administered, *3)* two computerized and one interviewer, *4)* two interviewer, one computerized; done at 0, 2, and 8 weeks and food records at 0 and 2 weeks (case-control trial)	Computerized assessments correlated better with food records (r = 0.16–0.52) compared with interviewer-administered assessments (r = 0.02–0.51)	Study conclusion: allowing patients to self-report food intake on a computer can increase RD counseling time with patients
Kattelmann 2009	n = 114 Northern Plains Indians with type 2 diabetes (n = 61 intervention group, n = 53 control group)/6 months	Evaluate if culturally adapted lessons based on the Medicine Wheel Model for Nutrition and usual nutrition education improves glycemic control more than usual care (RCT)	A1C: NS changes in either group; intervention group had modest weight loss ($P \le$ 0.05); no weight loss in control group; no differences in nutrition or physical activity behaviors	Author conclusions: more frequent contact of longer duration may be needed to improve glycemic control

Table 22.2 Studies Related to Nutrition Counseling for Diabetes Published After March 2008* (*continued*)

	Population/ Duration of Study	Intervention (type of study)	Major Findings	Comments
Mian 2009	n = 53 South Asians with diabetes (five focus groups by RDs)/ not applicable	Provide insights on diabetes nutrition education methods and resources (cross-sectional)	Clients preferred individual counseling; fasting was important and managing sweets around the holidays was crucial	Resources needed to target different client skill levels
Samuel-Hodge 2009	n = 24 churches (intervention = 13 churches, 117 participants; control = 11 churches, 84 participants)/1 year	Evaluate a church-based intervention (individual counseling and group education sessions by health professionals, peer support by phone and provider postcard contacts) to improve diabetes self-management (randomized trial)	At 8 months, 0.5% decrease in A1C in intervention vs. control (P = 0.009) and at 1 year nonsignificant between groups	High acceptability rates for the intervention; A1C at baseline was 7.8%, so intervention may have had more impact with higher A1C
Lieb-brandt 2010	n = 38 overweight patients with type 2 diabetes (22 at 1-year follow-up)/1 year	Pilot study: effect of PRISMA on dietary intake at 6 and 12 months (pre-/post-study)	6 months: ↓ energy and macronutrient intake; follow-up counseling needed to improve long-term outcomes; A1C ↓ 0.6% at 12 months (P = 0.11)	PRISMA: group sessions (~10 patients), 2 periods of 3.5 h over 2 weeks, led by RDs, RNs, or psychologist
Homenko 2010	n = 74 rural older adults with diabetes receiving nutrition counseling through telemedicine/not applicable	Evaluate differences related to presence or absence of food insecurity (telephone survey)	In both groups, 85% usually able to follow RD's advice when purchasing food and had similar adherence to advice and glycemic control	IDEATeli demonstration project; study conclusion: telemedicine effective

	Population/ Duration of Study	Intervention (type of study)	Major Findings	Comments
Huang 2010	$n = 154$ patients with type 2 diabetes in Taiwan ($n = 75$ intervention; $n = 79$ usual care)/1 year	Evaluated the effect of RD-led individualized nutrition counseling every 3 months and multidisciplinary diabetes education vs. routine care control group on glycemic control and macronutrient intake (RCT)	A total of 56 patients in the intervention with poor baseline control had greater ↓ in A1C (0.7%) than the 60 control subjects (0.2%) ($P = 0.034$); greater improvements in FBG ($P = 0.007$) and systolic blood pressure ($P = 0.012$); patients in the intervention (A1C ≥7%) had a mean ↓ 230 kcal/day; control had a mean ↑ 56 kcal/day ($P < 0.001$); association between ↓ in CHO intake and improvements in A1C ($P < 0.001$)	Conclusion: RD-led program in primary care clinics for patients with poorly controlled diabetes improves glycemic control; changes may be partially attributed to changes in CHO intake, emphasizing importance of CHO counting
Al-Sinani 2010	$n = 98$ patients with type 2 diabetes in Oman (43% illiterate)/3-year follow-up	Effectiveness of nutrition and lifestyle advice on diabetes management (cross-sectional)	Improvement in FBG; shifted patients from "poor" to "good" control (A1C, FBG, total cholesterol)	11 patients (11.6%) did not follow RD diet advice, 62 (63.2%) sometimes, 24 (25.2%) strictly followed; women were more likely than men to follow advice
Spahn 2010	$n = 87$ studies through March 2008 (12 targeted to diabetes management only)/not applicable	Effectiveness of behavior-change theories and strategies used in nutrition counseling (systematic review)	In diabetes studies, significant improvements in A1C, FBG, weight, and CVD risk factors at 6–12 months	Research controlling for pharmacotherapy needed to determine if positive outcomes can be sustained

Table 22.2 Studies Related to Nutrition Counseling for Diabetes Published After March 2008* (*continued*)

	Population/ Duration of Study	Intervention (type of study)	Major Findings	Comments
Naik 2011	$n = 87$ patients with diabetes ($n = 45$ intervention; $n = 42$ traditional education)/1-year follow-up	Traditional diabetes group education (diabetes and nutrition education) plus routine primary care vs. diabetes group intervention (diabetes and nutrition education) focused on training patients to integrate provider treatment plans into collaborative self-management goals and action plans (RCT)	Intervention patients had greater improvements in A1C immediately after the active intervention ($P = 0.03$), and these differences persisted at 1 year ($P = 0.05$); time-by-treatment interaction on A1C levels favoring intervention group ($P = 0.03$), which was partially mediated by diabetes self-efficacy ($P = 0.002$)	Author conclusions: primary care–based diabetes group clinics that use goal-setting approaches can significantly improve A1C
Vadstrup 2011	$n = 143$ patients with type 2 diabetes ($n = 70$ group education; $n = 73$ individual education)/6 months	Group diabetes education and supervised exercise in a primary care setting vs. individual counseling (diabetes nurse specialist, RD, and podiatrist) program in an outpatient clinic (RCT)	Mean A1C ↓ 0.3% in group and 0.6% in individual at 6 months ($P < 0.05$); nonsignificant differences between groups for CVD outcomes	Group program did not yield better results despite more contact time (57.5 vs. 6.75 h for individual counseling program)
Weinger 2011	$n = 222$ patients with diabetes ($n = 74$ group structured behavioral experimental intervention; $n = 75$ group education control; $n = 73$ individual control group)/1 year	Tested efficacy of a structured behavioral diabetes education program vs. a curriculum-based group education vs. 1:1 education with registered nurse (RN) and RD educators in patients with long-duration poorly controlled diabetes (RCT)	A1C: improved in all three groups ($P < 0.001$); structured behavioral arm had greater improvements than group and individual control arms ($P = 0.04$ for group × time interaction); patients with type 2 diabetes had greater improvements than type 1 diabetes patients ($P = 0.04$ for type of diabetes × time interaction)	All interventions improved A1C with the structured behavioral group arm (cognitive behavioral strategies) being most effective in improving and maintaining glycemic control at 1 year

CHO, carbohydrate; CVD, cardiovascular disease; FBG, fasting blood glucose; IDEATeli, Informatics for Diabetes Education and Telemedicine; PRISMA, PRo-active Interdisciplinary Self-MAnagement program; RCT, randomized controlled trial.

*Studies before March 2008 are included in Spahn 2010.

Intervention studies included community-based interventions delivered by both professionals and peers (Samuel-Hodge 2009) and peer-only education and counseling (Perez-Escamilla 2008). These interventions have modest effects on health outcomes and improvements in diabetes knowledge and self-care behaviors; however, more research is needed using randomized controlled trials to further assess their impact.

Nutrition and lifestyle advice provided modest improvements in health outcomes (Al-Sinani 2010). Structured group programs (Naik 2011; Vadstrup 2011; Weinger 2011), individualized education and counseling programs, or a combination of the two (i.e., individual *and* group interventions) (Huang 2010; Vadstrup 2011; Weinger 2011) had greater effects on health outcomes and/or self-care behaviors in most studies, but not all (Davies 2008; Liebbrandt 2010). In the systematic review by Spahn and colleagues (2010), the following question was addressed: Which is more effective: individual or group counseling? In the few studies that found group counseling was significantly more effective than individual counseling, attrition rates in most of the studies was high (>30%). In studies published since that review, one study observed greater improvements in a structured behavioral diabetes education program than the individual counseling (Weinger 2011), although the individual counseling program did still observe significant changes in A1C. However, in another study, the individual program observed greater decreases in A1C than the group program (Vadstrup 2011). More research is needed to address this question.

IMPLICATIONS FOR HEALTH CARE PROVIDERS

Diabetes educators and other health care providers who provide nutrition education and counseling are both educators and counselors. Initially, individuals with diabetes must first understand how their lifestyle behaviors affect key outcomes for their diabetes management (e.g., glycemic control, lipid levels, blood pressure level). In terms of nutrition, it is important that individuals with diabetes be educated on the fundamentals of their eating pattern and that they be given the skills, through training, to implement their food plan. Their readiness to change, learning style, health literacy, culture, and age are all factors that are important to consider in the nutrition education and counseling process.

Many of the current behavior-counseling models and strategies (Table 22.1) may require extensive time and training to fully implement. It is recommended that professionals providing nutrition education and counseling seek advanced training. Many organizations provide continuing education in these areas, such as the Academy of Nutrition and Dietetics (eatright.org), the American Association of Diabetes Educators (diabeteseducator.org), the American Diabetes Association (diabetes.org), the Institute for Healthcare Communication (healthcarecomm.org), and the Motivational Interviewing Network of Trainers (motivationalinterviewing.org).

A brief counseling approach that does not require a lot of training and offers a simple framework that can be integrated with other diabetes nutrition education and counseling resources is the 5As (Assess, Advise, Agree, Assist, Arrange). This concept was introduced by the National Cancer Institute as a guide to help physicians counsel their patients with smoking cessation (Glynn 1989). This framework has since been expanded to address broader issues of health-behavior change and to give diabetes educators and other health care providers the flexibility of addressing important lifestyle topics in a manner ranging from simple to in-depth (depending on time, training, and resources). Table 22.3 outlines how the 5As could work in diabetes nutrition education and counseling.

Table 22.3 Framework for Nutrition Education and Counseling Using the 5As

The 5As	Action Steps	Tools and Strategies
Assess	■ Review medical history. ■ Identify risk factors (genetic, biological, behavioral). ■ Evaluate blood glucose records. ■ Identify behavioral mediators (self-efficacy, stage of change, barriers, social support) and cultural beliefs.	■ Logbooks ■ Online or paper assessment tools ■ Verbal questions ■ Biological tests (A1C, lipid profiles)
Advise	■ Review nutrition recommendations and standards of care for diabetes patients. ■ Recommend a plan of care tailored to individual history and needs. ■ Recommend lifestyle changes (e.g., eating, activity, stress management) on the basis of readiness and willingness to change.	■ Give respectful, clear advice on the basis of assessments, and link advice to health concerns/beliefs. ■ Give rationale for suggested changes and education about likely outcomes. ■ Emphasize personal autonomy.
Agree	■ Set short-term goals (e.g., carbohydrate counting, glucose monitoring). ■ Set long-term goals (e.g., A1C). ■ Outline course of action for addressing medical needs. ■ Outline potential strategies for lifestyle change.	■ Recognize readiness for change. ■ Collaborate on acceptable approaches to lifestyle change. ■ Emphasize achievable goals, on the basis of client confidence and goal importance. ■ Agree on action steps and goals.
Assist	■ Discuss important personal skills (self-monitoring blood glucose, planning of meals, engaging in regular activity). ■ Assist with motivation and problem-solving. ■ Discuss other resources to find more in-depth or specific information.	■ Present treatment options highlighting what has worked well for others. ■ Provide skills training and modeling for identified lifestyle changes. ■ Use counseling techniques such as motivational interviewing, verbal encouragement, and cognitive reframing. ■ Provide educational handouts. ■ Refer to other specialty providers or programs.
Arrange	■ Schedule follow-up visits. ■ Provide contact information for future questions. ■ Make referrals.	■ Discuss follow-up options and agree on a feasible schedule. ■ Provide contact information for other providers.

Adapted from Glynn 1989 and VanWormer 2003.

SUMMARY

Nutrition therapy is one of the cornerstones of diabetes treatment. Nutrition education and counseling are necessary to ensure that individuals with diabetes have the knowledge, skills, and training required to effectively implement the lifestyle changes needed to achieve their health goals. Counseling strategies can be used by diabetes educators to make their interactions promote behavior change (Maurer 2005). Health care professionals working with individuals with diabetes are encouraged to learn how to integrate various behavior-change theories and strategies into their practice, so they can effectively plan and implement effective nutrition counseling interventions with their clients. These counseling interventions should be designed to promote and support health behavior change.

BIBLIOGRAPHY

2007 Roper U.S. Diabetes Patient Market Study, November 2007. By permission of GfK Market Measures

Academy of Nutrition and Dietetics: *International Dietetics & Nutrition Terminology (IDNT) Reference Manual*. 3rd ed. Chicago, IL, Academy of Nutrition and Dietetics, 2011

Al-Sinani M, Min Y, Ghebremeskel K, Qazaq HS: Effectiveness of and adherence to dietary and lifestyle counseling. *Sultan Qaboos Univ Med J* 10:341–349, 2010

Curry KR, Jaffe A: *Nutrition Counseling & Communication Skills*. Philadelphia, PA, WB Saunders, 1998

Davies MJ, Skinner TC, Campbell MJ, Carey ME, Cradock S, Dallosso HM, Daly H, Doherty Y, Eaton S, Fox C, Oliver L, Rantell K, Rayman G, Khunti K; Diabetes Education and Self Management for Ongoing and Newly Diagnosed Collaborative: Effectiveness of the Diabetes Education and Self Management for Ongoing and Newly Diagnosed (DESMOND) programme for people with newly diagnosed type 2 diabetes: cluster randomised controlled trial. *Br Med J* 336:491–495, 2008

Diabetes Prevention and Control Programs. Available at http://www.cdc.gov/diabetes/statistics/preventive/fy_class.htm. Accessed December 2011

Fiore M, Bailey W, Cohen SJ, Dorman SF, Goldstein MG, Gritz ER, Heyman RB, Jaen CR, Kottke TE, Lando HA, Mecklenburg RE, Mullen PD, Nett LM, Robinson L, Stitzer ML, Tommasello AC, Villejo L, Wewers ME: *Treating Tobacco Use and Dependence: Clinical Practice Guideline*. Washington, DC, U.S. Department of Health and Human Services, Public Health Service, June 2000

Funnell MM, Brown TL, Childs BP, Haas LB, Hosey GM, Jensen B, Maryniuk M, Peyrot M, Piette JD, Reader D, Siminerio LM, Weinger K, Weiss MA: National standards for diabetes self-management education. *Diabetes Care* 34 (Suppl. 1):89–96, 2011

Gary TL, Genkinger JM, Gualler E, Peyrot M, Brancati FL: Meta-analysis of randomized educational and behavioral interventions in type 2 diabetes. *Diabetes Educ* 29:488–501, 2003

Glynn TJ, Manley MW: *How to Help Your Patients Stop Smoking: A National Cancer Institute Manual for Physicians*. Bethesda, MD, National Cancer Institute, 1989, NIH publ. no. 89-3064

Hoerger TJ, Segel JE, Gregg EW, Saaddine JB: Is glycemic control improving in U.S. adults? *Diabetes Care* 31:81–96, 2008

Homenko DR, Morin PC, Eimicke JP, Teresi JA, Weinstock RS: Food insecurity and food choices in rural older adults with diabetes receiving nutrition education via telemedicine. *J Nutr Educ Behav* 42:404–409, 2010

Huang MC, Hsu CC, Wang HS, Shin SJ: Prospective randomized controlled trial to evaluate effectiveness of registered dietitian-led diabetes management on glycemic and diet control in a primary care setting in Taiwan. *Diabetes Care* 33:233–239, 2010

Kattelmann KK, Conti K, Ren C: The medicine wheel nutrition intervention: a diabetes education study with the Cheyenne River Sioux tribe. *J Am Diet Assoc* 109:1532–1539, 2009

Knowles M: Adult learning. In *The ASTD Training and Development Handbook*. Craig RL, Ed. New York, McGraw-Hill, 1996, p. 253–264

Kushner RF, Kushner N, Jackson Blatner D: *Counseling Overweight Adults: The Lifestyle Patterns Approach and Toolkit*. Chicago, IL, American Dietetic Association, 2009

Liebbrandt AJ, Kiefte-de Jong J, Hogeneist MHE, Snoek FJ, Weijs PJM: Effects of the PRo-active Interdisciplinary Self-MAnagement (PRISMA, Dutch DESMOND) program on dietary intake in type 2 diabetes outpatients: a pilot study. *Clin Nutr* 29:199–205, 2010

Maurer L, Mesznik S: Counseling strategies to promote behavior change. *On the Cutting Edge* 26:17–21, 2005

Mian SI, Brauer PM: Dietary education tools for South Asians with diabetes. *Can J Diet Pract Res* 70:28–35, 2009

Miller W: Rediscovering fire: small interventions, large effects. *Psychol Addict Behav* 14:6–8, 2000

Naik AD, Palmer N, Petersen NJ, Street RL, Rao R, Suarez-Almazor M, Haidet P: Comparative effectiveness of goal setting in diabetes mellitus group clinics. *Arch Intern Med* 171:453–459, 2011

Norris WL, Lau J, Smith SJ, Schmid CH, Engelgau MM: Self-management education for adults with type 2 diabetes: a meta-analysis of the effect on glycemic control. *Diabetes Care* 25:1159–1171, 2002

Perez-Escamilla R, Hromi-Fiedler A, Vega-Lopez S, Bermudez-Millan A, Segura-Perez S: Impact of peer nutrition education on dietary behaviors and health outcomes among Latinos: a systematic literature review. *J Nutr Educ Behav* 40:208–225, 2008

Probst YC, Faraji S, Batterham M, Steel DG, Tapsell LC: Computerized dietary assessments compare well with interviewer administered diet histories for patients with type 2 diabetes mellitus in the primary healthcare setting. *Patient Educ Couns* 72:49–55, 2008

Resnick HE, Foster GL, Bardsley J, Ratner RE: Achievement of American Diabetes Association clinical practice recommendations among U.S. adults with diabetes, 1999–2002: the National Health and Nutrition Examination Survey. *Diabetes Care* 29:531–537, 2006

Robbins JM, Thatcher GE, Webb DA, Valdmanis VG: Nutrition visits, diabetes classes, and hospitalization rates and charges: the Urban Diabetes Study. *Diabetes Care* 31:655–660, 2008

Samuel-Hodge CD, Keyserling TC, Park S, Johnsont LF, Gizlice Z, Bangdiwala SI: A randomized trial of church-based diabetes self-management program for African Americans with type 2 diabetes. *Diabetes Educ* 35:439–454, 2009

Spahn JM, Reeves RS, Keim K, Laquatra I, Kellogg M, Jortberg B, Clark NA: State of the evidence regarding behavior change theories and strategies in nutrition counseling to facilitate health and food behavior change. *J Am Diet Assoc* 110:879–891, 2010

Vadstrup ES, Frolich A, Perrild H, Birg E, Roder M: Effect of a group-based rehabilitation programme on glycaemic control and cardiovascular risk factors in type 2 diabetes patients: the Copenhagen Type 2 Diabetes Rehabilitation Project. *Patient Educ Counsel* 84:185–190, 2011

VanWormer JJ, Boucher JL: Counseling diabetic patients about weight management: a pragmatic approach. *Practical Diabetology* 22:30–35, 2003

Weinger K, Beverly EA, Lee Y, Sitnokov L, Ganda OP, Caballero E: The effect of a structured behavioral intervention on poorly controlled diabetes. *Arch Intern Med* 171:1990–1999, 2011

Zgibor JC, Peyrot M, Ruppert K, Noullet W, Siminerio LM, Peeples M, McWilliams J, Koshinsky J, DeJusus C, Emerson S, Charron-Prochownik D; AADE/UPMC Diabetes Education Outcomes Project: Using the American Association of Diabetes Educators Outcomes System to identify patient behavior change goals and diabetes educator responses. *Diabetes Educ* 33:839–842, 2007

Jackie Boucher, MS, RD, CDE, is Vice President, Education, at the Minneapolis Heart Institute Foundation, Minneapolis, MN.

Chapter 23

Health Literacy and Numeracy in Diabetes Nutrition Therapy and Self-Management Education

MARJORIE CYPRESS, PHD, CNP, CDE

Highlights
Health Literacy and Numeracy in Diabetes Nutrition Therapy and Self-Management Education

■ Approximately 36% of English-speaking American adults have limited literacy, which makes it difficult for them to use and understand basic health information.

■ Many people with diabetes have limited health literacy and numeracy, which affects their ability to effectively self-manage the disease and achieve goals for improved knowledge, behavior, and clinical outcomes.

■ Health literacy has been defined by the Institute of Medicine as "the degree to which individuals have the capacity to obtain, process, and understand basic health information and services needed to make appropriate health decisions."

■ Health numeracy is related to health literacy and is defined as the use of numbers in everyday life. Because diabetes self-management requires skills that include understanding and performing numerical calculations, health care professionals need to be attentive to people with limited skills and abilities.

■ It is frequently difficult to identify people with limited health literacy and numeracy. Although there are some predictors, many people with limited literacy may converse easily and be educated. Numerous assessment tools are available that can be administered in <5 min; some are specifically developed to assess skills needed for diabetes self-management.

■ Interventions in people with diabetes and low health literacy show that personalized approaches, adaptation of educational materials, and training of health care professionals to work with people with limited literacy and goal-setting are beneficial in improving knowledge, behavior, and other outcomes. A universal precautionary approach is recommended.

Health Literacy and Numeracy in Diabetes Nutrition Therapy and Self-Management Education

Research has focused on health literacy for many years, but more recently, health literacy in people with diabetes has been of particular interest. The most current information on health literacy comes from the 2003 National Assessment of Adult Literacy, which surveyed over 19,000 adults over the age of 16 years (Kutner 2006). Results indicate that only 12% of these adults demonstrated proficient health literacy. According to these estimates, limited health literacy affects 9 out of 10 English-speaking adults in the U.S. Other studies have confirmed that low health literacy is common among individuals with diabetes (Schillinger 2004; Williams 1998). Literacy may be thought of as simply reading and writing skills as well as educational background, age, type of employment, and income; however, this description does not adequately address health literacy. Health literacy includes both knowledge and skills including basic reading, understanding and acting upon health care information, and numerical tasks that may involve calculations or other quantitative skills that are required to function in the health care system. The Institute of Medicine defines health literacy as "the degree to which individuals have the capacity to obtain, process, and understand basic health information and services needed to make appropriate health decisions" (Institute of Medicine 2004). Having health literacy also requires the ability to understand technical or unfamiliar words. These skills may be needed when filling out medical or insurance forms, or even communicating with health care providers. Perhaps the most diabetes-relevant definition for health literacy is the proposed definition for the World Health Organization. This definition seems to speak specifically to those issues necessary for effective and successful diabetes self-management: "Health literacy represents the cognitive and social skills which determine the motivation and ability of individuals to gain access to, understand, and use information in ways which promote and maintain good health" (Nutbeam 1998). For health care professionals and health care systems, health literacy means to be sensitive to people with limited health literacy and develop materials for the public that can be more easily understood.

Numeracy is also an important component of health literacy that has simply been defined as the ability to understand and use numbers in everyday life. Health numeracy specifically divides numeracy into skills that people need to function in the health care system (Golbeck 2005). It includes those skills necessary to identify numbers and make sense of certain quantitative data. For example, basic health numeracy includes being able to identify the appropriate number of pills from a bottle of medication, whereas computational numeracy involves not only counting, but being able to quantify and do simple computations, such as determining the number of grams of carbohydrate in a serving from a nutrition label. Higher levels of health numeracy involve analytical concepts such as understanding percentages, estimations, and proportions, where the patient may need to pull information from a number of sources and infer, such as knowing whether glucose levels are within a normal range, and the ability to calculate macronutrient intake and adjust insulin dosage on the basis of glucose values and carbohydrate intake.

People with limited health literacy may be difficult to identify. They may be educated and have good conversational skills, but are not likely to discuss their inability to read or understand out of embarrassment or shame (Parikh 1996; Wolf 2007). For chronic conditions requiring ongoing self-management on the part of patients, limited literacy may act as a particularly powerful barrier to achieving optimal outcomes. People may be able to read the words, but if there is no attention to organization, layout, and design, the ability to comprehend words and numbers and apply that information to health situations can be difficult. Sometimes limited time with patients may result in attempts to create "sound bytes" during short office visits that can often result in misleading and difficult-to-understand statements.

Effective diabetes self-management requires mastery of a knowledge and skill set that is increasingly complex. With the advent of new medications, patients with diabetes may be taking three or more different medications just for their diabetes, not counting the antihypertensive and antihyperlipidemic agents that many providers prescribe. Figuring out when and how much medication to take can be a daunting experience for many of our patients. For example, some medications are taken before, during, or after meals. Some medications must be injected within a specific time frame to be effective. In addition, insulin dosages may require the determination of the grams of carbohydrate consumed at a meal as well as fairly elaborate calculations and computations using insulin-to-carbohydrate ratios and insulin correction factors based on personal target blood glucose levels. When we add that to inadequate health literacy and numeracy, and studies that remind us that all patients, regardless of literacy, forget 40–80% of what is discussed during an office visit, it is no wonder that patients are confused (Kessels 2003). It is important that health care professionals become more aware of the issues surrounding health literacy and numeracy, learn how to assess, and intervene to provide the best quality care.

This chapter will discuss the prevalence of health literacy and its complications and identify assessment tools that can be incorporated into practice. It will review how limited health literacy affects people with diabetes specifically, review intervention trials targeted at individuals with diabetes and low literacy, and offer strategies to health care professionals and diabetes educators.

PREVALENCE AND SCOPE OF THE PROBLEM

In 1995, one of the first studies to identify inadequate health literacy was published (Williams 1995). This study found that a high proportion of patients presenting for acute care were unable to read and understand basic medical instructions, such as reading prescription labels, understanding when next appointments were scheduled, and using medical consent forms. Among 2,659 predominately indigent and minority patients, 41.6% were unable to understand directions for taking medication on an empty stomach, and 26% could not comprehend when their next appointment was scheduled. Among the elderly in this study, poor health literacy was very prevalent. In people ≥60 years of age, 81.3% of English-speaking patients and 82.6% of Spanish-speaking patients had health literacy that was inadequate or marginal. In another study, among 3,260 Medicare enrollees aged ≥65 years, 33.9% of English-speaking and 53.9% of Spanish-speaking respondents had inadequate or marginal health literacy (Gazmarian 1999).

The results of the National Assessment of Adult Literacy showed that 53% of adults had intermediate literacy, 22% had basic literacy, and 14% had below-basic literacy; only 12% were proficient. Individuals who scored lower indicated below-basic health literacy skills and included individuals in vulnerable populations, who appear to suffer from the greatest health disparities: people ≥65 years of age, Hispanics, African Americans, American Indian and multiracial individuals, people with low income, people with low levels of education, and individuals less proficient in English. That being said, limited health literacy has also been seen in people with college degrees, white collar jobs, and individuals with good conversational skills. Some people tend to overestimate their own abilities. One study reported that 67.1% of people who scored at the lowest literacy level and 90% of people with low literacy said their reading skills were good or excellent (Roberts 1998).

People with limited health literacy may not participate in preventive medicine but instead deal with complications as they arise, which is particularly a problem for people with chronic illnesses (Scott 2002). The National Academy on an Aging Society (NAAS) reported that people with limited health literacy skills have longer hospital stays and use substantially more hospital resources than adults with higher health literacy skills (NAAS 1999). It is estimated that low health literacy skills increase annual health care expenditures by $73 billion. Limited health literary costs in the U.S. may range from $106 billion to $238 billion annually and may be closer to $1.6 trillion to $3.6 trillion when future costs of limited health literacy that result from action or lack of action are added (Vernon 2007). A new Agency for Healthcare Research and Quality (AHRQ) evidence report including data from 2004 to 2010 indicated that "more than 75 million English-speaking adults in the U.S. have limited literacy" and that low health literacy was linked to a higher risk of death and more emergency room visits and hospitalizations when compared to people with higher health literacy (AHRQ 2011). Therefore, improving health literacy could lead to personal, social, and economic benefits.

DIABETES AND HEALTH LITERACY/NUMERACY

People with diabetes and limited health literacy may have problems acquiring the appropriate knowledge and skills necessary for diabetes self-management, thus affecting health outcomes. In a study using a diabetes-specific numeracy test, nearly 70% of patients had less than a ninth-grade level of general numeracy skills, and 26% could not correctly identify, among a list of glucose values, which values fell within a target range of 60–120 mg/dL. Some patients with low literacy could not identify the correct dosage on an insulin syringe, 56% could not calculate the number of total carbohydrates in a snack-size bag of potato chips, and 59% could not calculate insulin dose requirements adjusted for carbohydrate and blood glucose level (Cavanaugh 2008; Rothman 2006).

Studies comparing people with limited health literacy to people with higher or adequate health literacy found that individuals with limited health literacy and numeracy had less knowledge about diabetes (Cavanaugh 2008; DeWalt 2007; Powell 2007; Gazmarian 1999; Williams 1998) and difficulty understanding food labels (Rothman 2006) and estimating portion sizes (Huizinga 2009). Poorer health outcomes in diabetes were associated with limited health literacy, more frequent hypoglycemia (Sarkar 2010a; Sarkar 2006), decreased self-efficacy (Sarkar 2006; Osborn 2010), increased mortality in end-stage renal disease (Cavanaugh 2010), and, in some studies, poor glycemic control and higher A1C levels (Cavanaugh 2008; Schillinger 2002; Williams 1998). In one study, poor diabetes numeracy skills were more likely to predict poor diabetes control than belonging to the high-risk African American race (Osborn 2009). In the age of Internet-based education, a recent study showed that patients with diabetes who had limited health literacy were less likely to access and navigate an Internet-based patient portal than people with adequate health literacy (Sarkar 2010b). Another study found that compared to people with adequate literacy, people with limited health literacy spent less time on a computer with health education that was placed in an office waiting room (Gerber 2005). These studies are of concern and should prompt us to identify patients with limited health literacy and numeracy skills so we can intervene.

ASSESSING/MEASURING HEALTH LITERACY AND NUMERACY

Many times, clinicians read about a survey tool that is designed for use in practice settings. In the research study, it appears to work well and has good psychometric properties. However, in the "real world" setting, it may not be practical. Several tools will be discussed that have been shortened for use in clinical practice and may help practitioners identify patients with limited literacy. Measuring health literacy includes the ability of people to read written materials, understand prose, and be able to conduct numerical calculations. Table 23.1 outlines some of the more widely used and well-known measures. Some measure general health literacy, some measure general medical terms, and several are diabetes specific.

The Rapid Estimate of Adult Literacy in Medicine (REALM) (Davis 1991) and the diabetes-specific Literacy Assessment for Diabetes (LAD) (Nath 2001) use word recognition to evaluate reading. The REALM lists common medical terms or layperson terms for body parts and illnesses. Patients are asked to pronounce as many words as they can. The shorter version of the REALM, the REALM-R (Bass 2003; Davis 1993), uses items from the REALM and correlates well with the shortened version of the Wide Range Achievement Test (WRAT). LAD is a diabetes-specific word recognition test that measures patients' ability to pronounce terms related to diabetes and health care. The Short Assessment of Health Literacy for Spanish Adults (SAHLSA) is based on the REALM and assesses the ability to read and pronounce health-related terms (Lee 2006).

The WRAT is primarily used in general education evaluations and assesses reading recognition and comprehension, spelling, and arithmetic (Jastak 1993). It

Table 23.1 Assessing Health Literacy and Health Numeracy: Assessment Tools

Name	Assessment	Time to Administer (min)	Language Available	Resources*
REALM	Ability to read and pronounce health-related terms	3	English	Terry C. Davis: tdavis1@lsuhsc.edu
REALM-R	Ability to read and pronounce health-related terms	<2	English	Terry C. Davis: tdavis1@lsuhsc.edu
LAD§	Ability to read and pronounce health-related terms	3–5	English	Charlotte Reese Nath: nathc@rcbhsc.wvu.edu
TOFHLA	Comprehension of written prose and numerical information	20–25	English and Spanish	http://www.peppercorn-books.com
S-TOFHLA	Comprehension of written prose	7	English and Spanish	http://www.peppercorn-books.com
WRAT	Reading, spelling, and computation	20–30; 5 if only reading recognition subtest	English and Spanish	http://www4.parinc.com
DNT§	Numeracy-related skills	30	English	http://www.mc.vanderbilt.edu/diabetes/drtc/preventionandcontrol/tools.php
DNT15§	Numeracy-related skills	15	English/Spanish	http://www.mc.vanderbilt.edu/diabetes/drtc/preventionandcontrol/tools.php
NVS	Ability to understand text and numbers	3	English and Spanish	http://www.clearhealth-communication.com
SAHLSA	Based on REALM	3–6	Spanish	sylee@email.unc.edu

*Sites accessed in October 2011. §Diabetes specific.

may be helpful for patients with diabetes because it includes the ability not only to read and understand, but to be able to make quantitative calculations that patients may need to count carbohydrates or determine insulin dosages. A shortened version (WRAT-R) is also available (Jastak 1993).

The Test of Functional Health Literacy in Adults (TOFHLA) (Parker 1995), used in the original 1995 study documenting the prevalence of health literacy (Williams 1995), is frequently the standard against which other health literacy assessments are measured. The TOFHLA consists of reading passages related to common health care scenarios and multiple-choice questions that assess reading comprehension and numeracy. A Short Test of Functional Health Literacy in Adults (S-TOFHLA) is available, retains much of the validity and reliability of the full version, and is highly correlated with tests used in general education (Baker 1999).

A diabetes-specific instrument that is useful for assessing a patient's ability for diabetes self-management is the Diabetes Numeracy Test (DNT) (Huizinga 2008). The DNT measures both knowledge and skills. Also available is a shortened version known as the DNT15 (15 items from original) and the DNT5 (consists of 5 questions). The DNT is also available in Spanish.

A useful instrument for diabetes educators is the "Newest Vital Sign," developed specifically as an easy screening tool for primary care physicians. It is available in English and Spanish, was validated against TOFHLA, and can be administered in 3 min (Weiss 2005). It consists of a nutrition label for a container of ice cream. After reading the label, the patient is asked six questions as to how they would act on the information. There is a scoring sheet (which includes correct responses) to record responses; low health literacy is suggested if patients are unable to answer four questions correctly. The questions involve the ability to understand and perform calculations. Sarkar found that one question was effective in identifying patients with low health literacy: "How confident are you filling out medical forms by yourself?" (Sarkar 2010c).

The AHRQ and the U.S. Department of Health and Human Services advocated for universal precautions for health literacy because it may be difficult to predict or recognize people with limited health literacy (AHRQ 2011; USDHHS 2011). A toolkit for health care professionals was developed that includes guidelines for interventions (DeWalt 2010).

Shame and embarrassment have also been associated with low health literacy (Parikh 1996; Wolf 2007). Because there is frequently a stigma associated with limited literacy, assessment of patients should be done sensitively in a nonthreatening and nonjudgmental way. Certain factors that may alert a practitioner to patients who may have limited health literacy include the following: nonadherence to medical regimens, frequently missed appointments, leaving medical and registration forms blank, patients who say they take their medications but it is obvious from laboratory tests that this cannot be the case, or patients who do not follow through with lab requests or referrals to specialties. Other clues of limited health literacy are patients who cannot name their medications but identify them by color and shape, patients who cannot tell you for what condition they take medication, and how patients take their medication. Individuals who comment, "I forgot my glasses; I'll read this when I get home," or those who look over instructions and say they understand or do not ask any questions may also have low health literacy (Weiss 2007). Self-efficacy has sometimes been found to be associated with health literacy (Osborn 2010; Sarkar 2006), although results are inconsistent and further research is needed. Some studies have linked low health literacy to a person's low self-rating of their health status (Bennett 2009; Jeppensen 2009). Health literacy and health numeracy should be included in the comprehensive needs assessment done on all patients with diabetes before an educational plan is developed and goals are established.

DIABETES INTERVENTION STUDIES IN LOW-LITERACY POPULATIONS

It is clear from numerous studies that a large number of people with diabetes have limited health literacy (Cavanaugh 2008; Rothman 2004a; Williams 1995). One of the biggest problems for practitioners when identifying low health literacy/numeracy in patients is what to do next. Over the past number of years, researchers have been examining what type of interventions will improve health outcomes in these populations. There have been differing results. Table 23.2 includes a number of randomized controlled trials and pre-/post-intervention studies among people with diabetes and limited literacy. Important outcomes in these studies included diabetes knowledge, glycemic control, self-management behavior change, and self-efficacy. Interventions included adaptation of diabetes materials so they are more literacy-sensitive (Wolff 2009; Cavanaugh 2009; Hill-Briggs 2008), group education (Ntiri 2009; Schillinger 2009; Hill-Briggs 2008), automated telephone calls (Schillinger 2009), health provider training (Cavanaugh 2008, 2009; Wallace 2009; Seligman 2005), multimedia educational tools (Gerber 2005; Kandula 2009), disease management programs (Rothman 2004a, 2004b; Schillinger 2008, 2009; Rothman 2005), goal-setting (DeWalt 2009; Schillinger 2009; Wallace 2009), and personalized teaching (Hill-Briggs 2008; Ntiri 2009; Schillinger 2008, 2009).

Improved diabetes knowledge was seen in most studies (Ntiri 2009; Wallace 2009; Kandula 2009; Rothman 2004b), and among people with below-average literacy, the knowledge gain was more pronounced (Hill-Briggs 2008; Kandula 2009; Rothman 2004b). The two studies that used multimedia interventions targeting individuals with low health literacy had differing results (Gerber 2005; Kandula 2009). This outcome may have been related to the fact that the individuals with low literacy were much less likely to use the computer kiosk in the waiting room than people with higher health literacy (Gerber 2005). Knowledge has not consistently been shown to change behavior. Behavior change was only seen in those studies targeting change in self-management behaviors by goal-setting and action-planning (Schillinger 2009; Wallace 2009; DeWalt 2009).

Self-efficacy is frequently seen as a predictor of behavior change, and in a number of health literacy/numeracy studies, the intervention proved beneficial. In a brief 15-min counseling intervention including low-literacy materials and two follow-up phone calls, self-efficacy scores improved significantly, regardless of literacy level, as did self-reported change in behavior (Wallace 2009). In two other studies, both intervention and control groups showed improved self-efficacy (Cavanaugh 2009; Schillinger 2009), but despite these improvements, the researchers did not see behavior change.

Glycemic control is a frequently examined outcome in most diabetes studies. In studies that used A1C as an outcome, there was little difference in glycemic control between intervention and control groups (Gerber 2005; Rothman 2004a; Schillinger 2008, 2009), except for one study, where there was improvement at 3 months but no difference at 6 months (Cavanaugh 2009), and another study that did show a significant decrease in A1C that was maintained at the 12-month follow-up (Rothman 2005). Some studies found that people with limited health literacy had greater improvements in outcomes regardless of whether they were in

Table 23.2 Intervention Studies of Diabetes and Health Literacy

	Population/ Duration of Study	Intervention (type of study)	Major Findings	Comments
Rothman 2004a	n = 159 adults with type 2 diabetes and A1C ≥8% stratified by literacy level; 55% at or below 6th grade level/1 year	Pre-/post-disease management with educational sessions, telephone reminders, assistance in overcoming barriers to care, communication techniques (cohort study)	A1C: ↓ of 1.9% (95% CI –1.2 to –2.5) in patients with low literacy; A1C: ↓ 1.8% (95% CI –1.0 to –2.5) in patients with higher literacy; nonsignificant difference in A1C between groups	Literacy level measured by REALM
Gerber 2005	n = 244 adults with type 2 diabetes (n = 183 completers)/1 year	C: standard care vs. I: audiovisual computer kiosk on diabetes self-care targeted for low literacy and low numeracy; no personal teaching (RCT)	No difference in knowledge, weight, self-efficacy, self-reported medical care, and BP; no difference in A1C except in people with lower literacy and A1C ≥9%; larger ↓ in A1C in I than in C (P = 0.036)	Kiosk was in waiting room; computer programs varied in length from 10 to 20 min, done before or after office visit
Rothman 2005, 2004b	n = 217 adults with type 2 diabetes and A1C ≥8.0%/12 months	I: diabetes disease management including education sessions, low literacy/low numeracy tools, treatment algorithms, telephone counseling and reminders vs. C: one management session (RCT)	Knowledge ↑ and improved systolic BP were similar across literacy levels; A1C: patients with low literacy had more improvement in A1C from baseline than C and more likely to achieve <7% at 12 months than C	Did not report patient self-management behavior change
Seligman 2005	n = 182 patients with type 2 diabetes and limited health literacy; 63 physicians/3 months	Physicians randomized to be notified if patients had low literacy (I and C groups) (RCT)	A1C and self-efficacy: no change at 3 months, and between groups, physicians and patients supported use of health literacy testing	Physicians received no formal training in health literacy interventions

	Population/ Duration of Study	Intervention (type of study)	Major Findings	Comments
Hill-Briggs 2008	$n = 30$ African Americans with type 2 diabetes; 15 with below-average literacy, 15 with average literacy/1 week	One 90-min education call and educational materials adapted for low literacy/low numeracy; personalized teaching (cohort study)	Knowledge: diabetes and cardiovascular knowledge ↑ for below-average literacy group ($P = 0.005$) and average literacy group ($P = 0.002$)	Small pilot study, 1 week duration
Schillinger 2008, 2009	$n = 339$ patients with diabetes/1 year	Weekly automated telephone management with tools specifically targeted for low numeracy/literacy, personal response by phone if needed, and creation of action plan vs. monthly group education with similar tools (RCT)	SMB: both interventions improved self-efficacy and diabetes-related behaviors and engaged patients in action planning; A1C and BP: no improvement in either group	Weekly automated telephone management yielded higher engagement among patients with lower literacy and limited English; randomization to group visits may have included unwilling participants
Cavanaugh 2009	$n = 198$ with type 2 diabetes, 18–80 years; A1C ≥7%; 35% male, 43% African American/3-month intervention and 6-month follow-up	Usual diabetes education vs. usual diabetes education plus literacy- and numeracy-sensitive diabetes education and management (RCT)	A1C at 3 months: improved in both groups; > in I (−1.50); control (−0.8); nonsignificant at 6 months; self-efficacy: improved in both groups; SMB and treatment satisfaction: nonsignificant	Used specific diabetes numeracy toolkit; no mention of goal-setting with participants
Kandula 2009	$n = 190$ patients with type 2 diabetes from federally qualified health centers (79% adequate literacy; 13% marginal literacy; 8% inadequate literacy)/1 session	Multimedia diabetes education program (observational study)	Knowledge increased among all literacy levels, $P < 0.001$; inadequate literacy learned less compared with adequate literacy	No personalized teaching

Table 23.2 Intervention Studies of Diabetes and Health Literacy
  (*continued*)

	Population/ Duration of Study	Intervention (type of study)	Major Findings	Comments
Ntiri 2009	*n* = 20 adults with type 2 diabetes/1 month	Six group educational sessions during 3 weeks using group education, tools targeted for low numeracy/low literacy, and personal teaching (cohort study)	Diabetes knowledge: ↑ immediately after the intervention (*P* < 0.01) and 1 month after intervention (*P* < 0.05)	Did not evaluate clinical or behavioral changes; small study; short time frame
Wallace 2009; DeWalt 2009	*n* = 250 patients with type 2 diabetes/4 weeks	*Living with Diabetes Guide*; brief behavior-change counseling session with goal-setting; telephone follow-up at 2 and 4 weeks; personalized teaching with tools targeted for low numeracy/literacy; creation of action plans (cohort study)	Knowledge: ↑ at 3 months; improvements similar across literacy levels; SMB: improvements in patient activation (33% met goals at follow-up); self-efficacy levels: Spanish speakers less improvement than English speakers but greater improvement in diabetes-related distress	Short time frame

BP, blood pressure; C, control group; I, intervention group; RCT, randomized controlled trial; SMB, self-management behaviors.

an intervention or control group (Gerber 2005; Rothman 2005). The interventions that appeared to show the best outcomes overall were those that specifically included goal-setting, action-planning, and personalized teaching.

It is evident that health care professionals also need education and training in dealing with low-literacy patients. A randomized trial was conducted that notified physicians about the health literacy level of their patient before the office visit to see if there was any change in physician behavior (Seligman 2005). When compared to physicians who did not receive the literacy level of their patient, it was found that the intervention physicians were more likely to refer the patient to a nutritionist or involve the patient's family in discussion. The intervention physicians were less satisfied with their visits than control physicians and felt less effective. Interestingly, 62% of physicians overestimated the health literacy level of their patients. These studies point to the difficulty in managing and educating patients with low health literacy and numeracy. More research needs to be done with a variety of patient interventions, along with training and evidence-based recommendations for health care providers and self-management support strategies.

IMPLICATIONS FOR DIABETES EDUCATORS

It is essential that diabetes educators and other health care providers incorporate the needs of people with low or limited health literacy into their practice. Think about all the tasks that are involved with a diabetes health care visit (DeWalt 2010). The patient needs to make an appointment, bring his or her glucose records and medications, and sometimes arrange for transportation to the office. Once there, patients are asked to complete forms, update their medical history, review glucose values, review food/eating pattern and physical activity history, set self-care goals, receive prescriptions, schedule an eye or podiatry appointment, check out, pay their bill, and set up the follow-up appointment. After the visit, they will need to go to the pharmacy to get their prescriptions filled, make recommended appointments, monitor their glucose levels daily, take medications as prescribed, work on adhering to the diet and exercise plan, and continue to deal with their other daily life activities (DeWalt 2010). Shopping for food requires the ability to plan meals, create a shopping list, read food labels, and fit costs into a budget. Individuals with limited health literacy may struggle to deal with these types of daily issues, in addition to dealing with family and job responsibilities, which can feel overwhelming.

Using the "universal precautions" approach, health care professionals may find the following strategies useful (Weiss 2007; DeWalt 2010; Joint Commission 2007).

- Assess barriers and facilitators to self-management. These may include an individual's health beliefs as well as issues such as finances or travel.
- Work on improving communication with the patient. By asking more open-ended questions, patients are better able to explain their concerns and ask questions. Active listening and empathy are skills that have been shown to improve communication among health care professionals and patients. Avoid using medical jargon. Use simple, plain, easy-to-understand words. For example, most people know what beans are but may not understand "legumes"; they will know what milk is but may not understand "dairy products."
- Elicit information about types of social support the patient has, such as spouses, children, friends, church, and other relationships. You may want a support person to come to the next visit or teach the patient how to approach family members for support.
- Limit educational messages to three key concepts and repeat them before the end of the visit.
- Use the teach-back, or feedback, approach. This process helps you to know what your patient understood from the visit and can help you to correct any misconceptions. There are a variety of ways to do this. "I want to make sure that we covered the important things today; can you repeat what we dis-

cussed?" "Can you tell me how you will take your medication, so I am sure I told you correctly?"
- Help patients develop behavioral goals that are SMART: Specific, Measurable, Attainable, Realistic, and Timely. A goal that is too unrealistic and not attainable may result in failure and feelings of hopelessness. Patients may give up because they do not know how to go about reaching the goal. Set goals into small manageable steps and assist patients so they know exactly what they will be doing when they leave your office. Goals can be as simple as calling the local gym to find out if there is a pool.
- AskMe3 is a program by the National Patient Safety Foundation that was designed to encourage patients to talk to their health care professionals and get the information they need to understand their health condition. It also promotes more patient-provider communication. The questions are: *1*) What is my main problem? *2*) What do I need to do? *3*) Why is it important for me to do this? (National Patient Safety Foundation 2011).

SUMMARY

Low health literacy is a prevalent problem that often results in poor health outcomes. In a chronic disease such as diabetes, where self-management is key to achieving glycemic control and improved health, low health literacy is a barrier to self-care. Health care professionals should include health literacy in their formal comprehensive assessment, intervene appropriately, and continually evaluate to ensure the best outcomes. Personalized teaching, goal-setting, and follow-up appear to be essential in changing behaviors, which helps lead to improved clinical outcomes. Unless the health care profession addresses the issue of limited health literacy and numeracy, providers and patients will hold on to inaccurate assumptions and fail in our efforts to help our patients. It behooves us as educators to screen our patients. Our ultimate goal is to improve clinical and behavioral outcomes and quality of life in our patients by helping them to actively participate in their care. This step can only be accomplished if the information we think we are providing is accurately and clearly understood, and acted upon.

ACKNOWLEDGMENTS

The author would like to acknowledge Andrea Wallace, Kerri Cavanaugh, Darren DeWalt, Russell Rothman, Erin Van Scoyoc, Robert White, and Kathleen Wolff for their knowledge and expertise, which helped in the writing of this chapter.

BIBLIOGRAPHY

Agency for Healthcare Research and Quality (AHRQ): *Health Literacy Interventions and Outcomes: An Updated Systematic Review*. Available at http://www.ahrq.gov/clinic/tp/lituptp.htm. Accessed on 25 May 2011

Baker DW, Williams MV, Parker RM, Gazmararian JA, Nurss J: Development of a brief test to measure functional health literacy. *Patient Educ Couns* 38:33–42, 1999

Bass PF, Wilson JF, Grifffith CH: A shortened instrument for literacy screening. *J Gen Intern Med* 18:1036–1038, 2003

Bennett IM, Chen Y, Soroui JS, White S: Contributions of health literacy to disparities in self related health status and preventive health behavior in older adults. *Ann Fam Med* 7:204–211, 2009

Cavanaugh K, Huizinga MM, Wallston KA, Gebretsadik T, Shintani A, Davis D, Gregory RP, Fuchs L, Malone R, Cherrington A, Pignone M, DeWalt DA, Elasy TA, Rothman RL: Association of numeracy and diabetes control. *Ann Intern Med* 148:737–746, 2008

Cavanaugh K, Wallston KA, Gebretsadik T, Shintani A, Huizinga MM, Davis D, Gregory RP, Malone R, Pignone M, DeWalt D, Elasy TA, Rothman RL: Addressing literacy and numeracy to improve diabetes care: two randomized controlled trials. *Diabetes Care* 32:2149–2155, 2009

Cavanaugh KL, Wingard RL, Eden S, Shintani A, Wallston KA, Huizinga MM: Low health literacy associates with increased mortality in ESRD. *J Am Soc Nephrol* 21:1979–1985, 2010

Davis TC, Crouch MA, Long SW, Jackson RH, Bates P, Gorge RB, Bairnsfather LE: Rapid assessment of literacy levels of adult primary care patients. *Fam Med* 23:433–435, 1991

Davis TC, Long SW, Jackson RH, Mayeaux EJ, George RB, Murphy PW, Crouch MA: Rapid estimate of adult literacy in medicine: a shortened screening instrument. *Fam Med* 25:391–395, 1993

DeWalt DA, Boone RS, Pignone MP: Literacy and its relationship with self efficacy, trust and participation in medical decision-making. *Am J Health Behav* 31:S27–S35, 2007

DeWalt DA, Callahan LF, Hawk VH, Boucksou KA, Hink A, Rudd R, Brach C: Universal precautions toolkit (prepared by the North Carolina network consortium, the Cecil G. Sheps Center for Health Services Research and University of North Carolina at Chapel Hill). AHRQ publ. no. 10-0046-EF, 2010

DeWalt DA, Davis TC, Wallace AS, Seligman HK, Bryant-Shilliday B, Arnold CL, Freburger JK, Schillinger D: Goal setting in diabetes self-management: taking the baby steps to success. *Patient Educ Couns* 77:218–223, 2009

Gazmarian JA, Baker DW, Williams MV, Parker RM, Scott TL, Green DC, Fehrenbach SN, Ren J, Koplin JP: Health literacy among Medicare enrollees in a managed care organization. *JAMA* 281:545–551, 1999

Gerber BS, Brodsky EG, Lawless KA, Smolin LI, Arozullah AM, Smith EV, Berbaum ML, Heckerling PS, Eiser AR: Implementation and evaluation of a low-literacy diabetes education computer multimedia application. *Diabetes Care* 28:1574–1580, 2005

Golbeck AL, Ahlers-Schmidt CR, Paschal AM: A definition and operational framework for health numeracy. *Am J Prev Med* 29:375–376, 2005

Hill-Briggs F, Renosky R, Lazo M, Bone L, Hill M, Levine D, Brancati FL, Peyrot M: Development and pilot evaluation of literacy-adapted diabetes and CVD education in urban diabetic African Americans. *J Gen Intern Med* 23:1491–1494, 2008

Huizinga MM, Carlise AJ, Cavanaugh KL, Davis D, Greg RP, Schulnt DG, Rothman RL: Literacy, numeracy and portion size estimation skills. *Am J Prev Med* 36:324–328, 2009

Huizinga MM, Elasy TA, Wallston KA, Cavanaugh K, Davis D, Gregory RP, Fuchs LS, Malone R, Cherrington A, DeWalt DA, Buse J, Pignone M, Rothman RL: Development and validation of the diabetes numeracy test (DNT). *BMC Health Serv Res* 8:96–104, 2008

Institute of Medicine: *Health Literacy: A Prescription to End Confusion.* Washington, DC, National Academies Press, 2004

Jastak S, Wilkinson GS: *Wide Range Achievement Test.* Revised 3rd ed. Wilmington, DE, Jastak Associates, 1993

Jeppensen KM, Coyle JD, Miser WF: Screening questions to predict limited health literacy: a cross sectional study of patients with diabetes. *Ann Fam Med* 7:24–31, 2009

Kandula NR, Nsiah-Kumi PA, Makoul G, Sager J, Zei CP, Glass S, Stephens Q, Baker DW: The relationship between health literacy and knowledge improvement after a multimedia type 2 diabetes education program. *Patient Educ Couns* 75:321–327, 2009

Kessels RP: Patients' memory for medical visit information. *Jr Soc Med* 96:219, 2003

Kutner M, Greenberg E, Jin Y, Paulsen C: *The Health Literacy of America's Adults: Results from the 2003 National Assessment of Adult Literacy.* U.S. Department of Education. National Center for Education Statistics, 2006. Available from http://nces.ed.gov/pubsearch/pubsinfo.asp?pubid=2006483. Accessed 4 April 2012

Lee SD, Bender DE, Ruiz RE, Cho YI: Development of an easy to use Spanish health literacy test. *Health Serv Res* 4:1392–1412, 2006

Nath CR, Sylvester ST, Yasek V, Gunel E: Development and validation of a literacy assessment tool for persons with diabetes. *Diabetes Educ* 27:857–864, 2001

National Academy on an Aging Society (NAAS): Low health literacy skills increase annual health care expenditures by $73 billion. 1999. Available at www.agingsociety.org/agingsociety/publications/fact/fact_low.html. Accessed on 29 October 2011

National Patient Safety Foundation: AskMe3. Available at http://www.npsf.org/for-healthcare-professionals/programs/ask-me-3. Accessed on 29 October 2011

Ntiri DW, Stewart M: Transformative learning intervention: effect on functional health literacy and diabetes knowledge in older African Americans. *Gerontol Geriatr Educ* 30:100–113, 2009

Nutbeam D: Health promotion glossary. *Health Promot Int* 13:349–364, 1998

Osborn CY, Cavanaugh K, Wallston KA, Rothman RL: Self-efficacy links health literacy and numeracy to glycemic control. *J Health Commun* 15 (Suppl. 2):146–158, 2010

Osborn CY, Cavanaugh K, Wallston KA, White RO, Rothman RL: Diabetes numeracy: an overlooked factor in understanding racial disparities in glycemic control. *Diabetes Care* 32:1614–1619, 2009

Parikh NS, Parker RM, Nurss JR, Baker DW, Williams MV: Shame and health literacy: the unspoken connection. *Patient Educ Couns* 27:33–39, 1996

Parker RM, Baker DW, Williams MV, Nurss JR: The test of functional health literacy in adults: a new instrument for measuring patients' literacy skills. *J Gen Intern Med* 10:537–541, 1995

Powell CK, Hill EG, Clancy DE: The relationship between health literacy and diabetes knowledge and readiness to take health actions. *Diabetes Educ* 33:144–151, 2007

Roberts P, Fawcett G: *International Adult Literacy Survey: At Risk: A Socioeconomic Analysis of Health Literacy Among Seniors.* Canada, Ministry of Canada, category number 89-552, no. 5, 1998

Rothman R, Malone R, Horten C, DeWalt D, Pignone M: The relationship between literacy and glycemic control in a diabetes disease-management program. *Diabetes Educ* 30:263–273, 2004a

Rothman RL, DeWalt DA, Malone R, Bryant B, Shintani A, Crigler B, Weinberger M, Pignone M: Influence of patient literacy on the effectiveness of a primary care-based diabetes disease management program. *JAMA* 292:1711–1716, 2004b

Rothman RL, Housam R, Weiss H, Davis D, Gregory R, Gebretsadik T, Shintani A, Elasy TA: Patient understanding of food labels: the goal of literacy and numeracy. *Am J Prev Med* 31:391–398, 2006

Rothman RL, Malone R, Bryant B, Shintani AK, Crigler B, DeWalt DA, Dittus R, Weinberger M, Pignone MP: A randomized trial of a primary care-based disease management program to improve cardiovascular risk factors and glycated hemoglobin levels in patients with diabetes. *Am J Med* 118:276–284, 2005

Sarkar U, Fisher L, Schillinger D: Is self-efficacy associated with diabetes self-management across race/ethnicity and health literacy? *Diabetes Care* 29:823–829, 2006

Sarkar U, Karter AJ, Liu JY, Adler NE, Nguyen R, Lopez A, Schillinger D: The literacy divide: health literacy and the use of an Internet-based patient portal in an integrated health system: results of the diabetes study of northern California (DISTANCE). *J Health Comm* 15 (Suppl. 2):183–196, 2010b

Sarkar U, Karter AJ, Liu JY, Moffet HH, Adler NE, Schillinger D: Hypoglycemia is more common among type 2 diabetes patients with limited health literacy: the diabetes study of northern California (DISTANCE). *J Gen Intern Med* 25:962–968, 2010a

Sarkar U, Schillinger D, Lopez A, Sudore R: Validation of a self-reported health literacy question among diverse English and Spanish speaking populations. *J Gen Intern Med* 26:265–271, 2010c

Schillinger D, Bindman A, Stewart A, Wang F, Piette JD: Functional health literacy and the quality of physician-patient interpersonal communication. *Patient Educ Couns* 52:315–323, 2004

Schillinger D, Grumbach K, Piette JD, Wang F, Osmond D, Daher C, Palacious J, Sullivan GD, Bindman AD: Association of health literacy with diabetes outcomes. *JAMA* 288:475–482, 2002

Schillinger D, Hammer H, Wang F, Palacious J, McLean I, Tang A, Youmans S, Handley M: Seeing in 3-D: examining the reach of diabetes self-management support strategies in a public health care system. *Health Educ Behav* 35:664–682, 2008

Schillinger D, Handley M, Wang F, Hammer H: Effects of self-management support on structure, process, and outcomes among vulnerable patients with diabetes: a three-arm practical trial. *Diabetes Care* 32:559–566, 2009

Scott TL, Gazmararian JA, Williams MV, Baker DW: Health literacy and preventive health care use among mediate enrollees in a managed care organization. *Med Care* 40:395–404, 2002

Seligman HK, Wang FF, Palacious JL, Wilson CC, Daher C, Piette JD, Schillinger D: Physician notification of their diabetes patients' limited health literacy: a randomized trial. *J Gen Intern Med* 20:1001–1007, 2005

The Joint Commission: "What Did the Doctor Say?" Improving Health Literacy to Protect Patient Safety. 2007. Available at http://www.jointcommission.org/What_Did_the_Doctor_Say. Accessed on 11 June 2011

U.S. Department of Health and Human Services, Office of Disease Prevention and Health Promotion (USDHHS): Fact Sheet: Health Literacy and Health Outcomes. http://www.health.gov/communication/literacy/quickguide/factsbasic.htm. Accessed 20 April 2011

Vernon J, Trujillo AA, Rosenbaum S, DeBuono B: *Low Health Literacy: Implications for National Health Policy.* Storrs, CT, University of Connecticut, 2007

Wallace AS, Seligman HK, Davis TC, Schillinger D, Arnold CL, Bryant-Shilliday B, Freburger JK, DeWalt DA: Literacy-appropriate educational materials and brief counseling improve diabetes self-management. *Patient Educ Couns* 75:328–333, 2009

Weiss BD: *Health Literacy and Patient Safety-Help Patients Understand: Manual for Clinicians.* 2nd ed. American Medical Association and American Medical Association Foundation, 2007

Weiss BD, Mays MZ, Martz W, Castro KM, Pignone MP, Mockbee JH, Hale FA: Quick assessment of literacy in primary care: the newest vital sign. *Ann Fam Med* 3:514–522, 2005

Williams MV, Parker RM, Baker DW, Nurss JR: Relationship of functional health literacy to patients' knowledge of their chronic disease. *Arch Intern Med* 158:166–172, 1998

Williams MV, Parker RA, Baker DB, Parikh NS, Pitkin K, Coates WC, Nurss JR: Inadequate functional health literacy among patients at two public hospitals. *JAMA* 274:1677–1682, 1995

Wolf MS, Williams MV, Parker RM, Parikh NS, Nowlan AW, Baker DW: Patients' shame and attitudes towards discussing the results of literacy screening. *J Health Comm* 12:1–12, 2007

Wolff K, Cavanaugh K, Malone R, Hawk V, Gregory BP, Davis D, Wallston K, Rothman RL: The diabetes literacy and numeracy education toolkit (DLNET): materials to facilitate diabetes education and management in patients with low literacy and numeracy skills. *Diabetes Educ* 35:233–245, 2009

Marjorie Cypress PhD, CNP, CDE, is a Nurse Practitioner and Diabetes Educator at ABQ Health Partners in Albuquerque, NM, and the 2014 President of Healthcare and Education for the American Diabetes Association.

Chapter 24
Cost-Effectiveness of Diabetes Medical Nutrition Therapy

Carolyn C. Harrington, RD, CDE

Highlights

Literature Review

Translation of Evidence into Nutrition Interventions

Reimbursement for MNT

Summary

Highlights
Cost-Effectiveness of Diabetes Medical Nutrition Therapy

■ Clinical trials and outcomes research have provided evidence on the cost-effectiveness of medical nutrition therapy (MNT) for diabetes care provided by registered dietitians.

■ MNT is cost-effective in reducing diabetes comorbidities by improving lipid levels and blood pressure and reducing the need for medications.

■ Because MNT results in cost-savings and improved outcomes, MNT should be adequately covered by insurance and other payers (American Diabetes Association 2012).

Cost-Effectiveness of Diabetes Medical Nutrition Therapy

In 2007, the national cost of diabetes in the U.S. exceeded $174 billion (American Diabetes Association [ADA] 2008). This estimate includes $116 billion in excess medical expenditures attributed to diabetes, as well as $58 billion in reduced national productivity. Medical costs attributed to diabetes include $27 billion for direct expenses to treat diabetes, $58 billion to treat diabetes-related chronic complications, and $31 billion in excess general medical costs. The largest components of medical expenditures attributed to diabetes are hospital inpatient care (50% of total cost), diabetes medication and supplies (12%), retail prescriptions to treat diabetes complications (11%), and physician office visits (9%). On average, people with diagnosed diabetes have medical expenditures that are ~2.3 times higher than people without diabetes. One in five health care dollars is spent caring for someone with diabetes, and one in ten dollars spent on health care is attributed to diabetes and its complications. Indirect economic costs include absenteeism, reduced productivity, and lost productive capacity due to early mortality. The actual cost likely exceeds this $174 billion estimate, since it omits the social cost of intangibles such as pain and suffering, care provided by non-paid caregivers, and excess medical costs associated with undiagnosed diabetes. The burden of diabetes is imposed on all sectors of society—higher insurance premiums paid by employees and employers, reduced earnings through productivity loss, and reduced overall quality of life for people with diabetes and their families (ADA 2008). It is projected that the incidence of diagnosed and undiagnosed diabetes will reach ~53 million Americans, at a cost of $514 billion by 2025 (Institute for Alternative Futures 2011). Without significant changes in public or private strategies, this population and cost growth is expected to add significant strain to an already-burdened health care system (Huang 2009). It is imperative that medical nutrition therapy (MNT) be provided early in the diabetes disease process to aid in reducing the costs and burdens of this devastating condition.

LITERATURE REVIEW

A literature search was conducted using the Academy of Nutrition and Dietetics Evidence Analysis Library and PubMed MEDLINE, with additional articles identified from reference lists (Table 24.1). The search identified 28 articles and all of these articles were retrieved for review. In addition, three articles were identified from reference lists. Seven articles met inclusion criteria and are listed in Table 24.1. Search criteria were specific to the cost-effectiveness of MNT. Articles

Table 24.1 Studies Reporting Cost-Effectiveness of MNT for Diabetes

	Population/ Duration of Study	Intervention (type of study)	Major Findings	Comments
Franz 1995	n = 179 adults with type 2 diabetes/6 months	Basic care vs. PGC (RCT)	Fasting plasma glucose and A1C ↓ more in PGC group; cost-effective because of ↓ use of medications	Short-term study; small sample size for economic evaluation
Sheils 1999	n = 12,308 adults ≥55 years of age with diabetes, 10,895 with cardiovascular disease, and 3,328 with renal disease/6 years	Outcomes from the implementation of MNT (review)	MNT associated with a ↓ in use of hospital services of 9.5% for patients with diabetes and ↓ use of physician services by 23.5%	
Wolf 2004, 2007, 2009 (one study)	n = 147 adults with type 2 diabetes and obesity/1 year	Lifestyle intervention by an RD vs. usual medical care by a physician (RCT)	Lifestyle intervention ↓ risk of lost workdays by 63% and disability days by 87.2% vs. individual receiving usual medical care	Short-term study; small sample size for economic evaluation; generalizable to insured population only
Cho 2008	n = 67 adults with type 2 diabetes/6 months/1 or 3 visits	Hospitals providing basic nutrition education (1 visit) vs. intensive nutrition education by RD (3 visits) (RCT)	MNT by RDs resulted in significant improvements in medical and clinical outcomes vs. basic nutrition education, reducing costs	Short-term study; small sample size
Robbins 2008	n = 18,404 people with any diabetes diagnosis/7 years, 10 months	Observational study of diabetes education classes vs. individual nutritionist visit(s)	Nutritionist visits more strongly associated with reduced hospitalizations than diabetes classes	

Population/ Duration of Study	Intervention (type of study)	Major Findings	Comments
Coppell 2010	$n = 93$ adults under age 70 years with type 2 diabetes/6 months	Intensive individualized MNT by RD vs. usual care by general practitioner (RCT)	Intensive MNT achieved ↓ in A1C ($P = 0.007$) and weight ($P = 0.032$); ↓ in insulin and hypoglycemic drugs and ↓ need to add new drugs led to cost savings	Short-term study, but the high retention rate and the use of internationally accepted nutrition guidelines were strengths
Bertram 2010	Epidemiological modeling approach/not applicable	Six interventions: three pharmaceutical therapies (acarbose, metformin, orlistat) and three lifestyle interventions (diet alone, exercise alone, diet and exercise) (time series)	Diet and exercise combined or metformin are the most cost-effective intervention; incremental addition of one intervention to the other is not cost-effective	

FPG, fasting plasma glucose; PGC, practice guidelines nutrition care; RCT, randomized controlled trial.

that focused primarily on the cost-effectiveness of diabetes self-management education/training were eliminated.

TRANSLATION OF EVIDENCE INTO NUTRITION INTERVENTIONS

MNT implemented by registered dietitians (RDs) results in reductions in A1C, ranging from 0.5 to 2.9% (average of ~1–2%), depending on the type and duration of diabetes. These results were similar to the effects of many glucose-lowering medications (Franz 2008). Multiple studies have demonstrated sustained improvements in A1C at 12 months and longer when nutrition therapy is provided in follow-up visits ranging from monthly to three sessions per year (see Chapter 1 for information on the effectiveness of nutrition therapy in diabetes).

In an econometric study of 12,308 patients with diabetes, the potential savings from MNT was measured and the net cost to Medicare of covering these services for Medicare enrollees was estimated. MNT was associated with a 9.5% reduction in use of hospital services and a 23.5% reduction in use of physician services for individuals with diabetes. The authors concluded that after an initial period of implementation, coverage for MNT can result in a net reduction in health services use and costs. In individuals aged ≥55 years, the savings will actually exceed the cost of providing the MNT benefit (Sheils 1999).

In a more recent review of the cost-effectiveness of diabetes education, nutritionist visits were more strongly associated with reduced hospitalizations than diabetes classes. Each nutritionist visit was associated with a substantial reduction in hospital charges, suggesting that providing these services in the primary care setting may be highly cost-effective for the health care system (Robbins 2008).

Absenteeism and disability are indirect indicators of health and are costly not only to patients but also to employers (Wolf 2009). Diabetes is associated with elevated rates of lost productivity and disability. In 2007, people with diabetes lost 15 million days of work because of diabetes, costing the U.S. economy approximately $2.6 billion (ADA 2008). Provision of an RD-led lifestyle intervention of six individual sessions, plus six 1-h small group sessions, along with brief monthly phone contacts over 1 year to people with diabetes was found to significantly reduce the risk of having lost workdays by 64.3% and disability days by 87.2% (Wolf 2009). People who received lifestyle case management by an RD also had substantially greater weight loss, decreased prescription medication use, and improved health-related quality of life compared to usual medical care (Wolf 2004). Case management participants also had fewer inpatient admissions, which substantially lowered medical costs (Wolf 2007).

When considering the comorbidities of diabetes, such as cardiovascular disease, prevention through the provision of MNT is also cost-effective. People with diabetes have twice the risk for coronary heart disease and stroke as people without diabetes (Centers for Disease Control and Prevention [CDC] 2002). Subjects who received group MNT by RDs in a 6-month randomized trial were reported to have a 6% decrease in total and LDL cholesterol levels compared with the group not receiving MNT. Results revealed a savings of $4.28 for each dollar spent on MNT compared with the cost of statin therapy (Delahanty 2001). An 8.6% reduction in hospital use and 16.9% reduction in physician visits associated with MNT was documented for patients with cardiovascular disease (Sheils 1999). In a study of 64 obese men with hypertension assigned to diet treatment (reduce weight by >5%, restrict sodium to <1,700 mg/day, and decrease alcohol intake if consuming >9 oz/week) or drug treatment (atenolol), the nutrition intervention was shown to be cost-effective (Johannesson 1992). Most diabetes-attributed costs are from the microvascular and macrovascular complications that increase the use of medical services. Studies such as these suggest that MNT can be a cost-effective strategy for reducing the long-term complications of diabetes.

REIMBURSEMENT FOR MNT

It is the position of the Academy of Nutrition and Dietetics (formerly the American Dietetic Association) that MNT is effective in treating disease and preventing disease complications, resulting in health benefits and cost-savings for the public. Therefore, MNT provided by RDs is an essential reimbursable component of comprehensive health care services (American Dietetic Association 1995). Current procedural terminology (CPT) codes and billing procedures for MNT within government-funded programs and private sector insurance plans have varied and have been widely interpreted by carriers and billing agencies. The regulations for billing Medicare Part B for MNT services are clearly defined by the Centers for Medicare & Medicaid Services (CMS) (www.cms.gov). Since 1 January 2002, RDs have been able to bill Medicare Part B for MNT provided to patients with diabetes and/or renal disease using CPT codes 97802, 97803, or

97804. This Medicare benefit allows 3 h of MNT in the first referral year and 2 h in each subsequent calendar year. At the time of publication, Medicare Part B does not cover MNT for prediabetes or cardiovascular disease. Many private payers recognize the MNT CPT codes for diagnoses such as prediabetes, diabetes, obesity, hyperlipidemia, and hypertension. Individuals with diabetes should be encouraged to contact their health plan provider to determine their benefits for MNT.

SUMMARY

Diabetes is a costly and devastating disease. Lifestyle modification (MNT plus exercise) in people with prediabetes is cost-effective and should be recommended to prevent or slow the onset of diabetes (Bertram 2010). Diabetes prevention is more cost-effective than diabetes treatment (Urbanski 2008). Clinical trials and outcomes research have provided evidence on the cost-effectiveness of MNT for diabetes care provided by RDs. When RDs are involved in active decision-making about interventions such as nutrition prescriptions, number of visits needed, and medication changes, cost-effectiveness is enhanced (Franz 1996). Health care costs such as hospitalizations, doctor visits, and medications can be reduced when people with diabetes receive MNT by an RD. MNT provided by RDs is vital early in the disease process to delay and prevent the costly complications of diabetes.

BIBLIOGRAPHY

American Diabetes Association: Economic costs of diabetes in the U.S. in 2007. *Diabetes Care* 31:596–615, 2008

American Diabetes Association: Standards of medical care in diabetes: 2012. *Diabetes Care* 35 (Suppl. 1):S11–S63, 2012

American Dietetic Association: Position of the American Dietetic Association: cost-effectiveness of medical nutrition therapy. *J Am Diet Assoc* 95:88–91, 1995

Bertram MY, Lim SS, Barendregt JJ, Vos T: Assessing the cost-effectiveness of drug and lifestyle intervention following opportunistic screening for pre-diabetes in primary care. *Diabetologia* 53:875–881, 2010

CDC Diabetes Cost-Effectiveness Group: Cost-effectiveness of intensive glycemic control, intensified hypertension control, and serum cholesterol level reduction for type 2 diabetes. *JAMA* 287:2542–2551, 2002

Cho Y, Lee M, Jang H, Rha M, Kim J, Park Y, Sohn C: The clinical and cost effectiveness of medical nutrition therapy for patients with type 2 diabetes mellitus. *Korean J Nutr* 41:147–155, 2008

Coppell KJ, Kataoka M, Williams SM, Chisholm AW, Vorgers SM, Mann JI: Nutritional intervention in patients with type 2 diabetes who are hyperglycaemic despite optimized drug treatment: Lifestyle Over and Above Drugs in Diabetes (LOADD) study: randomized controlled trial. *BMJ* 341:c3337, 2010

Delehanty LM, Sonnenberg LM, Hayden D, Nathan DM: Clinical and cost outcomes of medical nutrition therapy for hypercholesterolemia: a controlled trial. *J Am Diet Assoc* 101:1012–1023, 2001

Franz MJ, Boucher JL, Green-Pastors J, Powers MA: Evidence-based nutrition practice guidelines for diabetes and scope and standards of practice. *J Am Diet Assoc* 108:S52–S58, 2008

Franz MJ, Monk A, Bergenstal R, Mazze R: Outcomes and cost-effectiveness of medical nutrition therapy for non-insulin-dependent diabetes mellitus. *Diabetes Spectrum* 9:122–127, 1996

Franz MJ, Splett PL, Monk A, Barry B, McLain K, Weaver T, Upham P, Bergenstal R, Mazze R: Cost-effectiveness of medical nutrition therapy provided by dietitians for persons with non-insulin dependent diabetes mellitus. *J Am Diet Assoc* 95:1018–1024, 1995

Huang ES, Basu A, O'Grady M, Capretta JC: Projecting the future diabetes population size and related costs for the U.S. *Diabetes Care* 32:2225–2229, 2009

Institute for Alternative Futures: Diabetes 2025. Available at www.altfutures.org/diabetes2025. Accessed on 17 July 2011

Johannesson M, Fagerberg B: A health-economic comparison of diet and drug treatment in obese men with mild hypertension. *J Hypertens* 10:1063–1070, 1992

Robbins JM, Thatcher GE, Webb DA, Valdmanis VG: Nutritionist visits, diabetes classes and hospitalization rates and charges: the Urban Diabetes Study. *Diabetes Care* 31:655–660, 2008

Sheils JF, Rubin R, Stapleton DC: The estimated costs and savings of medical nutrition therapy: the Medicare population. *J Am Diet Assoc* 99:428–435, 1999

Urbanski P, Wolf A, Herman WH: Cost-effectiveness of diabetes education. *J Am Diet Assoc* 108 (Suppl. 1):6–11, 2008

Wolf AM, Conaway MR, Crowther JQ, Hazen KY, Nadler JL, Oneida B, Bovbjerg VE: Translating lifestyle intervention to practice in obese patients with type 2 diabetes: Improving Control with Activity and Nutrition (ICAN). *Diabetes Care* 27:1570–1576, 2004

Wolf AM, Siadaty MS, Crowther JQ, Nadler JL, Wagner DL, Cavalieri SL, Elward KS, Bovbjerg VE: Impact of lifestyle intervention on lost productivity and disability: improving control with activity and nutrition. *J Occup Environ Med* 51:139–145, 2009

Wolf AM, Siadaty M, Yaeger B, Crowther JQ, Conaway M, Nadler J, Bovberg VE: Effects of lifestyle intervention on health care costs: Improving Control with Activity and Nutrition (ICAN). *J Am Diet Assoc* 107:1365–1373, 2007

Carolyn C. Harrington, RD, CDE, is a Diabetes Education Specialist in Venice, FL.

Chapter 25
Nutrition Therapy and Prediabetes

Gretchen Youssef, MS, RD, CDE

Highlights
Nutrition Therapy and Prediabetes

■ In individuals with prediabetes, lifestyle interventions including modest weight loss (5–7% of body weight) and moderate physical activity (equivalent to 30 min brisk walking on most days of the week) are effective in decreasing the risk of converting to diabetes by 29–67%. The impact of this level of lifestyle intervention in preventing and/or delaying the onset of type 2 diabetes can persist for at least 10 years.

■ Large randomized controlled trials for preventing type 2 diabetes have repeatedly confirmed that lifestyle interventions are effective in all ethnic groups, different age-groups, and various social and cultural settings worldwide.

■ Physical activity should be recommended to prevent type 2 diabetes, not only for its weight-management benefits, but also for improving metabolic markers, including insulin sensitivity, an important factor in prevention. The recommendation of 2.5 h of physical activity per week is evidence-based, is generally considered feasible, and can be fulfilled by brisk walking and/or other equivalent forms of physical activity.

■ Evidence suggests that an eating pattern high in saturated and *trans* fatty acids is associated with increased markers of insulin resistance and risk for type 2 diabetes; therefore, saturated fat intake should be decreased.

■ At this time, there are no randomized clinical trials on the efficacy of low-carbohydrate diets in diabetes prevention. Conversely, epidemiological studies do not support the premise that dietary patterns high in carbohydrate cause insulin resistance and type 2 diabetes. It is more likely that overweight/obesity and the accompanying insulin resistance are the consequences of consuming excess energy from all nutrient sources, including carbohydrates and saturated fat.

■ Intake of sugar-sweetened beverages is associated with increased risk for type 2 diabetes. Individuals at risk for type 2 diabetes should be encouraged to limit their intake of sugar-sweetened beverages.

■ Adhering to a combination of healthy lifestyle habits (a healthy eating pattern, participating in regular physical activity, maintaining a normal body weight, moderate alcohol intake, and being a nonsmoker) can reduce the risk of developing type 2 diabetes by as much as 84% for women and 72% for men.

Nutrition Therapy and Prediabetes

Scientific evidence has demonstrated that type 2 diabetes is, to a large extent, a preventable disease. Yet, worldwide, type 2 diabetes is reaching epidemic proportions, with an estimated 366 million people currently having the disease, and projections are that >552 million people, representing fully 7.7% of the world's population, will have this disorder by 2030 (International Diabetes Federation 2011). Furthermore, impaired glucose tolerance (IGT), the precursor to diabetes, affected >280 million people worldwide in 2011, and that number is estimated to increase to 398 million by 2030. In the U.S., >26 million people have diabetes, and an additional 79 million individuals over the age of 20 years are estimated to have prediabetes. If current trends continue, a staggering one in three children born in 2000 in the U.S. will have diabetes by 2050 (Centers for Disease Control and Prevention [CDC] 2011). Also, disturbingly, type 2 diabetes, once considered an adult disease, is now being diagnosed with increasing frequency in children and adolescents. Prediabetes, indicating a high risk for diabetes, refers to individuals with impaired fasting glucose (fasting glucose of 100–125 mg/dL) and/or IGT (2-h post-glucose value during an oral glucose tolerance test of 140–199 mg/dL).

An epidemic of overweight and obesity parallels the type 2 diabetes epidemic. BMI, a risk factor for diabetes, increased 0.4 kg/m^2 per decade from 1980 to 2008 (Finucane 2011). In the U.S., males had the greatest increase in BMI at 1.1 kg/m^2 per decade compared to other high-income countries. In 2008, it was estimated that 1.46 billion adults worldwide have a BMI of ≥25 kg/m^2 and that 502 million of them are obese. Factors that play a role in overweight and obesity include the following: energy imbalance, physical inactivity, genetics, metabolism, behavior, environment, culture, and socioeconomic status (CDC 2011). As the rates of obesity and diabetes continue to grow, there is an urgent need to focus on evidence-based modifiable risk factors such as eating patterns, physical activity, and environmental changes that could halt the twin epidemics, thus preventing type 2 diabetes and its comorbidities and mortality.

This chapter begins with a summary of lifestyle and diabetes prevention from the 1999 book *American Diabetes Association Guide to Medical Nutrition Therapy for Diabetes* (Wing 1999) and reviews and updates the evidence on intensive lifestyle interventions, weight-loss interventions, physical activity, macronutrients, micronutrients, and eating patterns in the prevention of diabetes. A literature search was conducted using Ovid MEDLINE, and additional articles were identified from reference lists. Search criteria included diabetes prevention in human subjects and English language articles and publication after the completion of the 1999 chapter on lifestyle and the prevention of diabetes. Subject headings included in the online search were type 2 diabetes (prevention and control), lifestyle, diet, and physical activity/exercise. The initial search of potentially relevant articles identified 255 articles, of which 204 articles were excluded because titles or abstracts did not meet inclusion criteria. A total of 51 articles were retrieved for more detailed evaluation. Of these, 24 were included and 38 were added, making a total of 62 articles that met inclusion criteria. Twenty-five primary studies (14 randomized clinical trials, 11 epidemiological studies) and 14 systematic reviews or meta-analyses are included in the table.

The 1999 chapter concluded that modest amounts of weight loss (5–10%) and an increase in physical activity (500 to 1000 calories/week) may be sufficient to reduce the risk of diabetes. Intervention studies at that time supported the benefits of lifestyle interventions, but methodological limitations prevented the author from making definite conclusions. Since the 1999 book was published, large randomized controlled trials (RCTs) have been performed and have produced follow-up data, which will be discussed in this chapter.

INTERVENTION TRIALS TO PREVENT DIABETES

Results from large RCTs in the U.S., China, Finland, Japan, and India demonstrated that lifestyle interventions reduce the relative risk of developing diabetes (29–67% across the studies) in people with prediabetes (Pan 1997; Tuomilehto 2001; Diabetes Prevention Program [DPP] 2002; Kosaka 2005; Ramachandran 2006). The goals of modest weight loss (usually 5–7% of body weight) and moderate physical activity on most days of the week were consistent across the trials. The common components among all of the lifestyle interventions were increasing physical activity, decreasing energy and fat intake, and choosing more nutrient-rich foods.

Lifestyle Interventions for Diabetes Prevention

The U.S. DPP reduced the incidence of diabetes by 58% compared to metformin (31%) and placebo. At study end, 38% of the participants were at the 7% weight loss goal and 58% met the minimum goal of 150 min of physical activity per week. Mean weight loss at study end was significant (5.6 kg in the lifestyle group, 2.1 kg in the metformin group, and 0.1 kg in the placebo group) (DPP 2002). Of interest is the 10 years from baseline follow-up, in which the diabetes incidence rates were similar between treatment groups, but the cumulative incidence remained the lowest in the lifestyle intervention group (DPP 2009).

In the Finnish Diabetes Prevention Study at year 1, 43% of lifestyle intervention participants met the 5% weight loss goal, with a mean weight loss of 4.2 kg. At the end of the study, there was a 58% reduction of the conversion to diabetes compared to the control group, with cumulative incidence of diabetes being less than half that in the control group. At 7 years from baseline, follow-up revealed that participants in the intervention group continued lifestyle changes after the individual lifestyle counseling was stopped. Success in achieving intervention goals was related to continued reduction in diabetes incidence (Lindstrom 2006).

In the Da Qing IGT and Diabetes Study, 6 years of risk reduction in developing diabetes was 33% in the diet only group, 47% in the exercise group, and 38% in the diet plus exercise group (Pan 1997). In the longest follow-up at this time, the group-based lifestyle intervention over 6 years continued to prevent or delay diabetes for up to 14 years after the active intervention (Li 2008).

A Japanese trial using lifestyle intervention in males with IGT demonstrated a 67.4% risk reduction in diabetes. Weight loss in the control and lifestyle intervention groups was 0.39 and 2.18 kg, respectively. In both the control and intervention groups, there was a positive correlation to change in BMI and incidence of diabetes (Kosaka 2005).

The Indian Diabetes Prevention Program randomized young Asian Indians with IGT to a control group, lifestyle modification (LSM) group, or metformin plus LSM group. Cumulative incidence of diabetes in the control group (55%) was much higher than that seen in the other major diabetes prevention programs. Total relative risk reduction was 28.5% for LSM, 26.4% for metformin, and 28.2% for LSM and metformin. There was no added benefit to adding metformin to LSM. Weight loss was not significant in any of the groups (Ramachandran 2006). (See Table 25.1.)

Pharmacological Agents for Diabetes Prevention

Pharmacological agents including metformin, α-glucosidase inhibitors, orlistat, and thiazolidinediones have been shown to decrease the rate of diabetes (range: from 25 to 75%) (American Diabetes Association [ADA] 2012). At this time, the U.S. Food and Drug Administration has not approved any of these agents for the treatment of prediabetes. Because of cost, adverse events, and lack of persistent effect of the medications, metformin is the only drug recommended for use in prediabetes at this time (ADA 2012). The ADA recommends that people with prediabetes be counseled on lifestyle changes with goals similar to those of the DPP—7% weight loss and 150 min physical activity per week. Metformin therapy for prevention of diabetes might be reasonably recommended in individuals with IGT, IFG, or an A1C of 5.6–6.4%, especially for people with very high risk of diabetes, including individuals with a history of gestational diabetes, those who are very obese, and/or those with progressive hyperglycemia. As demonstrated in the DPP, individuals who would benefit least from metformin are individuals with a BMI <35 kg/m^2 and individuals >60 years of age (DPP 2002).

Conclusions

Trials to prevent type 2 diabetes have repeatedly confirmed that lifestyle interventions are effective in all ethnic groups and in various social and cultural settings worldwide. Furthermore, it appears that individuals who changed and maintained their lifestyle to a desirable level were protected the most against risk of diabetes. Lifestyle interventions are safe and they promote healthy behaviors that have multiple health benefits.

PHYSICAL ACTIVITY AND PREVENTION OF TYPE 2 DIABETES

Evidence that regular physical activity plays a key role in the prevention of type 2 diabetes was demonstrated in landmark clinical trials such as the DPP and the Finnish Diabetes Prevention Study (DPP 2001; Tuomilehto 2001). Nonetheless, the 2008 National Health Interview Survey revealed that, in the U.S., only 33% of adults engaged in leisure-time physical activity on a regular basis (three or more sessions per week of vigorous activity lasting at least 20 min or five or more sessions per week of light/moderate activity lasting at least 30 min in duration), 31% participated in

Table 25.1 Studies of Lifestyle Intervention Trials

	Population/ Duration of Study	Intervention (type of study)	Major Findings	Comments
Pan 1997	$n = 577$ adults from 33 clinics in China (age 45 years, BMI 25.8 kg/m², IGT)/6 years	Randomized by clinics: 1) control, 2) diet, 3) exercise, 4) diet + exercise; counseling by physician and then group counseling (RCT)	Cumulative diabetes incidence: 68% usual care, 44% diet, 41% exercise, 46% diet + exercise; reduction in diabetes: 33% in diet only ($P < 0.03$), 47% in exercise ($P < 0.005$), 38% in diet + exercise ($P < 0.005$)	Relative ↓ in rate of conversion to diabetes in all three treatment groups similar when patients stratified as lean or overweight
Tuomilehto 2001	$n = 522$ adults (age 40–60 years, BMI ≥25 kg/m², 100% IGT)/3.2 years	LI: individualized counseling (↓ weight 5%, <30% kcal fat, <10% saturated fat, ↑ fiber 15 g/1,000 kcal, 30 min/day moderate exercise) vs. control group; year 1, 17 sessions with nutritionist, every 3 months after year 1 (RCT)	LI group: 58% ↓ risk of type 2 diabetes ($P < 0.001$); cumulative incidence of diabetes 11% in IL and 23% in control	
Diabetes Prevention Program Research Group 2002	$n = 1,079$ adults (age ≥25 years, BMI ≥24 kg/m², 100% IGT)/2.8 years	LI: goal-based, frequent contact, individualized; goals (7% weight loss, ≥150 min/week physical activity) vs. metformin (850 mg two times daily) vs. control (RCT)	LI: twice as effective as metformin, ↓ type 2 diabetes by 58%; metformin: ↓ incidence by 31%; 38% in LI met the 7% weight loss goal	
Kosaka 2005	$n = 458$ males in Japan (BMI 24 kg/m², IGT)/4 years	LI (goal BMI ≤22 kg/m², smaller portions, ≤50 g fat/day, ↓ in alcohol, physical activity of 30–40 min/day) vs. control (RCT)	LI: 4-year incidence 3.0 vs. 9.3% in control; RR ↓ in LI group 67.4% ($P < 0.001$); weight ↓ 2.18 kg in LI and 0.39 kg in control ($P < 0.001$)	Authors noted that ↓ or ↑ of 2 kg weight associated with large difference in glucose tolerance
Ramachandran 2006	$n = 531$ Asian Indians (IGT, BMI 25.8 kg/m², 46 years)/30 months	Randomized by clinic: 1) control, 2) LSM, 3) metformin (250 mg BID), 4) LSM + metformin (LSM = brisk walking 30 min/day; diet ↓ in total kcal, refined carbohydrate, fats; avoidance of sugar; ↑ in high-fiber foods) (RCT)	Cumulative incidence of diabetes: 39.3% control, 40.5% metformin, 39.5% LSM + metformin, 55% control; RR ↓ of diabetes: LSM 29%, metformin 26.4%, LSM + metformin 28.2%	Younger, leaner, and more insulin resistant than patients in other trials; low dose of metformin due to adverse events

	Population/ Duration of Study	Intervention (type of study)	Major Findings	Comments
Lindstrom 2006	n = 475 participants in the Finnish Diabetes Prevention Study/3 years after the 4-year follow-up (7 years)	Participants still free of diabetes at 4 years assessed to determine diabetes risk reduction after discontinuation of active counseling (RCT)	LI maintained after the intervention; diabetes incidence rates were 4.6 and 7.2 per 100 person-years in LI vs. control (P = 0.0401), 36% ↓ in RR	Intervention group sustained lifestyle changes and reduction in diabetes incidence
Li 2008	n = 577 adults from 33 clinics in China/14 years follow-up (20 years)	Assessment of long-term effects of interventions (RCT)	Compared with control, combined LI groups had 51% ↓ incidence of diabetes at 6 years and 43% ↓ over 20 years	No significant differences between IL and control groups in reduced CVD and mortality
Diabetes Prevention Program Research Group 2009	n = 2,766 of 3,159 (88%) DPP participants/5.7 years follow-up (10 years)	Persistence of DPP 2.8-year effects long term (RCT)	LI group lost and then partly regained weight, weight loss with metformin maintained; 34% ↓ diabetes incidence in LI, 18% ↓ in metformin vs. placebo group	Prevention or delay of diabetes with LI or metformin can persist for at least 10 years

LI, lifestyle intervention.

some leisure-time physical activity (adults classified as having some leisure-time activity reported at least one session of light/moderate or vigorous physical activity of at least 10 min duration but did not meet the definition of regular leisure-time activity), and fully 36% were considered inactive (no sessions of light/moderate or vigorous leisure-time activity of at least 10 min duration) (Pleis 2009). In view of the burgeoning national obesity and diabetes epidemic, suboptimal levels of physical activity constitute an ongoing significant public health concern.

Regular physical activity enables prevention of type 2 diabetes, not only through promoting weight management, but also through reduction in insulin resistance, independent of weight loss, in both normal and insulin-resistant individuals (Duncan 2003; Laaksonen 2005). Mechanisms for improved insulin sensitivity are a twofold increase in insulin-stimulated glycogen synthesis in muscle due to an increase in insulin-stimulated glucose transport phosphorylation (Perseghin 1996). In addition, while initial weight loss may be accomplished in the individual with prediabetes through restriction of energy intake alone, the National Weight Loss Registry (NWLR) longitudinal follow-up of people who successfully lost and maintained ≥30 lb for 1 year or longer reported that 90% of these individuals exercised, on average, about 1 h/day (NWLR 2011). This suggests that maintenance of weight loss cannot be accomplished without regular physical activity.

A meta-analysis of 10 prospective cohort studies found that moderate physical activity reduced the risk of type 2 diabetes (Jeon 2007). Examples of moderate activities include a brisk walk of 3.5 miles/h, playing golf, or biking at 10 miles/h.

The U.S. Department of Health and Human Services (DHHS) 2008 Physical Activity Guidelines recommend 2 h and 30 min of moderate-intensity physical activity each week, which is equivalent to 30 min of brisk walking on most days of the week for adults (DHHS 2008). This recommendation is consistent with the interventions implemented in most of the lifestyle intervention trials. For additional health benefits, it is recommended that individuals increase to 5 h of moderate-intensity exercise per week or 2 h and 30 min of vigorous-intensity exercise per week. In addition, muscle-strengthening exercises (resistance training) are encouraged two or more times per week, since resistance training provides bone-strengthening and other health benefits (Dietary Guidelines Advisory Committee [DGAC] 2010).

In summary, physical activity should be recommended to prevent diabetes, not only for the weight-management benefits, but also for improving metabolic markers, including insulin sensitivity, an important factor in preventing type 2 diabetes. The recommendation of 2 h and 30 min of physical activity per week is evidence-based, would generally be considered feasible, and can be fulfilled by brisk walking and/or other equivalent forms of exercise. (See Table 25.2.)

Table 25.2 Studies Reviewing the Role of Physical Activity in the Prevention of Diabetes

	Population/ Duration of Study	Intervention (type of study)	Major Findings	Comments
Duncan 2003	n = 18 sedentary adults without diabetes/6 months	Walking 30 min at high intensity, high frequency, vs. high intensity, low frequency, vs. moderate intensity, high frequency/RCT	Exercise without weight loss increases S_i ($P <$ 0.005) and post-heparin plasma lipase ($P < 0.001$) activity in previously sedentary adults	Regular aerobic exercise increases S_i and markers of lipid metabolism, independent of weight loss
Laaksonen 2005	n = 487 adults with IGT (Finnish Diabetes Prevention Study)/4.1 years	Post hoc analysis of the role of LTPA in preventing type 2 diabetes (RCT)	↑ LTPA from moderate to vigorous or strenuous: 63–65% ↓ in type 2 diabetes; low-intensity PA and walking also of benefit	Author conclusions: LTPA ↓ diabetes risk through mechanisms beyond weight loss alone
Jeon 2007	n = 10 prospective cohort studies on PA (301,221 participants and 9,367 incident cases of diabetes)/not applicable	Association of PA of moderate intensity and risk of type 2 diabetes (systematic review)	Regular PA of moderate intensity (RR 0.69) vs. being sedentary; walking ≥2.5 h/ week (RR 0.70) vs. no walking	Association independent of BMI suggests moderate-intensity PA without achieving weight loss may still ↓ type 2 diabetes risk

LTPA, leisure-time physical activity; PA, physical activity; S_i, insulin sensitivity.

MACRONUTRIENTS AND PREVENTION OF TYPE 2 DIABETES

Carbohydrate

The role of carbohydrate in the prevention of diabetes is a popular topic in consumer publications, and recommendations are usually not evidence-based. This section will focus on the research that has been conducted investigating the role of carbohydrate intake and insulin resistance, consumption of sugar-sweetened beverages, glycemic index (GI) eating pattern, and the role of whole grains in the prevention of diabetes.

Carbohydrate and insulin resistance. Dietary carbohydrate is often discussed in the lay press and in many popular diets (e.g., Atkins Diet, South Beach Diet), suggesting that a high-carbohydrate content may be implicated in the development of insulin resistance, a metabolic disorder that predisposes to the onset of type 2 diabetes. However, at this time, there are no clinical trials on the efficacy of low-carbohydrate diets in diabetes prevention, and epidemiological studies do not support the premise that eating patterns high in carbohydrate cause insulin resistance and type 2 diabetes. It is more likely that overweight/obesity and accompanying insulin resistance are not simply a result of high-carbohydrate intake, but rather a combination of consumption of excess calories from all nutrient sources, including carbohydrates and saturated fat (Bessesen 2001; McClenaghan 2005; DGAC 2010).

Sugar-sweetened beverages. In the U.S., sugar-sweetened beverage intake has more than doubled, from 64.4 to 141.7 kcal/day in the past four decades. These beverages have been implicated as a contributing factor to the current obesity epidemic. Sugar-sweetened beverages include soft drinks, fruit drinks, iced tea, and energy and vitamin water drinks containing sucrose, high-fructose corn syrup, and/or fruit juice concentrates (Malik 2010). In a meta-analysis of eight prospective cohort studies (n = 310,819), a diet high in consumption of sugar-sweetened beverages was associated with the development of type 2 diabetes (n = 15,043). Individuals in the lowest quantile of sugar-sweetened beverage intake (0 or <1 serving per month) compared with the highest quantile (2 or more servings/day) had a 1.26 relative risk of diabetes or 26% greater risk of developing diabetes (Malik 2010).

Sugar-sweetened beverages have dense calorie volume, which when combined with low satiety value, can contribute to weight gain. Excessive consumption of sugar-sweetened beverages can lead to increased blood glucose and insulin levels, induction of glucose intolerance, and insulin resistance. These, in turn, are implicated in β-cell function decline. Sugar-sweetened beverages also contribute to visceral adiposity and increase in inflammatory markers, such as C-reactive protein, which are elevated in uncontrolled type 2 diabetes and implicated in the pathogenesis of atherosclerosis (Hu 2011; Malik 2010).

GI or glycemic load. GI is a numerical scale that has received attention as a tool that may be used to rank carbohydrate foods according to their effect on postprandial glucose. However, in a review of 10 longitudinal prospective observational studies published since 2000, the DGAC 2010 concluded that evidence is mixed as to whether there is an association between high-GI diets and type 2 diabetes. Five of the studies showed a positive association between GI and type 2 diabetes, four of the studies showed no association, and one demonstrated an inverse relationship. In addition, there is little evidence that a high glycemic load (grams of carbohydrate in a food serving × GI = glycemic load) is associated with type 2 diabetes (DGAC 2010). Although there is no evidence to support a low-GI eating pattern in diabetes prevention, the ADA recommends that low-GI foods rich in fiber and nutrient-dense foods should be encouraged (ADA 2008). Some examples of low-GI foods are oats, legumes, dairy products, and fruits.

Whole grains. Whole-grain foods are a source of fiber and other nutrients. Americans consume an average of 6.3 servings of refined grains per day. The DGAC recommends no more than 3 servings of refined grains per day, with at least half of all servings of grains coming from whole grains (U.S. Department of Agriculture [USDA] DHHS 2010). In the U.S., <95% of the 19- to 50-year-old individuals surveyed from 1999 to 2004 reported that they ate at least three servings of whole-grain foods per day, leaving at least 95% of people consuming inadequate amounts of whole-grain foods (O'Neil 2010).

Potential mechanisms for improvement in metabolic control provided by whole-grain foods include the following: modulation of secretion of certain gut hormones, improved insulin sensitivity, effects on metabolic and inflammatory markers, shift in the relation of gut microbiotic communities, and environmental/dietary influences on genetic risk (Nettleton 2010; Weickert 2008).

Several reviews of observational studies demonstrated an inverse relationship for the risk of type 2 diabetes and consumption of whole-grain foods (de Munter 2007; Priebe 2009; Sun 2010). The DGAC reviews of several studies demonstrated similar findings (USDA DHHS 2010).

Meta-analyses of 14 cohort studies demonstrated an inverse relationship between whole-grain intake and fasting glucose and insulin levels with incremental decreases with each serving of whole grains (Nettleton 2010). However, the WHOLEheart trial, a 4-month RCT, saw no improvement in insulin and glucose levels with intake of whole-grain foods (Brownlee 2010).

As in many of the macro- and micronutrients reviewed in this chapter, there are limited RCTs. The DGAC 2010 states that limited evidence shows that consumption of whole grains is associated with a reduced incidence of type 2 diabetes in large prospective cohort studies. Although there is limited evidence for type 2 diabetes risk reduction, overall health benefits of whole grains would warrant the DGAC whole-grain food intake recommendations. (See Table 25.3.)

Fatty Acids

Fatty acids influence glucose metabolism by altering cell membrane function, enzymatic activity, insulin signaling, and gene expression (Riserus 2009). Both epidemiological and clinical studies provide evidence that the type of fat plays a role in insulin resistance and the development of type 2 diabetes (DGAC 2010). Strong evidence suggests that a diet high in saturated fatty acids and *trans* fatty acids is associated with increased markers of insulin resistance and risk for type 2 diabetes, whereas unsaturated fatty acid intake is inversely associated with risk of diabetes.

Table 25.3 Studies Reviewing Whole-Grain Foods and Diabetes Prevention

	Population/ Duration of Study	Intervention (type of study)	Major Findings	Comments
de Munter 2007	n = 6 prospective cohort studies (286,125 participants)/not applicable	WG, bran, and germ intake and risk of type 2 diabetes (systematic review)	RR was 0.75 for highest vs. lowest WG quintile (P trend 0.03); two serving/day increment of WG associated with 21% ↓ in type 2 diabetes	Author conclusions: WG intake is inversely associated with type 2 diabetes risk
Priebe 2009	n = 11 prospective cohort studies (≥5 years duration) and 1 RCT (≥6 weeks)/not applicable	WG foods and/or cereal fiber and risk of type 2 diabetes (Cochrane review)	↓ Risk in type 2 diabetes with higher intake of WG foods (27–30%) or cereal fiber (28–37%)	Author conclusions: evidence too weak to draw conclusions about preventive effects of WG and type 2 diabetes
Brownlee 2010	n = 316 adults (BMI >25 kg/ m^2)/16 weeks	60 g WG/day for 16 weeks vs. 60 g WG/day for 8 weeks then 120 g WG for 8 weeks vs. control (<30 g WG/day) (RCT)	No differences in serum glucose or insulin and other CVD risk factors	4 months may not be long enough; ↑ WG intake linked to ↑ total kilocalories and sodium intake
Sun 2010	n = 3 prospective cohort studies (39,765 men and 157,463 women)/not applicable	White and brown rice intake and type 2 diabetes (review)	White rice (≥5 servings/week) vs. (<1/ month) associated with ↑ RR (1.17) of type 2 diabetes; brown rice (≥2 servings/week) vs. (<1/ month) associated with ↓ risk RR (0.89)	Author conclusions: substitution of WG, in this case brown rice for white rice, may lower the risk of type 2 diabetes
Nettleton 2010	n = 14 cohort studies (~48,000 adults of European descent)/not applicable	WG intake and genetic variation affects glucose and insulin levels (meta-analysis)	Each one serving/day greater intake WG: fasting glucose –0.2 mg/dL (P < 0.0001); fasting insulin –0.011 pmol/L (P < 0.0003); diet-gene interaction nonsignificant	

WG, whole grain.

Eating patterns that decrease saturated fatty acids by 5% of total calories and replace saturated fatty acids with monounsaturated fatty acids (MUFAs) or polyunsaturated fatty acids (PUFAs) (specifically long-chain n-6 fatty acids) are associated with improved insulin sensitivity and decreased risk of type 2 diabetes and are recommended (DGAC 2010). The linoleic acid (n-6 PUFA) is the specific PUFA that is associated with improved insulin sensitivity. Therefore, food sources high in linoleic acid should be recommended, including corn, sunflower, safflower, and soybean oils, as well as nuts and seeds (DGAC 2010).

Although it was reported that long-chain n-3 fatty acids, often called "marine oils" or "omega-3 fatty acids," do not have an impact on insulin sensitivity or glucose metabolism (Riserus 2009), two more recent studies reported a lower risk for type 2 diabetes associated with omega-3 fatty acids. In one study, of >3,000 older U.S. adults, in individuals with the highest blood levels of eicosapentaenoic acid and docosahexaenoic acid, 5% developed diabetes over the next 10 years compared to 6.5% with the lowest blood levels. The difference was greater for α-linolenic acid levels, with the highest blood levels, just under 4%, developing diabetes versus 8.5% of those with the lowest blood levels (Djousse 2011). In the other study, 43,176 Singapore adults were interviewed about their dietary habits and then followed for 10 years. Overall, 5% of subjects in the highest quartile for α-linolenic acid developed diabetes compared to 6% in the lowest quintile (Brostow 2011). RCTs are needed to determine the role of omega-3 fatty acids in diabetes prevention.

All of the large lifestyle intervention trials recommended decreasing fat intake. For example, the DPP protocol recommended consuming 25% of total calories from fat (DPP 2002), and the Japanese diabetes prevention trial recommended consuming ≤50 g fat/day (Kosaka 2005). The recommendation for the low fat intake in the DPP was based on epidemiological studies available at the time of writing the protocol and on the cardiovascular and general overall health benefits. The assumption was that by decreasing fat, total caloric intake would also decrease. At year 1, food frequency questionnaires indicated that 27.5% of the total caloric intake came from fat, down from 34.1% at baseline (DPP 2002).

Although the DPP protocol recommends 25% of calories from fat, higher-fat eating patterns, up to 35% fat, may be more realistic in terms of adherence because of satiety and palatability values. However, the majority of the fatty acids should be from PUFAs and MUFAs and caloric deficits must be achieved to promote weight loss.

Alcohol and Risk of Type 2 Diabetes

Comprehensive reviews and meta-analyses suggest a protective effect of moderate alcohol intake on the risk of developing diabetes compared to abstainers (Table 25.4). The association of moderate intake of alcohol and reduced incidence of type 2 diabetes could result from increased insulin sensitivity with ingestion of alcohol or be related to an overall healthy lifestyle by individuals who drink alcoholic beverages. Conversely, higher intake of alcohol may be related to obesity, specifically truncal obesity, which would not be beneficial.

The U.S. Dietary Guidelines for Americans define moderate alcohol consumption as up to one drink per day for women and up to two drinks per day for men. One drink is defined as 12 oz regular beer, 5 oz wine (12% alcohol), or 1.5

oz 80-proof distilled spirits, the equivalent of 13.7 g alcohol. Although moderate alcohol consumption appears to confer some health benefits, the U.S. Dietary Guidelines do not recommend that individuals commence alcohol consumption or increase alcohol intake solely based on these potential benefits (DGAG 2010).

A systematic review of 32 studies demonstrated a U-shaped relationship between alcohol consumption and incidence of diabetes compared with no alcohol use. Consumption of one to three drinks per day was associated with a 33–56% lower incidence of type 2 diabetes. Heavy consumption of alcohol, defined as three or more drinks per day, was associated with up to a 43% increased incidence of type 2 diabetes (Howard 2004).

In a meta-analysis of 20 cohort studies (n = 477,200), a U-shaped relationship between alcohol intake and diabetes was found in both men and women; however, the protective effects of moderate alcohol intake occurred more often in women. For men, alcohol intake had a protective effect for developing diabetes at 22 g/day (relative risk [RR] 0.87) and an increased risk for developing diabetes at >60 g/day (RR 1.01). In women, intake of 24 g/day alcohol demonstrated a protective effect with an increased risk shown at 50 g/day (RR 1.02) (Baliunas 2009).

Another meta-analysis of 15 prospective cohort studies (n = 369,862) demonstrated a 30% reduced risk of diabetes in moderate alcohol consumption ranging from 6 to 48 g/day compared to abstainers and heavy consumers (>48 g/day). The risk of diabetes was the same in the heavy consumers and the abstainers (RR 1.04). There also was no difference in risk reduction in the moderate-consumption group in individuals with a low and high BMI (Koppes 2005). (See Table 25.4.)

The Mediterranean Diet and Prevention of Diabetes

The Mediterranean-style eating pattern (MedDiet), so named for the components shared by countries in that region, is characterized by the following: high levels of monounsaturated fatty acids such as olive oil; high intake of plant-based foods (vegetables, legumes, grains, fruits, and nuts); moderate amounts of fish and wine; and a low intake of red and processed meat and whole-fat dairy products (Martínez-González 2008). The total fat composition ranges from 30 to 40% of the total calorie intake, with a high ratio of monounsaturated fatty acid to saturated fatty acids (Giugliano 2008). The benefits of this diet may be the combination of the foods consumed and the quality of the food rather than one food component.

The MedDiet is associated with lower rates of developing morbidity and mortality caused by cardiovascular disease (CVD), cancer, obesity, and type 2 diabetes (Giugliano 2008). Epidemiological studies have demonstrated that adherence to a MedDiet exerts a beneficial role in the development of diabetes (Kastorini 2009; InterAct Consortium 2011) and reduced risk of metabolic syndrome and its components (Kastorini 2011). In a prospective, post-infarct study, Italian patients on the MedDiet who did not have diabetes in the highest versus lowest quartile of MedDiet adherence had a 37% lower incidence of diabetes (Mozaffarian 2007). The intake of cheese, wine, and coffee was not found to be associated with the incidence of diabetes, and fish oil treatment did not reduce the incidence of prediabetes and diabetes. It was hypothesized that the benefits of the fish were likely not the n-3 fatty acids, but rather other components such as protein or selenium.

Table 25.4 Studies Reviewing Alcohol Consumption and Diabetes Incidence

	Population/ Duration of Study	Intervention (type of study)	Major Findings	Comments
Howard 2004	n = 18 prospective cohort studies (n = 304,636 adult men and women)/4–16.8 years	Effect of alcohol consumption on incidence of diabetes (systematic review)	Eight studies: U-shaped relationship between alcohol and diabetes; 1–3 drinks/day = 33–56% ↓ risk of diabetes; three studies: inverse relationship between alcohol and diabetes; moderate drinkers 43–46% ↓ risk; two studies: no association between alcohol use and diabetes; one study: ↑ risk with intake of alcohol two to three times/week; one study: ↑ risk for BMI <22 kg/m^2 and ↓ risk for normal BMI; two studies: + association with risk for diabetes in men but not in women; one study: no worsening of glucose tolerance in IGT or diabetes	Author conclusions: moderate alcohol consumption is associated with ↓ diabetes incidence; prevalence of heavy drinking in study was low (1–3%)
Koppes 2005	n = 15 prospective cohort studies (n = 369,862); 11,959 adult men and women with type 2 diabetes/mean 12 years	Relationship between alcohol consumption and type 2 diabetes (meta-analysis)	U-shaped relationship between average alcohol consumed/day and diabetes incidence; lowest risk intake of 6–48 g alcohol/day; intake of 48 g/day was equal to the risk of abstainers	Author conclusions: ~30% ↓ risk of type 2 diabetes in alcohol consumers of 6–48 g/day; no differences in risk in low or high BMI
Baliunas 2009	n = 20 prospective cohort studies (n = 477,200); 12,556 adult men and women with type 2 diabetes/ 6.2–19.8 years	Dose-responsiveness relationship between alcohol consumption and type 2 diabetes (review and meta-analysis)	Moderate alcohol consumption (22 g/day for men [RR 0.87] and 24 g/day for women [RR 0.60]) is protective for type 2 diabetes; higher intake (60 g/day for men [RR 1.01] and 50 g for women [RR 1.02]) ↑ risk	Author conclusions: U-shaped relationship between average alcohol consumed/day and type 2 diabetes incidence

In another large prospective cohort study of Spanish university graduates, the incidence of type 2 diabetes was significantly reduced in subjects with a moderate to high adherence to the MedDiet. The incident ratio for the moderate- and high-adherence group was 0.41 and 0.17, respectively. There was an inverse association of risk of diabetes and adherence to the MedDiet, with an 83% relative risk reduction in people with high adherence to the diet (Martínez-González 2008).

A clinical trial in Spain that included subjects with at least three CVD risk factors (hypertension, dyslipidemia, overweight, or family history of premature CVD) examined the effects of a MedDiet on the incidence of type 2 diabetes (Salas-Salvadó 2011). The study compared a control group (low fat [<35% fat]) to the MedDiet, supplemented with olive oil or with mixed nuts. The interventions were not restricted in calories, and weight change and physical activity did not differ in any of the three groups. After a mean follow-up of 4 years, diabetes incidence in the control group was 17.9%; the MedDiet plus olive oil, 10.9%; and the MedDiet plus nuts, 11.0%. A 52% risk reduction was seen when the MedDiet groups were combined.

It is hypothesized that the MedDiet exerts a protective mechanism on metabolic pathways for the prevention of diabetes and other chronic illnesses because of the antioxidant and anti-inflammatory properties of the foods within the MedDiet. Adherence to a MedDiet is associated with lower plasma concentrations of inflammatory markers and markers of endothelial dysfunction. Additionally, this eating pattern is associated with an increased production of glucagon-like peptide-1, which is low in people with diabetes, as well as high levels of adiponectin, which are associated with a reduced risk of diabetes (Martínez-González 2008). Olive oil, the main source of oil in the MedDiet, protects against insulin resistance and exerts a beneficial effect on proinflammatory cytokines (Giugliano 2008). However, when PUFAs were substituted for MUFAs in a large northern European cohort study, they were equally as effective in increasing survival among older people (Trichopoulou 2005).

The MedDiet appears to be a palatable alternative to the low-fat diets recommended in the landmark diabetes prevention trials noted at the beginning of this chapter. Health care providers can attempt to identify what patients are capable of following based on their income, access to food items, food preference, and readiness to change current food eating patterns. However, introducing the MedDiet can pose challenges to certain populations at risk for developing diabetes. Because some of the foods that are integral to this eating pattern are not commonly found in many American diets, a good option may be to recommend small changes based on this eating pattern. For example, suggesting lower levels of red meat and high-fat dairy products or introducing olive or other polyunsaturated oils, fish, and small amounts of nuts can be incremental approaches to introducing certain elements of the MedDiet. (See Table 25.5.)

MICRONUTRIENTS AND DIABETES PREVENTION

Over the past decade, there has been increased interest in the non-skeletal benefits of vitamin D and calcium. Low serum vitamin D levels have been associated with the development of several chronic conditions, including diabetes. Vitamin D deficiency often results from one or more of the following: a diet low in

Table 25.5 Studies Examining the Role of the Mediterranean Diet in the Prevention of Diabetes

	Population/ Duration of Study	Intervention (type of study)	Major Findings	Comments
Mozaffarian 2007	$n = 8,291$ patients after myocardial infarct/3.2 years	Adherence to a MedDiet based on a brief survey focusing on vegetables, fruit, fish, oil, butter, cheese, wine, and coffee (prospective cohort study)	37% ↓ incidence of diabetes in the highest vs. the lowest quartile in adherence to the MedDiet	Author conclusions: lifestyle changes including prevention of weight gain and MedDiet could lower the risk of diabetes
Martínez-González 2008	$n = 13,380$ Spanish university graduates without diabetes/4.4 years	Adherence to a MedDiet based on 136-item food frequency questionnaire and 9-point index (prospective cohort study)	Moderate and high adherence to the MedDiet, incident rate of diabetes of 0.41 and 0.17 vs. low adherence group 1.0; high adherence, 83% ↓ risk of diabetes	Author conclusions: adherence to MedDiet is associated with a ↓ risk of diabetes
Salas-Salvadó 2011	$n = 418$ without diabetes and CVD but at high CVD risk (three risk factors)/4 years	Three diet interventions: 1) low-fat diet (C), 2) MedDiet with olive oil (1 liter/week), 3) MedDiet with nuts (30 g/day) (RCT)	Diabetes incidence: C = 17.9%; MedDiet, olive oil = 10.1%; MedDiet, nuts = 11.0%; Med/diets pooled and vs. C, diabetes incidence ↓ 52%	Author conclusions: MedDiet without calorie restriction effective in the prevention of diabetes in subjects at high risk for CVD
InterAct Consortium 2011	$n = 15,798$ participants in the EPIC study/3.99 million person-years of follow-up	rMed (0–18) used to assess adherence to MedDiet based on nine dietary components (prospective case-cohort study)	Hazard ratios of type 2 diabetes with medium adherence to MedDiet (rMed 7–10) was 0.93, high adherence (11–18), 0.88, compared to low adherence (0–6)	In large European study, individuals with a high rMed were 12% less likely to develop diabetes

C, control; EPIC, European Prospective Investigation into Cancer and Nutrition Study; rMed, relative Mediterranean diet score.

vitamin D or poor absorption; lack of or low exposure to ultraviolet B radiation from sunlight, resulting in insufficient cutaneous synthesis; obesity; age; geographic location; or skin pigmentation (Liu 2009; Song 2010). Several potential mechanisms for the effects of vitamin D and calcium on developing diabetes have been suggested. These mechanisms are unclear and may involve insulin secretion, improvement on insulin action, and improvement in systemic inflammation (Pittas 2006; Pittas 2007).

The Institute of Medicine defines four categories of vitamin D status based on serum 25-hydroxyvitamin D [25(OH)D]: risk of deficiency (<30 nmol/L), risk of inadequacy (<30–49 nmol/L), sufficiency (50–125 nmol/L), and reason for concern (>125 nmol/L). Using the above categories, 2001–2006 National Health and Nutrition Examination Survey (NHANES) data indicated that 67% of the population had sufficient vitamin D status, 24% were at risk for inadequacy, and 8% were at risk for deficiency (Looker 2011).

Serum Vitamin D and Prevalence of Prediabetes and Type 2 Diabetes

Observational studies have shown an association between serum 25-hydroxyvitamin D [25(OH)D] or reported vitamin D intake and type 2 diabetes. Mitri and associates performed a meta-analysis of eight observational cohort studies and 11 randomized controlled trials (RCTs) (Mitri 2011). In five observational studies, individuals with the highest vitamin D status (>25 ng/mL) had a 43% lower risk of developing type 2 diabetes compared with those in the lowest group (<14 ng/ml). In three observational studies, vitamin D intake >500 IU/day decreased risk of type 2 diabetes by 13% compared with vitamin D intakes of <200 IU/day.

Examples of observational studies reporting an association between vitamin D status and risk of developing diabetes include the following. The Framingham Offspring Study (n = 808) found that 25(OH)D was inversely associated with fasting plasma glucose, insulin concentration, and homeostatic model assessment–insulin resistance (HOMA-IR) (Liu 2009). Compared with participants in the lowest tertile of the predicted 25(OH)D score, those in the highest tertile had a 40% lower risk of type 2 diabetes after multivariate adjustment (Liu 2010). In the NHANES 2001–2006 study, there was an increase in prediabetes in people with 25(OH)D levels ≤76 nmol/L compared to >76.3 nmol/L (Gupta 2011). The association between 25(OH)D and risk of incident diabetes was assessed in participants in the Diabetes Prevention Program (combined placebo and intensive lifestyle arms) (Pittas 2012). Higher 25(OH)D, assessed repeatedly during follow-up (median concentration, 30.1 ng/mL), was associated with lower risk for developing diabetes, after adjusting for lifestyle interventions, compared to lower values (median concentration, 12.8 ng/dL).

However, not all observational studies have shown a relationship between vitamin D status and risk of diabetes. For example, a post hoc analysis of a case-control substudy of the Women's Health Initiative Clinical Trials and Observation Study showed that lower serum 25(OH)D was not associated with type 2 diabetes development (Robinson 2011). Although the initial analysis of the Women's Health Study reported an association with lower risk of developing type 2 diabetes and higher intakes of vitamin D (Liu 2005), after adjusting for other dietary factors this association became attenuated and became nonsignificant (Pittas 2006).

In analyses from the 11 RCTs, in eight trials in participants with normal glucose tolerance, vitamin D supplementation with cholecalciferol or ergocalciferol had no effect on glycemic outcomes including fasting plasma glucose or A1C and insulin resistance (Mitri 2011). For example, studies did not find an inverse relationship between vitamin D supplementation and lower insulin resistance/type 2 diabetes development (Avenell 2009; De Boer 2008).

In three small trials (*n*=32–62) in which participants had type 2 diabetes there was no effect of vitamin D supplementation on glycemic outcomes (A1C or fasting glucose) (Sugden 2008; Jorde 2009; Witham 2010). In two of these three trials some patients had baseline glucose intolerance and vitamin D supplementation improved insulin resistance but not glycemic outcomes.

Therefore, to determine the role of vitamin D in the development and progression of type 2 diabetes, high-quality observational studies and RCTs that measure blood 25(OH)D concentration are needed (Mitri 2011).

Calcium Intake and Incidence of Prediabetes and Type 2 Diabetes

Several studies have attempted to demonstrate a correlation between calcium and/or vitamin D intake and insulin resistance and development of diabetes, or both (Pitas 2007; Song 2011). However, it has been widely noted that randomized clinical trials are needed to provide strong evidence of the role of calcium and vitamin D in the development of diabetes. The Nurses' Health Study found no relationship between total (dietary and supplemental) vitamin D intake and incidence of type 2 diabetes. The study did find that subjects taking a combination of calcium plus vitamin D supplements had a 33% lower incidence of diabetes (Pittas 2006). The National Institutes of Health American Association of Retired Persons (NIH AARP) Diet and Health Study found that use of multiple vitamins was not associated with diabetes risk, but daily users of calcium supplements had a lower rate of diabetes than nonusers (Song 2011). However, a substudy of the Women's Health Initiative found that ingesting calcium (1,000 mg/day) and vitamin D (400 IU vitamin D_3/day) did not reduce the risk of developing diabetes (De Boer 2008).

Guidelines for Vitamin D and Calcium Intake for Non-Skeletal Health

Confusion continues to grow among the public regarding the adequate intake of vitamin D. There has been an increase in the number of serum 25(OH)D tests performed using multiple cut points to interpret results. Without clear guidelines, laboratories are trending toward setting cut points higher than those presently recommended by the Institute of Medicine (Ross 2011). Randomized trials are needed to provide evidence-based recommendations for calcium and vitamin D intake and serum 25(OH)D levels in non-skeletal health. The Institute of Medicine Committee to Review Dietary Reference Intakes for calcium and vitamin D set forth to comprehensively review evidence of dietary reference intakes for vitamin D and calcium on health outcomes. The committee concluded that for non-skeletal outcomes, including diabetes, there is inconclusive and/or insufficient evidence to warrant the development of a dietary reference intake. Reference values are currently based on skeletal health.

Currently, the estimated average requirement for calcium intake (age 1 year and older) is 500–1,100 mg/day. The recommended daily allowance (RDA) is 700–1,300 mg/day. The estimated average requirement for vitamin D is 400 IU/day (age 1 year or over), and the RDA is 600 IU/day (800 IU for age 71 years and older) (Institute of Medicine 2010). The committee warns that the prevalence of vitamin D inadequacy is overestimated based on the serum 25(OH)D levels. Until evidence-based guidelines are available, health care practitioners need to assess patients' intake of vitamin D and calcium to ensure that the intake is meeting the RDA and intake is below the tolerable upper intake level of calcium (1,000–3,000 mg/day) and vitamin D (1,000–4,000 IU) (Ross 2011).

Other Micronutrients and Risk of Type 2 Diabetes

Other micronutrients have also been investigated in their role in the development of type 2 diabetes. In a Cochrane review, one study on the role of zinc and diabetes prevention was found. It demonstrated that an increase in zinc consumption did not affect any of the measured outcomes (including the primary outcome, i.e., incidence of type 2 diabetes, or secondary outcomes, such as decreased insulin resistance and cholesterol levels [HDL, LDL, and triglycerides]) (Beletate 2007). However, a later observational study reported that a higher zinc intake may be associated with a slightly lower risk of type 2 diabetes in women (Sun 2009).

Meta-analyses of chromium supplementation did not show significant effects on glucose and insulin levels or A1C levels (Althuis 2002; Balk 2007). Additionally, in a randomized, double-blind trial of subjects with some history of insulin abnormality, there was no significant benefit to the subjects treated with chromium (Gunton 2005).

Magnesium intake may have a direct effect on insulin resistance and the development of type 2 diabetes. A meta-analysis of 13 prospective cohort studies identified a significant inverse association between magnesium intake and risk of type 2 diabetes. The association was stronger in overweight individuals than in normal-weight individuals. In addition, there was a dose response, with positive results increasing with every additional 100 mg/day magnesium intake (Dong 2011). Because evidence is needed from RCTs before recommending magnesium supplementation, it is advisable to recommend diets rich in high-magnesium foods, including green leafy vegetables, whole grains, and nuts. (See Table 25.6.)

BARIATRIC SURGERY AND DIABETES PREVENTION

Although there is currently strong interest in the field of bariatric surgery and its potential role in the long-term management of morbid obesity, type 2 diabetes, and CVD risk, limited data exist regarding the effectiveness of bariatric surgery in preventing type 2 diabetes. Observational studies have demonstrated that bariatric surgery reduces the incidence of type 2 diabetes and "resolves" or substantially improves glycemic control in people with type 2 diabetes (Lautz 2011), but there are no RCTs on the role of bariatric surgery in the prevention of diabetes to date.

Surgical treatments of obesity produce weight losses of 30–40 kg, equivalent to 10–15 kg/m^2 reduction in BMI, and can be sustained over a 10- to 15-year period (Lautz 2011). In the Swedish Obese Subjects Study, a large prospective case-controlled study, participants underwent gastric surgery (gastric bypass, ver-

Table 25.6 Studies Examining the Role of Micronutrients and Diabetes Prevention

	Population/ Duration of Study	Intervention (type of study)	Major Findings	Comments
Chromium (Cr)				
Althuis 2002	n = 15 RCTs (193 patients with type 2 diabetes, 425 without diabetes or IGT/not applicable	Effect of Cr supplementation on glucose and insulin responses (meta-analysis)	Nonsignificant effect of Cr on glucose/insulin in subjects without diabetes; inconclusive for patients with diabetes	Only study to show benefit on A1C was in 155 subjects with diabetes in China
Balk 2007	n = 41 RCTs (1,198 subjects)/not applicable	Effect of Cr on glucose metabolism and lipids (systematic review)	No benefit of Cr in subjects without diabetes; in patients with type 2 diabetes, Cr ↓ A1C –0.6% but not lipids	Almost half of the studies had poor quality
Magnesium (Mg)				
Dong 2011	n = 13 prospective cohort studies (536,318 subjects)	Mg and risk of type 2 diabetes (meta-analysis)	Inverse relationship between Mg intake and risk of type 2 diabetes (RR 0.78)	Relationship observed in BMI ≥25 kg/m² not in BMI <25 kg/m²
Vitamin D and Calcium (Ca)				
Pittas 2006	n = 83,799 women from Nurses' Health Study/assessment every 2–4 years	Assessment of vitamin D and Ca and risk of type 2 diabetes (prospective cohort study)	Highest (>400 IU vitamin D) vs. lowest (≤100 IU vitamin D): RR 0.87 of diabetes; combined (>1,200 mg Ca and >800 IU vitamin D) vs. (<600 mg Ca and 400 IU vitamin D): RR 0.67 of diabetes, 33% ↓ risk of type 2 diabetes	Combined intake inversely associated with development of type 2 diabetes; benefits appear to be additive
Pittas 2007	n = 4 studies/not applicable	Association between 25(OH)D levels and prevalence of type 2 diabetes (systematic review)	Incidence of diabetes OR 0.54 for the highest (25–38 ng/mL) vs. the lowest (10–23 ng/mL) 25(OH)D levels	Observational studies are cross-sectional, and intervention studies are of short duration with few subjects
De Boer 2008	n = 33,951 women from Women's Health Initiative/7-year follow-up	Ca plus vitamin D vs. placebo (double-blind randomized trial)	No ↓ of risk of diabetes with vitamin D/Ca in 2,291 women newly diagnosed with diabetes (RR = 1.01)	

	Population/ Duration of Study	Intervention (type of study)	Major Findings	Comments
Liu 2009	n = 808 participants in the Framingham Offspring Study/not applicable	Association of plasma vitamin D levels and markers of insulin resistance (cross-sectional)	Highest tertile of plasma 25(OH)D vs. lowest: 1.6% lower FPG (P trend = 0.007), 9.8% lower fasting insulin (P trend = 0.001), and 12.7% lower HOMA-IR score (P trend = 0.001)	
Avenell 2009)	n = 2,649 older adults with vitamin D, n = 2,643 without vitamin D/24–62 months	Vitamin D_3 (800 IU) vs. 1,000 mg Ca vs. both vs. placebo on development of diabetes (RCT)	No evidence that vitamin D, with or without the Ca, prevents diabetes	CIs do not rule out protective effects
Gupta 2011	n = 1,711 disease-free adults in NHANES 2001–2006/ not applicable	Association between low vitamin D levels and prediabetes and prehypertension (cross-sectional)	Inverse relationship between risk of early-stage diabetes and hypertension and low vitamin D levels; OR for prediabetes 1.33 in people with vitamin D levels ≤76.3 vs. >76.3 nmol	
Robinson 2011	n = 5,140 participants in the Women's Health Initiative/followed 7.3 years	Association between low serum levels of 25(OH)D and incidence of diabetes (cross-sectional)	No association between low serum levels of 25(OH)D and diabetes risk	
Mitri 2011	n = 8 observational studies and n = 11 RCTs/not applicable	Association between vit D status and incident type 2 diabetes, and the effect of vit D supplementation on glycemic outcomes (systematic review and meta-analysis)	In 8 observational studies, vit D intake >500 IU/d ↓ risk of type 2 diabetes by 13% vs. vit D intake of <200 IU/d; highest vit D status (>25 ng/mL) had a 43% ↓ risk of developing type 2 diabetes vs. lowest group (<14 ng/mL). In 11 RCTs (8 with pts with normal glucose tolerance and 3 with pts with type 2 diabetes), vit D supplementation had no effect on glycemic outcomes.	Author's conclusion: high-quality observational studies and RCTs are needed to define the role of vit D in the development and progression of type 2 diabetes

Table 25.6 Studies Examining the Role of Micronutrients and Diabetes Prevention (*continued*)

	Population/ Duration of Study	Intervention (type of study)	Major Findings	Comments
Pittas 2012	*n* = 2,039 participants (combined placebo and intensive lifestyle arms) in the Diabetes Prevention Program/2.7 years	Association of 25(OH)D and risk of diabetes assessed in plasma samples from baseline, 6-month, 1-, 2-, 3-, 4-year visits (cohort study)	For every 5 ng/mL increase in 25(OH)D, a 13% ↓ risk of progression to diabetes (*P*<0.0001); after multivariate adjustment, participants in the highest tertile [25(OH)D, 30.1 ng/mL], hazard ratio of 0.72 for developing diabetes vs. lowest tertile (12.8 ng/mL)	Adjustments made for lifestyle interventions (dietary changes, physical activity, and weight loss)
Zinc (Zn)				
Beletate 2007	*n* = 1 study (56 women)/not applicable	RCT on Zn supplementation vs. placebo for adults with insulin resistance on FPG and lipids (Cochrane review)	Nonsignificant differences between Zn supplementation vs. placebo	
Sun 2009	*n* = 82,297 women in the Nurses' Health Study/24-year follow-up	Relationship of Zn intake and risk of diabetes (prospective cohort study)	Risk of type 2 diabetes in highest quartile compared to lowest quartile: 0.90	
Multiple Vitamin Use				
Song 2011	*n* = 232,007 older adults in NIH AARP Diet and Health Study/5 years	Relationship between multivitamin use and diabetes risk (prospective observational study)	Multivitamin use not associated with diabetes, but use of Ca (seven times/week) and vitamin C lowers risk of diabetes, OR of 0.85 and 0.91, respectively	

FPG, fasting plasma glucose.

tical banded gastroplasty, or banding). When compared to the control group, subjects in the intervention group at 2 and 10 years after surgery demonstrated statistically significant improvement in terms of weight loss, insulin, and glucose levels and incidence of diabetes. At 10 years, the gastroplasty group had the greatest improvement in insulin levels (Sjöström 2004). Lifestyle interventions with diet alone, studied in the DaQing Trial, demonstrated clearly that even modest weight loss decreases the conversion from prediabetes to type 2 diabetes; hence, it could be surmised that bariatric surgery procedures, by significantly lowering

Table 25.7 Studies Examining the Role of Bariatric Surgery in Diabetes Prevention

	Population/ Duration of Study	Intervention (type of study)	Major Findings	Comments
Sjöström 2004	*n* = 4,047 at 2 years, *n* = 1,703 at 10 years, adults with BMI = 41 kg/m² at baseline/10 years	Metabolic control and weight loss over 2 and 10 years from gastric surgery (gastric bypass, vertical banded gastroplasty, or banding) vs. control (prospective cohort study)	Statistically significant improvement in ↓ weight (P < 0.0001), ↓ energy intake, ↑ physical activity	Bariatric surgery resulted ↓ rates diabetes, ↓ triglycerides, ↓ hyperuricemia; no difference in blood pressure and cholesterol

weight, will lower type 2 diabetes risk. However, studies are needed to provide evidence that this is indeed the case. (See Table 25.7.)

While improvement in glycemic control seen in type 2 diabetes after bariatric surgery is attributed to dietary intake changes and weight loss, it is also now hypothesized that improved glycemic control is independent of weight loss, especially in individuals who have received the Roux-en-Y gastric bypass. Possible mechanisms for this weight-independent impact of bariatric surgery on glycemic control include enterohormonal changes and neurohormonal events resulting from the anatomical changes of the surgery (Lautz 2011).

COMBINING HEALTHY LIFESTYLE FACTORS

Studies, as reviewed above, show that a healthy eating pattern, participation in regular physical activity, maintenance of a normal body weight, and moderate alcohol intake lower risk of developing type 2 diabetes. Of additional interest is how each alone and in combination contribute to reduced risk. To answer this question, data were analyzed from 207,479 people who are part of a larger NIH AARP Diet and Health Study and who were between the ages of 50 and 71 years when the study began in 1995 (Reis 2011). At the start of the study, participants had no signs of diabetes, heart disease, or cancer and provided comprehensive data on lifestyle factors, including dietary intake, body weight and height, physical activity, smoking, and alcohol consumption. Eleven years later, 9.6% of men in the study and 7.5% of the women had developed diabetes.

Participants were grouped into categories depending on their lifestyle factors. People in the low-risk category had all five healthy lifestyle factors, whereas people in the high-risk category had none. Men and women with diet score, physical activity level, smoking status, and alcohol use all in the low-risk group had odds ratios (ORs) for diabetes of 0.61 and 0.43, respectively. When absence of overweight and obesity were added, the respective ORs were 0.28 and 0.16 for men and women. Furthermore, results did not differ by family history or level of adiposity.

BMI had the strongest association for diabetes risk, with normal-weight men being 70% less likely to develop diabetes than overweight or obese men and normal-weight women being 78% less likely to develop diabetes. In calculations of factors, consuming a healthy eating pattern (fruit and vegetable intake and amount and type of fat) and exercising three times a week reduced risk by 30%. Being a nonsmoker for at least 10 years reduced risk another 4% in both men and women, whereas moderate alcohol consumption in men reduced risk by another 7% and in women 24%. When BMI was added to the other healthy lifestyle factors, men were 72% less likely to develop diabetes, whereas women had an 84% lower risk. Although weight was one of the most important factors, the authors noted that even overweight people can lower their odds by adopting other healthy lifestyle habits (Reis 2011).

The relationship between several diet-quality scores designed for use in the U.S. population—Healthy Eating Index (HEI) 2005, the alternative HEI (aHEI), the Recommended Food Score, the alternative Mediterranean Diet (aMed) score, and the Dietary Approaches to Stop Hypertension (DASH)—was compared for association with CVD and incident type 2 diabetes (de Koning 2011). Scores were calculated from food frequency questionnaires completed by men from the Health Professional Follow-Up Study. There were 2,795 incident cases of type 2 diabetes, and after multivariate adjustments, aHEI, aMed, and DASH scores were significantly associated with a reduced risk ($P < 0.01$). They reflect a common eating pattern that is characterized by high intake of fruits, vegetables, whole grains, nuts, legumes, and unsaturated fats; moderate intake of alcohol; and low intake of red and processed meat, sodium, sugar-sweetened beverages, and *trans* fat. This pattern of eating was most effective in people who were overweight or obese.

CONCLUSION

Lifestyle intervention trials demonstrated that diabetes can be prevented or delayed in people with prediabetes through modest weight loss and moderate physical activity equivalent to brisk walking on most days of the week.

In general, the reviewed lifestyle intervention trials recommend intake of <25–30% of energy from fat and an energy deficit of 500–1,000 calories per day. However, observational studies and the Dietary Guidelines for Americans provide support that a higher intake of up to 35% fat (mainly MUFA and PUFA) may be considered while restricting the saturated fatty acid content. Intake of up to 35% of total energy from fat may be more easily adhered to because of the satiety and palatability value of fat. In addition, individuals should be encouraged to consume at least half of their grains as whole grains and limit intake of sugar-sweetened beverages. Adjusting macronutrient components to individual preferences may optimize adherence to the eating pattern recommended for weight loss and maintenance. Combining healthy lifestyle habits and a healthy eating pattern dramatically decreases risk of developing type 2 diabetes.

BIBLIOGRAPHY

Althuis MD, Jordan NE, Ludington EA, Wittes JT: Glucose and insulin responses to dietary chromium supplements: a meta-analysis. *Am J Clin Nutr* 76:148–155, 2002

American Diabetes Association: Nutrition recommendations and interventions for diabetes: a position statement of the American Diabetes Association. *Diabetes Care* 31 (Suppl. 1):S61–S78, 2008

American Diabetes Association: Standards of medical care in diabetes: 2012. *Diabetes Care* 35:S11–S63, 2012

Avenell A, Cook JA, MacLennan GS, McPherson GC for the RECORD Trial Group: Vitamin D supplementation and type 2 diabetes: a substudy of a randomized placebo-controlled trial in older people (RECORD Trial). *Age Ageing* 38:606–609, 2009

Baliunas DO, Taylor BJ, Irving H, Roerecke M, Patra J, Mohapatra S, Rehm J: Alcohol as a risk factor for type 2 diabetes: a systematic review and meta-analysis. *Diabetes Care* 32:2123–2132, 2009

Balk EM, Tatsioni A, Lichtenstein AH, Lau J, Pittas AG: Effect of chromium supplementation on glucose metabolism and lipids: a systematic review of randomized controlled trials. *Diabetes Care* 30:2154–2163, 2007

Beletate V, El Dib R, Atallah ÁN: Zinc supplementation for the prevention of type 2 diabetes mellitus. *Cochrane Database Syst Rev* CD005525, 2007

Bessesen DH: The role of carbohydrates in insulin resistance. *J Nutr* 131:2782S–2786S, 2001

Brownlee IA, Moore C, Charfield M, Richardson DP, Ashby K, Kunznesolf SA, Jebb SA, Seal CJ: Markers of cardiovascular risk are not changed by increased whole-grain intake: the WHOLEheart study, a randomised, controlled dietary intervention. *Br J Nutr* 104:125–134, 2010

Brostow DP, Odegarrd AO, Koh WP, Duval S, Gross MD, Yuan JM, Pereira MA: Omega-3 fatty acids and incident type 2 diabetes: the Singapore Chinese Health Study. *Am J Clin Nutr* 94:520–526, 2011

Centers for Disease Control and Prevention: National Diabetes Fact Sheet. Available at http://www.cdc.gov/diabetes/pubs/estimates11.htm#1. Accessed 15 June 2011

Centers for Disease Control and Prevention: Obesity and overweight. Available at http://www.cdc.gov/obesity/causes/index.html. Accessed 15 June 2011

De Boer IH, Tinker LF, Connelly S, Curb JD, Howard BV, Kestenbaum B, Larson JC, Manson JE, Margolis KL, Siscovick DS, Weiss NS; Women's Health Initiative Investigators: Calcium plus vitamin D supplementation and the risk of incident diabetes in the Women's Health Initiative. *Diabetes Care* 31:701–707, 2008 de Koning L, Chiuve SE, Fung TT, Willett WC, Rimm EB, Hu FB: Diet-qualtiy scores and the risk of type 2 diabetes in men. *Diabetes Care* 34:1150–1156, 2011

de Munter JS, Hu FB, Spiegelman D, Franz M, van Dam RM: Whole grain, bran, and germ intake and risk of type 2 diabetes: a prospective cohort study and systematic review. *PLoS Med* 4:e261, 2007

Diabetes Prevention Program Research Group: The diabetes prevention program (DPP): description of lifestyle intervention. *Diabetes Care* 25:2165–2171, 2001

Diabetes Prevention Program Research Group: Reduction in the incidence of type 2 diabetes with lifestyle intervention or metformin. *N Engl J Med* 346:393–403, 2002

Diabetes Prevention Program Research Group, Knowler WC, Fowler SE, Hamman RF, Christophi CA, Hoffman H: 10-year follow-up of diabetes incidence and weight loss in the Diabetes Prevention Program Outcomes Study. *Lancet* 374:1677–1686, 2009

Dietary Guidelines Advisory Committee (DGAC) on the Dietary Guidelines for Americans, 2010. Available at http://www.cnpp.usda.gov/dgas2010-dgacreport.htm. Accessed 1 July 2011

Djousse L, Biggs ML, Lemaitre RN, King IB, Song X, Ix JH, Mukamal KJ, Siscovick DS, Mozaffarian D: Plasma omega-3 fatty acids and incident diabetes in older adults. *Am J Clin Nutr* 94:527–533, 2011

Dong J, Xun P, He K, Qin L: Magnesium intake and risk of type 2 diabetes. *Diabetes Care* 34:2116–2122, 2011

Duncan GE, Perri MG, Teriaque DW, Hutson AD, Eckel RH, Stacpoole PW: Exercise training without weight loss, increases insulin sensitivity and postheparin plasma lipase activity in previously sedentary adults. *Diabetes Care* 26:557–562, 2003

Finucane MM, Stevens GA, Cowan G, Lin JK, Paciorek CJ, Singh GM, Gutierrez HR, Lu Y, Bahalim AL, Farzadfar F, Riley LM, Ezzati M, on behalf of the Global Burden of Metabolic Risk Factors of Chronic Diseases Collaborating Group: National, regional, and global trends in body-mass index since 1980: systematic analysis of health examination surveys and epidemiological studies with 960 country-years and 9.1 million participants. *Lancet* 377:557–567, 2011

Franz MJ, VanWormer JJ, Crain AL, Boucher JL, Histon T, Caplan W, Bowman J, Pronk NP: Weight-loss outcomes: a systematic review and meta-analysis of weight-loss clinical trials with a minimum of 1-year follow-up. *J Am Diet Assoc* 107:1755–1767, 2007

Giugliano D, Esposito K: Mediterranean diet and metabolic diseases. *Curr Opin Lipidol* 19:63–68, 2008

Gunton JE, Cheung NW, Hitchman R, Hams G, O'Sullivan C, Foster-Powell K, McElduff A: Chromium supplementation does not improve glucose tolerance, insulin sensitivity, or lipid profile: a randomized, placebo-controlled, double-blind trial of supplementation in subjects with impaired glucose tolerance. *Diabetes Care* 28:712–713, 2005

Gupta AK, Brashear MM, Johnson WD: Prediabetes and prehypertension in healthy adults are associated with low vitamin D levels. *Diabetes Care* 34:658–660, 2011

Howard AA, Amsten JH, Gourevitch MN: Effect of alcohol consumption on diabetes mellitus: a systematic review. *Ann Intern Med* 140:211–219, 2004

Hu FB: Globalization of diabetes: the role of diet, exercise and genes. *Diabetes Care* 34:1249–1257, 2011

Institute of Medicine: *Dietary Reference Intakes for Calcium and Vitamin D.* Washington, DC, Institute of Medicine of the National Academies, 2010

InterAct Consortium: Mediterranean diet and type 2 diabetes risk in the European Prospective Investigation Into Cancer and Nutrition (EPIC) study. *Diabetes Care* 34:1913–1918, 2011

International Diabetes Federation: 5th IDF Diabetes Atlas. Available at http://www.idf.org/diabetesatlas/news/fifth-edition-releases. Accessed 15 November 2011

Jeon CY, Lokken RP, Hu FB, van Dam RM: Physical activity of moderate intensity and risk of type 2 diabetes: a systematic review. *Diabetes Care* 30:744–752, 2007

Jorde R, Figenschau Y: Suplementation with cholecalciferol does not improve glycaemic control in diabetic subjects with normal serum 25-hydroxyvitamin D levels. *Eur J Nutr* 48:349–354, 2009

Kastorini C-M, Milionis HJ, Esposito K, Giugliano D, Goudevenos JA, Panagiotakos DB: The effect of Mediterranean diet on metabolic syndrome and its components: a meta-analysis of 50 studies and 534,906 individuals. *J Am Coll Cardiol* 57:1299–1313, 2011

Kastorini C-M, Panagiotakos DB: Dietary patterns and prevention of type 2 diabetes: from research to clinical practice: a systematic review. *Curr Diabetes Rev* 5:221–227, 2009

Koppes LLJ, Dekker JM, Hendriks HFJ, Bouter LM, Heine RJ: Moderate alcohol consumption lowers the risk of type 2 diabetes: a meta-analysis of prospective observational studies. *Diabetes Care* 28:719–725, 2005

Kosaka K, Noda M, Kuzuya T: Prevention of type 2 diabetes by lifestyle intervention: a Japanese trial in IGT males. *Diabetes Res Clin Pract* 67:152–162, 2005

Laaksonen DE, Lindstrom J, Lakka TA, Eriksson JG, Niskanen L, Wikstrom K, Aunola S, Keinanen-Kiukaaniemi S, Laakso M, Valle TT, Ilanne-Paarikka P, Louheranta A, Hamalainen H, Rastas M, Salminen V, Cepaitis Z, Hakumaki M, Kaikkonen H, Harkonen P, Sundvall J, Tuomilehto J, Uusitupa M: Physical activity in the prevention of type 2 diabetes: the Finnish Diabetes Prevention Study. *Diabetes* 54:158–165, 2005

Lautz D, Halperin F, Goebel-Fabbri A, Goldfine AB: The great debate: medicine or surgery. What is best for the patient with type 2 diabetes? *Diabetes Care* 34:763–770, 2011

Li G, Zhang P, Wang J, Gregg EW, Yang W, Gong Q, Li H, Li H, Jiang Y, An Y, Shuai Y, Zhang B, Zhang J, Thompson TJ, Gerzoff RB, Roglic G, Hu Y, Bennett PH: The long-term effect of lifestyle interventions to prevent diabetes in the China Da Qing Diabetes Prevention Study: a 20-year follow-up study. *Lancet* 371:1783–1789, 2008

Lindstrom J, Ilanne-Parikka P, Peltonen M, Aunola S, Eriksson JG, Hemio K, Hamalainen H, Harkonen P, Keinanen-Kiukanniemi S, Laakso M, Louheranta A, Mannelin M, Paturi M, Sundvall J, Valle TT, Uusitupa M, Tuomilehto J, on behalf of the Finnish Diabetes Prevention Study Group: Sustained reduction in the incidence of type 2 diabetes by lifestyle intervention: follow-up of the Finnish Diabetes Prevention Study. *Lancet* 368:1673–1679, 2006

Liu E, Meigs JB, Pittas AG, McKeown NM, Economos CD, Booth SL, Jacques PF: Plasma 25-hydroxyvitamin D is associated with markers of the insulin resistant phenotype in nondiabetic adults. *J Nutr* 139:329–334, 2009

Liu E, Meigs JB, Pittas AG, Economos CD, McKeown NM, Booth SL, Jacques PF: Predicted 25-hydroxyvitamin D score and incident type 2 diabetes in the Framingham Offspring Study. *Am J Clin Nutr* 91:1627–1633, 2010

Liu S, Song Y, Ford ES, Manson JE, Buring JE, Ridker PM: Dietary calcium, vitamin D, and the prevalence of metabolic syndrome in middle-aged and older US women. *Diabetes Care* 28:2926–2570, 2005

Looker AC, Johnson CL, Lacher DA, Pfeiffer CM, Schleicher RL, Sempos CT: Vitamin D status: United States, 2001–2006. *NCHS Data Brief* 59:1–8, 2011

Malik VS, Popkin BM, Bray GA, Despres JP, Willett WC, Hu FB: Sugar-sweetened beverages and risk of metabolic syndrome and type 2 diabetes. *Diabetes Care* 33:2477–2483, 2010

Martínez-González MÁ, de la Fuente-Arrilaga C, Nunez-Cordoba JM, Basterra-Gortari FJ, Beunza JJ, Vazquex Z, Benito S, Tortosa A, Bes-Rastrollo M: Adherence to Mediterranean diet and risk of developing diabetes: prospective cohort study. *BMJ* 336:1348–1351, 2008

McClenaghan NH: Determining the relationship between dietary carbohydrate intake and insulin resistance. *Nutr Res Rev* 18:222–240, 2005

Mitri J, Muraru MD, Pittas AG: Vitamin D and type 2 diabetes: a systematic review. *Eur J Clin Nutr* 54:1005–1915, 2011

Mozaffarian D, Marfise RM, Levantesi G, Sukketta MG, Tavazzi G, Valafussa F, Marchioli R: Incidence of new-onset diabetes and impaired fasting glucose in patients with recent myocardial infarction and the effect of clinical and lifestyle risk factors. *Lancet* 370:667–675, 2007

National Weight Loss Registry: NWCR Facts, 2011. Available at http://www.nwcr.ws/people/default.htm. Accessed 1 September 2011

Nettleton JA, McKeown NM, Kanoni S, Lemaitre RN, Hivert M-F, Ngwa J, van Rooij FJA, Sonestedt E, Wojczynski MK, Ye Z, Tanaka T, the CHARGE Whole Grain Foods Study Group: Interactions of dietary whole-grain intake with fasting glucose- and insulin-related genetic loci in individuals of European descent: a meta-analysis of 14 cohort studies. *Diabetes Care* 33:2684–2691, 2010

Nutrition Evidence Library (NEL) for Dietary Guidelines for American, 2010. Available at http://www.nutritionevidencelibrary.com/category.cfm?cid=21. Accessed 1 July 2011

O'Neil CE, Nickles TA, Zanovec M, Cho S: Whole-grain consumption is associated with diet quality and nutrient intake in adults: the National Health and Nutrition Examination Survey, 1999–2004. *J Am Diet Assoc* 110:1461–1468, 2010

Pan XR, Li GW, Hu YH, Wang JX, Yang WY, An ZX, Hu XX, Lin J, Xio JZ, Cao HB, Liu PA, Jiang XG, Jiang YY, Wang JP, Zheng H, Zhang H, Bennett PH, Howard BH: Effects of diet and exercise in preventing NIDDM in people with impaired glucose tolerance: the Da Qing IGT and Diabetes Study. *Diabetes Care* 20:537–544, 1997

Perseghin G, Price TB, Petersen KF, Roden M, Cline GW, Rothman DLL, Shulman GI: Increased glucose transport-phosphorylation and muscle glycogen synthesis after exercise training in insulin-resistant subjects. *N Engl J Med* 335:1357–1362, 1996

Pittas AG, Dawson-Hughes B, Li T, Van Dam RM, Willett WC, Manson JE, Hu FB: Vitamin D and calcium intake in relation to type 2 diabetes in women. *Diabetes Care* 29:650–656, 2006

Pittas AG, Lau J, Hu FB, Dawson-Hughs B: The role of vitamin D and calcium in type 2 diabetes: a systematic review and meta-analysis. *J Clin Endocrinol Metab* 92:2017–2029, 2007

Pittas AG, Nelson J, Mitri J, Hillmann W, Garganta C, Nathan DM, Hu FB, Dawson-Hughes B, The Diabetes Prevention Program Research Group: Plasma 25-hydroxyvitamin D and progression to diabetes in patients at risk for diabetes. *Diabetes Care* 35:565–573, 2012

Pleis JR, Lucas JW, Ward BW: Summary health statistics for U.S. adults: National Health Interview Survey, 2008. National Center for Health Statistics. *Vital Health Stat 10* 1–157, 2009

Priebe M, van Binsbergen J, de Vos R, Vonk RJ: Whole grain foods for the prevention of type 2 diabetes. Cochrane Library, DOI: 10.1002/14651858. CD006061 1.pub2. Published online 21 January 2009

Ramachandran A, Snehalatha C, Mary S, Mukesh B, Bhaskar AD, Vijay V, Indian Diabetes Prevention Programme (IDPP): The Indian Diabetes Prevention Programme shows that lifestyle modification and metformin prevent type 2 diabetes in Asian Indian subjects with impaired glucose tolerance (IDPP-1). *Diabetologia* 49:289–297, 2006

Reis JP, Loria CM, Sorlie PD, Park Y, Hollenbeck A, Schatzkin A: Lifestyle factors and risk of new-onset diabetes: a population-based cohort study. *Ann Intern Med* 155:292–299, 2011

Riserus U, Willett WC, Hu FB: Dietary fats and prevention of type 2 diabetes. *Prog Lipid Res* 48:45–51, 2009

Robinson JG, Manson JE, Larson J, Liu S, Song Y, Howard BV, Phillips L, Shikany JM, Allison M, Curb JD, Johnson KC, Watts N: Lack of association between 25(OH)D levels and incident type 2 diabetes in older women. *Diabetes Care* 34:628–634, 2011

Ross CR, Manson JE, Abrams SA, Aloia JF, Brannon PM, Clinton SK, Durazio-Arvizu RA, Gallagher JC, Gallo RL, Jones G, Kovacs CS, Mayne ST, Rosen CJ, Shapses SE: The 2011 dietary reference intakes for calcium and vitamin D: what dietetics practitioners need to know. *J Am Diet Assoc* 111:524–527, 2011

Salas-Salvadó J, Bulló M, Babio N, Martinez-Gonzálex MA, Ibarrola-Jurado N, Basora J, Estruch R, Covas MI, Corella D, Arós F, Ruiz-Gutiérrez V, Ros E, for the PREDIMED Study Investigators: Reduction in the incidence of type 2 diabetes with the Mediterranean diet: results of the PREDIMED-Reus nutrition intervention randomized trial. *Diabetes Care* 34:14–91, 2011

Sjöström L, Lindroos AK, Peltonen M, Torgerson J, Bouchard C, Carlsson B, Dahlgren S, Larsson B, Narbro K, Sjöström CD, Sullivan M, Wedel H, for Swedish Obese Subjects Study Scientific Group: Lifestyle, diabetes and cardiovascular risk factors 10 years after bariatric surgery. *N Engl J Med* 351:2683–2693, 2004

Song Y, Manson JE: Vitamin D, insulin resistance, and type 2 diabetes. *Curr Cardio Risk Rep* 4:40–47, 2010

Song Y, Xu Q, Park Y, Hollenbeck A, Schatzkin A, Chen H: Multivitamins, individual vitamin and mineral supplements, and risk of diabetes among older U.S. adults. *Diabetes Care* 34:108–114, 2011

Sugden JA, Davies JI, Witham MD, Morris AD, Struthers AD: Vitamin D improves endothelial function in patients with type 2 diabetes mellitus and low vitamin D levels. *Diabet Med* 25:320–325, 2008

Sun Q, Spiegelman D, van Dam RM, Holmes MD, Mali VS, Willet W, Hu F: White rice, brown rice, and risk of type 2 diabetes in US men and women. *Arch Intern Med* 170:1479–1481, 2010

Sun Q, van Dam RM, Willett WC, Hu FB: Prospective study of zinc intake and risk of type 2 diabetes in women. *Diabetes Care* 32:629–634, 2009

Trichopoulou A, Orfanos P, Norat T, Bueno-de-Mesquita B, Ocké M, Peeters PH, van der Schouw YT, Boeing H, Hoffmann K, Boffetta P, Nagel G, Masala G, Krogh V, Panico S, Tumino R, Vineis P, Bamia C, Naska A, Benetou V, Ferrari P, Slimani N, Pera G, Martinez-Garcia C, Navarro C, Rodriguez-Barranco M, Clavel-Chapelon F, Boutron-Ruault M-C, Berglund G, Wirfalt E, Hallmans G, Johansson I, Tjonneland A, Olsen A, Overvad K, Hundborg H, Riboli E,

Trichopoulos D: Modified Mediterranean diet and survival: EPIC-elderly prospective cohort study. *BMJ* 330:991–998, 2005

Tuomilehto J, Lindström J, Eriksson JG, Valle TT, Hamalainen H, Ilanne-Parikka P, Keinanen-Kiukaanniemi S, Laakso M, Louheranta A, Rastas M, Salminen V, Uusitupa M, for the Finnish Diabetes Prevention Study Group: Prevention of type 2 diabetes mellitus by changes in lifestyle among subjects with impaired glucose tolerance. *N Engl J Med* 344:1343–1350, 2001

U.S. Department of Agriculture, United States Department of Health and Human Service (USDA DHHS): Report of the Dietary Guidelines Advisory Committee on the Dietary Guidelines for Americans, 2010. Available at www.cnpp.usda.gov/DGAs2010-DGACReport.htm. Accessed 20 July 2011

U.S. Department of Health and Human Services (DHHS). *2008 Physical Activity Guidelines for Americans.* Available at www.health.gov/PAGuidelines/factsheet-prof. Accessed 1 July 2011

Weickert MO, Pfeiffer AFH: Metabolic effect of dietary fiber consumption and prevention of diabetes. *J Nutr* 138:439–442, 2008

Wing RR: Lifestyle and the prevention of diabetes. In *American Diabetes Association Guide to Medical Nutrition Therapy for Diabetes.* Franz MJ, Bantle JP, Eds. Alexandria, VA, American Diabetes Association, 1999, p. 369–386

Witham MD, Dove FJ, Dryburgh M, Sugden JA, Morris AD, Struthers AD: The effect of different doses of vitamin D(3) on markers of vascular health in patients with type 2 diabetes: a randomized controlled trial. *Diabetologia* 53:2112–2119, 2010

Gretchen Youssef, MS, RD, CDE, is the Program Manager at the MedStar Diabetes Institute, MedStar Health, Washington, DC.

Chapter 26

Integrating Nutrition Therapy into Community-Based Diabetes Prevention Programs

Ann Albright, PhD, RD, and Heather Devlin, MA

Highlights

Highlights
Integrating Nutrition Therapy into Community-Based Diabetes Prevention Programs

■ People with prediabetes face an annual risk of developing diabetes that is 5–10 times higher than people with normal blood glucose levels. Interventions that address individual lifestyle change to prevent type 2 diabetes should focus on individuals at high risk.

■ Program interventions should have the goal of achieving 5–7% weight loss through improved nutrition and ≥150 min of moderate physical activity per week, such as brisk walking.

■ Community-based programs can be effectively delivered by clinical and nonclinical staff. Programs should use a mixture of personnel that is feasible, effective, and cost-effective in their setting.

■ Population-wide policies hold promise for supporting type 2 diabetes prevention and warrant further study.

Integrating Nutrition Therapy into Community-Based Diabetes Prevention Programs

The national estimates from 2010 indicate that ~79 million people ≥20 years of age in the U.S. have prediabetes (based on fasting plasma glucose or A1C levels) (Centers for Disease Control and Prevention [CDC] 2011). People with prediabetes have an increased risk of developing type 2 diabetes and cardiovascular disease. Between 5 and 10% of people with prediabetes (impaired fasting glucose or impaired glucose tolerance [IGT]) will develop type 2 diabetes each year, compared to <1% of people with normal blood glucose (Gerstein 2007).

The number of new cases of diabetes has doubled during the past decade (CDC 2008). Factors associated with this increase are 1) increasingly sedentary lifestyles and poor nutrition practices, resulting in a rise in overweight and obesity; 2) increases in racial and ethnic populations in the U.S. that have a higher diabetes prevalence; and 3) aging of the population. Projections from the CDC indicate that as many as one in three people could have diabetes in 2050 if current trends continue (Boyle 2010). These data make it clear that there is an urgent need to prevent new cases of diabetes.

Prevention of type 2 diabetes requires complementary and shared public health and clinical approaches (Figure 26.1). The clinical sector is important in assessing patients' risk for type 2 diabetes. Roles for this sector also include discussing risk status with patients and their support network; recommending that high-risk patients participate in effective, community-based, structured lifestyle programs and providing medical nutrition therapy or nutrition therapy; and, as appropriate, prescribing medications for people at high risk. The services provided by the public health sector include monitoring diabetes risk; mobilizing partnerships to reduce new cases of diabetes; linking people to proven diabetes prevention services; assuring quality of prevention programs; and developing policies that support individual risk reduction and community change that makes it easier to practice healthy behaviors. As reflected in Figure 26.1, public health can facilitate partnerships that enable the clinical and community sectors to be connected and articulated to work synergistically to achieve type 2 diabetes prevention.

Since diabetes risk progresses from low risk to high risk, it is important that effective interventions exist along the continuum. Most of the evidence currently available for diabetes prevention involves people at high risk for type 2 diabetes. Some evidence also provides insights into broader population risk reduction that may help people at high risk maintain healthy behaviors and prevent others from moving to high-risk status.

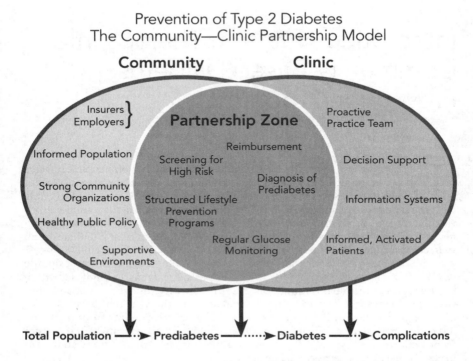

Figure 26.1 Provided by the Centers for Disease Control and Prevention, Division of Diabetes Translation. Elements in the clinical component are adapted from the Chronic Care Model, MacColl Institute for Healthcare Innovation. The elements listed are not intended to be all-inclusive, but to provide information on the kinds of elements contributed by each sector and shared across sectors.

This chapter begins with a brief review of the key efficacy trials that have informed the community translation studies. The evidence from translation studies provides direction for delivering lifestyle interventions in real-world settings, and the National Diabetes Prevention Program describes local implementation on a national scale. Population-wide policy level interventions are also briefly described, since obesity is a major driver of type 2 diabetes. It is highly likely that population-wide policies are necessary to address obesity, since its primary drivers—poor nutrition and physical inactivity—are rooted in modern lifestyles.

KEY EFFICACY TRIALS INFORMING COMMUNITY TRANSLATION STUDIES

Of the major randomized controlled trials (RCTs) of lifestyle interventions to prevent type 2 diabetes, only one—the Da Qing Impaired Glucose Tolerance and

Diabetes Study—had been published as of 1999 and was thus included in the 1999 *American Diabetes Association Guide to Medical Nutrition Therapy for Diabetes* (Wing 1999). Since then, at least six additional rigorous, large-scale RCTs have demonstrated the efficacy of lifestyle changes that include both exercise and nutrition for reducing incidence of type 2 diabetes among people at high risk (Baker 2011; Gillies 2007; Orozco 2008).

Gillies and colleagues reviewed pharmacological and lifestyle interventions to prevent type 2 diabetes, concluding that both can reduce progression to type 2 diabetes (Gillies 2007). The review identified 10 studies of lifestyle interventions for type 2 diabetes prevention: one tested exercise alone, three tested nutrition alone, and eight tested a combination of nutrition and exercise. In this meta-analysis, the pooled effect for all forms of lifestyle intervention was a relative 49% reduction in the risk of developing type 2 diabetes. Nutrition changes, exercise, and a combination of both showed similar and significant reductions in risk.

Orozco and colleagues conducted a Cochrane review of exercise and/or nutritional interventions to prevent type 2 diabetes among individuals at high risk. This review identified eight studies described in 25 publications: all eight examined exercise and nutrition combined; two (Pan 1997; Wing 1998) also tested exercise alone and nutrition alone, as well as exercise and nutrition combined. This review concluded that interventions targeting both nutrition and exercise can decrease the incidence of diabetes in people with IGT or metabolic syndrome (Orozco 2008).

Baker and colleagues reviewed the behavioral strategies used in RCTs of lifestyle changes to reduce the incidence of type 2 diabetes among those at high risk (Baker 2011). This review identified seven trials described in 95 publications and concluded that "a behavioral change strategy that focuses on achievable, modest changes across multiple lifestyle goals may be the key to diabetes prevention" (Baker 2011). In this review, the two studies demonstrating the largest reductions in diabetes incidence were the Swedish Diabetes Prevention Program and the Italian Diabetes Prevention Program, with relative risk reductions of 74 and 75%, respectively; the smallest reduction (29%) was seen in the Indian Diabetes Prevention Program. Greater success in achieving lifestyle modification goals was significantly related to reduced risk of type 2 diabetes in both the U.S. Diabetes Prevention Program (DPP) and the Finnish Diabetes Prevention Study (DPS), suggesting a dose-response relationship for type 2 diabetes prevention programs.

All seven studies used intensive modes of delivery, including highly trained staff. The DPP and DPS relied primarily on registered dietitians (RDs) to oversee the program, and all seven studies incorporated structured exercise. Three included supervised exercise sessions. The number of face-to-face contacts ranged from six in the Japanese Diabetes Prevention Program to over 22 in the Swedish Diabetes Prevention Program and DPP. Attrition was low across all the studies, ranging from 6.9 to 13.4% (Baker 2011).

Two RCTs, in particular, provide the foundation for a majority of community-based translation efforts: the DPP and the DPS (DPP 2002b; Tuomilehto 2001). Despite being conducted independently on different continents, both achieved substantial and identical relative risk reductions of 58%. Both showed that achieving ≥5% weight loss can reduce type 2 diabetes incidence. Further, the DPP curriculum was developed for a diverse study group (45% racial and ethnic minorities) and achieved similar success in reducing type 2 diabetes incidence regardless of racial or ethnic background (DPP 2002b).

Details of the behavioral intervention for both the DPP and DPS have been extensively published. Baker's review found that the DPP and DPS had generated 41 and 39 publications each, respectively, as of February 2009, compared with publication numbers ranging from one to five for each of the other five trials (Baker 2011).

COMMUNITY-BASED TRANSLATION FOR TYPE 2 DIABETES PREVENTION

The typical RCT relies on precisely defined, resource-intensive interventions among highly selected participants compared to control conditions that may not reflect standard practice in real-world conditions (Kessler 2011). The challenges of translating this type of evidence into practice are well documented (Glasgow 2007). Translation research has been defined as "… applied research that strives to translate the available knowledge and render it operational in clinical and public health practice" (Narayan 2010).

Lifestyle interventions that have proven efficacious tend to be intensive and time-consuming for both participants and staff (Baker 2011). Translation research is needed to determine the minimum intensity required to produce meaningful change in real-world practice settings (Glasgow 2007). For diabetes prevention, there must be a focus on how best to use limited resources to deliver lifestyle intervention of sufficient intensity to produce the levels of weight loss required to prevent type 2 diabetes. It must also be logistically and economically feasible to spread the resources broadly across diverse settings.

To make the results of RCTs relevant to real-world settings, additional types of evidence are needed, including feasibility and implementation data, process evaluation results, documentation of unintended or unanticipated outcomes, and contextual information, including local knowledge (Glasgow 2007). Different research designs are also needed, including practical trials, well-designed observational studies, and alternative experimental and quasi-experimental designs. Translation research should also examine multiple outcomes with relevance for policymakers, practitioners, and the public, including cost, generalization, and quality of life.

Modified versions of the lifestyle interventions developed by the DPP or DPS have been implemented in real-world settings and are rendering new types of evidence for diabetes prevention. To identify published literature describing these studies, we conducted a search using PubMed MEDLINE. Criteria were as follows: English language publications on community-based diabetes primary prevention interventions modeled on the DPP or the DPS and/or community-based studies that directly assessed the incidence of type 2 diabetes. We used the MeSH (Medical Subject Headings) terms "Diabetes Mellitus," "Type 2" and "Primary Prevention" in combination with the English words "diabetes prevention" and "community".

An initial search identified 337 articles published since 1999, of which 302 were excluded because they did not report results from a diabetes prevention intervention. A total of 36 articles were retrieved for more detailed evaluation; 26

were excluded after review because interventions were not modeled on the DPP or DPS and/or the study did not assess incidence of type 2 diabetes as an outcome.

The "related citations" function was used to identify articles similar to the 10 included articles; the first 20 related citations (i.e., those with the highest link rankings) were searched for each article. This process identified a total of six additional articles meeting criteria. Reference lists of all included articles were reviewed; this strategy identified one additional article. One new article meeting criteria was added to PubMed while the review was underway. The DPP and DPS efficacy trials and a total of 18 observational studies meeting inclusion criteria are included in Table 26.1.

Translation research studies have used diverse approaches relevant to wide-scale implementation of type 2 diabetes prevention. Factors relevant for broad and effective implementation of prevention programs include the following: participants' diabetes risk; the lifestyle intervention's format, duration, and intensity; attendance; body weight, nutrition, and physical activity monitoring; type of intervention staff; program costs; and weight loss achieved.

Basic Study Characteristics

Of the 18 studies identified by our review, 13 translated the DPP, 4 translated the DPS, and 1 was not based on a prior RCT; the community-based Tehran Lipid and Glucose Study (TLGS) examined diabetes incidence of type 2 diabetes as a primary outcome (Harati 2010). All of the DPP-based translations took place in the U.S., whereas the DPS-based studies took place in Australia, Finland, and Greece. Our review did not identify any U.S. translations of the DPS.

Study settings included community-based organizations such as Ys (also known as Young Men's Christian Association [YMCA]) and churches, worksites, neighborhoods, health care settings such as primary care and cardiac rehabilitation clinics, and health maintenance organizations (Table 26.1). One study (Vadheim 2010a) compared remote delivery of the intervention via telehealth with an in-person format already shown to be effective.

Intervention sample sizes ranged from 8 to 2,798 participants, with half of the studies having fewer than 100 participants. Evaluation periods (elapsed time between first and last outcome measurement) ranged from 3 months to 3.5 years, with two-thirds following participants for ≤12 months. For some studies, the evaluation period was the same as the duration of the lifestyle intervention; for others, the evaluation period was substantially longer. Proportions of participants lost to follow-up ranged from 0 to 43%, with over half of the studies losing ≤20% of their participants.

The typical participant was a woman in her mid-50s with a BMI >30 kg/m². As in most weight-loss research, men were underrepresented in nearly all the studies, despite there being similar risk of developing type 2 diabetes among men and women. The proportion of men ranged from 7 to 50%, with men comprising less than one-third in a majority of the study populations.

Factors Important for Broad and Effective Implementation

Participants' diabetes risk. Successful public health translation of diabetes prevention requires that biologically effective lifestyle programs be provided at a sustainable economic cost. Third-party payers such as private health insurers,

Table 26.1 Studies of the Effectiveness of Community-Based Diabetes Prevention Programs in Translating the DPP and DPS Lifestyle Interventions

	Population/ Duration of Study	Intervention (type of study)	Major Findings	Comments
DPP Research Group 2002	n = 1,079 adults (32% men) ≥25 years old, BMI ≥24 kg/m²; 100% IGT; six sessions (24 weeks)/2.8 years	Lifestyle: goal-based, frequent contact with lifestyle coaches; flexible, individualized approach; goals (>7% weight loss; <25% of kcal fat; 1,200–1,800 kcal/day; ≥150 min/ week moderate PA); metformin: 850 mg twice daily (RCT)	Lifestyle intervention: about twice as effective as metformin; lifestyle ↓ type 2 diabetes incidence by 58%; metformin ↓ incidence by 31% vs. placebo; 7% weight loss by lifestyle	Efficacy trial providing foundation for community-based translation studies; $1,399 first year cost/participant
Tuomilehto 2001	n = 522 adults (33% men) 40–60 years old, BMI ≥25 kg/m²; 100% IGT; three sessions first 6 weeks, then every 3 months/3 years	Tailored nutrition advice and supervised exercise to achieve five goals: <30% total kcal from fat; <10% total kcal saturated fatty acids; ≥15 g fiber/1,000 kcal; ≥4 h/week moderate-level PA; and >5% weight loss (RCT)	Lifestyle intervention ↓ type 2 diabetes incidence by 58% vs. placebo; 4.7% weight loss participants vs. 0.9% controls	Efficacy trial providing foundation for community-based translation studies
Aldana 2006	n = 35 adults (34% men); 89% IGT, remainder type 2 diabetes; 16 sessions (24 weeks)/1 year	Closely modeled on DPP; delivered by RNs and certified health educator; individual and group training in diet, PA, and behavior modification, including nutrient tracking cards; dietary fat addressed first; calorie goal added if no weight loss (cohort study)	Mean 2.9 kg (3.3%) weight loss; improved glucose tolerance; 12 of 22 normal glucose after 2 years; mean attendance 67%	Delivered by existing health care staff of local worksite; OGTT at baseline and 6, 12, and 24 months; small sample size but no one lost to follow-up
Davis-Smith 2007	n = 10 adults (30% men), ADA risk score ≥10; 100% IFG; six sessions (7 weeks)/1 year	Modeled on DPP; compressed, group-based curriculum by volunteer health care provider; three themes (nutrition, PA, and behavior change) in two vs. four sessions each; medical volunteers and space provided at no cost (cohort study)	Mean 4.0 kg (3.8%) weight loss; improved BMI, fasting glucose and BP; ↓ in weight, BMI, and fasting glucose at 1 year; mean attendance 78%	Group-based program economically feasible and acceptable in rural African-American church; fasting capillary BGT used for Dx; very small sample size

	Population/ Duration of Study	Intervention (type of study)	Major Findings	Comments
Laati-kainen 2007	*n* = 237 adults (27% men) 40–75 years old, FINDRISC score ≥12; 34% prediabetes; six sessions (8 months)/1 year	Modeled on DPS; group-based to achieve five goals of DPS; delivered by RNs, RDs, and physiotherapists; key components included goal-setting, regular self-assessment, and social support (cohort study)	Mean 2.5 kg (2.7%) weight loss; ↓ in IGT, total and LDL cholesterol, TG, WC, and DBP at 12 months; mean attendance not reported; completion defined as attending baseline and 12-month clinical tests and one or more group session	Feasible in Australian primary care settings; fasting plasma BGT and OGTT at baseline and 1 year; 24% attrition; non-completers (*n* = 74) had fewer years of education and higher psychological distress
Acker-mann 2008	*n* = 46 adults (50% men) BMI ≥24 kg/m², ADA risk score ≥10; 100% IFG; 16 sessions (20 weeks)/1 year	Closely modeled on DPP; group-based program delivered by YMCA staff; core curriculum focused on goal-setting, self-monitoring, and problem-solving (matched-pair, group randomized study)	Mean 5.5 kg (6.0%) weight loss in intervention group vs. 1.8% in controls; −13.5 vs. +11.8 mg/dL total cholesterol; ↓ weight and total cholesterol sustained at 1 year; mean attendance 57%	Low-cost program designed for sustainable delivery via YMCAs; Dx by random capillary BGT; $275–$325 1-year cost/participant
Boltri 2008	*n* = 8 adults (% men not reported) ≥18 years, ADA risk score ≥10; 100% IFG; 16 sessions (16 weeks)/1 year	Closely modeled on DPP; group-based curriculum delivered by volunteer medical personnel; emphasized group interaction and incorporated prayer (cohort study)	Mean 3.4 kg (3.6%) weight loss; improved BMI, fasting glucose, SBP, and DBP and sustained at 1 year; mean attendance 62%	Translated 16-session DPP for African-American church setting; very small sample size but no one lost to follow-up; Dx fasting capillary BGT
McBride 2008	*n* = 37 adults (41% men) 25–75 years old and ≥3 CVD or type 2 diabetes risk factors (elevated fasting glucose in diabetes range, if <6 months); 8% IFG; 12 sessions (12 weeks)/11 months	Modified DPP; compressed, group-based curriculum delivered by RD and clinical exercise physiologist; food and exercise records reviewed weekly; $250 "commitment fee" refunded upon completion with good attendance; local HMOs referred participants (cohort study)	Mean 5.0 kg (4.6%) weight loss; improvements in all metabolic measurements (except DBP), caloric intake, total and saturated fatty acids consumed, and PA sustained at 11 months; mean attendance not reported	Delivery via cardiac rehabilitation center positively received by sponsoring HMOs; Dx by fasting plasma BGT

Table 26.1 Studies of the Effectiveness of Community-Based Diabetes Prevention Programs in Translating the DPP and DPS Lifestyle Interventions (*continued*)

	Population/ Duration of Study	Intervention (type of study)	Major Findings	Comments
Seidel 2008	n = 88 adults (16% men) ≥18 years, BMI ≥25 kg/m², ≥3 of 5 components of the metabolic syndrome; 42% IFG; 12 sessions (12 weeks)/3 months	Modified DPP delivered by RD and exercise specialist; compressed group-based curriculum focused on healthy food choices; emphasized fat intake and kilocalories; encouraged pedometer use (cohort study)	Mean weight loss not reported; 46% lost 5% and 26% lost 7% of weight; 43% improved one or more component of metabolic syndrome; 73% sustained improvements at 6 months; reduced WC, BP; mean attendance 52%	Successful delivery in 11 low-income, medically underserved urban neighborhoods; Dx by fasting plasma BGT; 43% attrition
Absetz 2009	n = 352 adults (25% men) 50–65 years with FINDRISC score ≥12; 26% IGT; 6 sessions/8 months	Modeled on DPS; group-based program delivered by public health nurses within existing work schedule, supported by project RD and municipal sports officers; model included information provision, group discussions, self-monitoring, goal-setting, and planning (cohort study)	Mean 0.8 kg (0.9%) weight loss; 12% met weight ↓ goal of >5%; 20% met four of five DPS objectives; ↓ in weight and BMI at 1 year maintained at 3 years; 12% conversion from IGT to type 2 diabetes; mean attendance 89%	Translated DPS for delivery via primary health care centers; fasting plasma BGT and OGTT at baseline, 1 year and 3 years; 9% attrition at 1 year, 24% at 3 years; dropout more likely among the unemployed
Amundson 2009	n = 295 adults (20% men), BMI ≥25 kg/m², ≥1 risk factor for type 2 diabetes or CVD; 52% prediabetes; 16 sessions (16 weeks)/1 year	Closely modeled after DPP; delivered by RDs; interactive nutrition and PA demonstrations; readiness-to-change assessment (cohort study)	Mean 6.7 kg (6.7%) weight loss; 45% lost ≥7%; 67% lost ≥5%; weight loss sustained at 1 year; mean attendance 83%	Successful delivery via four health care facilities, one in a frontier county; Dx by primary care provider; limited gender diversity

	Population/ Duration of Study	Intervention (type of study)	Major Findings	Comments
Kramer 2009	n = 93 adults (19% men) 25–74 years old, BMI ≥25 kg/m^2, without diabetes and with metabolic syndrome; 46% IGT; 12 sessions (14 weeks)/1 year	Modified DPP; compressed, group-based curriculum by RNs, RD, health educators, and exercise specialist; focused on healthy food choices, kilocalorie and fat intake; emphasized self-monitoring tools, pedometer use (cohort study)	Mean 3.4 kg (3.5%) weight loss; 24% lost ≥7%; 52% lost ≥5%; improvements in WC, BMI, HDL cholesterol, non-HDL cholesterol, SBP, and DBP; weight loss sustained at 6 months; mean attendance 67%	Demonstrated feasibility of translation model in urban and rural primary care practices; Dx by fasting plasma BGT; 22% attrition; $300 cost per participant
Whittemore 2009	n = 31 adults (10% men) ≥65 years old, BMI ≥25 kg/m^2 or ≥21 years and ≥1 other risk factor for type 2 diabetes; 11 sessions (6 in-person, 5 phone)/6 months	Modeled after DPP; delivered by nurse practitioners and study nutritionists; compressed curriculum reduced number of in-person sessions; nutrition content emphasized healthy choices, kilocalorie balance, regular eating, eating slowly (group-randomized)	Mean 0.4 kg (1.1%) weight loss; 25% met weight-loss goal of ≥5% among intervention group vs. 11% among controls; mean attendance 98%	Demonstrated feasibility of delivery in nurse practitioner–led primary care sites serving low- and moderate-income adults; Dx by OGTT; low attrition (12%)
Harati 2010	n = 1,754 adults (40% men) ≥20 years; 25% IGT; 3.6 years	Community-based Tehran Lipid and Glucose Study focused on nutrition and dietary pattern, PA, and cigarette smoking; nutrition classes held 4 days/week; volunteer "health liaisons" delivered training at public sites; RDs and general practitioners provide counseling on nutrition and smoking, respectively, via clinics (large-scale cluster-controlled trial nested within a population-based prospective cohort)	65% ↓ relative risk for type 2 diabetes in intervention group vs. controls; intervention more effective for women than men; mean attendance in educational sessions was 70% among women (not reported for men)	Very high attrition, but rates were similar across intervention (43%) and control (41%)

Table 26.1 Studies of the Effectiveness of Community-Based Diabetes Prevention Programs in Translating the DPP and DPS Lifestyle Interventions (*continued*)

	Population/ Duration of Study	Intervention (type of study)	Major Findings	Comments
Makrila-kis 2010	*n* = 191 individuals (40% men), mean 56.3 years; FIN-DRISC score ≥15, 68% with prediabetes; six sessions/1 year	Modeled on DPS; recruitment at primary care sites and workplaces; group sessions by RDs near participant's home or workplace; five DPS prevention goals were intervention core; exercise counseling provided; no formal exercise sessions (cohort study)	Mean 1.0 kg (1.1%) weight loss; improved BMI, SBP, FPG, total and LDL cholesterol; glucose dysregulation improved in *n* = 125 who had a follow-up OGTT; mean attendance 64%	Individuals screened at workplaces were nearly five times more likely to participate and had better attendance and retention than those screened via primary care; fasting plasma BGT and OGTT at baseline and 1 year; 35% attrition for 1-year OGTT
Saaristo 2010	*n* = 2,798 individuals (33% men), mean 54.7 years; FIN-DRISC score ≥15 or prediabetes coronary heart disease or gestational diabetes history; 25% with prediabetes; six sessions/1 year	Modeled on DPS; recruitment at primary care clinics and occupational health outpatient sites; combined individual, "self-acting," and group interactions and readiness-to-change assessment, patient empowerment principles, peer support, and positive feedback (cohort study)	Mean 1.1 kg (1.3%) weight loss; ↓ WC and BP and improved lipid profile; 69% ↓ in risk of diabetes incidence over 1 year in individuals who lost ≥5% vs. those who maintained weight; mean attendance not reported	Large-scale study demonstrating feasibility of preventing type 2 diabetes in primary health care settings; fasting capillary or plasma BGT and OGTT at baseline and 1 year; attrition not reported
Vadheim 2010a	*n* = 84 adults (12% men), ≥1 risk factor for type 2 diabetes or CVD; 13% had prediabetes; 16 sessions (16 weeks)/6 months	Closely modeled on DPP; interactive guided training on PA and nutrition delivered by RD and nurse staff of the site's ADA-recognized DSME program; readiness-to-change assessment; emphasized fat, healthy choices, and portion control (cohort study)	Mean 7.0 kg (6.9%) weight loss; 62% lost ≥7%; 78% lost ≥5%; weight loss sustained at 6 months; mean attendance 77%	Demonstrated feasibility of delivery in a rural community; 23% attrition; some PA and food intake measures self-reported; Dx by primary care provider; $557 cost per participant

	Population/ Duration of Study	Intervention (type of study)	Major Findings	Comments
Vadheim 2010b	n = 16 adults (7% men), ≥1 risk factor for type 2 diabetes or CVD; 50% had prediabetes; 16 sessions (16 weeks)/6 months	Modeled on DPP; group-based curriculum delivered via trained lifestyle coaches (RD and nurse staff of the site's ADA-recognized DSME program); telehealth group simultaneously participated with on-site group in the weekly and monthly sessions; all involved could see and hear each other (cohort study)	Mean 6.7 kg weight loss among telehealth group; no differences in weight loss between on-site and telehealth groups; 45% of groups met 7% weight-loss goal; no difference in participation between on-site and telehealth groups	Delivery via telehealth video conferencing to members of a remote frontier community as successful as in-person sessions; self-reported PA and diet measures; Dx by primary care provider; $470 cost per participant
Vander-wood 2010	n = 816 (20% men), ≥1 risk factor for type 2 diabetes or CVD; 53% had prediabetes; 16 sessions (16 weeks)/1 year	Closely modeled on DPP; interactive guided training on PA and nutrition delivered by RDs; readiness-to-change assessment; emphasized fat, healthy choices, and portion control (cohort study)	Mean 6.8 kg (6.9%) weight loss; 45% met 7% weight-loss goal, 66% had 5% weight loss, and 66% met PA goal; improvements in SBP and DBP, FBG, LDL cholesterol, and HDL cholesterol; mean attendance 77%	Demonstrated feasibility of state-coordinated delivery in eight health care facilities; 42% attrition, analyses included only completers; some PA and food intake measures self-reported; Dx by primary care provider
Katula 2011	n = 151 individuals (43% men), ≥21 years; 100% with prediabetes; 24 sessions/24 weeks	Modeled on DPP; delivered by trained CHWs supervised by RDs; focused on nutrition and PA basics, kilocalorie balance, healthy eating; PA goal ≥180 vs. ≥150 min/week; contacts (group, individual, and phone counseling); behavioral strategies (goal-setting and incentives, problem-solving, and self-efficacy); CHWs had 36 h of training over 6–9 weeks (RCT)	Mean 7.3 kg weight loss; fasting glucose ↓ 4.3 mg/dL in intervention vs. 0.4 mg/dL in controls; mean attendance 68%	Demonstrated feasibility of delivery by CHWs in community settings such as parks and recreation centers; fasting glucose was primary outcome; Dx by prediabetes on two occasions with confirmatory fasting glucose 95–125 mg/dL; 10 CHWs paid $100/week during core, $200/month during follow-up

ADA, American Diabetes Association; BGT, blood glucose testing; BP, blood pressure; CHW, community health worker; CVD, cardiovascular disease; DBP, diastolic blood pressure; DSME, diabetes self-management education; Dx, diagnosis; FINDRISC, Finnish Diabetes Risk Score; HMO, health maintenance organization; IFG, impaired fasting glucose; OGTT, oral glucose tolerance test; PA, physical activity; SBP, systolic blood pressure; TG, triglycerides; WC, waist circumference.

employers, or federal, state, and local governments are unlikely to pay for diabetes prevention without the confidence that the intervention will at least pay for itself through future health care cost reductions. For this reason, participants' risk status is crucially important.

Annual risk of developing diabetes among people who have prediabetes is 5–10 times higher than that among individuals with normal glucose levels (Gerstein 2007). People with normal glucose levels are a less efficient target for diabetes prevention because their future risk for diabetes and diabetes-related health costs is low. Thus, even when effective, diabetes prevention programs that include participants with normal glucose levels are much less likely to save money (Narayan 2010).

An important translation challenge is that most people with prediabetes do not know they have it (Geiss 2010). Because the preferred method of diagnosing prediabetes requires access to a health professional and medical laboratory, effective partnerships with the clinical sector are needed to facilitate accurate and convenient identification of potential lifestyle intervention participants with prediabetes.

Only four of the studies in Table 26.1 reported having 100% of participants with prediabetes. Four studies (all from the same translation group) relied on a physician-reported diagnosis of prediabetes. The remaining 14 performed their own diagnostic tests: three used capillary (fingerstick) blood tests (one nonfasting), four administered fasting plasma blood tests, three used the oral glucose tolerance test, and four (all DPS translations) administered fasting capillary or plasma blood glucose tests plus an oral glucose tolerance test. All of the studies administering their own diagnostic tests first used risk factor screening to reduce the number of participants who required the more costly and less convenient blood tests.

Lifestyle curriculum and intervention format. All of the translation studies identified by this review sought the same weight-loss goals as the original RCT on which they were modeled; a few studies modified slightly the physical activity and nutrition-related goals. Some studies implementing a modified DPP curriculum made minor adjustments to the curriculum while maintaining the same goals. These studies typically emphasized energy balance and healthy food choices. Some also emphasized pedometer use.

All but four studies offered group sessions only. Three (Aldana 2006; Katula 2011; Saaristo 2010) offered both individual and group sessions. One (Whittemore 2009) offered predominantly individual sessions, although they were shorter in duration than other studies (20 vs. 60–120 min). About half the studies reported group size, which ranged from 5 to 34 people; a majority of those reported group sizes of 8–12.

Intervention duration and intensity. Intervention periods in both the DPP and DPS research trials had "core" and "post-core" phases. The core phase of both interventions consisted of intensive group sessions, often held weekly. The post-core phase consisted of less intensive group sessions, typically held monthly. The purpose of the post-core phase was to help participants improve and maintain lifestyle changes implemented during the core phase.

Among studies implementing a modified DPP, the number of core sessions ranged from 6 to 24 over 7–36 weeks. Among the DPP translation studies: one study offered 24 core sessions in 24 weeks; seven offered 16 over 16–24 weeks; three offered 12 over 12–15 weeks; one offered 6 over 7 weeks; and one offered 11 sessions (six in-person and five phone contacts) over 16 weeks. All but three of the DPP translation studies offered post-core sessions, typically extending 6–9 months after the core. Studies implementing a modified DPS curriculum held four to eight sessions over 8–12 weeks, with at least one follow-up session within 12 months. If more than one follow-up was offered, intervals were typically monthly.

The optimum frequency of post-core sessions for achieving and maintaining weight loss at sustainable economic cost has yet to be determined. Also, translation research has not yet explored the utility or economic implications of extending post-core sessions beyond the initial year of lifestyle intervention.

Attendance. Among studies translating the DPP, the average number of core sessions that participants attended ranged from 5 to 16; two studies did not report attendance. Two of the four DPS translations reported attendance, which averaged four and five sessions, respectively.

If fewer sessions proved more convenient for the participants and were thus associated with increased session attendance, it is possible that weight-loss outcomes could be improved. However, among the studies reported in Table 26.1, the *proportion* of sessions attended did not differ between studies offering 11–12 versus 16 sessions; if anything, attendance ratios were better among individuals offered ≥16 sessions (70% average attendance) versus those offered <16 sessions (63% average attendance). This result means that, in general, the total number of sessions attended is greater when a greater number of sessions are offered.

Self-monitoring of body weight, diet, and physical activity. In behavioral interventions, self-monitoring is correlated with weight loss and includes participants completing food intake and exercise logs and self-weighing (Burke 2011). Self-monitoring was one of the components most strongly emphasized in the original DPP trial lifestyle intervention (DPP Research Group 2002). In addition to self-monitoring, weighing participants at each class was also important.

All but three of the DPP translation studies reported that the lifestyle intervention incorporated self-monitoring of weight, food intake, and physical activity; three studies used pedometers along with paper logs for physical activity monitoring. Self-monitoring was not emphasized as strongly in the DPS. Only one of the four DPS translation studies (Laatikainen 2007) reported self-monitoring. The TLGS did not report self-monitoring (Harati 2010).

Intervention staff and program costs. Health care professionals—including physicians, certified diabetes educators (CDEs), RDs, registered nurses (RNs), and exercise specialists—have key roles to play in diabetes prevention among high-risk people, as described above. These include risk assessment and communication, active referral to prevention programs, and provision of medical nutrition therapy and/or initiation of pharmacotherapy as appropriate.

Cost-effectiveness of the DPP lifestyle intervention has been substantially improved by offering the intervention in a group format rather than individually

(Herman 2003). Further cost reductions are possible when less expensive staff deliver the intervention. All original DPP trial staff had at least a master's degree in a clinical discipline. In contrast, one of the DPP translation studies in this review used employees of a local Y who had associate or bachelor's degrees in health-related areas and whose hourly wage was approximately half that of behavioral experts in the DPP (Ackermann 2008). Another used community health workers under the supervision of an RD (Katula 2011).

Academic or clinical certification may be less important than empathy and group leadership skills for being an effective lifestyle coach (Katula 2010). If so, program cost could be further reduced without harming effectiveness by training lifestyle coaches without clinical qualifications or college degrees as intervention staff. A majority of the studies in this review (12 of 18) reported training staff to deliver the intervention. Training duration ranged from a single 60-min session to 36 h delivered over 6–9 weeks. In 7 of the 13 DPP translation studies, expert staff from the original DPP study conducted the training.

Only four of the DPP translation studies in this review reported per-participant program costs. All four were substantially lower than the DPP and three of the four achieved the ≥5% weight loss needed to prevent or delay type 2 diabetes. The greatest weight loss reported in this review was achieved using community health workers supervised by RD/CDEs with access to exercise and behavioral experts (Katula 2011). The program included 24 core sessions, and costs have not yet been reported, but this RCT may demonstrate a lower-cost strategy for delivering an effective DPP-based intervention.

Weight loss achieved. Subanalyses of the DPP trial showed that weight loss was the key mediating variable between improvements in nutrition and physical activity and reduced diabetes incidence. After statistically adjusting for changes in eating pattern and physical activity, the DPP found that, for every 1 kg weight loss, there was a 16% reduction in risk of developing type 2 diabetes, but the impact of nutrition and physical activity was not statistically significant after adjusting for weight loss.

The DPS ranked participants by their success in achieving the intervention's behavior-change goals, one of which was >5% weight loss; the DPS showed that attaining four or more of the five study goals was sufficient to reduce diabetes incidence. The DPS translation studies did not distinguish the core phase as clearly nor did they emphasize weight loss as strongly, focusing instead on achieving all five study goals, of which one is weight loss. However, a recent DPS translation examined reduction in type 2 diabetes risk by weight loss and found a clear, nearly stepwise relationship between weight loss and incidence of diabetes. Weight loss of ≥5% was associated with a 69% reduction in the risk of developing diabetes over 1 year compared with intervention participants who maintained weight (Saaristo 2010).

In the DPP, physical activity still had an impact on diabetes risk in the absence of significant weight loss, albeit less than losing ≥5 kg body weight. Among people who lost <3.5 kg *and* reported meeting the 150 min/week physical activity goal (30% of participants), there was a 44% reduction in 3-year diabetes incidence (Hamman 2006). In the DPS, reduction in diabetes incidence was still significant among participants who met the physical activity goal of ≥4 h/week but did not lose weight. This result underscores the importance of lifestyle intervention programs emphasizing physical activity goals for all participants. In the DPP, brisk walking was the recommended form of physical activity. The DPS included exercise components designed to improve both cardiorespiratory fitness and muscle strength.

Among studies identified by this review, the time periods over which weight loss was measured varied widely. Therefore, for purposes of comparison, Table 26.1 identifies the weight losses achieved during each study's core intervention phase, which ranged from 3 to 6 months in duration. An initial weight loss of ≥5% is predictive of longer-term weight maintenance (Anderson 2001). Most people reach their maximum weight loss 5–6 months after starting a lifestyle program (Jeffery 1998). Programs with ≥16 core sessions were the most likely to report achieving the recommended 5–7% weight loss. Among the 16 translation research studies that reported sufficient weight-loss information, 7 reported losses of 5 kg (5%) during the core phase; 5 of those had 16 or more core sessions.

Studies varied in mean BMI, proportion of male participants, losses to follow-up, and proportion of participants who had prediabetes, as well as other potentially important characteristics that could confound the association between number of core sessions and achieved weight loss.

U.S. National Diabetes Prevention Program

Although questions remain about how to maximize prevention of type 2 diabetes, the rapidly growing type 2 diabetes incidence demands urgent action to implement what is already known to be effective. Population-scale reduction in the incidence of type 2 diabetes in the U.S. will require collaboration with community-based organizations with sufficient infrastructure, health-payers, health professionals, public health, academia, and others.

In 2009, the CDC began to plan for how the proven DPP intervention can be taken to scale, from the RCT results to translation study findings and then to widespread community-based implementation. Indiana University, the CDC, and the National Institutes of Health convened a group that included third-party payers, state public health officials, community-based organizations, and other federal health officials to examine how to overcome barriers to implementing diabetes prevention on a national scale. This meeting established the beginning of important partnerships with third-party payers and community-based lifestyle intervention providers.

The CDC-led National Diabetes Prevention Program developed out of this collaborative planning process. The goal of the program is to systematically scale the translated model of the DPP for high-risk individuals to reduce the incidence of type 2 diabetes in the U.S. The strategic approach of the CDC to the National Diabetes Prevention Program has four components:

1. **Training,** to build a workforce that can implement the lifestyle intervention cost-effectively. CDC has established the Diabetes Training and Technical Assistance Center at Emory University to provide workforce training coordination and assistance.
2. **Program recognition,** to provide quality assurance for participants, funders, and individuals making referrals. The CDC Diabetes Prevention

Recognition Program will assure program quality and consistency, provide a registry of recognized programs, and implement standardized reporting on performance of recognized programs.

3. **Intervention sites,** to deliver the intervention. The Y, UnitedHealth Care, and Medica have stepped up as inaugural organizations in the National Diabetes Prevention Program—the Y to deliver the program and United-Health Care and Medica to provide third-party reimbursement. As the Diabetes Prevention Recognition Program is implemented, more organizations will become involved in both program delivery and reimbursement.

4. **Health marketing,** to raise awareness among both health care providers and high-risk populations to increase referral and use of the intervention. CDC conducted focus tests and interviews with various groups—including individuals at risk for diabetes, family members of people at risk, and health care professionals—to help develop messages and tools that will facilitate program referral and participation.

In March 2010, Congress passed legislation that specifically addresses diabetes prevention through H.R. 3590—the Patient Protection and Affordable Care Act, SEC. 3999V-3 National Diabetes Prevention Program. This legislation authorizes the CDC to manage the National Diabetes Prevention Program and establish a network of evidence-based lifestyle intervention programs for people at high risk of developing type 2 diabetes (U.S. Government Printing Office 2010).

Population-Wide Policy Level Nutrition Interventions

The magnitude and persistence of the increases in obesity and type 2 diabetes indicate that these problems will not be solved by the individual or by one sector and that population-wide policy to change behaviors and living environments is also necessary. Individuals with prediabetes who participate in evidence-based diabetes prevention programs may be more successful in making and sustaining lifestyle changes if the environments in which their choices are made support healthful options. Healthier environments might also prevent some people from developing prediabetes, thus reducing the number of people who require intensive individual intervention in the future to avert progression to type 2 diabetes.

Sacks and colleagues suggested a systematic approach to identifying areas amenable to policy interventions by considering policy opportunities for each level of governance (local, state, national, and organizational), in each sector of the food system (primary production, food processing, distribution, marketing, retail, catering, and food service), and in each sector that influences physical activity environments (infrastructure and planning, education, employment, transportation, and recreation) (Sacks 2008).

Evaluating the impact of population-wide policies is more difficult than evaluating the impact of individual-based interventions and often requires the use of quasi-experimental designs, which may yield evidence of modest strength. As noted above, policies with the potential to influence nutrition, physical activity, or both may be relevant for diabetes prevention. A thorough review of the literature on policy interventions is beyond the scope of this chapter. In the context of this volume's focus on nutrition, the evidence is described for nutrition-related policies that have been receiving increased attention. These include menu labeling at point-of-purchase, removal of *trans* fats, and food pricing (including sugar-sweetened beverages).

Menu labeling. Because eating away from home comprises ~50% of food expenditures in the U.S. (Stewart 2004), provision of caloric and other nutrition information at the point-of-purchase has garnered attention as a way of improving the public's nutrition choices. Harnack and French conducted a literature review on the effect of point-of-purchase calorie labeling on restaurant and cafeteria food choices (Harnack 2008). They concluded that the effect is weak or inconsistent, likely because of the multiple levels of influence, such as prices and other promotional activities at point-of-purchase. Two studies published since this review (Elbel 2009; Finkelstein 2011) also found no significant effect of menu-labeling policies on caloric intake.

Questions remain about how well consumers understand or internalize the information posted on menus and whether mandatory menu labeling encourages supply-side changes such as in-store promotions or reformulation of existing products, which could improve food choices. It is likely that multiple levels of influence must be targeted to have a more substantial impact.

Trans *fat*. Consumption of *trans* fatty acids is an important modifiable risk factor for coronary heart disease, and emerging data suggest *trans* fatty acids might also cause metabolic dysfunction and increase type 2 diabetes risk (Micha 2009). If effective, policies to reduce exposure to *trans* fat could potentially reduce the number of people who develop prediabetes and in turn the need for intensive individual intervention to prevent type 2 diabetes.

The major dietary sources of *trans* fat in the U.S. and other developed countries are partially hydrogenated vegetable oils used in bakery products, deep-fried foods, packaged snacks, margarines, and crackers (Micha 2008). The Dietary Guidelines for Americans, the Academy of Nutrition and Dietetics, the Institute of Medicine, and the National Cholesterol Education Program all recommend consumption of *trans* fat should be as low as possible, and the American Heart Association recommends limiting *trans* fat to <1% total energy intake (Remig 2010).

As of January 2006, in the U.S., nutrition labels for all conventional foods and supplements were required to list the content of *trans* fat. Foods with <0.5 g *trans* fat per serving can be listed as having zero content. Some food manufacturers have now reformulated their products to reduce *trans* fat. In New York City, food service establishments can no longer fry with fats that contain >0.5 g *trans* fatty acids per serving or serve foods with >0.5 g *trans* fatty acids per serving. The health impact of these policies has not been directly measured, but the negative impact of *trans* fat on health is well established.

Food pricing. Groups with higher education and incomes tend to consume higher-quality food, and higher-quality eating patterns are associated with higher costs (Aggarwal 2011). Pricing strategies are being proposed as a way to increase more nutritious food/beverage selections and reduce consumption of less nutritious options.

Andreyeva and colleagues reviewed 160 studies on price elasticity to estimate the effect of price changes on consumer demand for major commodity foods included in the Dietary Guidelines for Americans food categories (Andreyeva 2010). It was estimated that a 10% tax on soft drinks could lead to an 8–10% reduction in these beverage purchases. Conversely, a 10% reduction in the price of fruits and vegetables would increase purchases on average by 7.0 and 5.8%, respectively. However, price changes likely would need to be combined with other interventions to increase fruit and vegetable intake to levels recommended by the Dietary Guidelines for Americans.

Powell and Chaloupka found that small taxes or subsidies are not likely to produce significant changes in BMI or obesity prevalence, but "nontrivial" pricing may have some measureable effects on weight outcomes, particularly for youth and people with low socioeconomic status (Powell 2009).

SUMMARY GUIDELINES FOR COMMUNITY-BASED DIABETES PREVENTION

Preventing type 2 diabetes involves individuals, families/support networks, organizations (e.g., worksites and health care systems), and communities. In fact, the health of individuals is inseparable from the health of communities (U.S. Department of Health and Human Services 2010). As a result, individuals, families/support networks, organizations, and communities must all contribute to prevention efforts. Structured programs that focus on individual lifestyle change, where there is group support and ready accessibility in communities, show the strongest evidence for preventing or delaying type 2 diabetes in high-risk individuals. Because the bulk of prediabetes cases remain undiagnosed, strong partnerships between community-based programs and the clinical sector are necessary.

Program interventions should have the goal of achieving 5–7% weight loss through improved nutrition and ≥150 min moderate physical activity per week, such as brisk walking. Programs should include a strong self-monitoring component and emphasize energy reduction in the context of a balanced eating pattern. Whereas head-to-head comparisons of the impact of varying number of core sessions have not been studied, the currently available literature indicates that, in the U.S., 16 core sessions (delivered approximately weekly) are most likely to deliver the weight loss that is required to prevent or delay type 2 diabetes. Post-core sessions (maintenance phase) are important, but the optimal number and duration requires further study. Community-based programs can be effectively delivered by clinical and nonclinical staff. Until stronger evidence becomes available regarding optimal staffing, programs should use the staff mix that is feasible, effective, and cost-effective in their setting.

Individual change is more likely to be facilitated and sustained if the environment in which choices are made supports healthful options. However, population-wide policies such as point-of-purchase menu labeling, removal of *trans* fats, and food pricing, among others, require further investigation to more clearly determine their value for supporting prevention of type 2 diabetes and improving the health of the broader population.

BIBLIOGRAPHY

Absetz P, Oldenburg B, Hankonen N, Valve R, Heinonen H, Nissinen A, Fogelholm M, Talja M, Uutela A: Type 2 diabetes prevention in the real world: three-year results of the GOAL lifestyle implementation trial. *Diabetes Care* 32:1418–1420, 2009

Ackermann RT, Finch EA, Brizendine E, Zhou H, Marrero DG: Translating the Diabetes Prevention Program into the community: the DEPLOY Pilot Study. *Am J Prev Med* 35:357–363, 2008

Aggarwal A, Monsivais P, Cook AJ, Drewnowski A: Does diet cost mediate the relation between socioeconomic position and diet quality? *Eur J Clin Nutr* 65:1059–1066, 2011

Aldana S, Barlow M, Smith R, Yanowitz F, Adams T, Loveday L, Merrill RM: A worksite diabetes prevention program: two-year impact on employee health. *AAOHN J* 54:389–395, 2006

Amundson HA, Butcher MK, Gohdes D, Hall TO, Harwell TS, Helgerson SD, Vanderwood KK; Montana Cardiovascular Disease and Diabetes Prevention Program Workgroup: Translating the diabetes prevention program into practice in the general community: findings from the Montana Cardiovascular Disease and Diabetes Prevention Program. *Diabetes Educ* 35:209–223, 2009

Anderson JW, Konz EC, Frederich RC, Wood CL: Long-term weight-loss maintenance: a meta-analysis of US studies. *Am J Clin Nutr* 74:579–584, 2001

Andreyeva T, Long MW, Brownell KD: The impact of food prices on consumption: a systematic review of research on the price elasticity of demand for food. *Am J Public Health* 100:216–222, 2010

Baker MK, Simpson K, Lloyd B, Bauman AE, Singh MA: Behavioral strategies in diabetes prevention programs: a systematic review of randomized controlled trials. *Diabetes Res Clin Pract* 91:1–12, 2011

Bassett MT, Dumanovsky T, Huang C, Silver LD, Young C, Nonas C, Matte TD, Chideya S, Frieden TR: Purchasing behavior and calorie information at fast-food chains in New York City, 2007. *Am J Public Health* 98:1457–1459, 2008

Boltri JM, Davis-Smith YM, Seale JP, Shellenberger S, Okosun IS, Cornelius ME: Diabetes prevention in a faith-based setting: results of translational research. *J Public Health Manag Pract* 14:29–32, 2008

Boyle JP, Thompson TJ, Gregg EW, Barker LE, Williamson DF: Projection of the year 2050 burden of diabetes in the US adult population: dynamic modeling of incidence, mortality, and prediabetes prevalence. *Popul Health Metr* 8:1–29, 2010

Burke LE, Wang J, Sevick MA: Self-monitoring in weight loss: a systematic review of the literature. *J Am Diet Assoc* 111:92–102, 2011

Centers for Disease Control and Prevention: *National Diabetes Fact Sheet: National Estimates and General Information on Diabetes and Prediabetes in the United States, 2011.* Atlanta, GA, U.S. Department of Health and Human Services, Centers for Disease Control and Prevention, 2011

Centers for Disease Control and Prevention: State-specific incidence of diabetes among adults-participating states, 1995–1997 and 2005–2007. *MMWR Morb Mortal Wkly Rep* 57:1169–1173, 2008

Davis-Smith YM, Boltri JM, Seale JP, Shellenberger S, Blalock T, Tobin B: Implementing a diabetes prevention program in a rural African-American church. *J Natl Med Assoc* 99:440–446, 2007

de Vegt F, Dekker JM, Jager A, Hienkens E, Kostense PJ, Stehouwer CD, Nijpels G, Bouter LM, Heine RJ: Relation of impaired fasting and postload glucose with incident type 2 diabetes in a Dutch population: The Hoorn Study. *JAMA* 285:2109–2113, 2001

Diabetes Prevention Program Research Group: The Diabetes Prevention Program (DPP): description of lifestyle intervention. *Diabetes Care* 25:2165–2171, 2002a

Diabetes Prevention Program Research Group, Knowler WC, Barrett-Connor E, Fowler SE, Hamman RF, Lachin JM, Walker EA, Nathan DM: Reduction in the incidence of type 2 diabetes with lifestyle intervention or metformin. *N Engl J Med* 346:393–403, 2002b

Elbel B, Kersh R, Brescoll VL, Dixon LB: Calorie labeling and food choices: a first look at the effects on low-income people in New York City. *Health Aff (Millwood)* 28:1110–1121, 2009

Finkelstein EA, Strombotne KL, Chan NL, Krieger J: Mandatory menu labeling in one fast-food chain in King County, Washington. *Am J Prev Med* 40:122–127, 2011

Geiss LS, James C, Gregg EW, Albright A, Williamson DF, Cowie CC: Diabetes risk reduction behaviors among U.S. adults with prediabetes. *Am J Prev Med* 38:403–409, 2010

Gerstein HC, Santaguida P, Raina P, Morrison KM, Balion C, Hunt D, Yazdi H, Booker L: Annual incidence and relative risk of diabetes in people with various categories of dysglycemia: a systematic overview and meta-analysis of prospective studies. *Diabetes Res Clin Pract* 78:305–312, 2007

Gillies CL, Abrams KR, Lambert PC, Cooper NJ, Sutton AJ, Hsu RT, Khunti K: Pharmacological and lifestyle interventions to prevent or delay type 2 diabetes in people with impaired glucose tolerance: systematic review and meta-analysis. *BMJ* 334:299, 2007

Glasgow RE, Emmons KM: How can we increase translation of research into practice? Types of evidence needed. *Annu Rev Public Health* 28:413–433, 2007

Hamman RF, Wing RR, Edelstein SL, Lachin JM, Bray GA, Delahanty L, Hoskin M, Kriska AM, Mayer-Davis EJ, Pi-Sunyer X, Regensteiner J, Venditti B,

Wylie-Rosett J: Effect of weight loss with lifestyle intervention on risk of diabetes. *Diabetes Care* 29:2102–2107, 2006

Harati H, Hadaegh F, Momenan AA, Ghanei L, Bozorgmanesh MR, Ghanbarian A, Mirmiran P, Azizi F: Reduction in incidence of type 2 diabetes by lifestyle intervention in a middle eastern community. *Am J Prev Med* 38:628–636, 2010

Harnack LJ, French SA: Effect of point-of-purchase calorie labeling on restaurant and cafeteria food choices: a review of the literature. *Int J Behav Nutr Phys Act* 5:51–56, 2008

Herman WH, Brandle M, Zhang P, Williamson DF, Matulik MJ, Ratner RE, Lachin JM, Engelgau MM; Diabetes Prevention Program Research Group: Costs associated with the primary prevention of type 2 diabetes mellitus in the diabetes prevention program. *Diabetes Care* 26:36–47, 2003

Jeffery RW, Wing RR, Mayer RR: Are smaller weight losses or more achievable weight loss goals better in the long term for obese patients? *J Consult Clin Psychol* 66:641–645, 1998

Katula JA, Vitolins MZ, Rosenberger EL, Blackwell CS, Espeland MA, Lawlor MS, Rejeski WJ, Goff DC: Healthy Living Partnerships to Prevent Diabetes (HELP PD): design and methods. *Contemp Clin Trials* 31:71–81, 2010

Katula JA, Vitolins MZ, Rosenberger EL, Blackwell CS, Morgan TM, Lawlor MS, Goff DC Jr: One-year results of a community-based translation of the Diabetes Prevention Program: Healthy-Living Partnerships to Prevent Diabetes (HELP PD) Project. *Diabetes Care* 34:1451–1457, 2011

Kessler R, Glasgow RE: A proposal to speed translation of healthcare research into practice: dramatic change is needed. *Am J Prev Med* 40:637–644, 2011

Kramer MK, Kriska AM, Venditti EM, Miller RG, Brooks MM, Burke LE, Siminerio LM, Solano FX, Orchard TJ: Translating the Diabetes Prevention Program: a comprehensive model for prevention training and program delivery. *Am J Prev Med* 37:505–511, 2009

Laatikainen T, Dunbar JA, Chapman A, Kilkkinen A, Vartiainen E, Heistaro S, Philpot B, Absetz P, Bunker S, O'Neil A, Reddy P, Best JD, Janus ED: Prevention of type 2 diabetes by lifestyle intervention in an Australian primary health care setting: Greater Green Triangle (GGT) Diabetes Prevention Project. *BMC Public Health* 7:249–256, 2007

Leth T, Jensen HG, Mikkelsen AA, Bysted A: The effect of the regulation on trans fatty acid content in Danish food. *Atheroscler Suppl* 7:53–56, 2006

Makrilakis K, Liatis S, Grammatikou S, Perrea D, Katsilambros N: Implementation and effectiveness of the first community lifestyle intervention programme to prevent type 2 diabetes in Greece: the DE-PLAN study. *Diabet Med* 27:459–465, 2010

McBride PE, Einerson JA, Grant H, Sargent C, Underbakke G, Vitcenda M, Zeller L, Stein JH: Putting the Diabetes Prevention Program into practice: a program for weight loss and cardiovascular risk reduction for patients with metabolic syndrome or type 2 diabetes mellitus. *J Nutr Health Aging* 12:745S–749S, 2008

Micha R, Mozaffarian D: Trans fatty acids: effects on cardiometabolic health and implications for policy. *Prostaglandins Leukot Essent Fatty Acids* 79:147–152, 2008

Micha R, Mozaffarian D: Trans fatty acids: effects on metabolic syndrome, heart disease and diabetes. *Nat Rev Endocrinol* 5:335–344, 2009

Narayan KM, Williamson DF: Prevention of type 2 diabetes: risk status, clinic, and community. *J Gen Intern Med* 25:154–157, 2010

Orozco LJ, Buchleitner AM, Gimenez-Perez G, Roqué I, Figuls M, Richter B, Mauricio D: Exercise or exercise and diet for preventing type 2 diabetes mellitus. *Cochrane Database Syst Rev* 3:CD003054, 2008

Pan XR, Li GW, Hu YH, Wang JX, Yang WY, An ZX, Hu ZX, Lin J, Xiao JZ, Cao HB, Liu PA, Jiang XG, Jiang YY, Wang JP, Zheng H, Zhang H, Bennett PH, Howard BV: Effects of diet and exercise in preventing NIDDM in people with impaired glucose tolerance: the Da Qing IGT and Diabetes Study. *Diabetes Care* 20:537–544, 1997

Powell LM, Chaloupka FJ: Food prices and obesity: evidence and policy implications for taxes and subsidies. *Milbank Q* 87:229–257, 2009

Remig V, Franklin B, Margolis S, Kostas G, Nece T, Street JC: Trans fat in America: a review of their use, consumption, health implications, and regulation. *J Am Diet Assoc* 110:585–592, 2010

Saaristo T, Moilanen L, Korpi-Hyövälti E, Vanhala M, Saltevo J, Niskanen L, Jokelainen J, Peltonen M, Oksa H, Tuomilehto J, Uusitupa M, Keinänen-Kiukaanniemi S: Lifestyle intervention for prevention of type 2 diabetes in primary health care: one-year follow-up of the Finnish National Diabetes Prevention Program (FIN-D2D). *Diabetes Care* 33:2146–2151, 2010

Saaristo T, Peltonen M, Keinänen-Kiukaanniemi S, Vanhala M, Saltevo J, Niskanen L, Oksa H, Korpi-Hyövälti E, Tuomilehto J; FIN-D2D Study Group: National type 2 diabetes prevention programme in Finland: FIN-D2D. *Int J Circumpolar Health* 66:101–112, 2007

Sacks G, Swinburn BA, Lawrence MA: A systematic policy approach to changing the food system and physical activity environments to prevent obesity. *Aust New Zealand Health Policy* 5:13–20, 2008

Seidel MC, Powell RO, Zgibor JC, Siminerio LM, Piatt GA: Translating the Diabetes Prevention Program into an urban medically underserved community: a nonrandomized prospective intervention study. *Diabetes Care* 31:684–689, 2008

Stewart H, Blisard N, Bhuyan S, Nayga R: *The Demand for Food Away from Home: Full Service or Fast Food?* Washington, DC, USDA, Economic Research Service, 2004

Tuomilehto J, Lindström J, Eriksson JG, Valle TT, Hämäläinen H, Ilanne-Parikka P, Keinänen-Kiukaanniemi S, Laakso M, Louheranta A, Rastas M, Salminen V, Uusitupa M; Finnish Diabetes Prevention Study Group: Prevention of type 2 diabetes mellitus by changes in lifestyle among subjects with impaired glucose tolerance. *N Engl J Med* 344:1343–1350, 2001

U.S. Department of Health and Human Services: Healthy People 2010. http://www.healthypeople.gov. Accessed 6 June 2011

U.S. Government Printing Office. 2010. Public Law 111-148: March 23, 2010. http://www.gpo.gov/fdsys/pkg/PLAW-111publ148/pdf/PLAW-111publ148. pdf. Accessed 6 June 2011

Vadheim LM, Brewer KA, Kassner DR, Vanderwood KK, Hall TO, Butcher MK, Helgerson SD, Harwell TS: Effectiveness of a lifestyle intervention program among persons at high risk for cardiovascular disease and diabetes in a rural community. *J Rural Health* 26:266–272, 2010b

Vadheim LM, McPherson C, Kassner DR, Vanderwood KK, Hall TO, Butcher MK, Helgerson SD, Harwell TS: Adapted diabetes prevention program lifestyle intervention can be effectively delivered through telehealth. *Diabetes Educ* 36:651–656, 2010a

Vanderwood KK, Hall TO, Harwell TS, Butcher MK, Helgerson SD; Montana Cardiovascular Disease and Diabetes Prevention Program Workgroup: Implementing a state-based cardiovascular disease and diabetes prevention program. *Diabetes Care* 33:2543–2545, 2010

Whittemore R, Melkus G, Wagner J, Dziura J, Northrup V, Grey M: Translating the diabetes prevention program to primary care: a pilot study. *Nurs Res* 58:2–12, 2009

Wing RE: Lifestyle and the prevention of diabetes. In *American Diabetes Association Guide to Medical Nutrition Therapy*. Franz MJ, Bantle JP, Eds. Alexandria, VA, American Diabetes Association, 1999, p. 351–368

Wing RR, Venditti E, Jakicic JM, Polley BA, Lang W: Lifestyle intervention in overweight individuals with a family history of diabetes. *Diabetes Care* 21:350–359, 1998

Ann Albright, PhD, RD, is the Director of the Division of Diabetes Translation, Centers for Disease Control and Prevention, Atlanta, GA. Heather Devlin, MA, is a Health Scientist in the Division of Diabetes Translation, Centers for Disease Control and Prevention, Atlanta, GA.

The findings and conclusions in this chapter are those of the authors and do not necessarily represent the official position of the Centers for Disease Control and Prevention.

Index

Note: Page ranges in **bold** indicate an in-depth discussion of the topic. Page numbers followed by an *f* indicate a figure. Page numbers followed by a *t* indicate a table.